AF566828

DIAGNOSTIC RADIOLOGY

Gastrointestinal and Hepatobiliary Imaging

PIONEERS OF AIIMS-MAMC-PGI IMAGING COURSE SERIES

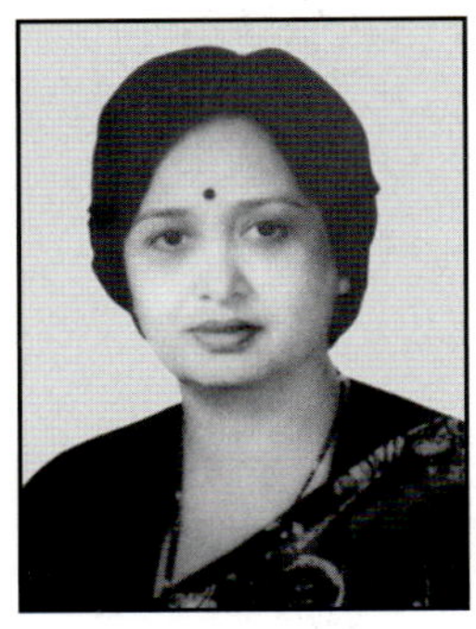

Manorama Berry

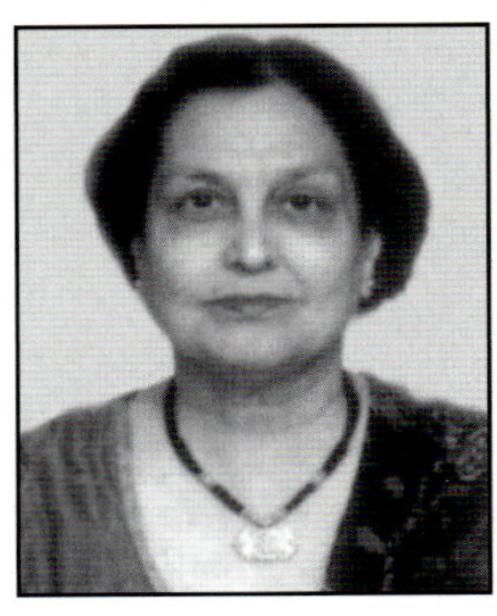

Sudha Suri

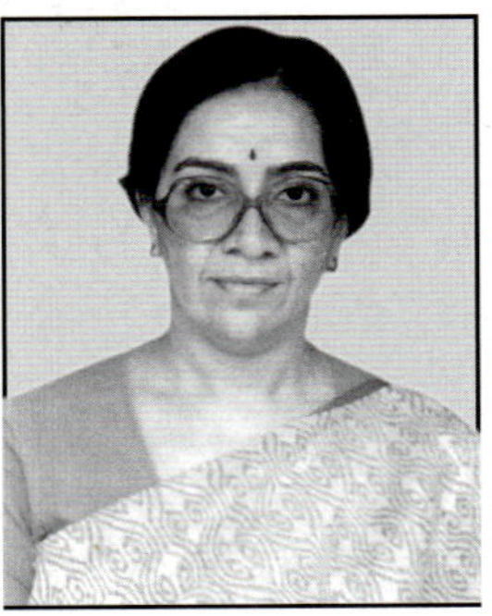

Veena Chowdhury

PAST EDITORS

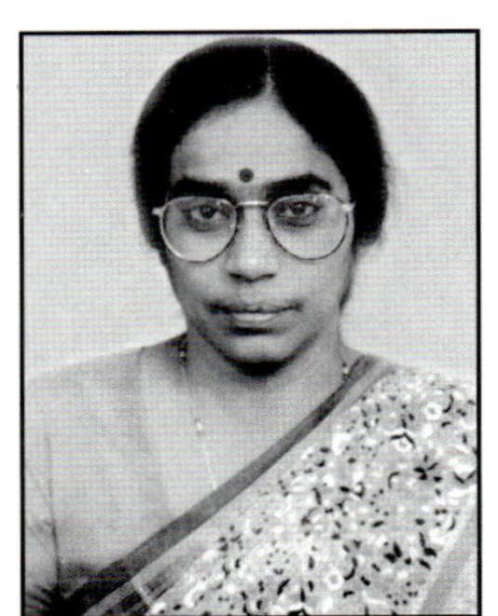

Sima Mukhopadhyay

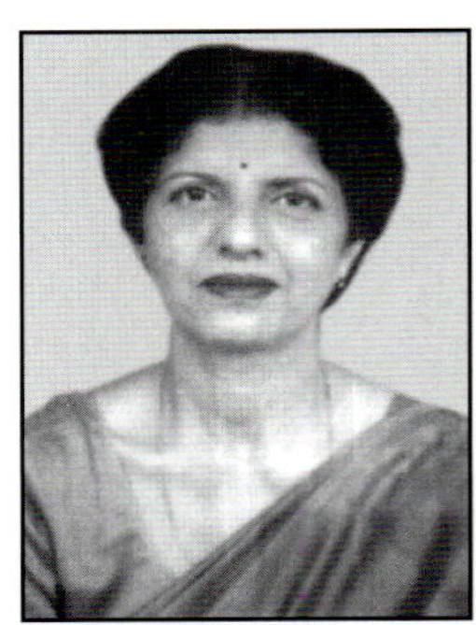

Sushma Vashisht

AIIMS-MAMC-PGI IMAGING COURSE SERIES

DIAGNOSTIC RADIOLOGY

Gastrointestinal and Hepatobiliary Imaging

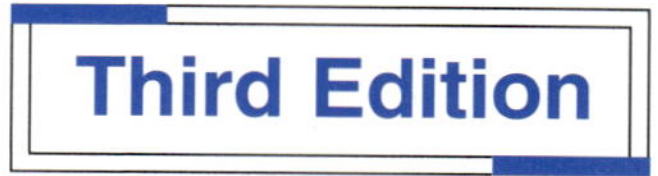

Third Edition

Editors

Arun Kumar Gupta MD MAMS
Professor and Head
Department of Radiodiagnosis
All India Institute of Medical Sciences
New Delhi, India

Veena Chowdhury MD
Director Professor and Head
Department of Radiodiagnosis
Maulana Azad Medical College
New Delhi, India

Niranjan Khandelwal MD DNB FICR
Professor and Head
Department of Radiodiagnosis
PGIMER, Chandigarh, India

Associate Editors

Deep Narayan Srivastava MD MAMS
Professor
Department of Radiodiagnosis
All India Institute of Medical Sciences
New Delhi, India

Raju Sharma MD
Additional Professor
Department of Radiodiagnosis
All India Institute of Medical Sciences
New Delhi, India

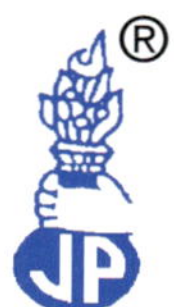

JAYPEE BROTHERS MEDICAL PUBLISHERS (P) LTD

New Delhi • St Louis • Panama City • London

Published by
Jaypee Brothers Medical Publishers (P) Ltd

Corporate Office

4838/24, Ansari Road, Daryaganj, **New Delhi** 110 002, India
Phone: +91-11-43574357, Fax: +91-11-43574314

Offices in India

- **Ahmedabad**, e-mail: ahmedabad@jaypeebrothers.com
- **Bengaluru**, e-mail: bangalore@jaypeebrothers.com
- **Chennai**, e-mail: chennai@jaypeebrothers.com
- **Delhi**, e-mail: jaypee@jaypeebrothers.com
- **Hyderabad**, e-mail: hyderabad@jaypeebrothers.com
- **Kochi**, e-mail: kochi@jaypeebrothers.com
- **Kolkata**, e-mail: kolkata@jaypeebrothers.com
- **Lucknow**, e-mail: lucknow@jaypeebrothers.com
- **Mumbai**, e-mail: mumbai@jaypeebrothers.com
- **Nagpur**, e-mail: nagpur@jaypeebrothers.com

Overseas Offices

- **North America Office, USA**, Ph: 001-636-6279734
  e-mail: jaypee@jaypeebrothers.com, anjulav@jaypeebrothers.com
- **Central America Office, Panama City, Panama**, Ph: 001-507-317-0160
  e-mail: cservice@jphmedical.com, Website: www.jphmedical.com
- **Europe Office, UK**, Ph: +44 (0) 2031708910
  e-mail: info@jpmedpub.com

Diagnostic Radiology: Gastrointestinal and Hepatobiliary Imaging

First Edition: 1997
Second Edition: 2004
Third Edition: 2009
Reprint: 2011

ISBN 978-81-8448-434-2

Typeset at JPBMP typesetting unit
Printed at Replika Press Pvt. Ltd.

List of Contributors

Anjali Prakash DMRD DNB MNAMS
Assistant Professor
Department of Radiodiagnosis
Maulana Azad Medical College
New Delhi

Anju Garg MD
Professor
Department of Radiodiagnosis
Maulana Azad Medical College
New Delhi

Anupam Lal MD
Associate Professor
Department of Radiodiagnosis
PGIMER, Chandigarh

Arun Kumar Gupta MD MAMS
Professor and Head
Department of Radio-diagnosis
All India Institute of Medical Sciences
New Delhi

Ashu Seith Bhalla
Associate Professor
Department of Radio-diagnosis
All India Institute of Medical Sciences
New Delhi

Atin Kumar
Assistant Professor
Department of Radio-diagnosis
All India Institute of Medical Sciences
New Delhi

Birinder Nagi MD MNAMS
Professor (Section of Radiology)
Department of Gastroenterology
PGIMER, Chandigarh

Chandan J Das MD DNB MNAMS
Pool Officer
Department of Radio-diagnosis
All India Institute of Medical Sciences
New Delhi

Deep Narayan Srivastava MD MAMS
Professor
Department of Radio-diagnosis
All India Institute of Medical Sciences
New Delhi

Gaurav S Pradhan DMRD DNB
Professor
Department of Radiodiagnosis
Maulana Azad Medical College
New Delhi

Harsh Kandpal
Pool Officer
Department of Radio-diagnosis
All India Institute of Medical Sciences
New Delhi

Madhusudhan KS
Senior Resident
Department of Radio-diagnosis
All India Institute of Medical Sciences
New Delhi

Mahesh Prakash MD
Assistant Professor
Department of Radiodiagnosis
PGIMER, Chandigarh

Mandeep Kang MD
Associate Professor
Department of Radiodiagnosis
PGIMER, Chandigarh

Manphool Singhal MD
Pool Officer
Department of Radiodiagnosis
PGIMER
Chandigarh

Naveen Kalra MD
Associate Professor
Department of Radiodiagnosis
PGIMER, Chandigarh

Niranjan Khandelwal MD DNB FICR
Professor and Head
Department of Radiodiagnosis
PGIMER
Chandigarh

Raju Sharma MD
Additional Professor
Department of Radio-diagnosis
All India Institute of Medical Sciences
New Delhi

Rashmi Dixit MD
Professor
Department of Radiodiagnosis
Maulana Azad Medical College
New Delhi

Sanjay Thulkar MD
Associate Professor
Department of Radio-diagnosis
(IRCH)
All India Institute of Medical Sciences
New Delhi

Sapna Singh MD DNB MNAMS
Assistant Professor
Department of Radiodiagnosis
Maulana Azad Medical College
New Delhi

Shashi Bala Paul
Scientist
Department of Radio-diagnosis
All India Institute of Medical Sciences
New Delhi

Shivanand Gamanagatti
Assistant Professor
Department of Radio-diagnosis
All India Institute of Medical Sciences
New Delhi

Smriti Hari
Assistant Professor
Department of Radio-diagnosis
All India Institute of Medical Sciences
New Delhi

Subrat Kumar Acharya
Professor and Head
Department of Gastroenterology
All India Institute of Medical Sciences
New Delhi

Sumedha Pawa MD
Professor
Department of Radiodiagnosis
Maulana Azad Medical College
New Delhi

Veena Chowdhury MD
Director Professor and Head
Department of Radiodiagnosis
Maulana Azad Medical College
New Delhi

Veenu Singla MD
Assistant Professor
Department of Radiodiagnosis
PGIMER
Chandigarh

Preface to the Third Edition

The first edition of Diagnostic Radiology on 'Hepatobiliary and Gastrointestinal Imaging' was published in 1997. Rapid advances in the field of imaging necessitated revision and therefore the second edition was published in 2004.

Encouraged by the response to the previous editions and to keep up with the pace of advances in imaging we decided to update the second edition, delete some and add few new chapters to make the third edition a very comprehensive, updated reference book for postgraduates, practicing radiologists, gastroenterologists and GI surgeons.

We hope that the readers will find this book informative and that in the long run it will serve to improve patient care.

We wish to take this opportunity to thank our faculty from AIIMS, MAMC and PGIMER for their active contribution and support without which this endeavor would not have been possible.

We would also like to thank Shri Jitendar P Vij, Chairman and Managing Director of M/s Jaypee Brothers Medical Publishers (P) Ltd., Mr. Tarun Duneja, Director Publishing, Ms. Samina Khan and other staff for their professional help and cooperation in publishing this book in a very short time.

Arun Kumar Gupta
Veena Chowdhury
Niranjan Khandelwal
Deep Narayan Srivastava
Raju Sharma

Preface to the First Edition

There has been a tremendous change in the approach to the diagnosis of abdominal diseases in the last decade, making the imaging of hepatobiliary and gastrointestinal system as one of the most interesting and challenging specialities to the radiologists. New imaging and therapeutic techniques, that have revolutionised the diagnosis and treatment of many abdominal diseases, have also given us the added responsibility of defining the proper role of these techniques, evaluating their efficacy against earlier and more established methods, and providing guidance to clinicians through the judicious use of newer technology.

It is with this goal in mind, the faculty of Departments of Radiodiagnosis at the All India Institute of Medical Sciences, New Delhi, Maulana Azad Medical College, New Delhi and Postgraduate Institute of Medical Education and Research, Chandigarh present this third book in the series of Diagnostic Radiology, devoted to Hepatobiliary and Gastrointestinal Imaging.

The book comprises of twenty-nine chapters covering the radiological and imaging aspects of Hepatobiliary and Gastrointestinal systems in detail. In spite of advancements in various imaging techniques, conventional radiology still remains the mainstay as the initial imaging modality for many abdominal disorders and its interpretation continues to be a great challenge. The importance of plain radiography and barium studies has been described in depth. Techniques of US, CT and the potential role of MRI in evaluation of these disorders have also been explicitly elaborated upon. There are separate sections dedicated to imaging of the liver, biliary tract and pancreas. Clinicopathological aspects with radiological correlation have been discussed in the section on liver with special reference to focal and diffuse, benign and malignant lesions. Biliopathy and pancreatic disorders have been covered at length, with two separate chapters dealing with interventions. Portal hypertension has been discussed in great detail with authors explaining the role of various radiological modalities including US, colour Doppler, angiography and newer imaging techniques. The status of conventional techniques and advances in imaging have been described in an attempt to provide a comprehensive overview of all regions of the GI tract involved by infective, benign, and malignant lesions with special reference to the evaluation of the patients with GI bleed.

We hope the reader shall find this book both instructive and informative for the improved use of imaging resources which will help to serve the common goal of good health care and management of patients everywhere.

We wish to take this opportunity to thank our faculty colleagues from AIIMS, MAMC and PGIMER for their active support, co-operation and timely submission of the manuscripts. We owe immense gratitude to Prof K Subbarao, Prof A Gajaraj, Prof Ratni B Gujral and Prof B Nagi who have been very kind to contribute their experience into this book. We specially like to thank Dr Sumedha Pawa, Dr Mona Bhatia, Dr Anju Garg, Dr Sima Mukhopadhyay and Dr Sushma Vashisht for their help and untiring efforts in bringing out this volume. We also express our sincere thanks to the publishers of the series of these books, M/s Jaypee Brothers for timely publication of this volume, as always, in the present form.

Manorama Berry
Veena Chowdhury
Sudha Suri

Contents

PART ONE
GASTROINTESTINAL IMAGING

IMAGING TECHNIQUES

THE ACUTE ABDOMEN

INFECTIONS, INFLAMMATION AND NEOPLASMS

PART TWO
HEPATOBILIARY AND PANCREATIC IMAGING

LIVER AND BILIARY TRACT

PANCREAS

HEPATIC VASCULAR DISEASES

INTERVENTIONS

Plate 1

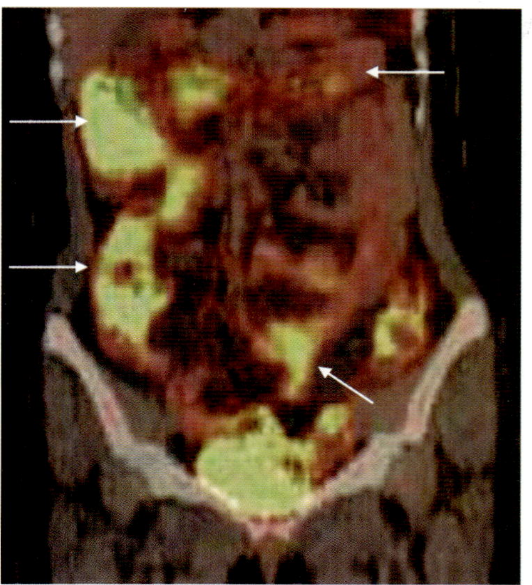

Fig. 1.4: PET-CT enteroclysis: Coronal PET-CT enteroclysis image in a patient with Crohn's disease showing diffuse uptake of FDG in small bowel (arrows)

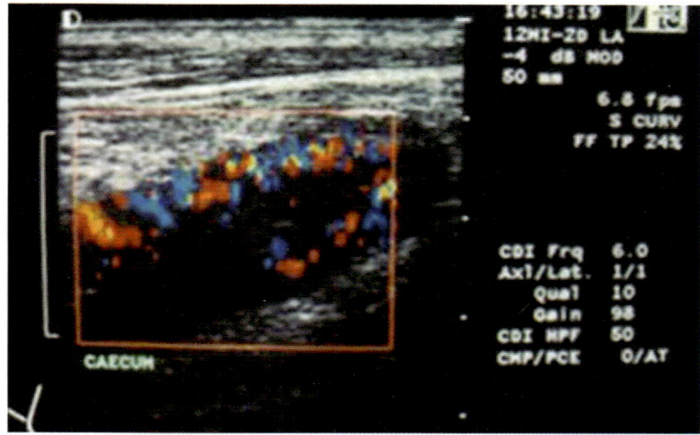

Fig. 7.39: CDFI. Shows a thick walled caecum with increased submuscosal vascularity

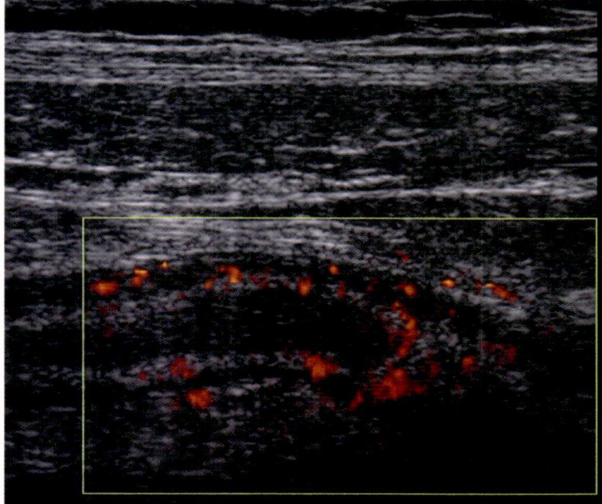

Fig. 8.34: Color Doppler showing increased vascularity in wall of appendix

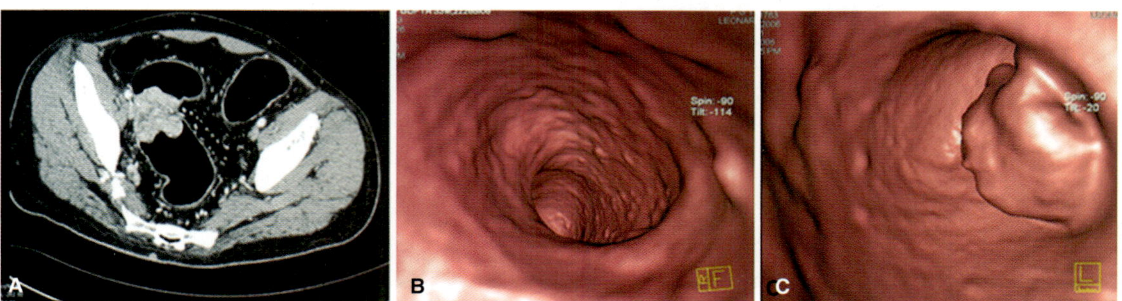

Figs 9.8A to C: (A) Axial CECT section shows a large polypoidal obstructive growth in the colon with increased vascularity in the adjacent mesentery. No pericolonic lymph nodes or stranding is seen. Actual colonoscopy was not possible in this patient, (B) CT colonography shows multiple pseudopolyps suggestive of ulcerative colitis and (C) The polypoidal growth in the sigmoid colon

Plate 2

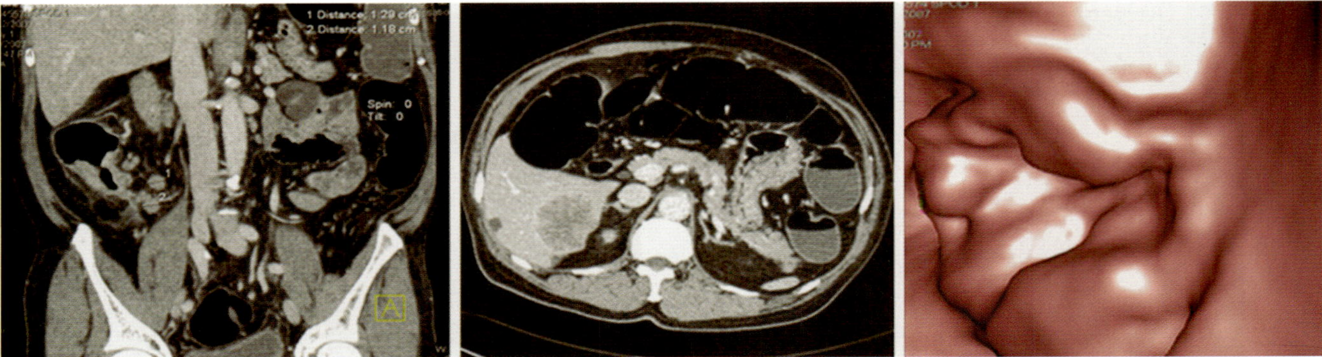

Figs 9.9A to C: (A) Coronal MPR image shows concentric mural thickening with a polypoidal component in the cecum. Pericolonic stranding and multiple enlarged pericolonic lymph nodes are also seen, (B) Axial CECT section of the upper abdomen shows hypodense lesions in segment VI of liver suggestive of metastases, (C) CT colonography endoluminal image shows the intraluminal irregular polypoidal growth

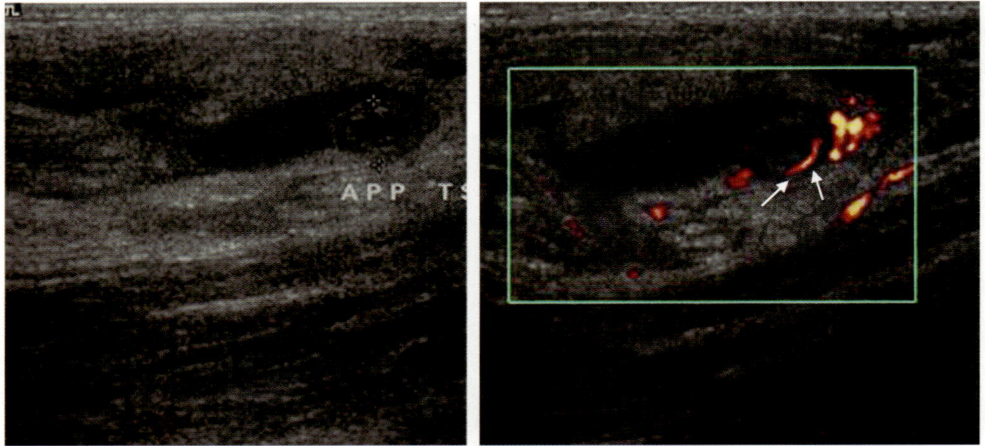

Fig. 11.12: Color Doppler in acute appendicitis. Doppler demonstrates focally increased flow in the appendiceal wall and in the adjacent inflamed fat

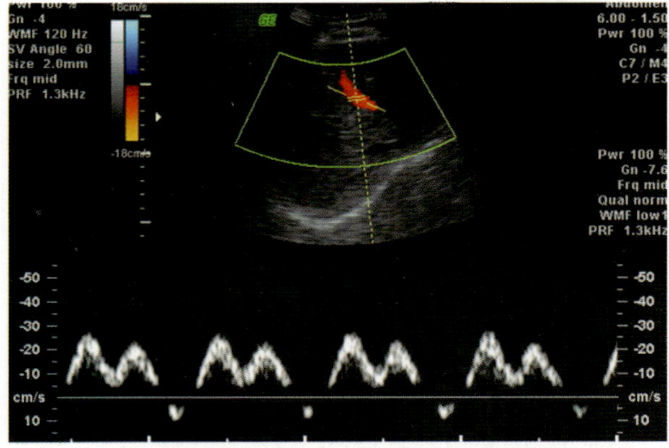

Fig. 12.2D: Color Doppler flow imaging of hepatic vein showing normal triphasic flow pattern with a short phase of reversed flow

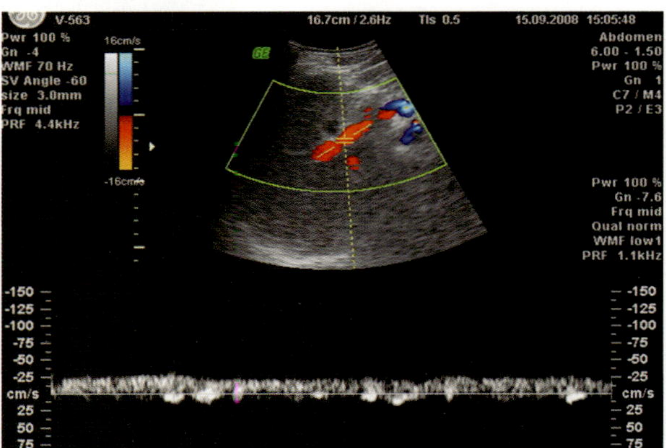

Fig. 12.2E: Color Doppler flow imaging of portal vein showing continuous antegrade flow with minimal phasicity

Plate 3

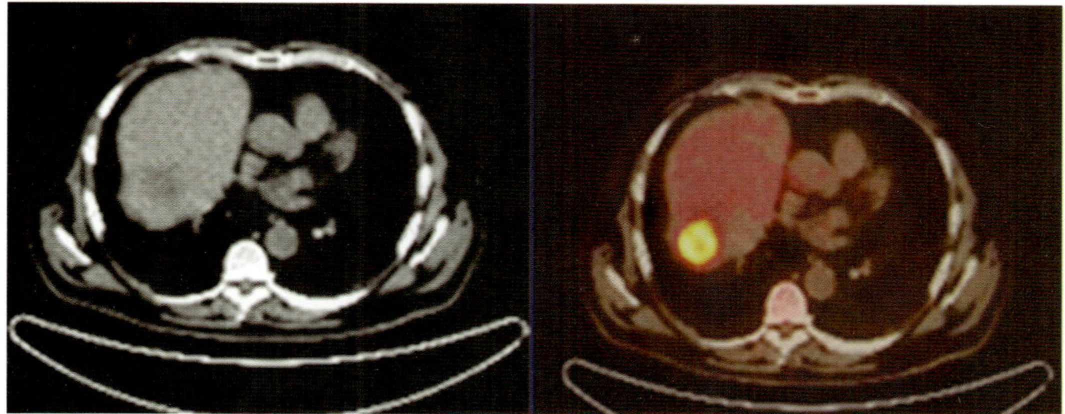

Fig. 12.12: FDG PET image showing a metastatic lesion in the segment 8 of liverin a newly diagnosed case of carcinoma colon

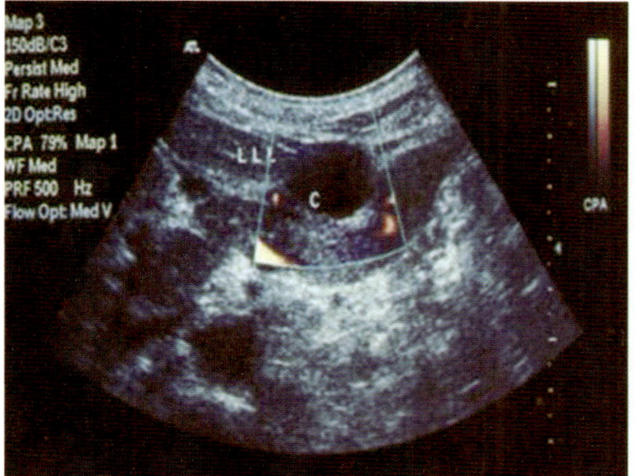

Fig. 13.2: Simple liver cyst seen as an anechoic lesion on color Doppler imaging

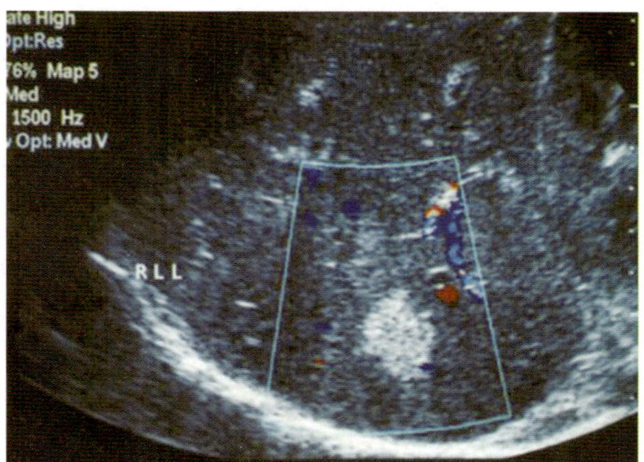

Fig. 13.7: Color flow imaging showing lack of internal vascularity in a hemangioma

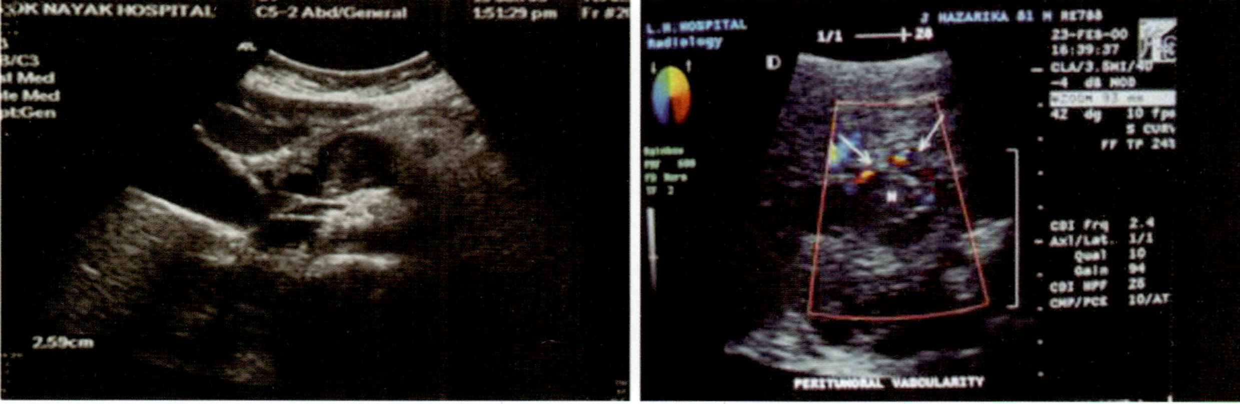

Figs 19.7A and B: Transverse sonogram showing a hypoechoic mass in the pancreatic head (A). On CDFI peritumoral vascularity and absence of internal vascularity seen. No vascular invasion was seen in this case

Plate 4

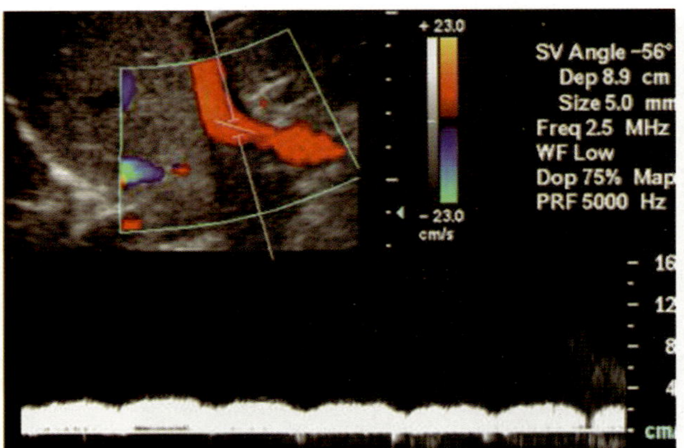

Fig. 20.5: CDFI of the main portal vein showing hepatopedal flow with a normal spectral trace

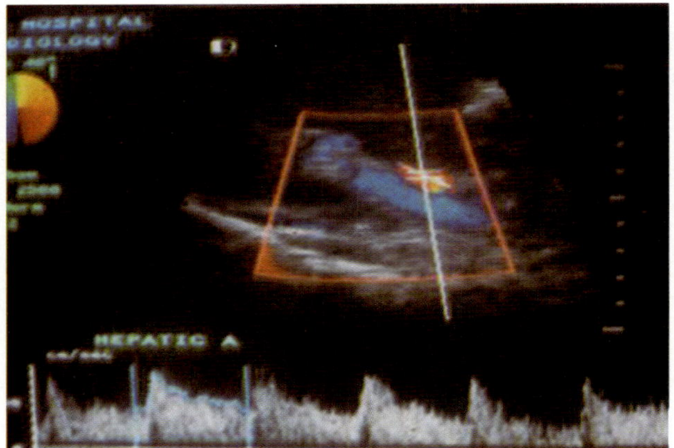

Fig. 20.6: CDFI in a patient of cirrhosis showing hepatofugal flow in the main portal vein. Note portal vein and hepatic artery show flow in opposite directions. Spectral trace from the hepatic artery is shown

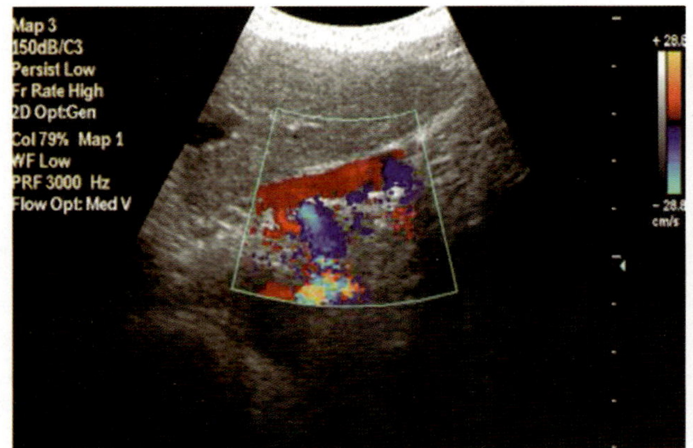

Fig. 20.7: Color Doppler study showing a tortuous coronary collateral with prominent varices at the gastroesophageal junction

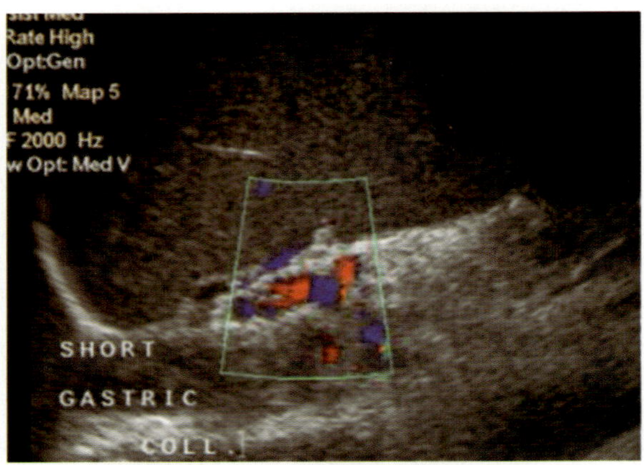

Fig. 20.8: Collateral vessels between upper pole of spleen and stomach consistent with short gastric collaterals

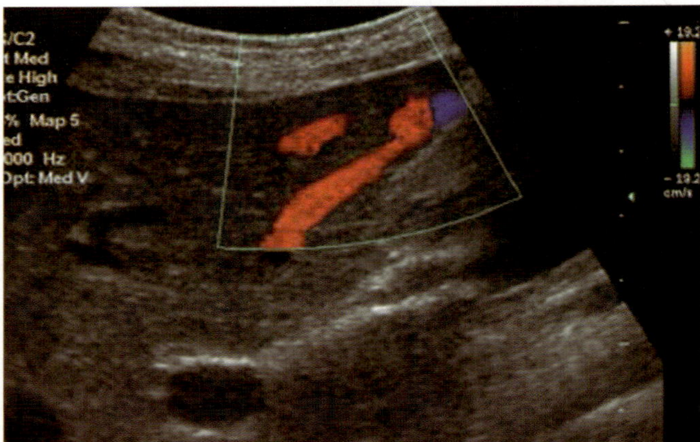

Fig. 20.9: Color Doppler study showing a paraumbilical collateral running in the ligamentum teres to the hepatic surface with hepatofugal flow

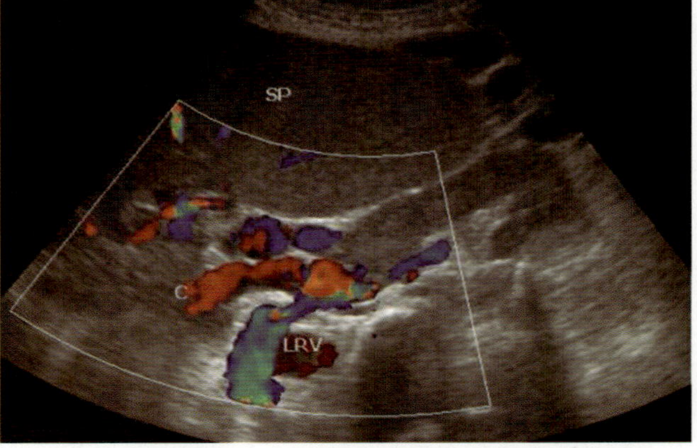

Fig. 20.10: CDFI showing a large lieno renal collateral draining into an enlarged renal vein

Plate 5

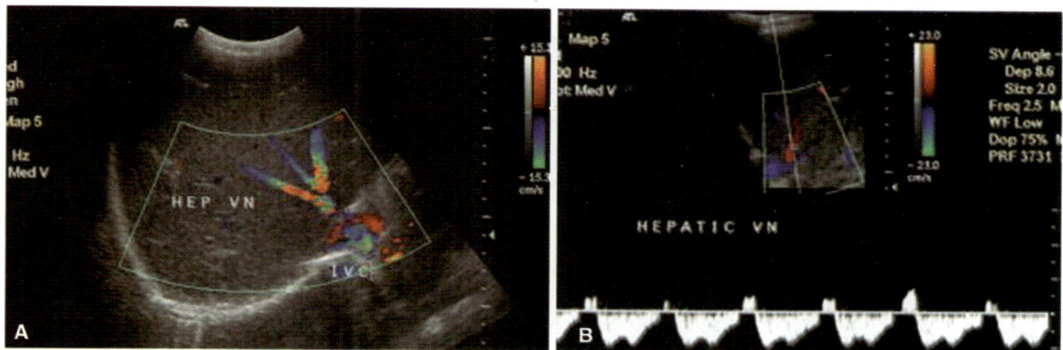

Figs 20.11 A and B: CDFI study showing the normal hepatic veins with the triphasic flow pattern

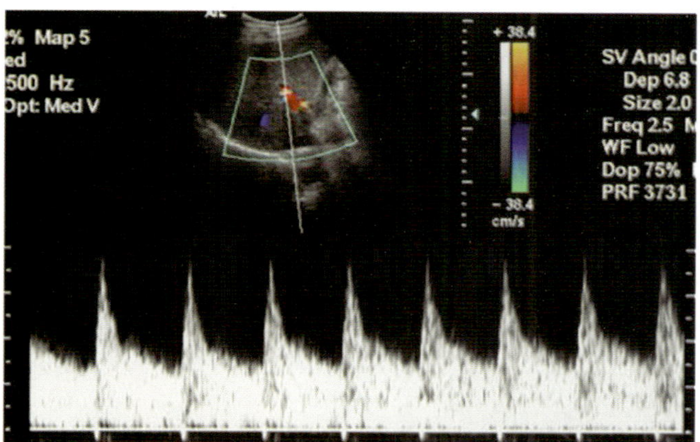

Fig. 20.12: Spectral Doppler trace from a normal hepatic artery

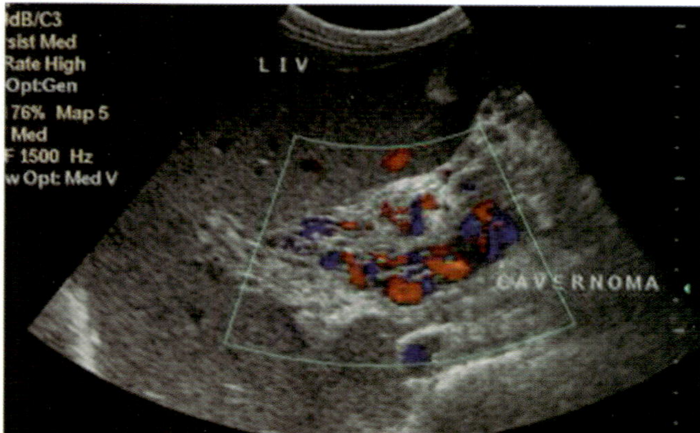

Fig. 20.16: Power Doppler study showing absence of color fill in the main portal vein due to anechoic thrombus

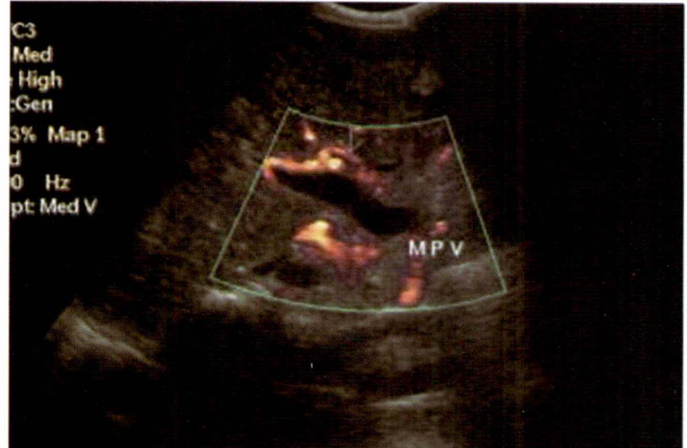

Fig. 20.17: Color Doppler showing absence of MPV with a tangle of vessels at the porta hepatis suggestive of cavernous transformation

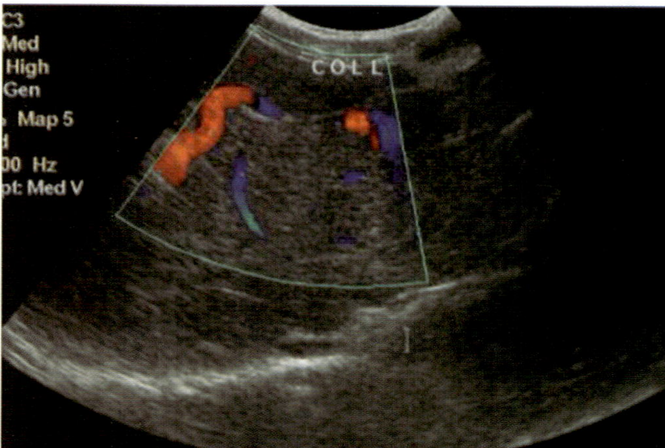

Fig. 20.18: Tortuous intrahepatic collateral coursing from the right to the left lobe in a patient of EHPO

Plate 6

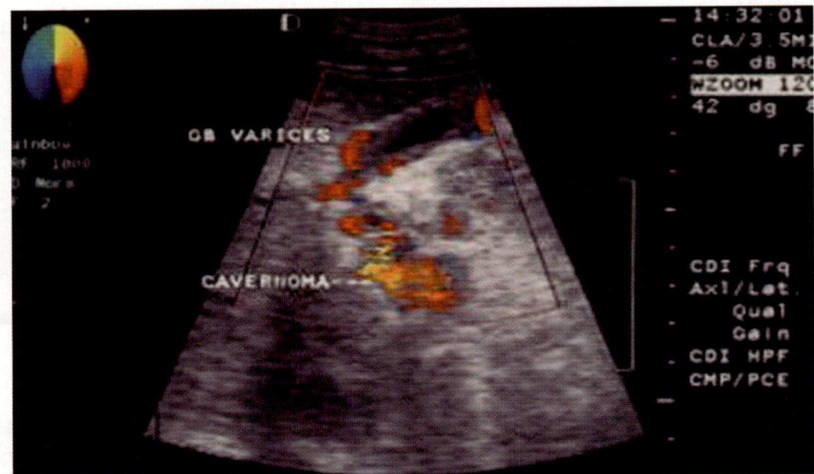

Fig. 20.19: Gallbladder varices in a case of EHPO seen as multiple rounded/tubular structures filling with color on CDFI

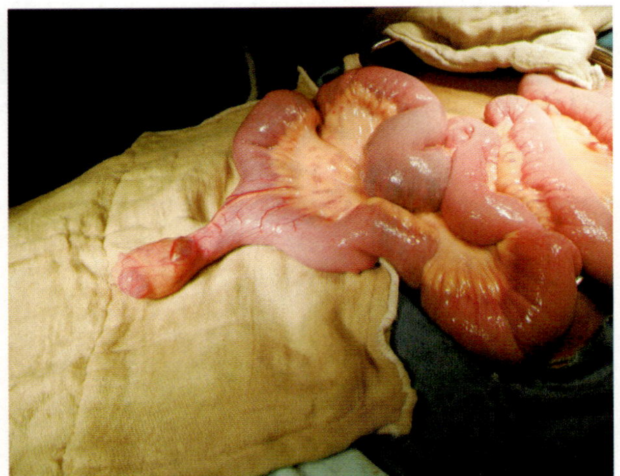

Fig. 22.10E: The diagnosis of Meckel's diverticulum was confirmed at surgery

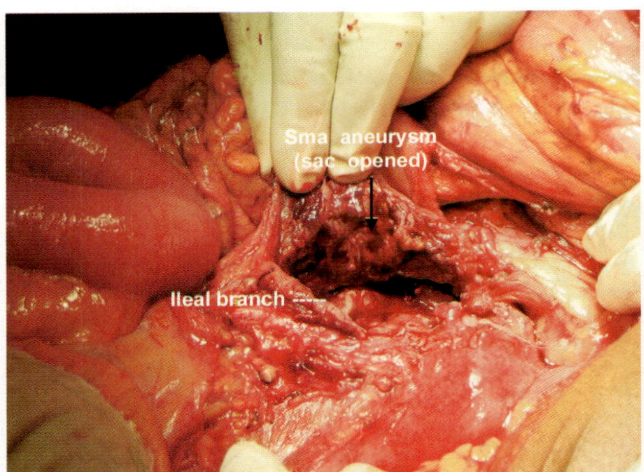

Fig. 22.14C: Later on surgically removed (C)

Plate 7

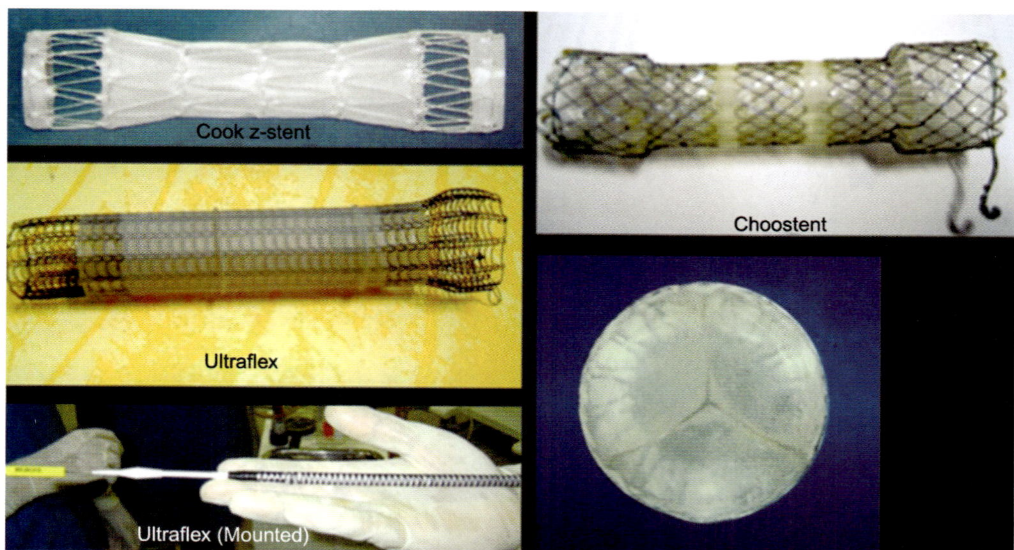

Fig. 25.2: Showing various designs of stents: Gianturco-Z stent (Cook). This is made from stainless steel and a polyethylene covering with barbs on the outside or uncoated flared ends to prevent migration. Ultraflex (Boston Scientific Ltd). This stent is made from a knitted Nitinol mesh and is available in both uncovered and covered. It has the weakest radial force but greater flexibility. These stents may be best for tortuous and upper third strictures

Choo Stent (Diagmed). This is a polyurethane-covered stent made from Nitinol and has a retrievable attached thread. These stents also come with an internal distal anti-reflux valve

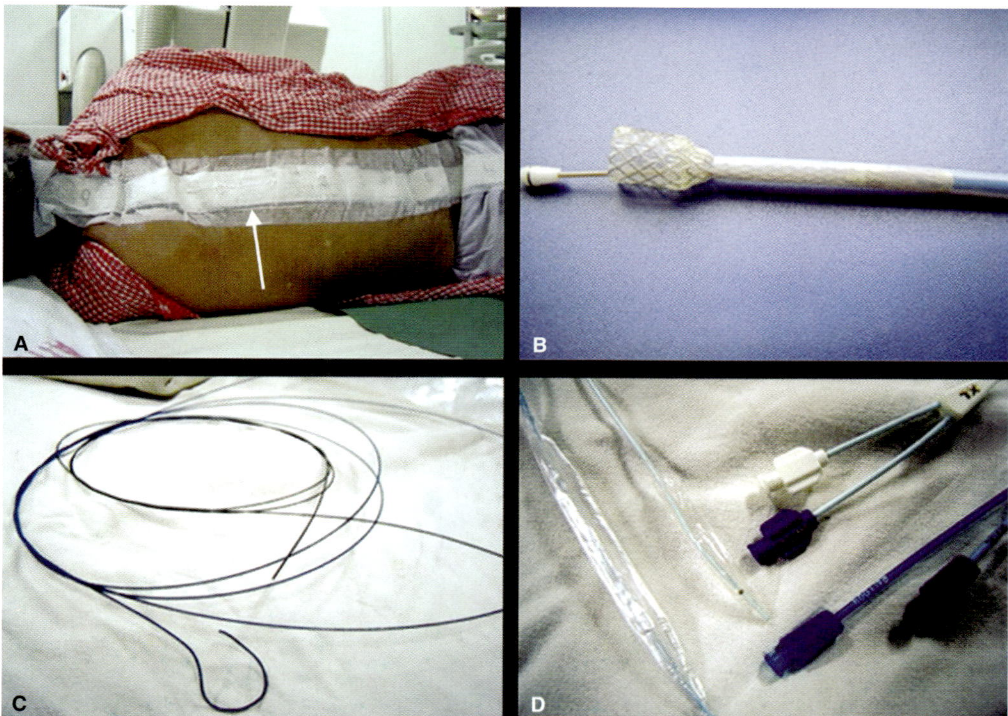

Fig. 25.3: Showing the preparation of esophageal stenting: Metallic marker pasted over the back of the patient (A) (arrow), Delivery system loaded with self expandable fully covered metallic stent (partially released) (B), Metallic and terumo guide wire (C) and Balloon catheter (D)

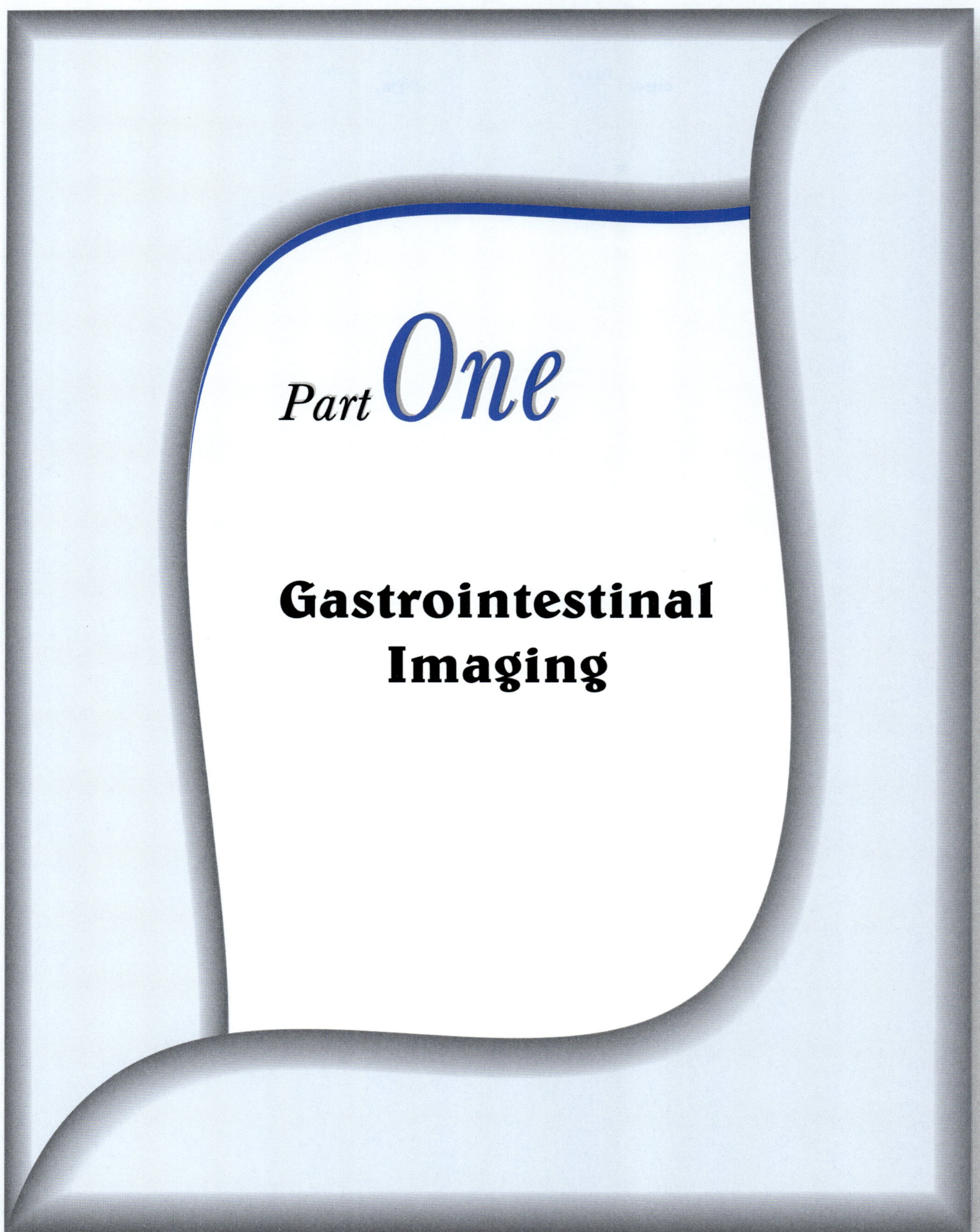

Part One

Gastrointestinal Imaging

Chapter One

Current Status of Conventional Techniques and Advances in GIT Imaging

Arun Kumar Gupta, Atin Kumar, Chandan Jyoti Das

INTRODUCTION

Gastrointestinal radiology has its true beginning less than a year after the exciting discovery of X-rays in 1895 and has been at the forefront of radiology, combining physiologic and anatomic informations right from its very inception. Over the years, with advances in instrumentation and techniques, gastrointestinal radiology has extended beyond conventional radiography, fluoroscopy and barium examinations. The imaging modalities of high resolution real time sonography, computerised tomography and to some extent magnetic resonance imaging have provided increasingly sophisticated and accurate diagnostic studies. However, these modalities have been primarily complementary to barium examinations and particularly helpful in assessing abnormalities of the wall and extraluminal spread of the disease. In spite of these high-tech modalities, barium contrast examination continued to be the best technique for evaluation of the mucosal surface of the gastrointestinal tract.[1] With the availability of flexible oesophagoscopy, gastroduodenoscopy and colonoscopy instrumentations, endoscopy emerged as an initial technique in the late 1980s and early 1990s in patients with upper gastrointestinal or colonic symptoms with resultant decline in the number of barium contrast studies. With the advent of capsule endoscopy even small bowel endoscopic images can be obtained which were earlier inaccessible to the endoscopists.

Development of Gastrointestinal Radiology

On reviewing the history of development of gastrointestinal radiology, conventional radiography consisting mainly of X-ray abdomen, fluoroscopy and single contrast barium study was the mainstay of technique till 1950s. With the development of image intensifiers and refinement in barium preparations, double contrast barium study became popular in 1960s for detection of small ulcers, early carcinoma or small colonic polyps. In the mid-1970s, development of flexible endoscopes made it possible to visualise directly the lumina of esophagus, stomach, duodenum and colon with the added advantage of biopsy facility for the suspected lesion. Thus, the evaluation of esophagus, stomach and colon no longer remained a domain of the radiologist and even with further improvements in technique and barium preparation for double contrast technique, radiological evaluation was taken away to a large degree by the endoscopists by the close of 1980s. However, the radiologist continued to have a primary responsibility in the evaluation of small bowel because of its unique anatomy and location. The endoscopists did not find a place in small bowel evaluation except for few inches of jejunum through upper gastrointestinal endoscopy or terminal ileum through colonoscopy. But recently capsule endoscopy has emerged as a promising technique to visualize small bowel beyond the reach of fibreoptic endoscopes. However it has the disadvantages of long hours of patient preparation time, small bowel transit and subsequent analysis of images. Also when a pathology is visualized, localizing it to a particular segment of bowel can be a problem with capsule endoscopy images. When a barium meal follow through examination is performed for a specific clinical problem indicating small bowel disease, the yield of positive study is higher. Also, this study provides more physiologic information about the antegrade flow and the natural response of the bowel to fluid bolus. However, barium meal follow through study is a lengthy examination, carries high false negative rate due to overlapping of bowel loops, peristalsis and poor distensibility of the segments.

The technique of enteroclysis, a dedicated small bowel study was introduced by Miller in 1982 which represented a significant improvement in ease of performance, speed of examination, optimal visualisation of the mucosal surface pattern and relationship of adjacent loops (Fig. 1.1). This has been accepted as a perferred technique for morphological demonstration of small lesions with other imaging techniques of US and CT giving an added dimension which is usually complementary.

In 1980s, in addition to the widespread use of endoscopy for gastrointestinal tract evaluation, the major development that influenced gastrointestinal radiology was further improvement in US and CT techniques for visualisation of endoluminal, intramural and perienteric components of the disease process. US and CT definitely score over double contrast techniques in the evaluation of the inflammatory disease affecting small and large bowel and staging of neoplasm involving gastointestinal tract.[2]

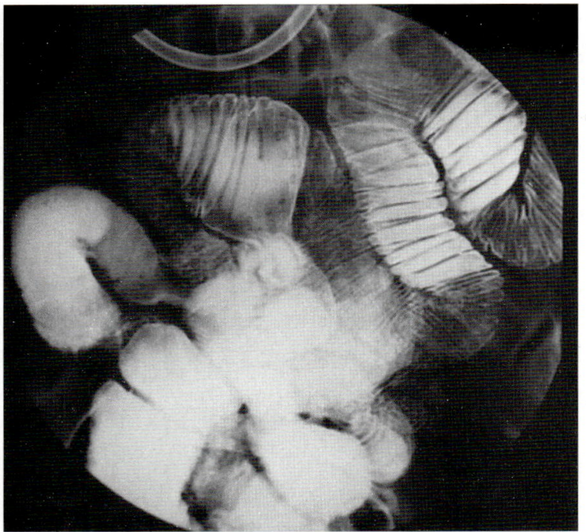

Fig. 1.1: Conventional small bowel enteroclysis showing normal distended jejunal and ileal loops

If the clinical history suggests primary mucosal disease process, barium study or endoscopy is an appropriate first choice but when the disease is suspected in which the information about extraluminal extension of the disease process is more critical than the changes in the mucosal surfaces, CT becomes the first investigation of choice.

With advances in CT technology, the role of CT has increased in evaluating patients with acute abdominal symptoms. CT can demonstrate intestinal and vascular changes and other ancillary abdominal features, hence it is considered the procedure of choice in clinically suspected intestinal obstruction or mesenteric ischaemia. Recently, MR imaging has also been reported to be comparable to CT in demonstrating these changes.

CT enteroclysis and more recently MR enteroclysis have emerged as techniques for small bowel imaging that combine advantages of barium enteroclysis with those of cross sectional imaging. Multidetector CT (MDCT) scanner with its capability of multiplanar reconstruction, can delineate the extent of the bowel disease and its complications. It can image the entire small and large bowel consistently which cannot be always achieved with barium study. MDCT is reliable, well tolerated, accurate and a fast imaging alternative technique to barium study for initial evaluation of small bowel and to assess extraenteric abnormalities especially in inflammatory bowel disease. The disadvantages of MDCT over barium study are increased radiation dose and the need for intravenous contrast. Nevertheless, information gained from MDCT justifies the increased radiation dose compared with barium study.[3]

Colonoscopy is a standard procedure for colonic evaluation both for diagnosis and biopsy as it visualises directly the mucosa and it may also be used in the treatment for removal of polyps. Virtual colonoscopy in recent years is emerging as a practical clinical technique for detection of colonic polyp or mass, both for colorectal cancer screening and for evaluation of patients with incomplete colonoscopy.[4]

Currently research is directed towards improving speed of image analysis, use of computer aided methods for detection of polyps, MR colonography, oral contrast tagging of faecal contents to avoid the need for rigorous bowel preparation, thereby improving patient compliance.

Conventional Techniques: Present Scenario

Since the year 2000, conventional radiological techniques for the evaluation of gastrointestinal tract have shown considerable decline. Plain radiograph of the abdomen has been limited mostly for bedside evaluation and for initial evaluation of abdominal distension for small bowel obstruction, intestinal ischaemia and perforation. In many centres CT is done as an initial technique replacing X-ray abdomen in acute abdominal conditions like acute appendicitis, intestinal obstruction, perforation, blunt trauma etc.

For evaluation of the esophagus, endoscopy is the first line investigation with fluoroscopic barium studies being complimentary for esophagitis and tumors. However the fluoroscopic barium studies still have a role in the assessment of motility disorders.

For evaluation of the stomach and the duodenum, fluoroscopic barium meal study is only complimentary to endoscopy for most cases of dyspepsia and abdominal pain. However it is superior to endoscopy for functional abnormalities like reflux, delayed emptying and sub-mucosal masses and infiltrative processes. The barium/ gastrograffin oral contrast study is also the technique of choice for evaluation in early postoperative period following gastric surgery, and in late postoperative period to define the anatomy.

For radiological evaluation of small bowel, enteroclysis has proven to a better technique than barium small bowel follow through examination.[5,6] It has been well accepted that enteroclysis is the technique of choice for demonstration of proximal disease, skip lesions, subtle strictures and mucosal abnormalities. The conventional enteroclysis has the advantages of shorter examination time, better distension of small bowel and better visualization of pathology but has drawbacks of more radiologist time, greater technical skill, more radiation dose to patient and operator and patient discomfort. CT enteroclysis and MR enteroclysis in addition have the advantage of cross-sectional studies like evaluation of wall and adjacent structures. Small bowel follow through study has the advantages of patient preference, ease to perform and ability to judge transit time. However the drawback of inadequate distension of small bowel coupled with dilution of barium renders it less useful as compared to enteroclysis and more recently capsule endoscopy. Capsule endoscopy is being increasingly used in clinical practice to visualize lesions of small bowel.[5,6] It is competing with enteroclysis as the modality of choice for evaluating small bowel. It has been shown to be very sensitive in detecting mucosal lesions and angiodysplasias but suffers from limitations of long hours of patient preparation time, small bowel transit and subsequent analysis of images. Other limitations include difficulty in localizing the pathology and inability to work in cases of intestinal obstruction. A small bowel follow through or enteroclysis may be required prior to capsule endoscopy in cases of clinical suspicion of small bowel obstruction.

Evaluation of colorectal diseases has been taken over by colonoscopy as an initial technique, double contrast barium enema being reserved as a second line of investigation in situtation with incomplete colonoscopy.[7] Also barium contrast enema is preferred in patients with question of large bowel obstruction, need for localisation of colonic disease preoperatively or to assess the status of colon anastomosis.

Advances in GIT Imaging

In recent years, advances in imaging technology of US, CT and MRI have contributed significantly in the imaging of various gastrointestinal diseases. Much interest has been focused on CT enteroclysis in recent times to overcome the individual deficiencies of CT (no distention of the small intestine) and conventional enteroclysis (no extraluminal information). CT enteroclysis has become a successful alternative imaging method for small-bowel evaluation and is reported to be highly accurate in depicting mucosal abnormalities and extraintestinal complications in patients with inflammatory diseases of the intestine. MR Enteroclysis (MRE) has the dual advantage of MRI (excellent soft-tissue contrast and multiplanar imaging capabilities) and enteroclysis (enables optimal distention of the small bowel) and could be the optimal imaging method for evaluation of the bowel. With the availability of ultra fast sequences, robust breath-hold sequences and adequate use of contrast media, a combined morphologic and functional imaging method for the small bowel, has now become possible with MRE. PET-CT scan has been the latest addition to the armoury.[8]

Ultrasonography (US) in GIT

Earlier, the inherent bowel gas was considered as an obstacle to useful US imaging but recently its role in intrinsic gastrointestinal diseases has been well recognized. The development of endoscopic US (EUS) has rendered upper gastrointestinal tract amenable to US examination. Also EUS instrument incorporating biopsy channel within the endoscope is available for fine needle aspiration of intramural or extramural lesions under US guidance. Intraoperative US using high frequency transducers can provide similar degree of resolution as EUS techniques.

Technique of endosonography can stage the tumor by depicting all layers of bowel wall and it has become a practical technique for staging carcinoma of the esophagus and the stomach in many centers. Transrectal ultrasonography using a high frequency rotating transducer is a valuable method, permits staging of colorectal carcinoma which can be correlated well with endoscopy. Anal endosonography is a modification of transrectal sonography that provides radial images of the anal canal and its sphincters. It has proven to be particularly useful for mapping traumatic defects of the external anal sphincter in patients with faecal incontinence.

Sonoenteroclysis is a useful technique in the evaluation of small bowel.[9] The diagnostic accuracy of sonoenteroclysis for detecting small bowel lesions is comparable to that of barium enteroclysis. This new, widely available, inexpensive, and undemanding technique can be used as an initial investigation in the evaluation of patients with small bowel disorders.[9] The application of color Doppler imaging and power Doppler may allow differentiation of active bowel thickening (increased blood flow) from chronic wall thickening/ fibrosis (no increased flow).[10] Similarly, Doppler ultrasound can also demonstrate hemodynamic changes in patients with active IBD which are not present in those with quiescent disease.[11] In a study by Hata[12] et al, ultrasound had a reported sensitivity of 86% for CD and 89% for UC. Although recent work is promising, ultrasound continues to be very operator dependent and adversely affected by factors such as obesity and intraluminal gas.

CT Enteroclysis (Fig. 1.2)

CT depicts mural and extraluminal abnormalities and CT Enteroclysis combines the advantages of both CT with IV contrast and enteroclysis with enteral contrast.[13] The contrast agent should allow imaging with homogeneous luminal enhancement, high contrast between the lumen and bowel wall, minimal mucosal absorption, absence of artifact formation, and without significant adverse effects. Enteral Contrast Agents can be neutral (0.5% methylcellulose, Water, Low density Barium (VoLumen and Polyethylene glycol) or positive (4-15% water soluble contrast, Dilute 6% Barium). Barium as contrast is preferred for CT Enterography and to demonstrate sinus tracts and fistulae. Patterns of abnormality that have to be observed on CT Enteroclysis are mural enhancement pattern (Target, homogenous, heterogeneous and diminished), length of involvement, degree of thickening, symmetric vs asymmetric thickening, location (proximal vs distal), location in the wall (mucosal/submucosal/ serosal) and associated abnormalities in the mesenteric vasculature.

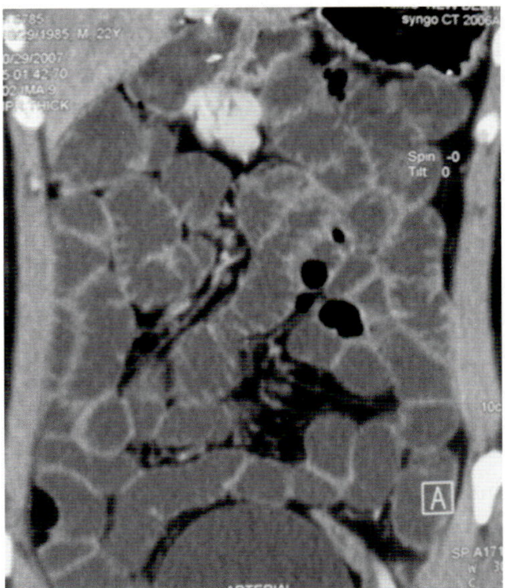

Fig. 1.2: Coronal CT enteroclysis showing nodular normal distension of the small bowel

Technique of CT Enteroclysis

Fluoroscopic Phase–Small bowel catheter used (12 F Frekka tube 120 cm)-positioned to the left of midline OR in proximal descending duodenum to evaluate obscure GI bleed or anemia.

CT Phase–Infusion of 2.5 L water with methyl cellulose or dilute barium infused at 80-100 ml/min-rate, Infuse 1.5 L of water at 100 ml/min; 2 L for large patients or when colon evacuation is important followed by 1 ampoule Buscopan given IV and IV contrast (100ml/min). CT images are acquired at 50 sec delay in the late arterial/ early portal venous phase. CT enteroclysis parameters for a 40 channel CT are source: 40 * 0.625 mm, reformat: 2.0 mm, width 1.0 mm reconstruction interval, window width = 360 HU and window level = 40HU (for negative contrast).

Indications

- Unexplained GI bleed or anemia
- Staging of known Crohn's disease
- Unexplained pain abdomen with no e/o significant small bowel distension on plain X-rays
- Alternate examination before/after capsule endoscopy or when CO_2 double contrast Ba enteroclysis is not technically possible.

CT Enterography

CT enterography has rapidly gained acceptance as a method for visualizing the small bowel lumen, wall and mesentery for a variety of clinical indications like CD and vascular and neoplastic small bowel masses.[14] CT enterography is similar to CT enteroclysis except for the fact that naso-jejunal tube is not used and only oral contrast is used to distend the small bowel loops. Patient preparation include nil per orally for 4 hrs prior to scan. Oral contrast of choice is 0.1% w/v barium solution mixed with sorbitol-attenuation 20 HU (volume-900–1800 ml over 30 min to 2 hrs before CT) followed by 1 amp buscopan (i/m, i/v). Scanning techniques include single phase imaging in "Enteric phase" with scan delay of 45 sec especially for evaluation of Crohn's disease and obstruction. Multiphasic imaging can also be performed with bolus triggered arterial phase with scan delay of 6 sec, enteric phase in 20-25 sec and delayed phase in 70-75 sec. This is important especially for obscure GI bleed.

MRI and MR Enteroclysis (MRE)

The mesenteric small bowel has remained a grey zone for enteroscopists despite the advances in various endoscopic techniques. MRE can be used as the initial imaging method for small-bowel diseases (Fig. 1.3). MRE has the potential to change the way how we assess the small bowel because of its capability to provide functional information, excellent soft-tissue contrast, and multiplanar imaging capabilities. TruFISP, HASTE, and post-gadolinium VIBE images can be employed in a comprehensive and integrated MRE examination protocol.[15-17]

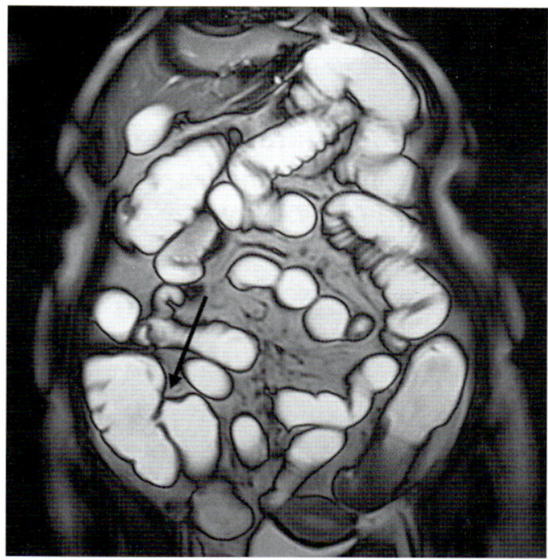

Fig. 1.3: T2W MRI coronal view showing stricture at ileocecal junction (arrow) with proximal dilation in intestinal TB

Distention of the small-bowel lumen with methylcellulose solution and intravenously administered gadopentetate dimeglumine provides optimal contrast between the bowel wall and lumen. This technique enables optimal distention of the small bowel and facilitates identification of wall abnormalities resulting in accurate visualization of stenoses and obstructions. MRE scores over other imaging modalities because of its excellent soft-tissue contrast, direct multiplanar imaging capabilities, lack of ionizing radiation and functional information of disease activity. MRE has shown excellent correlation with conventional enteroclysis in grading small bowel obstruction, visualization of transmural and extramural pathology and also provides functional information regarding disease activity status. Although superficial abnormalities are better seen on conventional enteroclysis, the characteristic transmural abnormalities of Crohn's disease such as bowel wall thickening, linear ulcers, and cobblestoning are better seen with MRE, especially with the TrueFISP sequence. MRE is comparable to conventional enteroclysis in the detection of the number and extent of involved small bowel segments and in the delineation of stenosis or prestenotic intestinal dilatation. MRE findings correlate well with disease activity in both active and chronic form of Crohn's disease.

PET-CT Enteroclysis and PET CT Colonography

Although CT enteroclysis and MR Enteroclysis provide excellent anatomical information, they fail to show the metabolic status of disease activity. Small intestinal endoscopic techniques such as capsule endoscopy and double balloon enteroscopy holds a lot of promise for evaluation of intestinal lumen. However, they fail to provide information on the intestinal wall and surrounding structures. Therefore, they are combined with a cross-sectional imaging technique such as CT enteroclysis or more often MR enteroclysis.[18] Therefore, we conceptualized a fusion of a metabolic imaging technique like positron emission tomography (PET) and an anatomical imaging modality like CT enteroclysis to derive information both on the morphological details and the functional activity of the lesions at the same time. PET is now a well-established functional imaging technique and is widely used in the management of various cancers.[19-21] Fusion of PET with CT (PET-CT) provides morphological localization of the metabolically active focus/foci. This technique exploits the property of viable malignant cells, which have higher uptake and metabolism of glucose.[22] Increase in the glucose utilization is not specific for cancer cells, various cytokines and growth factors increase the affinity of glucose transporters for deoxyglucose in inflammatory conditions also.[22] PET has been used for assessment of various inflammatory disorders and has shown encouraging results.[23-25] The interpretation of abdominal PET images is often difficult due to physiologic uptake of FDG in a variety of abdominal/pelvic organs, which makes it difficult to distinguish normal from abnormal uptake. As the intestine remains in a collapsed state, the resolution of the intestine remains very poor on PET-CT. Therefore, distension of the intestine is required for better resolution on imaging.[26] PET-CT scan can be acquired sixty minutes after intravenous injection of 10 mCi of IV 18 fluoro-deoxyglucose (FDG) radiotracer injection and infusion of 2 l of 0.5% methylcellulose through a naso-jejunal catheter just before the study. We in a pilot study including 17 patients with inflammatory diseases of intestine such as intestinal tuberculosis and CD showed that as a single investigation, PET-CT enteroclysis detects a significantly higher number of lesions both in small and large intestine in comparison to that detected by conventional barium and colonoscopy combined together (Fig. 1.4). This technique is non-invasive, feasible and very promising.[8] PET-CT enteroclysis may be used not only in the evaluation of IBD but also in the follow-up of patients non-invasively. PET-CT colonography is a similar technique like PET-CT enteroclysis and has the potential for non-invasive evaluation of patients with UC. PET-CT colonography is performed after ingestion of 2.5 liter of polyethylene glycol solution to distend colon and PET-CT scan was obtained 60 min after injection of 10 mCi of FDG. In an ongoing study, we found PET-CT colonography to be a novel non-invasive technique for assessment of disease extent in UC.[27]

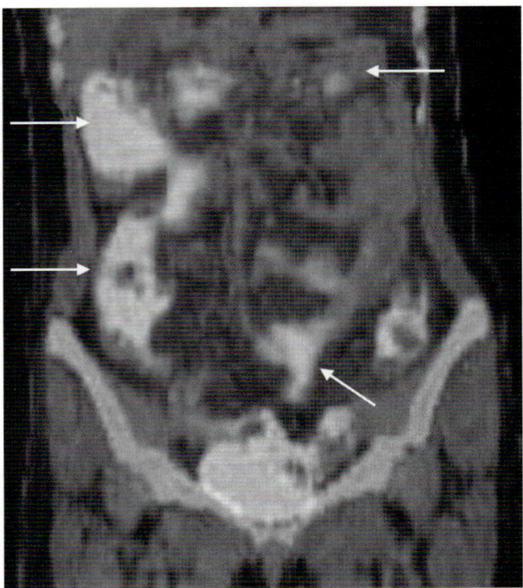

Fig. 1.4: PET-CT enteroclysis: Coronal PET-CT enteroclysis image in a patient with Crohn's disease showing diffuse uptake of FDG in small bowel (arrows) (*For color version see plate 1*)

NUCLEAR SCINTIGRAPHY

With the availability of radionuclide-labeled white blood cells (WBC) scintigraphy is quickly emerging as a promising technique for visualizing actively inflamed bowel. In the past, the major radionuclide used in evaluating patients with active IBD was gallium-67.[28-30] Now-a-days new radionuclide like indium and technetium are used to label WBCs. In these studies, blood is removed from the patient and the white blood cells are separated and labeled, then reinjected. The radionuclide accumulates at sites of acute inflammation or infection. Imaging is performed at 6,12 and 24 hours and any focal bowel or intra-abdominal activity is suggestive of active inflammation/infection. Published literature shows good correlation between the results of indium-labeled white cell studies and colonoscopy, barium enema and clinical symptoms in patients with active IBD.[31-34] With the advent of selective radionuclide, the role of nuclear scintigraphy in the evaluation of patients with IBD is expanding. The strength of these radionuclides lies in the ability to screen patients for disease and to differentiate active from inactive disease. However, because of the limited spatial resolution and current difficulty in differentiating between inflammatory and infectious bowel diseases, the scintigraphy is used as a problem solving modality when other tests are equivocal.

Characteristic imaging finding of common bowel disorders are discussed below.

Tuberculosis

CT may show mural thickening of IC area-concentric, low density areas in the bowel wall, skip areas, enlarged mesenteric lymph nodes with central low attenuation areas and obstruction. CT or MR enteroclysis can delineate the stricture and MRE specifically can tell about the activity of the stricture (Fig. 1.3). In addition, extraluminal findings like lymph nodes and peritoneal involvement can be seen.

Crohn's Disease

Complications of CD like stricture and fistulas are well seen on enteroclysis. Strictures are reported to occur in 21% of patients with small bowel CD and may result in high grade bowel obstruction necessitating surgical intervention in some cases. Enteroclysis is useful in differentiating fibrotic strictures which may require surgery from active ulcerated stenotic disease and luminal narrowing as a result of spasm. Resistance to lumen distension during enteroclysis confirms the presence of a fibrous stricture. Fistulas in CD occur in 6–33% cases. Most commonly these are ileo-ileal or ileo-caecal and are often multiple.

Specific advantages of cross-sectional imaging include demonstration of the transmural extent of inflammation; skip lesions without significant severe stenosis, intraperitoneal or extraintestinal complications and in assessment of the disease activity. CT is the modality of choice for evaluation of the bowel although recently MRI has also been shown to be as effective. A prerequisite for optimal evaluation of the small bowel with CT or MRI is adequate distension of the bowel loops. This can be achieved by administering 1-2 liters of contrast orally or better still via a naso-jejunal catheter. Bowel wall thickening usually ranging from 1-2 cm is the most consistent feature of Crohn's disease on cross-sectional imaging. The number of lesions, presence of luminal narrowing, prestenotic dilatation and pseudodiverticulum formation are easily recognized on the cross-sectional images. Fibrofatty proliferation in the adjacent mesentery is commonly seen in Crohn's disease. Cross-sectional imaging modalities especially CT or MRI can also depict complications like abscesses close to the involved bowel and fistulous communication (with adjacent bowel, skin or urinary bladder) and also the blind ending sinus tracts. Small mesenteric lymph nodes ranging from 3–8 mm in size can be seen in Crohn's disease. Knowledge of the inflammatory activity of the disease is important to institute appropriate treatment. CT and MRI are very useful in this regard. The findings which suggest active disease include: thickened bowel wall with marked contrast enhancement (Fig. 1.5), mural stratification, pericolic or perienteric hypervascularity (Coomb's sign) (Fig. 1.6), hyperintensity of the bowel on T2 weighted images, lymph node enlargement and exramural complications such as phlegmon and abscess.

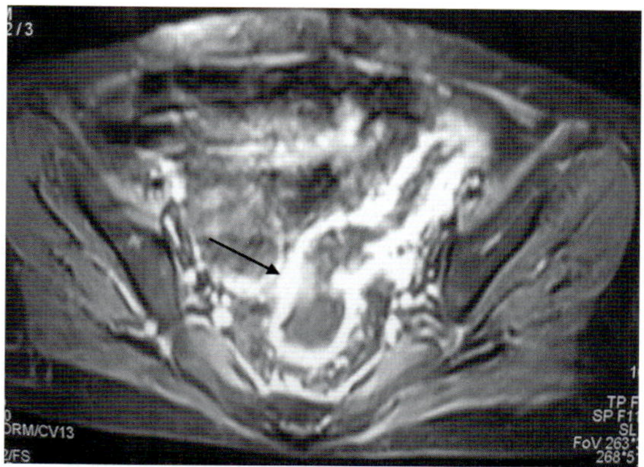

Fig. 1.5: Crohn's disease: Contrast-enhanced T1W MRI shows marked enhancement and wall thickening of the rectosigmoid (arrow) with positive Coombs' sign

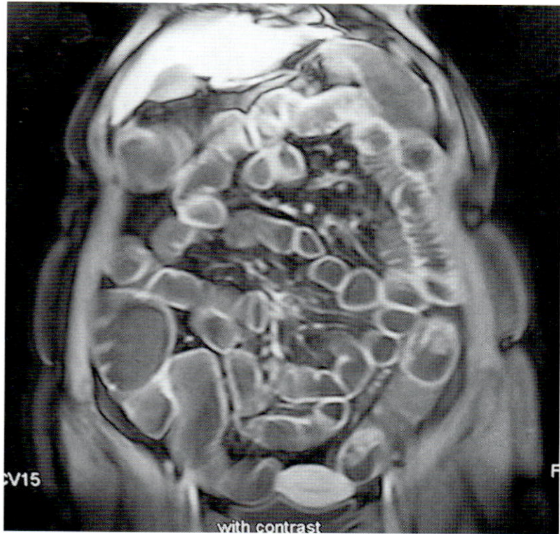

Fig. 1.6: Crohn's disease: Post Gad T1W coronal image showing enhancement of whole of small bowel

Imaging in Small Bowel Obstruction

Enteroclysis is the method of choice in low grade/intermittent obstruction, unsuspected closed loop obstruction, h/o laparotomy for malignancy, radiation enteropathy and strictures in Crohn's disease. Enteroclysis is contraindicated in acute and complete or high grade obstruction, suspicious strangulated obstruction and suspected perforation. CT has high sensitivity of 94-100% and accuracy of 90-95%. CT is the method of choice in acute, complete obstruction, adynamic ileus, prolonged high grade obstruction, suspicion of strangulation, and suspicion of inflammatory process (Figs 1.7 and 1.8). Common extrinsic causes include adhesions, closed loop obstruction, strangulation (circumferential wall thickening with increased attenuation, target sign, congestion/hemorrhage in the mesentery, pneumatosis intestinalis and ascites), hernias and tumors (carcinoid, lymphoma, peritoneal carcinomatosis, and diverticulitis). Intrinsic causes include adenocarcinoma, inflammatory conditions (Tuberculosis, CD), radiation enteropathy and intussusception.

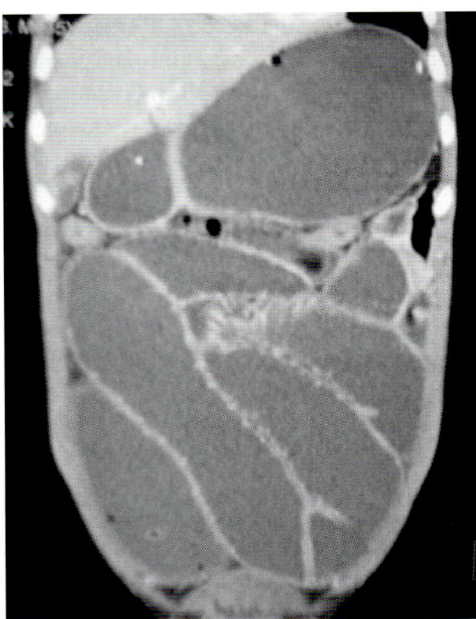

Fig. 1.8: Intestinal obstruction: Coronal CT enteroclysis showing gross dilatation of jejunal loops in a case of adhesion

Mesenteric Ischemia

Mesenteric ischemia results from major artery occlusion (SMA) or mesenteric vein thrombosis. Plain X-rays may show thickened valvulae conniventes, dilated gas filled bowel loops, thickening of bowel wall, thumb printing and occasionally air in intestinal wall/hepatic veins. Barium studies reveal thickened valvulae thumb-printing of mesenteric border, luminal narrowing and wall thickening with separation of bowel loops. CT findings include bowel wall thickening more than 8 mm, transmural infarction causing paper thin wall bowel dilatation, low density bowel wall, pneumatosis/ portomesenteric venous gas complete absence of enhancement, mesenteric edema. Vascular findings include thrombus, embolus, vasculitis, dissection, aneurysm and venous thrombosis.

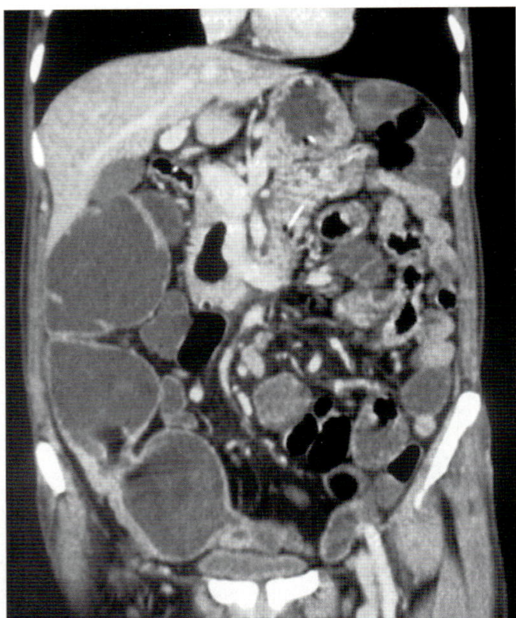

Fig. 1.7: Intestinal obstruction: Coronal CT enteroclysis showing multiple stenoses of jejunal loop with gross dilatation of intervening jejunal loops in a case of adhesion

Neoplasms Malignant

Forty percent of malignant small bowel tumors are adenocarcinomas. Barium shows narrowing and CT may show eccentric focal mass, circumferential asymmetric thickening and metastasis to lymph node and mesentery. Lymphoma is equally common. Barium may show aneurysmal, constrictive, nodular, ulcerative, mesenteric and endoexoenteric type of lesions. CT may show circumferential wall thickening, cavitary and mesenteric lymph nodal masses. Bulky, eccentric lesion with calcification, significant enhancement with IV contrast and metastasis to liver, omentum may be seen in leiomyosarcoma. Carcinoid may show characteristic crowding of folds with kinking of bowel wall on barium studies. In CT, it appears as a mesenteric mass with curvilinear strands extending to bowel loops (Stellate appearance) with adenopathy, calcification and liver metastasis. Angiography may show stellate arterial configuration at tumor periphery.

CONCLUSION

Advances in imaging technology of US, CT and MRI provide a clear understanding of the true extent of a gastrointestinal lesion. The rapid dissemination of MDCT provides faster and more accurate imaging. With robust computer processing power and larger set of data storage capacity will make image rendering faster, simpler and more affordable. It is quite likely that gastrointestinal imaging will continue to expand till it reaches its zenith due to further technical advances. In conclusion, judicious use of available modalities may lead to timely and prompt diagnosis of various intestinal disorders.

REFERENCES

1. Goldberg HI, Margulis AR. Gastrointestinal radiology in the United states: An overview of the past 50 years. Radiology 2000;216:1-7.
2. Thomas M, Gluecker C, Daniel J, et al. Colorectal cancer screening with CT colonography, colonoscopy and double contrast barium enema examinations: Prospective assessment of patient perceptions and preferences. Radiology 2003;227:378-84.
3. Jamieson DH, Shipman PJ, Israel DM, et al. Comparison of multidetector CT and barium studies of the small bowel: Inflammatory bowel disease in children. Am J Roentgenol 2003;180:1211-16.
4. Dachman AH and Yoshida H. Virtual colonoscopy past, present and future. RCNA 2003;41:377-93.
5. Maglinte DDT, Sandrasegaran K, Chiorean M, Dewitt J, McHenry L, Lappas JC. Radiologic investigations complement and add diagnostic information to capsule endoscopy of small-bowel diseases. AJR 2007;189: 306-12.
6. Maglinte DDT. Capsule imaging and the role of radiology in the investigation of diseases of the small bowel. Radiology 2005;236:763-67.
7. Rosman AS, Korsten MA. Meta-analysis comparing CT colonography, air contrast barium enema, and colonoscopy. Am J Med 120(3):203-210.e4.
8. Das CJ, Makharia G, Kumar R, Chawla M, Goswami P, Sharma R, Malhotra A. PET-CT enteroclysis: A new technique for evaluation of inflammatory diseases of the intestine. Eur J Nucl Med Mol Imaging. 2007;34(12): 2106-14.
9. Nagi B, Rana SS, Kochhar R, Bhasin DK. Sonoenteroclysis: A new technique for the diagnosis of small bowel diseases. Abdom Imaging 2006;31:417-24.
10. Sarrazin J, Wilson SR. Manifestations of Crohn disease at US. Radiographics 1996;16(3):499-520; discussion 520-1
11. Maconi G, Imbesi V, Bianchi Porro G. Doppler ultrasound measurement of intestinal blood flow in inflammatory bowel disease. Scand J Gastroenterol 1996;31(6):590-3.
12. Hata J, Haruma K, Suenaga K, Yoshihara M, Yamamoto G, Tanaka S, Shimamoto T, Sumii K, Kajiyama G. Ultrasonographic assessment of inflammatory bowel disease. Am J Gastroenterol 1992;87(4):443-7.
13. Engin G. Computed tomography enteroclysis in the diagnosis of intestinal diseases. J Comput Assist Tomogr 2008;32(1):9-16.
14. Hara AK, Swartz PG. CT enterography of Crohn's disease. Abdom Imaging 2008;23 [Epub ahead of print].
15. Malagò R, Manfredi R, Benini L, D'Alpaos G, Pozzi Mucelli R. Assessment of Crohn's disease activity in the small bowel with MR-enteroclysis: Clinico-radiological correlations. Abdom Imaging 2008;29:[Epub ahead of print]
16. Masselli G, Casciani E, Polettini E, Gualdi G. Comparison of MR enteroclysis with MR enterography and conventional enteroclysis in patients with Crohn's disease. Eur Radiol 2008;18(3):438-47.
17. Ryan ER, Heaslip IS. Magnetic resonance enteroclysis compared with conventional enteroclysis and computed tomography enteroclysis: A critically appraised topic. Abdom Imaging 2008;33(1):34-7.
18. Lewis PJ, Salama A. Uptake of fluorine-18-fluorodeoxyglucose in sarcoidosis. J Nucl Med 1994;35: 1647-49.
19. Annovazzi A, Peeters M, Maenhout A, Signore A, Dierckx R, Van De Wiele C. 18-Fluorodeoxyglucose positron emission tomography in nonendocrine neoplastic disorders of the gastrointestinal tract. Gastroenterology 2003;125:1235-45.
20. Palmer WE, Rosenthal DI, Schoenberg OI, et al. Quantification of inflammation in the wrist with gadolinium-enhanced MR imaging and PET with 2-[F-18]-fluoro-2-deoxy-D-glucose. Radiology 1995;196:647-55.
21. Neurath MF, Vehling D, Schunk K, et al. Noninvasive assessment of Crohn's disease activity: A comparison of 18F-fluorodeoxyglucose positron emission tomography, hydromagnetic resonance imaging, and granulocyte scintigraphy with labeled antibodies. Am J Gastroenterol 2002;97:1978-85.
22. Lemberg DA, Issenman RM, Cawdron R, et al. Positron emission tomography in the investigation of pediatric inflammatory bowel disease. Inflamm Bowel Dis 2005;11:733-38.
23. Loffler M, Weckesser M, Franzius C, et al. High diagnostic value of F-FDG-PET in pediatric patients with chronic inflammatory bowel disease. Ann NY Acad Sci 2006; 1072:379-85.
24. Antoch G, Saoudi N, Kuehl H, et al. Accuracy of whole-body dual modality fluorine-18-2-fluoro-2-deoxy-D-glucose positron emission tomography and computed tomography (FDG-PET/CT) for tumor staging in solid

tumors: Comparison with CT and PET. J Clin Oncol. 2004;22:4357-68.

25. Lebiedz P, Maaser C, Fanzius C, et al. Pet-CT—A new diagnostic tool for differentiation between inflammatory and fibromatous stenosis in Crohn's disease? Gastroenterology 2005;128(Suppl 2):A-310.
26. Louis E, Ancion G, Colard A, Spote V, Belaiche J, Hustinx R. Noninvasive assessment of Crohn's disease intestinal lesions with (18)F-FDG PET/CT. J Nucl Med 2007;48: 1053-9.
27. Das CJ, Makharia G, Kumar R, Goswami P, Sharma R, Malhotra A. PET-CT colonography: A novel technique for evaluation of ulcerative colitis. Journal of Gastroenterology and Hepatology 2008;(suppl. 5):A109.
28. Holdstock G, Ligorria JE, Krawitt EL. Gallium-67 scanning i patients with Crohn's disease: An aid to the diagnosis of abdominal abscess. Br J Surg 1982;69(5): 277-8.
29. Jones B, Abbruzzese AA, Hill TC, Adelstein SJ. Gallium-67-citrate scintigraphy in ulcerative colitis. Gastrointest Radiol 1980;5(3):267-72.
30. Rheingold OJ, Tedesco FJ, Block FE, Maldonado A, Miale A Jr. [67Ga]citrate scintiscanning in active inflammatory bowel disease. Dig Dis Sci 1979;24(5):363-8
31. Saverymuttu SH, Peters AM, Hodgson HJ, Chadwick VS, Lavender JP. Indium-111 autologous leucocyte scanning: comparison with radiology for imaging the colon in inflammatory bowel disease. Br Med J (Clin Res Ed). 1982;285(6337):255-7.
32. Saverymuttu SH, Peters AM, Hodgson HJ, Chadwick VS, Lavender JP.111Indium leukocyte scanning in small-bowel Crohn's disease. Gastrointest Radiol 1983;8(2): 157-61.
33. Segal AW, Ensell J, Munro JM, Sarner M. Indium-111 tagged leucocytes in the diagnosis of inflammatory bowel disease. Lancet. 1981;2(8240):230-2.
34. Stein DT, Gray GM, Gregory PB, Anderson M, Goodwin DA, McDougall IR. Location and activity of ulcerative and Crohn's colitis by indium 111 leukocyte scan. A prospective comparison study. Gastroenterology 1983;84(2):388-93.

Chapter Two

Non-traumatic Acute Abdomen

Mandeep Kang, Veenu Singla

Acute abdomen is defined as a clinical syndrome characterized by acute pain abdomen of sudden onset.[1] Patients with an acute abdomen comprise the largest group presenting to the surgical emergency.[2] Identification of patients who require surgery is crucial for timely management. Acute abdomen may be due to variety of diseases which may involve the gastrointestinal system, biliary tree, solid viscera or genitourinary system. Acute appendicitis is the most common cause of acute abdomen, particularly in young adults. In a review of 10,682 patients presenting with acute abdomen, acute appendicitis accounted for 28% of cases, followed by acute cholecystitis (9.7%), small bowel obstruction (4.1%), gynaecologic disorders (4%), acute pancreatitis (2.9%), renal colic (2.9%), peptic ulcer disease (2.5%), cancer (1.5%), diverticular disease (1.5%) and a variety of less common conditions (9%).[3] On account of the considerable overlap of symptoms and signs in an acute abdomen, the clinical accuracy for the specific diagnosis is low, ranging from 50-65%.[4] This limitation emphasizes the importance of imaging investigations in the diagnostic work-up of the acute abdomen.

The various imaging modalities available for investigating the acute abdomen include plain films, contrast studies, ultrasound (US), computed tomography (CT), and magnetic resonance imaging (MRI). The choice of the initial modality to be used should be guided by the disease suspected on clinical grounds, for example, plain radiographs continue to be initial imaging modality in cases of intestinal obstruction and perforation.[2] Contrast examinations have a limited role. An upper GI series with water soluble contrast may be performed in cases of suspected perforation or a contrast enema may be required to confirm a colonic obstruction.

US is the ideal screening modality for suspected hepatobiliary disease or for suspected pelvic pathology such as ectopic gestation or acute pelvic inflammatory disease (PID). It is also indicated for the initial evaluation of a patient with right lower quadrant pain especially in young women. In cases of suspected intestinal obstruction, it may at times be difficult to differentiate between mechanical obstruction and paralytic ileus on plain radiographs. US is of special value in such a situation as it demonstrates increased peristalsis in cases of mechanical obstruction, whereas presence of dilated, atonic loops suggest the diagnosis of paralytic items. US is also helpful in localizing intra-abdominal abscesses, particularly in the solid viscera.

The introduction of multidetector CT (MDCT) has impacted imaging of all organs of the body, especially the abdomen.[6] Because of the greater speed of coverage and thinner sections with 3D reconstruction now available, MDCT has become the imaging modality of choice for evaluation of the acute abdomen. It provides a comprehensive view of all the intra-abdominal solid and hollow viscera, as well as the peritoneum, mesentery, lymph nodes and retroperitoneum. Data can be acquired in different phases making MDCT an ideal modality for evaluation of suspected mesenteric ischemia or vascular disorders such as abdominal aortic aneurysms. Low dose unenhanced CT has replaced excretory urography as the screening method of choice for the evaluation of renal colic in most centers.[6] Recent improvements in resolution and development of faster breath-hold sequences have drastically increased the utility of MRI in evaluation of the gut.[7] However, MRI is still not routinely used for evaluation of an acute abdomen except in situations where iodinated contrast cannot be administered or in pregnant patients.

CT Technique

The technique used for acquisition of the image data set is of paramount importance for accurate diagnosis and should be tailored according to the most likely clinical diagnosis. Oral contrast is routinely administered to all patients in the form of 800-1000 ml of 2% iodinated contrast or dilute barium solution over a period of 45 minutes prior to the study. Negative oral contrast (plain water) is preferred in suspected mesenteric ischemia to adequately distend the bowel lumen. Oral contrast is withheld in patients with renal, ureteric or biliary calculi or patients in whom CT angiography is contemplated such as aortic dissection, aneurysm rupture etc. Per rectal contrast is given in patients with suspected pelvic or large bowel pathology. Intravenous contrast, preferably non-ionic iodinated contrast helps in better depiction of inflammatory as well as neoplastic pathology, enables differentiation of lymph nodes from vessels and detection of vascular complications. 100-120 ml of contrast is injected at a rate of 2.8-3.5 ml/second and images routinely obtained in the portal venous phase at 70 seconds delay.

Particular attention should be paid to the scanning parameters. Using a lower slice collimation with MDCT results in a higher radiation dose to the patient as compared to a single-slice CT.[6] Scanning should be performed from the domes of the diaphragm to the pubic symphysis using a slice thickness of 5-10 mm with a pitch of 0.75 (MDCT) or one (single-slice CT). The data can be retrospectively reconstructed to thinner sections for various 3D reconstructions.

Plain Radiographs in Evaluation of the Acute Abdomen

Plain radiographs still remain an important initial investigation in the evaluation of a patient with acute abdomen. Interpretation of these radiographs represents a formidable challenge to the radiologist, as the findings may be non-specific, confusing or at times even misleading.[2] Abdominal plain films are of greatest value in cases of hollow viscus perforation and intestinal obstruction.

Perforation

In the past, a minimum three film radiographic series was recommended for evaluation of an acute abdomen.[8] This includes a supine film of the abdomen and erect radiographs of the abdomen and chest (Figs 2.1A to C). More recently, it has been demonstrated that the erect film of the abdomen can be eliminated from the initial series without significant loss of the diagnostic infor-

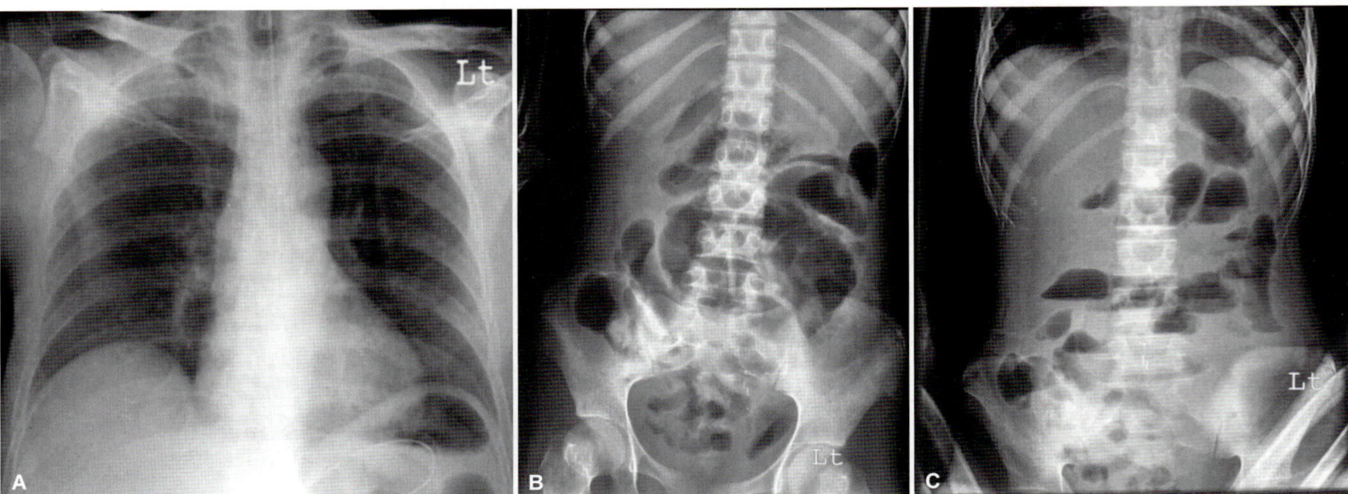

Figs 2.1A to C: Abdominal series (Three views of the abdomen) A. Chest X-ray reveals absence of free air under the domes of diaphragm. B. Supine film shows dilated jejunal and ileal loops with no air in the large bowel. C. Erect film demonstrates multiple air-fluid levels in a case of distal small bowel obstruction

mation.[9] The upright chest film is ideal for demonstrating free air as the X-ray beam strikes the hemidiaphragms tangentially at their highest point. Classical studies have shown that as little as 1 ml of free air can be detected below the right hemidiaphragm provided the patient has been in an erect position for at least 10-15 minutes prior to obtaining the radiograph.[10] The chest radiograph may also reveal chest diseases such as pneumonia, pulmonary or myocardial infarction which may mimic an acute abdomen. If the patient cannot sit or stand up a left lateral decubitus film will demonstrate air between the opacity of the liver and the abdominal wall. If the patient is too ill to roll over, a cross-table lateral view of the abdomen is obtained (Fig. 2.2).

Various signs of pneumo-peritoneum can be seen even on supine films if carefully searched for. The signs include "Rigler's" or "double wall" sign describing visualization of both the mucosal and serosal aspect of the bowel wall due to presence of intra and extra-luminal air (Fig. 2.3). The falciform ligament may be outlined by air in the upper abdomen. The "football" sign is due to presence of large quantity of air which fills the peritoneal cavity. The lateral umbilical ligaments may be visualized in the lower abdomen known as the "inverted V" sign. Free air in Morrison's pouch may be seen as an oval radiolucency in the sub-hepatic region. The right upper quadrant may appear radiolucent due to air collecting between the anterior surface of liver and the abdominal wall. The under surface of the central part of the diaphragm may be visualized - the "cupola" sign.[11] Retroperitoneal perforation of a duodenal ulcer results in air outlining the renal or psoas shadows (Fig. 2.4). Large bowel may also perforate into the retroperitoneal space resulting in mottled extra-luminal air lucencies.

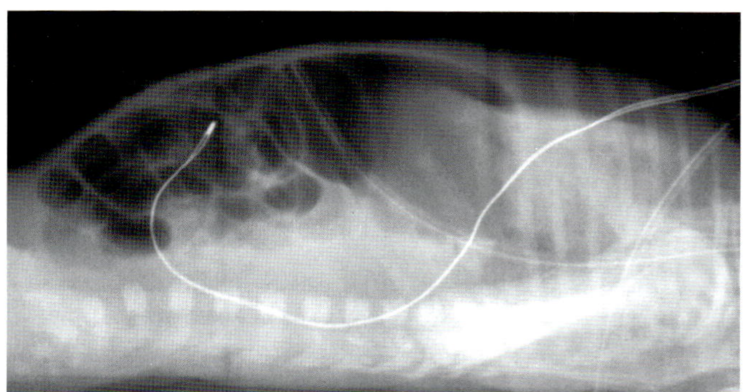

Fig. 2.2: Cross-table lateral view of a premature neonate reveals free intra-peritoneal air in a case of necrotizing enterocolitis

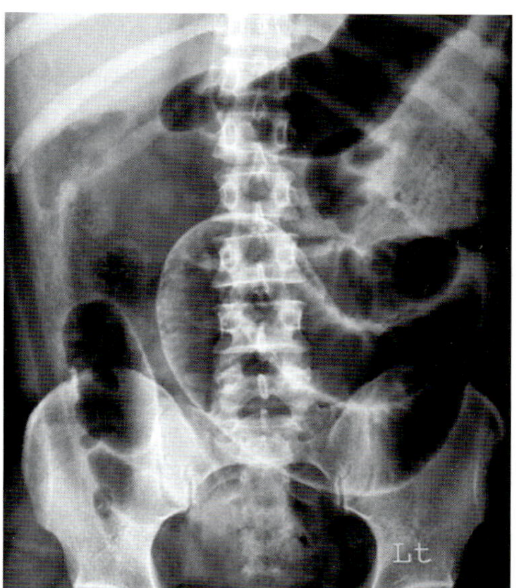

Fig. 2.3: X-ray abdomen, supine film. Both the inner and outer walls of the small bowel loop are visualized due to the presence of intra-peritoneal air. Air is also seen in the sub-hepatic region (Morrison's pouch)

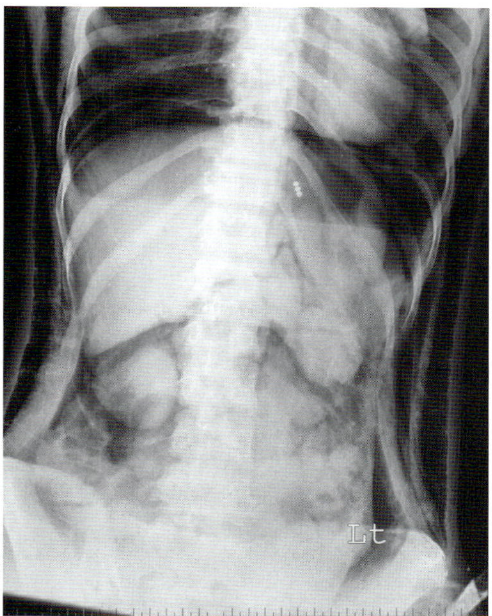

Fig. 2.4: Plain radiograph abdomen, erect film shows large amount of free air in the upper abdomen. In addition, air is also seen outlining the right kidney signifying retroperitoneal perforation of a duodenal ulcer

Plain films are inferior to CT for the detection of free intraperitoneal air. Supine abdominal films may detect free air in only about 60% of the cases, therefore CT has been proposed as the initial radiological investigation in patients with acute abdomen.

Intestinal Obstruction

The diagnosis of intestinal obstruction may be correctly suggested on the basis of plain films alone in nearly 80% of the cases. Additional imaging with US and CT is required in equivocal causes and also to determine the level and cause of obstruction.

In mechanical obstruction, plain films reveal dilated, gas-filled bowel loops with air-fluid levels proximal to the obstruction with collapsed loops with absence of air distal to the obstruction (Figs 2.1A to C). Dilatation of both small and large bowel loops from stomach to rectum indicates a diagnosis of paralytic ileus (Fig. 2.5). It may not always be possible to differentiate between mechanical obstruction and paralytic ileus. A lateral view to look for air in the rectum may aid in the differentiation, however US or contrast studies may be required in equivocal cases.[2,8]

Distinction between small and large bowel loops on plain films is based on the central position of the small bowel, presence of valvulae conniventes in the jejunum and tubular featureless appearance of ileum. The dilated loop measures between 3-5 cm. The valvulae conniventis form thin, 1-2 mm complete rings at intervals of 1 mm. In contrast, the large bowel loops are located peripherally, measure more than 5 cm in diameter and display haustral markings that are incomplete, 2-3 mm wide and occurring at intervals of 1cm.[12] The erect film in a normal person usually displays 2-3 fluid levels in the small bowel which does not exceed 3 cm in caliber. Dilated fluid-filled loops of small bowel may be identified as oval or round soft tissue densities.[2] At times the bowel loops proximal to the site of obstruction may get completely filled with fluid resulting in a gasless abdomen. When a tiny amount of gas accompanies a large amount of intra-luminal fluid, small gas bubbles get trapped between the valvulae conniventis resulting in the "string-of-beads" sign. This appearance is virtually diagnostic of mechanical obstruction as it is never seen with paralytic ileus.

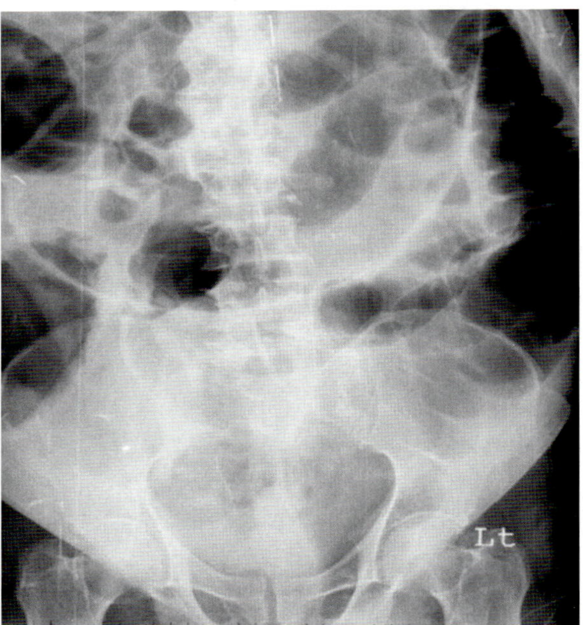

Fig. 2.5: X-ray abdomen, supine view shows gaseous distension of both the small and large bowel loops including the rectum in a case of paralytic ileus

Strangulating obstruction is a mechanical obstruction caused when two limbs of a loop are incarcerated within a hernia so as to cause vascular compromise by compression of the mesenteric vessels. Presence of thumb-printing due to submucosal edema or hemorrhage should suggest ischemia in the loops. If left untreated, the ischemia may progress causing breach of the mucosa, intramural air, air in the mesenteric and portal veins and frank perforation which are all ominous signs.

Intramural air in the form of parallel streaks of gas along the bowel wall or as rings may also be seen in infants with necrotizing enterocolitis. This appearance should not be confused with the bubbly appearance of *pneumatosis coli* which is a benign condition affecting the colon in adults.

The causes of intestinal obstruction vary with the age of the patient. In neonates and infants, the usual causes of obstruction are congenital conditions such as hypertrophic pyloric stenosis, duodenal stenosis or atresia, ileal atresia etc. Duodenal atresia shows the typical "double-bubble" sign. In young children, intussusception or Ladd's bands are common causes of obstruction. Intussusception may be seen as a mass-like soft tissue shadow with a crescent of gas surrounding the leading edge. A barium examination will reveal the coil-spring appearance of the intussuscepiens with the "claw" sign (Fig. 2.6).

In adults, adhesions and hernias account for more than 80% of small bowel obstructions. Other causes include an intraluminal obturation by neoplasm, gall stone or bezoar or a volvulus due to twisting of the gut around its mesentery. Sigmoid volvulus is generally seen

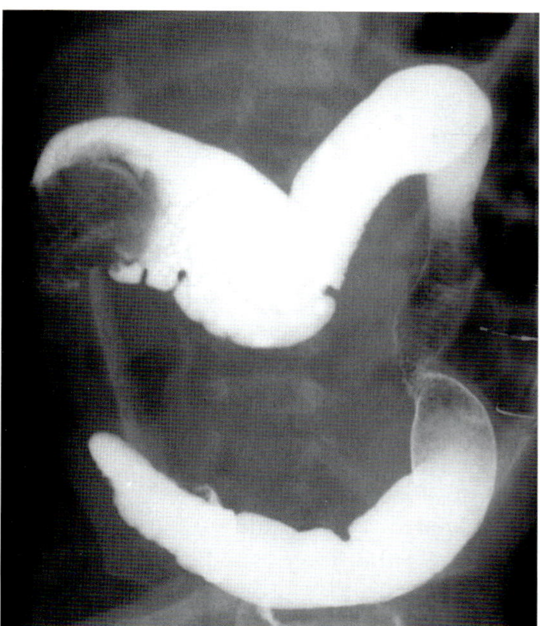

Fig. 2.6: Barium enema in a case of large bowel obstruction shows a crescentric intraluminal filling defect in the hepatic flexure with a soft tissue mass due to ileo-colic intussusception

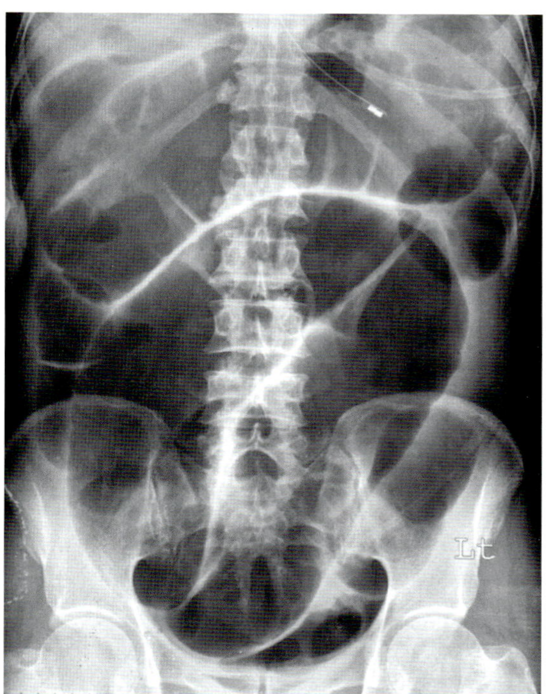

Fig. 2.7: X-ray abdomen, supine view shows a hugely dilated ahaustral loop arising from the pelvis with the "coffee-bean" sign in a case of sigmoid volvulus

in the older age group. The distended ahaustral sigmoid loop assumes an inverted "U" shape with its apex under either dome. The opposed inner walls of the loops appear as a single line giving the "coffee bean" appearance (Fig. 2.7). Cecal volvulus generally occurs in younger individuals. The cecum twists and inverts so that its pole and appendix lie in the left upper quadrant.

In mechanical large bowel obstruction, the small bowel loops also dilate if the ileo-cecal valve is incompetent. However, if the ileo-cecal valve is competent, it can result in gross gaseous distension of the cecum with the attendant dangers of ischemia and perforation.

Miscellaneous Conditions

Apart from perforation and intestinal obstruction, plain films may sometimes reveal important findings which may clinch the diagnosis or indirectly suggest the possible diagnosis such as:

a. Presence of intramural and intraluminal gas in patients of gangrenous cholecystitis.
b. Presence of air in the biliary tree with small gut obstruction due to gallstone ileus caused by erosion of the gallstone into the duodenum.
c. Presence of localized duodenal ileus (sentinel loop), dilated transverse colon with "colon cut off" in case of acute pancreatitis.
d. Presence of extraluminal mottled gas in patients of abdominal abscess.
e. Presence of soft tissue mass with obliteration of properitoneal fat line in the right lower quadrant and scoliosis with convexity to the left in patients of acute appendicular abscess.
f. Presence of gas in the perinephric region in cases of emphysematous pyelonephritis.
g. Presence of intestinal pneumatosis or porto-mesenteric air in mesenteric ischemia.

Role of Cross-sectional Imaging in Specific Disease Entities

Acute Appendicitis

In the majority of patients, the clinical picture is typical and patients undergo laparotomy without any imaging. Imaging is needed only in equivocal cases or when the clinical diagnosis is in doubt. In about one third of patients, presentation of acute appendicitis is atypical. Conversely, other conditions may also mimic appendicitis resulting in a false negative laparotomy rate of 20% which rises to 35-45% in young women of reproductive age in whom distinction from acute PID and other gynecological conditions such as torsion of ovarian cyst is difficult on clinical grounds alone.[13] On plain radiography, although the presence of an appendicolith strongly suggests appendicitis, it is visualized on properly exposed radiographs in only 14% of all patients with appendicoliths.[8] At barium enema, lack of appendiceal visualization and presence of a cecal mass impression are nonspecific findings and not definitely diagnostic of appendicitis. Filling of the appendix up to its bulbous tip virtually excludes appendicitis, however, the appendix may not fill completely in up to one third of normal individuals.[14] US is the screening modality of choice for initial evaluation in suspected appendicitis, followed by CT in selected cases. Graded compression sonography using high frequency linear transducers is a highly accurate technique with a sensitivity of 80-93%, specificity of 94-100% and an accuracy of 95-97% for the diagnosis of acute appendicitis.[15] Another technique for improving visualization of retrocecal appendix in obese or muscular patients is posterior manual compression of right lower quadrant in anterior or anteromedial direction using the left hand with simultaneous anterior graded compression by transducer. Turning the patient from supine position to left oblique lateral decubitus position also displaces cecum, terminal ileum and appendix medially onto the psoas muscle and reduces the depth of the lateral portion of the retrocecal area, thereby improving visualization of retrocecal appendix.[16]

The US criteria for a normal appendix are presence of a compressible, tubular, blind-ending structure filled with fluid, gas or feces, originating from the base of the cecum having a wall thickness of 2 mm or less and diameter of 6 mm or less. The sonographic diagnosis of acute appendicitis is based on one or more of the following: direct visualization of a concentrically layered, aperistaltic, non-compressible appendix with an anteroposterior diameter > 6 mm, or echogenic incompressible peri-appendicular inflamed fat with or without an appendicolith (Fig. 2.8). On color doppler, increased flow signals in the appendiceal wall or peri-appendicular space allow confirmation of the diagnosis. Perforation should be suspected if there is loss of symmetry of the concentric layers of the wall or a right lower quadrant fluid collection without visualization of inflamed appendix. However, inconclusive US studies may be seen in a right lower quadrant phlegmon or abscess without a visible appendix, retrocecal inflamed appendix, cecal edema or terminal ileum thickening, distal or tip appendicitis with a normal proximal appendix, obesity and if there is pain limiting compression. A false-positive sonogram may be seen in Crohn's disease, cecal diverticulosis and salpingitis.

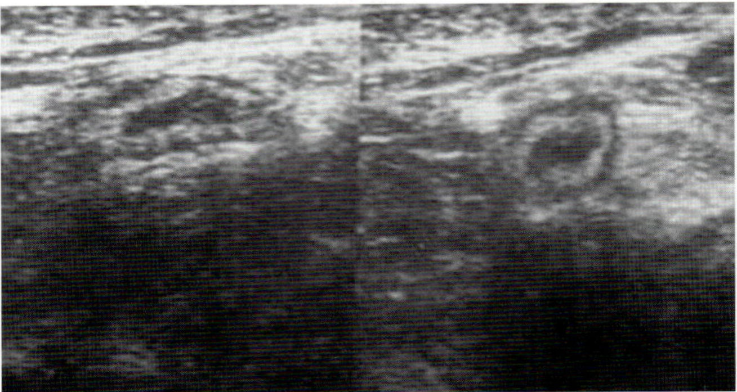

Fig. 2.8: Longitudinal and transverse sonograms showing the classical target lesion in the right iliac fossa due to inflamed, incompressible appendix with thickened walls

Helical CT using thin sections (4-5 mm) has a higher reported sensitivity of 90-100%, specificity of 91-99% and accuracy of 94-98% compared to US.[17] CT signs of appendicitis include visualization of an abnormal appendix with a distended lumen, thickened and enhancing wall or an appendicolith, peri-appendicular inflammatory changes in the form of fat stranding, phlegmon, fluid, abscess or adenopathy, cecal changes like circumferential mural thickening of cecum and terminal ileum, cecal apical thickening or the "arrow head" sign which results due to funneling of contrast medium on both sides of the inflamed cecal apex coming to a point at the occluded orifice of the appendix (Figs 2.9A and B). As the "arrow head" sign highlights extension of inflammation to the upper portion of cecum, it may identify patients who require more than standard ligation appendectomy. CT is also of special value in suggesting alternative diagnosis in patients who do not have appendicitis.

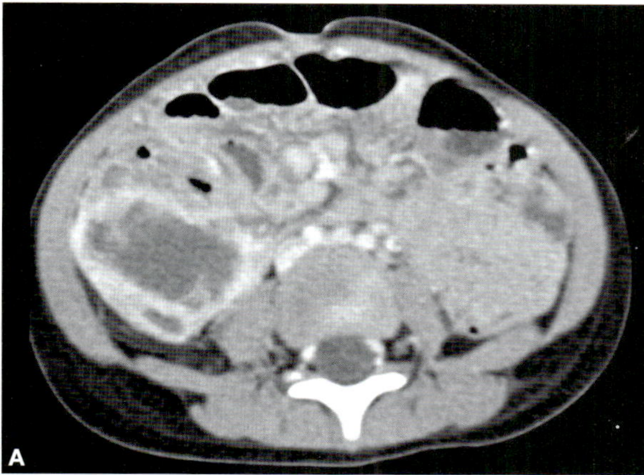

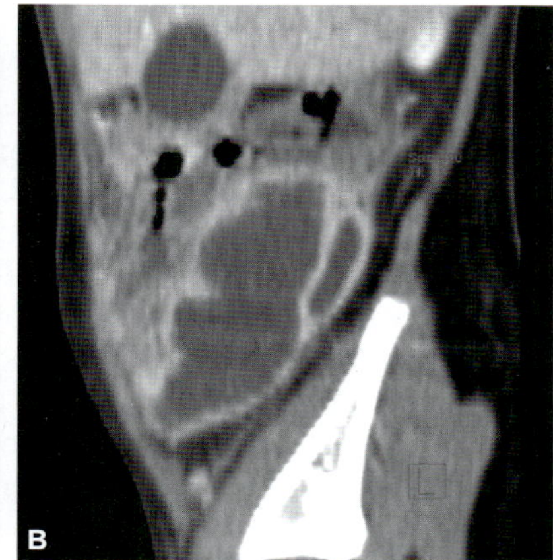

Figs 2.9A and B: Acute appendicitis. Axial and sagittal reconstructed CT images demonstrating a large, irregular collection with thick enhancing walls in the right iliac fossa posterior to cecum which is displaced anteromedially. A tubular structure with enhancing walls is seen posterior to this collection representing the inflamed appendix

Acute Cholecystitis

Sonography is the primary imaging modality of choice for evaluating the gallbladder. Acute cholecystitis is associated with gall stones in 90-96% of patients with a calculus causing cystic duct obstruction being the commonest cause. Sensitive sonographic features are positive Murphy's sign (in 96% of patients with acute cholecystitis), calculi (in 95%) and a thickened gallbladder wall (in 73%).[18] However these signs are not specific and may be encountered in other conditions such as chronic cholecystitis, pancreatitis, cirrhosis or hepatitis. Other sonographic signs include distension of the gallbladder (GB), edematous wall, mucosal irregularity, intramural gas and/or pericholecystic collection (Fig. 2.10). Doppler sonography improves diagnostic confidence in acute cholecystitis by revealing mural hypervascularity. CT is not the imaging modality of choice but may be used as an adjunct to US if sonography is inconclusive, especially in acalculous cholecystitis or when complications such as perforation or emphysematous cholecystitis are suspected.[19] CT findings of acute cholecystitis include wall thickening, pericholecystic stranding, GB distension, pericholecystic fluid, subserosal edema, high attenuation bile and sloughed membranes, gas or septations within the gallbladder (Fig. 2.11).[20] As the inflammatory response in calculous and acalculous cholecystitis is similar, the CT appearance of inflammation is similar in both. MRI can be a valuable complement to US and CT

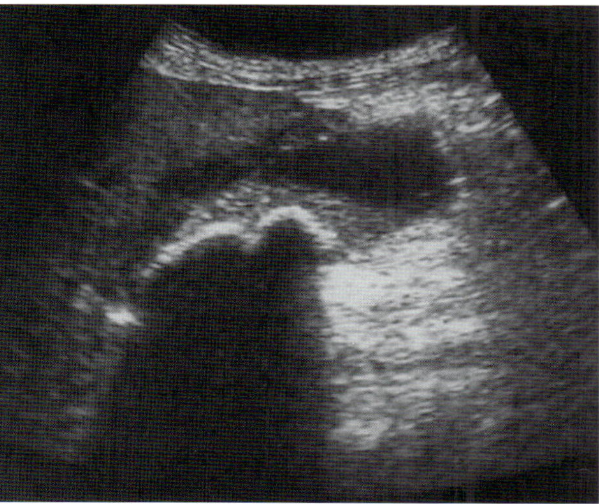

Fig. 2.10: Acute calculous cholecystitis. Ultrasonogram shows calculi and debris in the lumen of the GB which has thick irregular walls. US Murphy's sign was positive

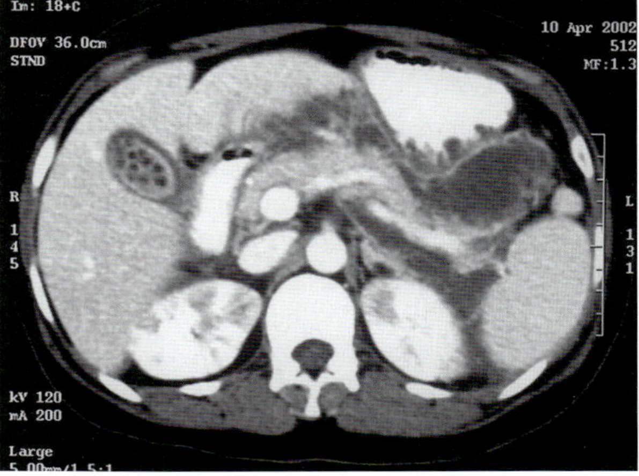

Fig. 2.11: Axial CECT abdomen. The GB has thick, enhancing walls with a hypodense rim of peri-cholecystic fluid. The lumen is filled with high density bile resulting in the calculi appearing as filling defects. Note the loss of peripancreatic fat planes with a large collection in the lesser sac due to associated pancreatitis

in demonstrating impacted calculi in the gallbladder neck or cystic duct which are often difficult to detect on US. Also, conditions causing acalculous cholecystitis like adenomyomatosis, gall bladder polyp, malignant neoplasm or other cancers can be depicted on MR.[21]

Complications of acute cholecystitis include empyema, gangrenous cholecystitis, gallbladder perforation and emphysematous cholecystitis. Empyema occurs when pus fills the distended and inflamed GB, typically in diabetic patients. On US and CT, pus resembles sludge. Heavily T2-weighted images are sensitive in demonstrating purulent bile as a dependent hypointense layer relative to normal bile.

Gangrenous cholecystitis is an advanced, severe form of acute cholecystitis, seen more common in elderly men. It results from marked distension of the GB with resultant increase in tension in the wall. Associated inflammation leads to ischemic necrosis. US reveals heterogenous or striated thickening of GB wall or intraluminal membranes representing desquamated mucosa. US findings typical of uncomplicated acute cholecystitis may be absent in this subset of patients: GB wall thickness may be less than 3 mm or Murphy's sign may be absent due to denervation of the GB wall.[22] CT features consist of intraluminal membranes, irregular wall, pericholecystic fluid/abscess and lack of mural enhancement.

Gall bladder perforation is most often a complication of acute gangrenous cholecystitis. As blood supply is poor in the region of fundus, this is the most common site of perforation. Perforation can be classified into 3 types: a) acute free perforation into peritoneal cavity, b) subacute perforation with pericholecystic abscess and c) chronic perforation with a cholecystoenteric fistula.[23] Subacute perforations are the most common. Following perforation, US, CT and MR show complex pericholecystic fluid collections and the wall of GB can appear focally disrupted.[7]

Emphysematous cholecystitis is a rare form of acute cholecystitis seen in patients with diabetes and peripheral atherosclerotic disease. The majority of patients are between 50-70 years. US demonstrates intraluminal and intramural gas as highly echogenic foci. CT is the most sensitive and specific imaging modality to identify gas in the lumen or wall.[24]

Acute Pancreatitis

Acute pancreatitis is an acute inflammatory process of the pancreas which may range in severity from a mild parenchymal edema to severe necrotizing pancreatitis with variable involvement of other regional tissues or remote organ systems. Most of the patients with the mild form of the disease have an uneventful recovery, however the cases with severe pancreatitis show significant mortality and morbidity with development of failure of various organ systems and require aggressive management.

The diagnosis of acute pancreatitis is usually made on clinical grounds supported by laboratory data. The role of imaging is to confirm the diagnosis, stage the severity of disease and detect complications such as infection, pseudocyst formation or vascular involvement. Ultrasound may reveal an enlarged, hypoechoic pancreas in the early stages with presence of peripancreatic fluid. It may also detect the presence of cholelithiasis or choledocholithiasis which is a major etiological factor for acute pancreatitis. It can also be used in the follow-up of acute fluid collections or pseudocysts particularly after percutaneous catheter drainage.

Contrast enhanced CT is the modality of choice not only to confirm the diagnosis or detect extra-pancreatic intra-abdominal disease, but also to stage the severity of disease which is required for prognostication. It is also highly accurate for the detection of necrosis and complications.

Balthazar et al[25] described five grades of pancreatitis on CT:

1. Grade A: Radiologically normal pancreas.
2. Grade B: Focal or diffuse enlargement of the pancreas with or without contour irregularities or non-homogenous attenuation of the gland with no evidence of peri-pancreatic disease.
3. Grade C: Peri-pancreatic fat inflammation (Fig. 2.12).

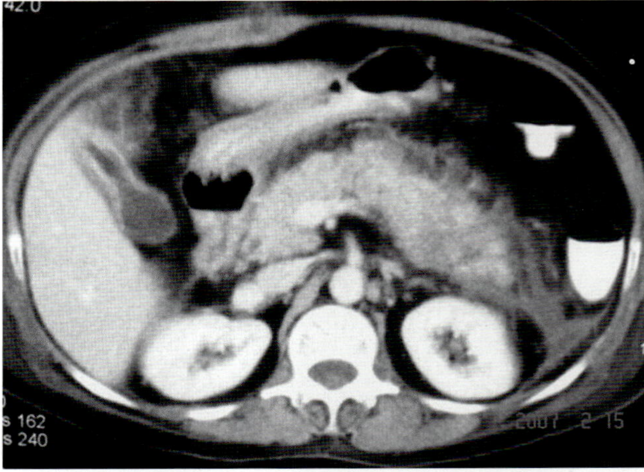

Fig. 2.12: Acute pancreatitis. Axial CECT section shows a bulky pancreas with a heterogenous attenuation and loss of the peripancreatic fat planes. Note the enhancing mural thickening of the GB due to cholecystitis

4. Grade D: Single, intra- or extra-pancreatic, ill-defined fluid collection.
5. Grade E: Two or more intra- or extra-pancreatic, poorly defined collections or presence of gas in or adjacent to the pancreas.

Patients with grade A or B disease usually run a mild, uncomplicated course, whereas patients with grade D and E disease often exhibit a protracted clinical course with increased incidence of complications and mortality.

The presence of hypodense areas in the pancreatic parenchyma which do not show any evidence of enhancement implies pancreatic necrosis which is a harbinger of severe disease (Fig. 2.13). The Balthazar's CT severity index (CTSI)[26] introduced in 1990 takes the presence and degree of pancreatic necrosis into account and has been found to be a more reliable prognostic indicator of disease than the CT grading or the clinical scoring systems such as Ransons or the APACHE II.

A score of 0-3 denotes mild pancreatitis, 4-6 is moderate pancreatitis while a CTSI score above 7 denotes severe pancreatitis.

Recently a modified CTSI has been proposed which takes into account the presence of extrapancreatic complications such as vascular involvement, bowel or extrapancreatic parenchymal involvement, pleural effusion and ascites while calculating the CTSI.[27] The authors have also simplified the degree of pancreatic involvement into three grades from five. The degree of pancreatic necrosis has also been simplified to just three

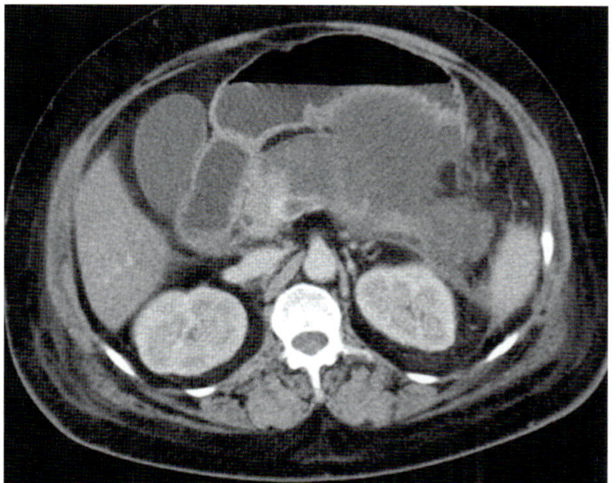

Fig. 2.13: Acute necrotising pancreatitis grade E. The body and tail of the pancreas are hypodense with only a small amount of normally enhancing parenchyma seen in the head of pancreas. There are extra-pancreatic collections with a hypodense filling defect in the portal vein due to thrombosis. CTSI-10

Table 2.1 CT Severity index (Balthazar)

Findings	*Points*
Normal pancreas	0
Focal or diffuse pancreatic enlargement	
Plus peripancreatic inflammatory changes	1
Plus single fluid collection	2
Plus > 2 fluid collections/gas in or adjacent to pancreas	3
Area of pancreatic necrosis	
< 30 percent	2
31-50 percent	4
>50 percent	6
Maximal score:10	

grades as no necrosis, less than or more than 30% necrosis, the rationale being that there is no significant difference in the morbidity and mortality between patients with 30-50% necrosis or more than 50% necrosis. The modified CTSI is claimed to correlate more significantly with the clinical outcome but awaits ratification.

Vascular complications may occur in 10% of patients with acute pancreatitis and are classified as thrombotic, inflammatory and destructive.[28] Thrombosis may involve the arterial or venous system but most commonly involves the splenoportal axis (Fig. 2.13). Inflammatory changes are seen as spasm/luminal irregularity or narrowing in the peripancreatic vasculature and are generally reversible once the pancreatic inflammation subsides. Destructive changes are in the form of pseudo-aneurysms, which may involve the pancreaticoduodenal, gastroduodenal and splenic arteries. MDCT angiography may reliably detect vascular complications and guide appropriate management.

MR has also been reported to have similar accuracy to MDCT for the diagnosis of acute pancreatitis and assigning a severity index. The presence of hyperintensity in the pancreatic parenchyma on non-contrast T1 and T2 weighted images signifies the presence of hemorrhagic pancreatitis. Fat suppressed non-contrast sequences are used to detect hemorrhagic peri-pancreatic collections, both these situations signify a more severe form of pancreatitis.[29]

Intra-abdominal Abscess

A localized collection of pus can occur anywhere in the abdomen: in the parenchyma of solid organs, in the peritoneal or extra-peritoneal spaces. Early detection,

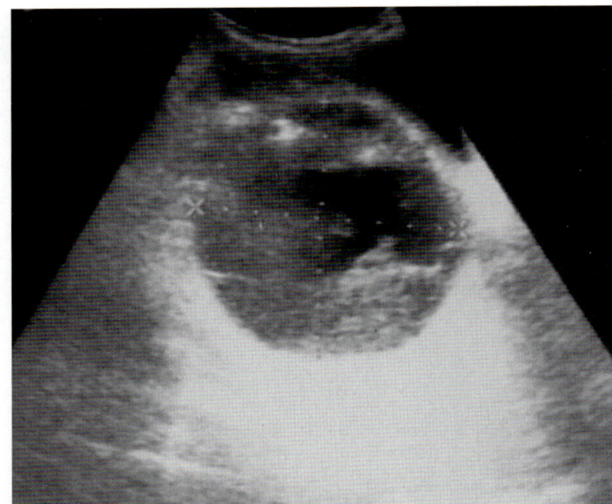

Fig. 2.14: Ultrasound of the pelvis shows a rounded fluid collection with internal echoes, debris and septations with posterior acoustic enhancement in a case of postoperative abdominal abscess

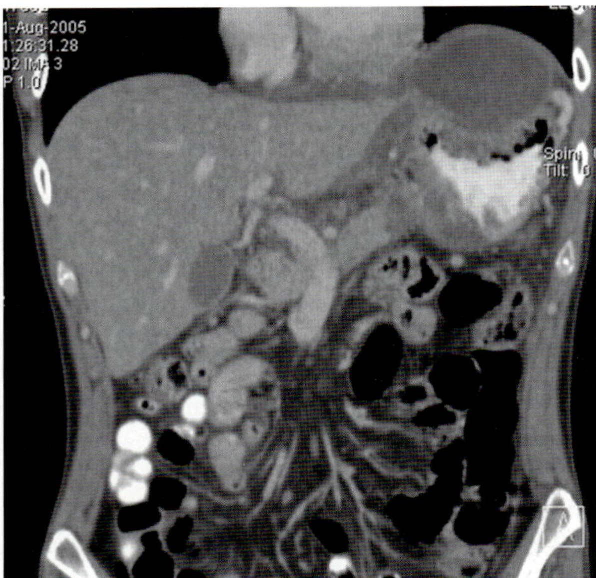

Fig. 2.15: Coronal MPVR image shows a large, left subphrenic, low attenuation fluid collection elevating the left hemi-diaphragm. The transpleural approach had to be employed for percutaneous drainage of this abscess

accurate localization and prompt drainage are the mainstay of successful management. US is an excellent modality for the detection of visceral abscesses and is also useful for screening for intra-peritoneal abscesses, e.g. in the postoperative patient.[30] Abscesses appear as a rounded, complex fluid collection with irregular walls, posterior acoustic enhancement, low level internal echoes, septations or debris (Fig. 2.14). A fluid-fluid level may be seen. At times, the abscess may have a solid appearance. Color Doppler demonstrates peripheral hypervascularity.

CT has a high sensitivity and specificity with an overall accuracy of 95% for the detection of intra-abdominal abscesses.[31] CT will show a low attenuation fluid collection with mass effect and peripheral rim enhancement with or without gas bubbles or an air-fluid level. MDCT allows accurate delineation of the complex anatomy which may exist in intra-abdominal collections and thus enables proper planning of a safe approach route for percutaneous catheter drainage (Fig. 2.15).

Intestinal Obstruction

Imaging studies such as US and CT are required to confirm the clinical diagnosis of obstruction (made on the basis of clinical findings and plain X-ray appearance), differentiate between mechanical obstruction and paralytic ileus and for determining the level and cause of mechanical obstruction. CT is also useful for detecting an obstruction not visualized on plain films, e.g., closed loop obstruction. More importantly, CT can detect complications like strangulation which require emergent surgery.

CT diagnosis of bowel obstruction is based on the presence of dilated loops (small bowel > 2.5 cm, large bowel > 5 cm) with air-fluid levels proximal to a transition zone with collapsed distal bowel. Minimal mural thickening with enhancement may at times be seen at the transition zone in cases of adhesions (Fig. 2.16).[32] The "small bowel feces sign" refers to the presence of gas bubbles mixed with particulate matter in dilated loops

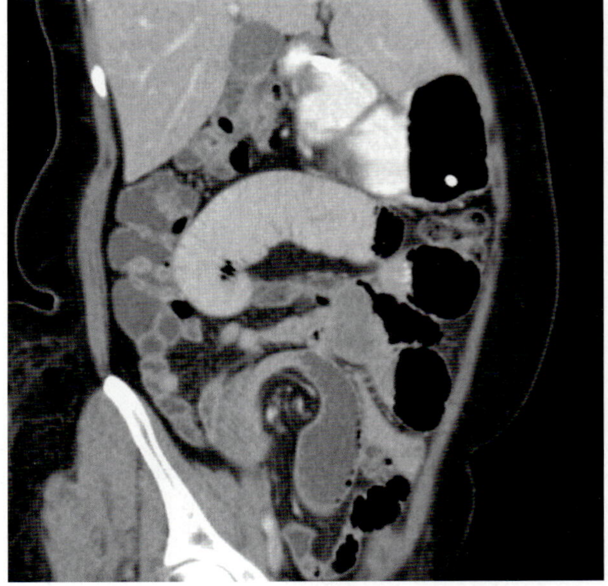

Fig. 2.16: CT Enteroclysis. Oblique MPR image showing abrupt angulation of an ileal loop with minimal mural thickening at the site of postoperative adhesion in a case of small bowel obstruction

proximal to the site of obstruction. This is a less common but reliable indicator of mechanical obstruction. Gas filled loops, mesenteric vessels and fat may be seen in the inguinal canal or other sites of external hernias. Circumferential mural thickening of the dilated bowel loops with increased attenuation in the mesentery or bowel wall denotes the presence of strangulation. An internal hernia can be diagnosed if a cluster of dilated small bowel loops which appears to be enclosed in a sac is seen in an ectopic location (e.g. lesser sac or anterior to transverse colon) with crowding and twisting of the mesenteric vessels. A markedly dilated, fluid filled bowel segment with abrupt tapering ends denotes a closed loop obstruction. These show relatively little dilatation of the proximal bowel and are at greater risk for strangulation. Fixed radial distribution of several dilated small bowel loops with stretched and prominent mesenteric vessels converging towards the point of torsion (whirl sign) with mesenteric edema indicates a small bowel volvulus (Fig. 2.17). A target appearance in cross-section with a bowel-within-bowel appearance on longitudinal scans suggests a diagnosis of intussusception. Mesenteric fat and vessels can be identified within the mass as can the lead point if present (Fig. 2.18). Entero-enteric intussusceptions without proximal dilatation that are less than 3.5 cm in length are probably not significant in adults. Intussusceptions involving the colon that are 4 cm in length or longer, have proximal dilatation or mural thickening should be carefully evaluated for an underlying neoplasm. Foreign bodies, gallstones and bezoars can all cause obstruction and can be readily identified on CT. CT has a sensitivity of 90-96%, specificity of 91-96% and overall accuracy of 90-95% for the diagnosis of high grade obstruction.[1,33] CT enteroclysis is a new technique which has a sensitivity of 89% and specificity of 100% in the diagnosis of low grade obstruction involving the small bowel (Figs 2.19A and B).[34] Fast MRI has also been shown to be sensitive (95%), specific (100%) and accurate (96%) in the setting of small bowel obstruction.[35]

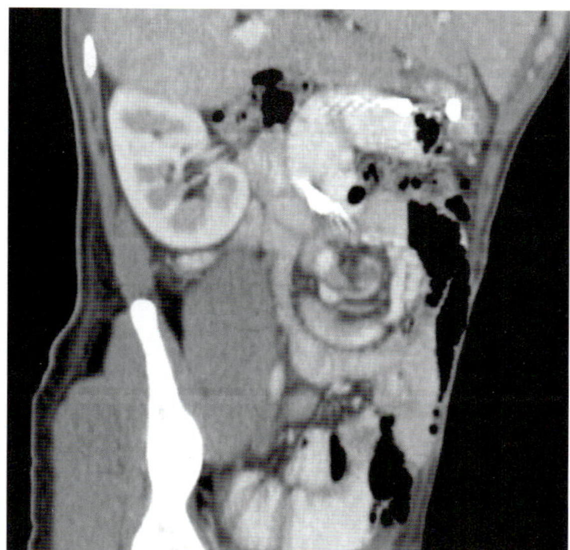

Fig. 2.17: CT Enteroclysis: Oblique MPR image showing midgut volvulus with presence of whirl sign

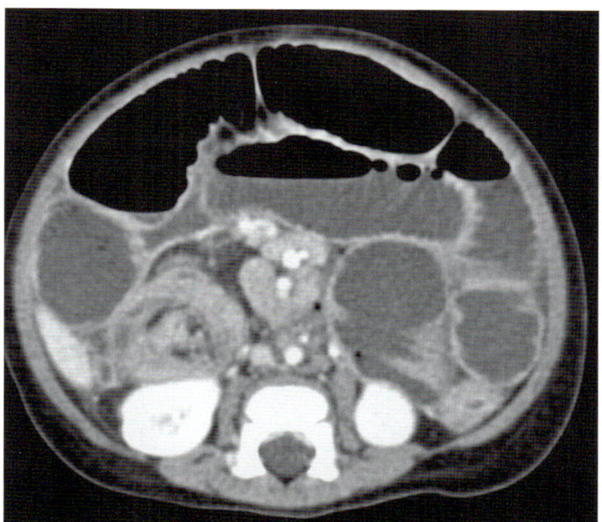

Fig. 2.18: Axial CECT section demonstrates a 4 x 5 cm, heterogenous mass in the right lumbar region showing a target appearance with mesenteric fat and vessels within the lesion suggestive of intussusception. The proximal small bowel loops are dilated

Bowel Perforation

Gastrointestinal (GI) tract perforation can be caused by peptic ulcer disease, foreign body, appendicitis, bacterial enteritis, Crohn's disease, diverticulitis, bowel ischemia, obstruction or malignant neoplasms. Some studies have reported USG to be a more sensitivity modality than plain radiography for the diagnosis of pneumoperitoneum.[36] Sonographic findings of perforated hollow viscus include demonstration of free air as echogenic spots or lines with posterior ring-down artifacts that shift with change in patient position, enhancement of the peritoneal stripe, echogenic free peritoneal fluid and decreased peristalsis.[37] When patient is in supine position, the reverberations are seen between anterior surface of left lobe of liver and anterior abdominal wall. Shifting phenomenon is seen on rolling the patient to left lateral position as free air rises to the highest portion of right hypochondrium. Enhancement of peritoneal stripe refers to increased echogenicity and thickening of the peritoneal stripe due to free intraperitoneal air with associated dirty shadowing.

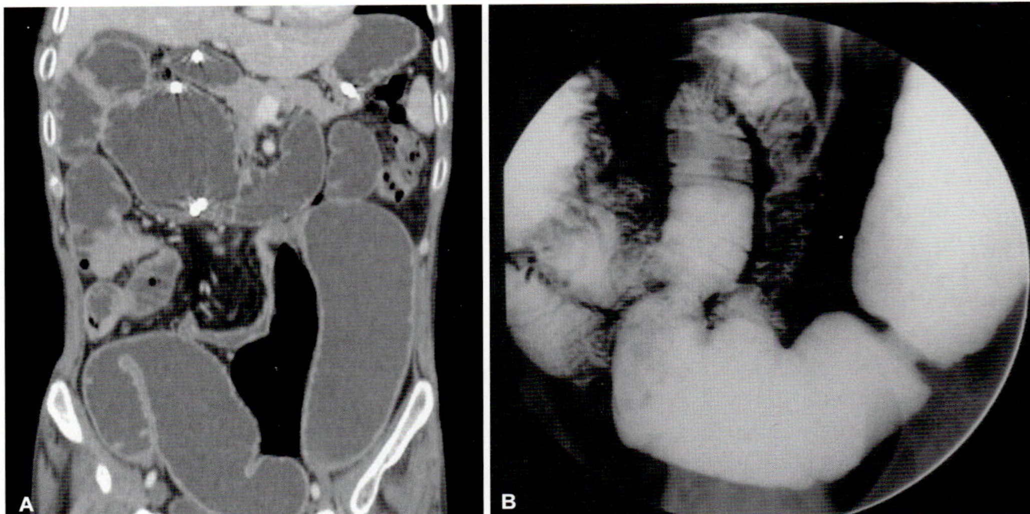

Figs 2.19A and B: (A) CT Enteroclysis coronal MPR image showing a long segment distal ileal stricture causing obstruction with dilatation of the proximal small bowel loops, (B) Barium enteroclysis done subsequently confirms the stricture in a case of tuberculosis

CT is superior to both plain films and US for the detection of presence, cause and site of perforation. Pre-operative localization of the site of perforation is beneficial for the surgeon, with the laparoscopic approach currently being used for most surgical procedures instead of open surgery. Extraluminal contrast extravasation, when seen, is pathognomonic. Other direct signs are the presence of extraluminal air or discontinuity of the bowel wall. Inflammatory changes may also be seen at the site of perforation. CT images should be assessed in wide window settings to distinguish free air from fat density. Careful analysis of anterior peritoneal surfaces of liver and mid-abdomen as well as of peritoneal folds should be done, so as not to overlook a small amount of extraluminal air. The site of colonic perforation may be predicted by the site of extraluminal contrast leakage, concentrated bubbles of air in close proximity to the bowel wall, focal interruption of bowel wall, segmental bowel wall thickening, ill-defined mass, adjacent fat stranding and extraluminal fluid (Figs 2.20A and B). A large amount of intraperitoneal air usually indicates gastroduodenal perforation, except for bowel perforation caused by obstruction or an endoscopic

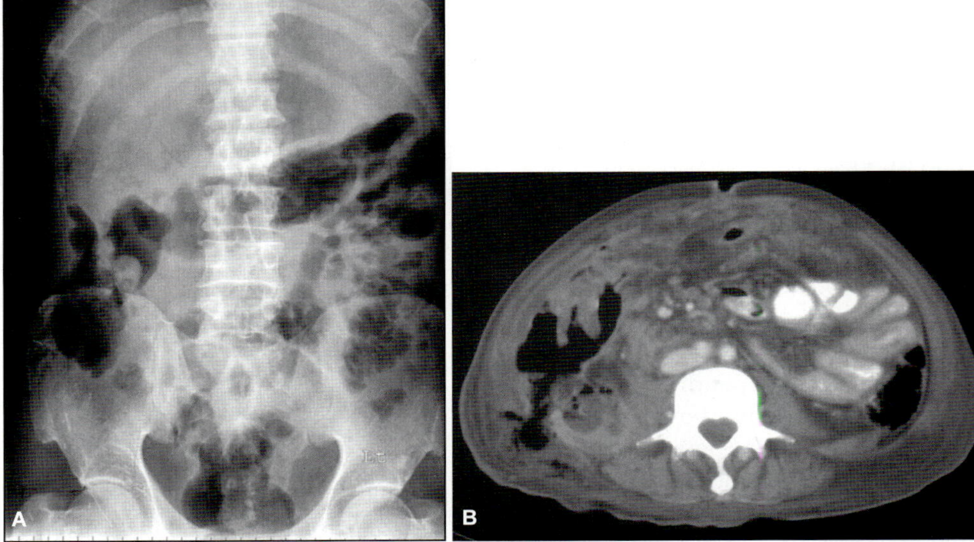

Figs 2.20A and B: (A) Plain radiograph of the abdomen shows extraluminal, mottled air lucencies in the right iliac region denoting perforation of a hollow viscus (B) Axial CECT section reveals an ill-defined mass involving the cecum with discontinuity of the lateral cecal wall. A large amount of extraluminal air is seen adjacent to the perforation with extension of inflammation into the right gluteal region and formation of an abscess. This was a case of carcinoma cecum with perforation

procedure.[38] The location of air also helps in determining the site of perforation. Air in the lesser sac can be seen in posterior perforation of stomach or duodenum, or less commonly, from perforation of transverse colon. Free air confined to the intra-hepatic ligamentum teres is commonly due to gastroduodenal perforations. Air trapped in the mesenteric folds is found in colon and small bowel perforation, but seldom in gastric perforation. Retroperitoneal air is caused by perforation of extraperitoneal sites of gastrointestinal tract viz. descending and horizontal parts of duodenum, ascending and descending colon, sigmoid colon and rectum.

Mesenteric Ischemia

Bowel ischemia or infarction is a common but complex disorder with a plethora of primary causes and a wide range of clinical and pathological manifestations. Acute mesenteric ischemia is therefore a diagnostic challenge particularly in view of its high mortality rate which ranges from 50-90% depending upon the cause and degree of bowel wall damage. Acute occlusion of the superior mesenteric artery (SMA) due to embolus is the most common cause of mesenteric ischemia accounting for nearly 50% of cases.[39] Thrombosis of the SMA or the superior mesenteric vien (SMV) are responsible for another 10-20% of cases. Occlusion of the arteries may be due to atherosclerosis, various types of vasculitis and thrombotic microangiopathies or the antiphospholipid antibody syndrome. Venous occlusions may be caused by infiltrative, neoplastic or inflammatory conditions or hypercoagulable states. Non-occlusive ischemia is seen in low-flow states when there is decreased cardiac output such as cardiogenic or septic shock. The manifestation may range from a self-limiting superficial ischemia involving the watershed zones to a diffuse ischemic injury to the entire bowel - "shock bowel".[40] Other causes of bowel ischemia include neoplasms, bowel obstruction, abdominal inflammatory conditions, trauma, drugs, chemotherapy, radiation and corrosive injury.

There are three stages of acute mesenteric ischemia. In the first stage, there is mucosal involvement with necrosis, ulcerations and/or hemorrhage. The injury is superficial and will eventually heal completely. In stage II, there is necrosis of the deep submucosal and muscular layers which may lead to the development of fibrotic strictures. Stage III ischemia represents transmural bowel necrosis which requires immediate surgical intervention. The imaging appearance in a given case will therefore depend on the etiology as well as the degree of ischemia. Plain films reveal the characteristic thick-walled dilated loops with thumb-printing in only 20-30% of cases.[41] Intramural air or porto-mesenteric air is also rarely visualized on the plain radiograph.

MDCT angiography is the modality of choice for the evaluation of bowel ischemia with a sensitivity approaching that of angiography (82%). The arterial occlusion/narrowing as well as the venous occlusion can be readily detected. Involvement of the vasa recta (Coombs' sign) may be seen in small vessel vasculitis. In addition, involvement of a long segment of bowel or both small and large bowel with skip segments are features of small vessel disease. The most common finding of mesenteric ischemia is bowel wall thickening though this feature strongly depends on the degree of bowel distension. Mural thickening is commoner with ischemic colitis and with veno-occlusive disease but is rare in arterio-occlusive disease where the involved segment of bowel may show dilated, fluid-filled loops with paper-thin walls. The bowel wall may show a striated appearance due to the presence of sub-mucosal edema or hemorrhage. In complete arterial occlusion, there can be absence of the normal enhancement of the bowel wall. Conversely, in non-occlusive ischemia there can be abnormal persistent mural enhancement. The target sign is seen when there is hyperenhancement of the mucosa and submucosa due to hyperemia and hyperperfusion with mural edema (Figs 2.21A and B).

Luminal dilatation with air-fluid levels can be seen in 56-91% of cases.[40] Mesenteric fat stranding, fluid and/or ascites are non-specific CT findings. Some authors have postulated that presence of stranding or fluid in the mesentery when there is isolated involvement of the small bowel signifies transmural necrosis. However, in large bowel ischemia, peri-colonic streakiness may be due to super-infection of the ischemic segment.

Pneumatosis and portomesenteric gas are less common but more specific findings of ischemia being present in 6-28% and 3-14% of cases respectively (Figs 2.22A and B).[39,40] The presence of pneumoperitoneum or focal peritonitis signifies perforation.

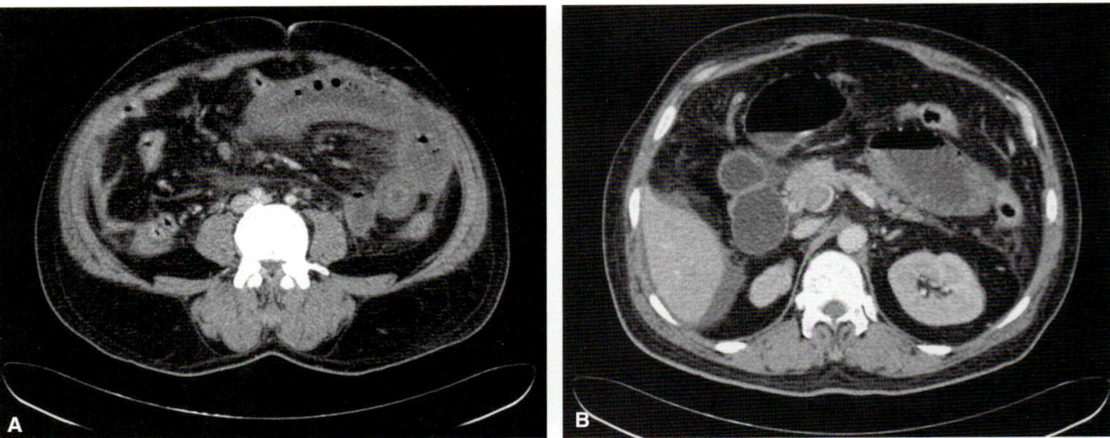

Figs 2.21A and B: CECT abdomen, venous phase images. A. There is dilatation with mural thickening of the small bowel with a striated pattern giving a target appearance on transverse sections. Note the increased density of the subtending mesentery. B. A large hypodense filling defect is seen in the superior mesenteric vein as the cause of mesenteric ischemia

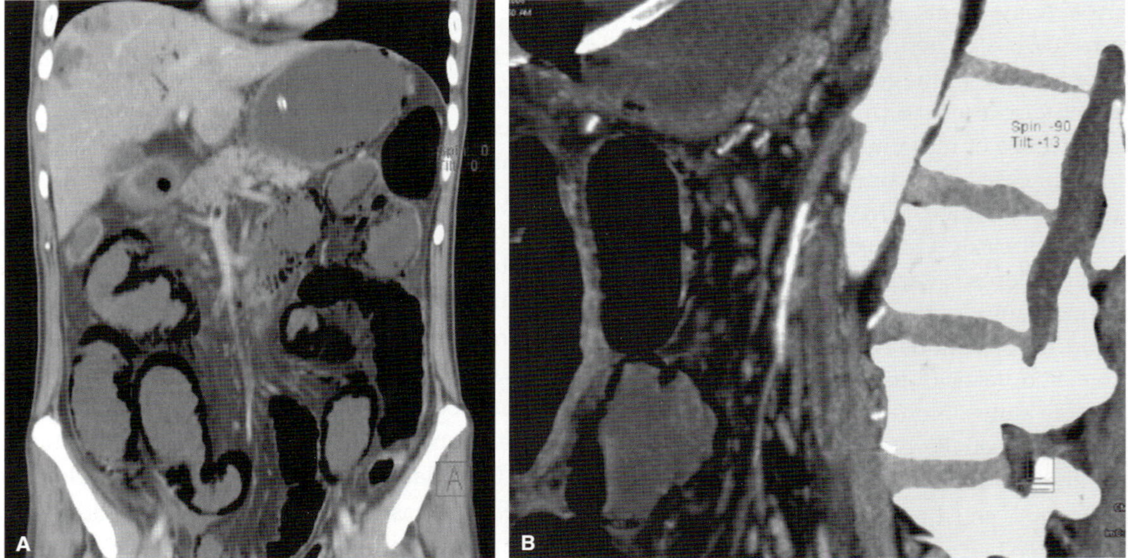

Figs 2.22A and B: Mesenteric ischemia, CT angiography. (A) The small bowel loops are dilated with thinned-out walls and gross pneumatosis. Air is also seen in the mesenteric veins and the portal radicles in the liver. Note the irregular, non-enhancing hypodense areas in the periphery of the liver due to infarcts (B) Sagittal MIP image demonstrates the occlusion of the proximal superior mesenteric artery

Vascular Causes

Vascular conditions that may present as acute abdomen include rupture of an aortic aneurysm, spontaneous aortic occlusion, acute hemorrhage and hepatic or splenic vascular occlusion. Aneurysmal dilatation of the abdominal aorta is rare before the age of 50 with average age at the time of diagnosis being 65-70 years. Most abdominal aortic aneurysms are true aneurysms and occur below the level of renal arteries. An abdominal aortic aneurysm is defined as an aortic diameter of 3 cm or more[42] while a diameter of 5.5 cm or more warrants urgent intervention. Presence of a pulsatile mass and sudden hypotension in the clinical setting of acute pain abdomen suggests the diagnosis of a ruptured aortic aneurysm. Although US may detect the aneurysm as well as the associated thrombus and hematoma, frequently the entire

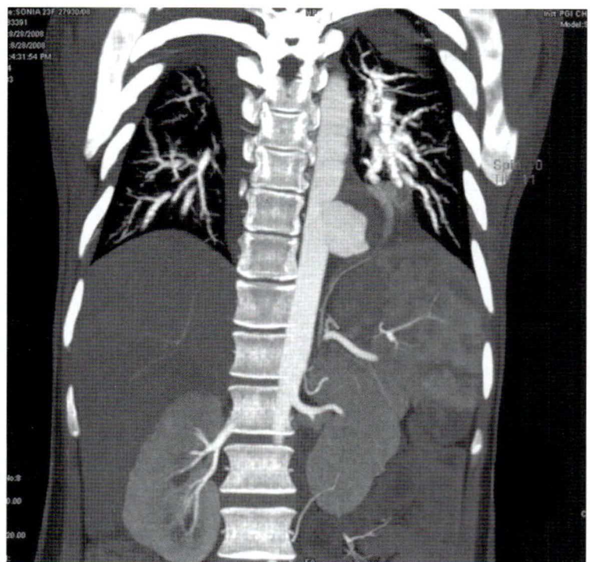

Fig. 2.23: CT angiography. MIP image shows an irregular, sac-like lobulated outpouching from the wall of the thoraco-abdominal aorta due to a mycotic pseudoaneurysm in a case of infective endocarditis. There is associated thrombus as well as a peripheral rim of hyperdensity because of the surrounding hematoma

aorta cannot be evaluated due to overlying bowel gas or body habitus. Multidetector CT is the modality of choice for evaluation of acute aortic syndrome. The most common finding of rupture of aortic aneurysm is a retroperitoneal hematoma adjacent to the aneurysm (Fig. 2.23). Other CT features may include active extravasation of contrast, extension of periaortic blood into perirenal or pararenal spaces or the psoas muscle or peritoneal cavity. Signs predictive of impending rupture are:

a. Draped aorta sign – Seen with contained leak. The posterior wall of aorta cannot be defined due to close application and lateral 'draping' of the aneurysm around the adjacent vertebral bodies.[43]
b. Increase in aneurysm size – A patient with a very large aneurysm (> 7cm diameter) who presents with acute aortic syndrome has a high likelihood of aneurysm rupture. Also, a rate of enlargement of >10 mm per year warrants surgical repair.
c. Thrombus-to-lumen ratio - This ratio decreases with increasing aneurysm size. A thick circumferential thrombus is protective against rupture.
d. Focal discontinuity in intimal calcification.
e. Hyperattenuating crescent sign due to hemorrhage in either the peripheral thrombus or aneurysm wall.

Acute abdominal hemorrhage may result due to ruptured aneurysm in a case of polyarteritis nodosa, ruptured tumor (usually renal cell carcinoma) or in a patient on anticoagulant therapy. Non-contrast CT demonstrates a hyperdense collection at the site of hemorrhage. MDCT angiography can accurately delineate the site and cause of hemorrhage.

Rare causes of acute abdomen include hepatic vein thrombosis (acute Budd-Chiari syndrome) and portal vein thrombosis. US in the acute phase may show liver enlargement, partial or complete inability to visualize hepatic veins, intraluminal hepatic vein echogenicity or thrombosis, marked narrowing of intrahepatic IVC and ascites. Color Doppler is the technique of choice for initial evaluation. Absence of flow or flow in an abnormal direction in all or part of the hepatic veins may be seen. CT and MR are complimentary techniques for definitive diagnosis which provide a more complete evaluation of the hepatic parenchyma, hepatic veins and IVC.

Pelvic Disease

The various entities that have to be additionally thought of while evaluating a young female in the reproductive age group presenting with acute abdomen are ruptured ectopic pregnancy, PID, twisted ovarian cyst and complications of early pregnancy, etc.

a. Signs of a ruptured ectopic pregnancy on ultrasound include an inhomogeneous adnexal mass, pelvic fluid or hematoma, decidual reaction without intrauterine gestation sac, in the presence of a positive pregnancy test. Visualization of an echogenic adnexal ring separate from the ovary that has prominent peripheral flow on color Doppler is highly suggestive of ectopic gestation. Corpus luteum is a useful guide while looking for an ectopic pregnancy and is usually seen in the ipsilateral ovary in 70-85% cases.[44] Using transvaginal ultrasound, the live embryo can be detected in upto 17% of all ectopic pregnancies.
b. Fibroids may present with acute pain if there is torsion or degeneration of a submucosal or subserosal fibroid. On imaging, uterine enlargement with a focal mass or contour deformity are seen. Degenerated fibroids may have a cystic appearance.
c. Ovarian torsion usually occurs in children and is attributed to excessive mobility of the ovary. In adults, a cyst or mass, frequently a cystic teratoma, is present in the ovary undergoing torsion. Sonographic findings include an enlarged ovary with peripherally

distributed follicles, an associated cyst or mass, with diminished or absent central venous flow on Doppler. On CT, deviation of the uterus to the twisted side, obliteration of fat planes and an enlarged ovary displaced from its adnexal location is seen. Contrast enhanced CT may show surrounding enhancing blood vessels due to congestion.

d. Hemorrhage into a corpus luteal or follicular cyst may manifest with abrupt onset of pelvic pain. If the cyst ruptures, associated hemoperitoneum can be life threatening. On imaging, hemorrhagic ovarian cysts can mimic a variety of solid and mixed solid-cystic masses. A fluid-fluid level may be present. On CT, high attenuation components are usually seen due to hemorrhage.

e. Pelvic inflammatory disease (PID) is among the common causes of acute pain in young women. In the early stage of PID, US may demonstrate a small amount of fluid in the cul-de-sac or endometrial canal. On CT, there may be stranding in the parapelvic fat, thickening of uterosacral ligament and ovarian enlargement with oophoritis. In advanced stages, there is development of pyosalpinx or tubo-ovarian abscess.

f. Ovarian vein thrombosis (OVT) should be suspected as a cause of abdominal pain in the postpartum period, in women with PID, recent abdominal surgery, malignancy or known hypercoagulable state. Pregnancy increases the risk for venous thrombosis due to stasis, alteration in coagulation factors and by nearly tripling the diameter of the ovarian veins. In 90% of cases, the right ovarian vein is involved due to dextrotorsion of the uterus.[45] OVT may be diagnosed by US, CT or MRI, however, CT is the modality of choice and demonstrates a low attenuation thrombus in lumen of ovarian vein.[45]

MISCELLANEOUS

Diverticulitis

The tetrad of left lower quadrant pain and tenderness, fever and leukocytosis is the classic presentation of diverticulitis. Diverticular disease of the colon affects 65% of the Western population by the age of 65 years, and diverticulitis eventually develops in up to 25% of individuals with diverticulosis.[46] Findings on barium enema include diverticulae, muscular wall hypertrophy, intramural or extramural mass effect on the barium column, colonic obstruction or peritoneal extravasation of contrast material, such as with fistula or sinus tract formation. The full extent of peritoneal involvement cannot be estimated on barium examination, hence it has largely been replaced by CT for imaging of suspected diverticulitis. Findings on CT include diverticulae, muscular wall hypertrophy, symmetrical mural thickening > 4 mm, pericolonic fat stranding, phlegmon, extraluminal gas bubbles, extravasation of contrast in case of perforation and paracolic abscess formation. Adequate distension and opacification of the colon by contrast material administered per-rectally is the cornerstone of an optimal CT evaluation and helps to distinguish true inflammatory wall thickening from apparent wall thickening due to incomplete luminal distension. Differential diagnosis includes carcinoma. Presence of enlarged lymph nodes, mural thickening > 1.5 cm and an abrupt change from normal to abnormal colon favors carcinoma over diverticulitis.[47]

Toxic Megacolon

Toxic megacolon is an acute transmural fulminant colitis which can occur as a complication of any colitis but is most commonly seen with ulcerative colitis (1.6-13% of cases). Plain radiographs show marked colonic dilatation (> 8 cm) particularly of the transverse colon as this is the least dependent part of the large bowel in the supine position. The wall has a shaggy appearance with mucosal islands or pseudopolyps with absence of haustra due to profound inflammation and ulceration (Fig. 2.24). There may be air-fluid levels and small bowel dilatation. CT

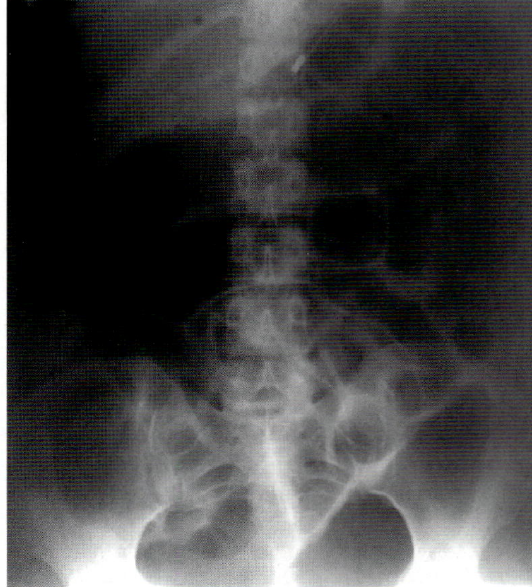

Fig. 2.24: Toxic megacolon. Plain radiograph, supine film shows dilatation of the large bowel loops particularly the transverse colon which has thick, shaggy walls due to mucosal islands

shows the distended colon filled with air, fluid and blood with a distorted or absent haustral pattern and irregular, nodular wall.[48] There may be presence of intra-mural air or blood. The prognosis is poor in the presence of perforation and complications.

Acute Pyelonephritis

Acute pyelonephritis is the bacterial or fungal infection of the renal parenchyma and collecting system. Presenting features include flank pain, dysuria and high grade fever with rigors. On US, renal enlargement, decreased visualization of sinus fat secondary to compression, loss of corticomedullary differentiation, focal poorly marginated hypoechoic areas representing interstitial edema or complications like abscesses may be seen. CT is the imaging modality of choice and can reveal calculi, obstruction, renal enlargement, striated nephrogram, ill-defined wedge-shaped areas of decreased attenuation radiating from the papillae to the cortical surface, abscess, thickening of Gerota's fascia and perinephric stranding (Fig. 2.25). Emphysematous pyelonephritis usually occurs in patients with poorly controlled diabetes with the most common infecting organism being *Escherichia coli*. Presence of air in the renal parenchyma is pathognomonic of this condition.

Acute Urinary Colic

Impacted ureteric stone is the commonest cause of acute post-renal obstruction. US is useful for the detection of small/radiolucent calculi missed on plain films. Secondly, direct visualization of the effects of these calculi on the urinary tract is also possible. However, because pelvicaliectasis may be mild to negligible in acute obstruction, US may miss up to one-third of acute obstructions. Color Doppler US helps demonstrate absence of the normal urinary jet on the obstructed side. Unenhanced helical CT has emerged as an attractive modality in the diagnostic workup of urinary tract disease. NCCT KUB is performed rapidly, without patient preparation and without risk of contrast reaction. It can provide information about size, localization and chemical composition of the stone. In addition to direct stone visualization, secondary CT signs of urinary obstruction, including ureteral dilatation, perinephric or periureteric fat stranding, blurring of renal sinus fat and ureteral wall edema, are usually present to confirm the diagnosis even after recent stone passage.[49]

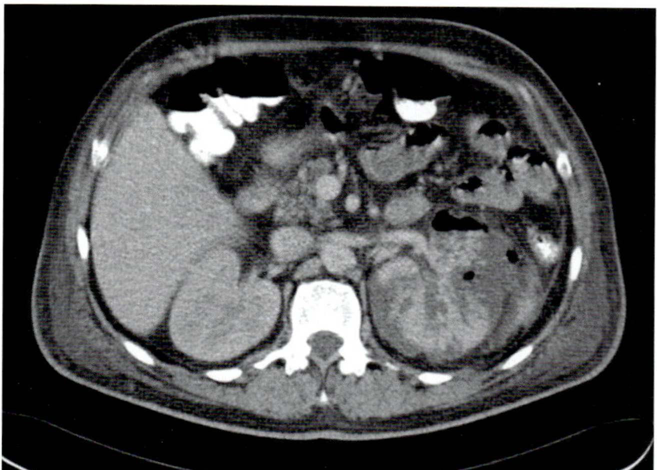

Fig. 2.25: Axial CT image shows multiple, irregular, linear, hypodense areas in the left kidney due to pyelonephritis. A hypodense area with an air-fluid level is seen in anterior cortex suggestive of renal abscess. In addition, perinephric collection with air is also visualized

Acute Epiploic Appendagitis, Omental Infarction

Epiploic appendages are fat-containing peritoneal outpouchings that arise from cecum to rectosigmoid junction, along the serosal surface of the colon. These are 0.5-5.0 cm long and contain fat and small vessels. Epiploic appendagitis is due to torsion of an epiploic appendage leading to venous occlusion and ischemia. It is usually associated with obesity, hernia and unaccustomed exercise. The condition manifests as acute left lower quadrant pain, predominantly in males in the 4th-5th decades of life. On US, a hyperechoic, incompressible mass delineated by a hypoechoic ring is seen at the point of maximum tenderness. The lesions are hyperechoic due to their fat content or hemorrhagic necrosis. CT features include an oval, fat attenuation lesion less than 5 cm in diameter that abuts the anterior or anterolateral serosal aspect of the colonic wall, surrounded by inflammatory changes.[50] A hyperattenuating rim corresponding to the hypoechoic ring on US is seen on CT due to swollen serosa covered by fibrinoleukocyte exudate.

Omental infarction commonly involves the inferior aspect of right side of omentum. It is characteristically situated between the anterior abdominal wall and the transverse or ascending colon, corresponding in location to the greater omentum. Predisposing factors include obesity, strenuous activity, congestive heart failure, digitalis administration, recent abdominal surgery and abdominal trauma. Pain is localized to the right lower or upper quadrant and the presumptive diagnosis is usually appendicitis. Both US and CT show an ovoid, soft tissue mass just beneath the anterior abdominal wall. The infarcted omental fat is hyperechoic on ultrasound and appears heterogeneous with no enhancement on CT.

Although omental infarction may resemble acute epiploic appendagitis on CT, it lacks the hyper-attenuating ring seen in the latter. Moreover, omental infarction is larger than epiploic appendagitis which is often less than 5 cm. Omental infarction is commonly located next to the cecum and ascending colon whereas acute epiloic appendagitis is usually located adjacent to sigmoid colon.[50]

REFERENCES

1. Silen W. Cope's early diagnosis of the acute abdomen (19th Ed) Oxford University Press, New York, 1996.
2. Field S. The plain abdominal radiograph—The acute abdomen. In Grainger RG, Allison DJ (Eds): Diagnostic Radiology (3rd edn), Churchill Livingstone, Edinburgh, 1997.
3. de Bombal FT. Introduction. In de Bombal FT (Ed). Diagnosis of acute abdominal pain (2nd Ed) Churchill Livingstone, Edinburgh 1991.
4. Balthazar EJ, Chako AC. Computerized tomography in acute gastrointestinal disorders. Am J Gastroenterol 1990;85:1445-52.
5. Macari M, Balthazar EJ. The acute right lower quadrant: CT evaluation. Radiol Clin N Am 2003;41:1117-36.
6. Kundra V, Silverman PM. Impact of mutlislice CT on imaging of acute abdominal disease. Radiol Clin N Am 2003;41:1083-93.
7. Lomas DJ. Technical developments in bowel MRI. Eur Radiol 2003;13:1058-71.
8. Mindelzun RE, McCort JJ. Acute abdomen. In Margulis AR, Burhenne HJ (Eds): Alimentary Tract Radiology (4th Edn) CV Mosby Co., St. Louis, Mo 1983.
9. Mirvis SE, Young JWR, Keramati B, et al. Plain film evaluation of patients with abdominal pain: Are three radiographs necessary? AJR Am J Roentgenol 1986; 147:501-03.
10. Miller RE, Nelson SW. The roentgenological demonstration of tiny amounts of free intra-peritoneal gas: Experimental and clinical studies. AJR Am J Roentgenol 1971;112:574-85.
11. Rubesin SE, Levine MS. Radiologic diagnosis of gastrointestinal perforation. Radiol Clin N Am 2003; 41:1095-1115.
12. Messmer JM. Gas and soft tissue abnormalities. In Gore RM, Levine MS (Eds): Textbook of Gastrointestinal Radiology (2nd Edn). WB Saunders company 2000.
13. Bongard F, Landers DV, Lewis F. Differential diagnosis of appendicitis and pelvic inflammatory disease. Am J Surg 1985;150:90-96.
14. Rao PM, Rhea JT, Novelline RA, et al. Helical CT technique for the diagnosis of appendicitis: Prospective evaluation of a focused appendix CT examination. Radiology 1997;140:139-44.
15. Gaitini D, Beck-Razi N, Mor-Yosef D, et al. Diagnosing acute appendicitis in adults: Accuracy of color Doppler sonography and MDCT compared with surgery and clinical follow-up. AJR Am J Roentgenol 2008;190:1300-1306.
16. Lee JH, Jeong YK, Park KB, et al. Operator dependent techniques for graded compression sonography to detect the appendix and diagnose acute appendicitis. AJR Am J Roentgenol 2005;184:91-7.
17. Poortman P, Lahle PNM, Schoemaker CMC, et al. Comparison of CT and sonography in the diagnosis of acute appendicitis: A blinded prospective study. AJR Am J Roentgenol 2003;181:1355-9.
18. Uggowitzer M, Kugler C, Schramayer G, et al. Sonography of acute cholecystitis: Comparison of color and power Doppler sonography in detecting a hypervascularized gallbladder wall. AJR Am J Roentgenol 1997;168:707-12.
19. Blankenberg F, Wirth R, Jeffry BR Jr, et al. Computed tomography as an adjunct to ultrasound in the diagnosis of acute acalculous cholecystitis. Gastrointestinal Radiol 1991;16:149-53.
20. Fidler J, Paulson EK, Layfield L. CT evaluation of acute cholecystitis: Findings and usefulness in diagnosis. AJR Am J Roentgenol 1996;166:1085-8.
21. Watanabe Y, Nagayama M, Okumura A, et al. MR imaging of acute biliary disorders. Radiographics 2007;27:477-95.
22. Bennett GL, Rusinek H, Lisi V, et al. CT findings in acute gangrenous cholecystitis. AJR Am J Roentgenol 2002; 178:275-81.
23. Morris BS, Balpande PR, Morani AC, et al. The CT appearances of gallbladder perforation. BJR 2007;80:898-901.
24. Gore RM, Yaghmai V, Newmark GM, et al. Imaging benign and malignant disease of the gallbladder. Radiol Clin North Am 2002;40:1307-23.
25. Balthazar EJ, Ranson JHC, Naidich DP, Megibow AJ, Caccavak R, Cooper MM. Acute pancreatitis: Prognostic value of CT. Radiology 1985;156:767-72.
26. Balthazar EJ, Robinson DL, Megibow AJ, Ranson JHC. Acute pancreatitis: Value of CT in establishing prognosis. Radiology 1990;174:331-6.
27. Mortele KJ, Wiesner W, Intreire L, et al. A modified CT severity index for evaluating acute pancreatitis: Improved correlation with patient outcome. AJR Am J Roentgenol 2004;183:1261-5.
28. Dorffel T, Wruck T, Ruckert R, Romanivk P, Dorffel Q. Vascular complications of acute pancreatitis assessed by color duplex ultrasonography. Pancreas 2000;21:126-33.
29. Stimac D, Miletic D, Radic M. The role of NEMRI in early assessment of acute pancreatitis. Am J Gastroenterol 2007;102(5):997-1104.

30. Joseph AEA, MacVicar D. Ultrasound in the diagnosis of abdominal abscess. Clin Radiol 1990;42:154-6.
31. Go Hl, Baarslaq HJ, Vermeulen H, Laméris JS, Legemate DA. A comparative study to validate the use of ultrasonography and computed tomography in patients with post-operative intra-abdominal sepsis. Eur J Radiol 2005; 54(3):383-7.
32. Federle MP, Anne VS. Small bowel obstruction. In Federle MP (Ed): Diagnostic imaging—Abdomen (1st Edn). Amirsys Inc, Utah 2004.
33. Canon CL. Gastrointestinal Tract. In Lee JKT, Sagel SS, Stanley RJ, Heiken JP, (Eds): Computed body tomography with MRI correlation (4th edn). Lippincott Williams and Wilkins, Philadelphia PA 2006.
34. Bondiaf M, Jaff A, Soyer P, Bouhnik Y, Hamzi L, Rymer R. Small bowel diseases: Prospective evaluation of multi-detector row helical CT enteroclysis in 107 consecutive patients. Radiology 2004;233:338-44.
35. Beall DP, Fortman BJ, Lawler BC, et al. Imaging bowel obstruction: A comparison between fast magnetic resonance imaging and helical computed tomography. Clin Radiol 2002;57(8):719-24.
36. Chen SC, Wang HP, Chen WJ, et al. Selective use of ultrasonography for the detection of pneumo-peritoneum. Acad Emerg Med 2002;9:643-5.
37. Jones R. Recognition of pneumo-peritoneum using bedside ultrasound in critically ill patients presenting with acute abdominal pain. Am J Emerg Med 2007;25:838-41.
38. Furukawa A, Sakoda M, Yamasaki M, et al. Gastro-intestinal tract perforation: CT diagnosis of presence, site and cause. Abdom Imaging 2005;30:524-34.
39. Rha SE, Ha HK, Lee S, et al. CT and MR imaging findings of bowel ischemia from various primary causes. Radiographics 2000;20:29-42.
40. Wiesner W, Khurana B, Ji H, Ros PR. CT of acute bowel ischaemia. Radiology 2003;226:635-50.
41. Ha HK, Rha SE, Kim AY, et al. CT and MR diagnosis of intestinal ischaemia. Seminars in US, CT and MRI 2000 21(1):40-55.
42. Scott RA, Ashton HA, Kay DN. Abdominal aortic aneurysm in 4,237 screened patients: Prevalence, development and management over 6 years. Br J Surg 1991;78:1122-5.
43. Rakita D, Newatia A, Hines JJ, et al. Spectrum of CT findings in rupture and impending rupture of abdominal aortic aneurysms. Radiographics 2007;27:497-507.
44. Condous G, Okaro E, Khalid A, et al. The accuracy of transvaginal ultrasonography for the diagnosis of ectopic pregnancy prior to surgery. Hum Reprod 2005;20:1404-9.
45. Heavrin BS, Wrenn K. Ovarian vein thrombosis: A rare cause of abdominal pain outside the peripartum period. J Emerg Med 2007;34:67-69.
46. Rao PM, Rhea JT, Novelline RA, et al. Helical CT with only colonic contrast material for diagnosing diverticulitis: Prospective evaluation of 150 patients. AJR Am J Roentgenol 1998;170:1445-9.
47. Chintapalli KN, Esola CC, Chopra S, et al. Pericolic mesenteric lymph nodes: An aid in distinguishing diverticulitis from cancer of the colon. AJR Am J Roentgenol 1997;169:1253-5.
48. Imbriaco M, Balthazar EJ. Toxic megacolon: Role of CT in evaluation and detection of complications. Clin Imaging 2001;25:349-54.
49. Sourtzis S, Thibeau JF, Damry N, et al. Radiologic investigation of renal colic: Unenhanced helical CT compared with excretory urography. AJR Am J Roentgenol 1999;172:1491-4.
50. Singh AK, Gervais DA, Halin PF, et al. Acute epiploic appendagitis and its mimics. Radiographics 2005;25: 1521-34.

Chapter Three

Imaging in Abdominal Trauma

Atin Kumar, Sanjay Thulkar

INTRODUCTION

Blunt abdominal trauma in isolation represents 5% of trauma mortality and further contributes 15% to mortality as part of polytrauma.[1] Excessive bleeding accounts for 80-90% of acute deaths from abdominal injury. In recent years advances in cross-sectional imaging coupled with image-guided interventional therapies have made significant contributions in enabling nonsurgical management of blunt abdominal trauma in hemodynamically stable patients.

A radiologist must have a detailed understanding of the patterns of injury, image appearances of traumatic injuries, assessment of hemodynamic status, and common image artifacts. The patient evaluation must take place within the context of systematic and orderly resuscitation of the patient.

Abdominal trauma could be blunt or penetrating. Blunt trauma occurs in approximately two-thirds of abdominal injury patients. Motor vehicle accidents account for up to 80% of blunt trauma with the remainder being caused by falls, assault and industrial accidents. Penetrating injuries commonly result due to gunshot injuries and stab wounds.

The incidence of organ injury in both categories of trauma as observed by Anderson et al[2] is given in Table 3.1.

Up to two-thirds of the abdominal trauma patients have a significant injury to other systems as well and these injuries may take precedence in terms of diagnosis and treatment.

Table 3.1 Incidence of organ injury in blunt and penetrating trauma

Blunt		*Penetrating*	
Spleen	25%	Liver	37%
Kidney	12%	Small bowel	26%
Intestine	15%	Stomach	19%
Liver	15%	Colon	16.5%
Retroperitoneum	13%	Vascular retro-peritoneum	11.0%
Mesentery	5%	Mesentery	7.0%
Pancreas	3%	Diaphragm	5.5%
Diaphragm	2%	Kidney	5.0%
Vascular	2%	Pancreas	3.5%
		Duodenum	2.5%
		Biliary system	1.0%
		Others	1.0%

Prompt and accurate clinical assessment is essential in the initial evaluation of an abdominal trauma patient. Unfortunately, the clinical evaluation is often unreliable. Neurological impairment due to traumatic event itself or to concomitant factors such as intoxication or inebriation significantly limits the usefulness of clinical examination. The most reliable signs in conscious patients are pain and tenderness with guarding. Twelve to 16% of patients with abdominal trauma present in a state of shock.[3] After initial evaluation and resuscitation, subsequent management depends on hemodynamic stability of the patient. As per the ACR guidelines/

appropriateness criteria[4] the patients are divided into following categories:

Category A: This category includes hemodynamically unstable patients following clinically obvious major abdominal trauma and with unresponsive profound hypotension need rapid clinical evaluation and immediate resuscitation with volume replacement. If such unstable patients do not respond to resuscitation (become hemodynamically stable), and if they have clear clinical evidence of abdominal injury, they should go immediately to the operating room without imaging. During resuscitative efforts if time and circumstances permit, conventional radiographs of the chest and abdomen are often obtained as part of trauma protocols. This may help identify a pneumothorax, pneumoperitoneum, or significant bone injury. Ultrasound performed by an experienced sonologist to check for intraperitoneal free fluid may quickly provide information that can support a decision to operate immediately, with the caveat that the false negative rate is at least 15%. More detailed ultrasound to check for organ injury takes too long in this setting and suffers from poor sensitivity. There is now general agreement that routine diagnostic peritoneal lavage (DPL) is obsolete because of its invasive nature, lack of specificity, and inability to predict the need for therapeutic surgery.

Category B: This category includes hemodynamically stable patients, patients with mild to moderate responsive hypotension presenting to the emergency room after blunt abdominal trauma, and unstable patients who stabilize after initial resuscitation. These patients typically have a history of significant trauma and have at least moderate suspicion of intra-abdominal injury based on clinical signs and symptoms. These patients should be evaluated by imaging. In patients with clinical evaluation suggesting a lesser index of suspicion for significant intraabdominal injury, chest and abdominal radiographs, hematocrit with blood chemistries and a urinalysis should be performed. If these tests are unremarkable in the setting of a reliable clinical abdominal exam, a period of clinical observation may all be that is needed. However, if a reliable abdominal exam cannot be performed (patient is unconscious or prolonged nonabdominal surgery is anticipated) or if a clinical evaluation suggests organ injury, hemoperitoneum, or peritonitis, further imaging is needed. The need for initial radiographs may be obviated if the clinical condition at initial evaluation merits a computed tomography.

Ultrasound is not a good modality for further imaging because it is relatively much less sensitive than computed tomography for liver and spleen injuries and highly insensitive for renal, pancreatic, mesenteric, gut, bladder and retroperitoneal injuries. If due to circumstances, a negative ultrasound is the sole imaging modality used to triage a patient, for safety reasons it must be followed by a 12-24 hour period of in-hospital observation. A negative ultrasound alone may be adequate to release the patient from observation only in a separate subcategory of stable patients with trivial trauma, a low clinical index of suspicion, and no signs or symptoms of intraabdominal injury. Any positive findings on ultrasound would however warrant computed tomography.

In contrast, computed tomography is an excellent modality for detecting solid organ and gut injuries together with even small amount of hemoperitoneum. The findings of computed tomography in combination with clinical status of the patient plays an important role in deciding whether a patient needs urgent therapeutic surgery or therapeutic angiography or whether he can be managed conservatively. Identification of active hemorrhage, parenchymal blush or pseudoaneurysm in spleen, gut perforation, diaphragmatic injury and pancreatic injury tilt the scales towards surgical or angiographic management. Selected stable patients with negative computed tomography can be discharged without observation whereas patients with positive computed tomography findings in which surgical intervention is not required may be managed conservatively under observation with imaging follow up.

Category C: This category includes patients with hematuria which require some modification to imaging workup. Patients with microscopic hematuria (less than 35 red blood cells per high power field) do not need specific urinary tract imaging. All patients with microscopic hematuria greater than 35 red blood cells per high power field, with macroscopic hematuria, or with fracture/ diastasis of the symphysis pubis and its rami plus any hematuria need imaging of the urinary tract. If the urethral meatus has gross blood, if there is a floating prostate, or if a Foley catheter cannot be passed, a retrograde urethrogram should first be performed to rule out urethral injury. However, if clinical evaluation or the urethrogram indicates no urethral injury, a computed tomography cystogram should be added to the abdominal computed tomography.

DIAGNOSTIC IMAGING

Plain Radiography

Stable patients and those who respond to initial fluid therapy should undergo radiographic studies of the cervical spine, chest and pelvis because of the relatively high incidence and potentially devastating injuries to these areas. The plain radiographs may reveal fractures. The upright chest X-ray is a relatively sensitive means of detecting pneumoperitoneum. Small amount of air may not be initially seen on upright chest radiograph as it may take up to 10 minutes to rise to the highest point in the peritoneal cavity. It is possible with optimal radiographic technique to demonstrate upto 1.0 cc of free air on upright chest radiograph.

Plain radiographs of the abdomen are insensitive for the detection of hemoperitoneum. Intraperitoneal volume of greater than 800 cc is usually necessary for the demonstration of classic plain radiographic signs, e.g. "dog ear" or "bladder ear" sign when there is accumulation of intraperitoneal blood in the pouch of Douglas. In the true abdomen the most dependent intraperitoneal areas are paracolic gutters. Blood tracking from liver and spleen will collect in the respective gutter appearing as a soft tissue haze. This collection of blood displaces the right or left colon medially.

Ultrasonography (US)

Sonography is commonly used for the initial assessment of abdominal trauma. Abdominal ultrasound in cases of major trauma is usually performed with a FAST (*F*ocussed *A*ssessment with *S*onography in *T*rauma) examination. It provides a fast overview of abdomen to detect free fluid which indicates hemoperitoneum and visceral organ injury in this setting. The FAST scan should be completed within few minutes with an aim to primarily search for free intraperitoneal fluid and screen organs for injury. While parenchymal organ injuries may be detected, search for such injuries should not delay the examination specially in the setting of suspicion of hemorrhage. Following standard views are recommended:

1. Transverse view of epigastrium to detect pericardial fluid and injury to left lobe of liver.
2. Longitudinal view of right upper quadrant for right lobe of liver, right kidney and Morrison's pouch and perihepatic free fluid.
3. Longitudinal view of left upper quadrant for spleen, left kidney and perisplenic free fluid.
4. Longitudinal views of bilateral flanks to look for free fluid in paracolic gutters
5. Transverse and longitudinal views of suprapubic region for urinary bladder and free fluid in pelvis and pouch of douglas.
6. Bilateral longitudinal thoracic views for pleural effusion.

The reported sensitivity of FAST for detection of free intraperitoneal fluid ranges from 0.64-0.98 and specificity from 0.86-1.00.[5] So false negative rate of FAST is average 15% for free fluid detection. Negative FAST should be interpreted as indicating the absence of hemoperitoneum, not the absence of intra-abdominal injury. However it should be remembered that the sensitivity of FAST for free fluid is less than that of CT. A negative FAST should be viewed with suspicion if the finding is not commensurate with patient's clinical presentation. On the other hand, a positive FAST does not necessarily mandate laparotomy. Hemodynamically stable patients with positive FAST should have their injuries staged with CT, giving them the benefit of non-operative management whenever possible. FAST is not reliable for assessment of retroperitoneum.

The sensitivity of ultrasound for detection of liver injury ranges from 0.15-0.88[5] and it misses average 15% injuries to liver. The sensitivity for splenic injuries is reported to be between 0.37-0.85[5] with a average false negative rate of more than 50%. Sensitivity for renal and pancreatic injuries is less than of liver and spleen and even lesser for bowel and mesenteric injuries. The sensitivity for pericardial effusion is high (0.97-1.00).[5]

In a technically successful examination, hemoperitoneum (Fig. 3.1) is visualised as a lenticular collection in the subphrenic space, triangular in Morison's pouch and ovoid in the pelvis. Solid organ injury can be recognised by subcapsular or intraparenchymal hematoma. US appearance of hematoma depends on multiple factors, especially on its duration. The early hematoma is echogenic but gradually progresses to sonolucency over 96 hours.

Ultrasound has certain limitations as the technique is operator dependent and may be limited by excessive bowel gas (especially in post-traumatic paralytic ileus). It may also be limited by open wounds and bandages and by cutaneous emphysema.

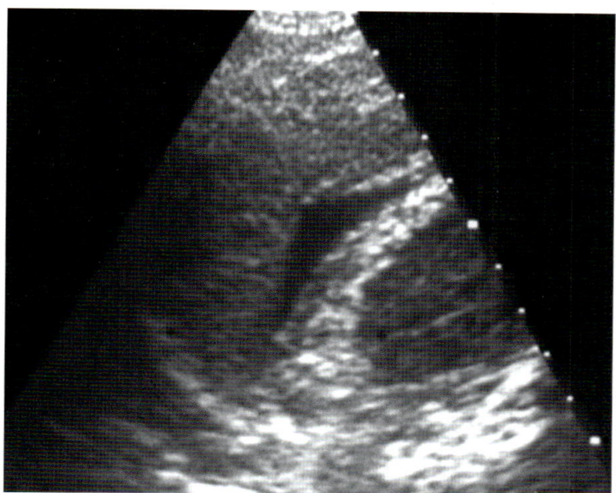

Fig. 3.1: Axial ultrasound image shows free fluid in hepatorenal pouch

Radionuclide Scanning

Nuclear medicine studies are generally not used in the screening evaluation of abdominal trauma. Although (Tc^{99m}) sulphur colloid may detect liver and spleen injury but this technique does not assess the entire abdomen and pelvis and cannot differentiate the defects specific to traumatic injuries. Serial nuclear scans can be used to follow known liver or splenic injuries. In the setting of hepatic injury involving the biliary tree, the use of a biliary scanning agent such as Tc^{99m}-HIDA can demonstrate a biloma or bilious fluid leakage or fistula. In certain circumstances, radionuclide angiography can demonstrate small vascular injuries and may exceed the sensitivity of conventional angiography. This technique uses either Tc^{99m} sulphur colloid, or more sensitive Tc99m labeled RBC study, that may demonstrate bleeding as low as 1 ml/mt.[6]

Magnetic Resonance Imaging (MRI)

Currently, MRI does not play a role in the initial evaluation of the acutely injured patient. MRCP may be specifically useful in detecting biliary leaks. MR imaging is useful only in doubtful cases and in hemodynamically stable patients.

Angiography

With recent trends towards non-operative management of abdominal trauma patients, angiography with embolisation has been increasingly used in the management. Angiographic embolisation is indicated when CT shows evidence of vascular injury (pseudoaneurysm, arteriovenous fistula) and in active contrast extravasation as an alternative to surgery. It has also been used in controlling bleeding in patients with high grade (IV and V) liver and spleen injuries specially in hemodynamically stable patients with known visceral injury of high grade (IV and V) but falling hematocrit to determine the presence of active bleeding requiring embolisation or surgical intervention.

Computed Tomography (CT)

Computed tomography is now firmly established as the principal imaging modality for diagnostic evaluation of abdominal trauma. It is useful in detecting otherwise occult injuries to both intra-abdominal and retroperitoneal structures and grading severity of specific parenchymal injury. Associated injuries of head and chest etc. can also be evaluated. CT is as accurate as DPL in detecting blunt abdominal injuries. CT offers a number of advantages over DPL, including detailed anatomic evaluation of injuries, quantification of associated hemorrhage and detection of active arterial extravasation. CT excels in detection of retroperitoneal injuries that are not picked up by DPL or ultrasound. With these advantages of CT, DPL has now almost become obsolete. Following a negative abdominal CT study using helical scanner, trauma patients could be safely discharged from the emergency department without a period of observation.[7]

CT Technique

Attention to scanning technique is essential. Scans should be done expeditiously and care should be taken to avoid artifacts and repeat scanning. Helical CT is preferred over the conventional CT as it offers optimal intravenous contrast enhancement, avoids respiratory misregistration, is less prone to motion artifacts and reduces scan time. MDCT is very useful in this setting as excellent quality reconstructions can be obtained in coronal and saggital planes. Administration of intravenous iodinated contrast material is mandatory as it makes detection and location of parenchymal contusions and hematoma more conspicuous, identifies great vessels and provides information regarding integrity of organs or extent of the injury. MDCT protocols vary from institution to institution but typically involve imaging at sub-mm slice thickness 60-70 seconds after initiating an injection of 100-120 ml of 300 mg/dl low osmolar IV contrast medium at 2.5-3.0 ml per second. Successful breath holding is often not possible and image acquisition during shallow and quiet breathing is often necessary. Use of oral contrast is highly desirable. It is helpful in defining pancreas, integrity of bowel and free intraperitoneal fluid from fluid filled bowel. Administration of 500 ml of 2-5% iodinated water soluble contrast is generally sufficient. It is given orally or through the nasogastric tube and allowed to travel as far as possible through the gastrointestinal tract. Rectal contrast is used occasionally to detect colorectal injuries in patients with perineal lacerations and penetrating flank or back wounds. Delayed scanning of kidneys during urographic phase is essential to detect collecting system injuries. Delayed imaging is also useful in specific situations for differentiating between active contrast extravasation from vascular injuries.[8] Viewing with bone window for subtle fractures and upper sections with lung windows for unsuspected pneumothorax, lung contusion or free peritoneal gas should be done.[9]

CT Signs in Blunt Abdominal Trauma[10]

Sentinel Clot Sign

Clotted blood adjacent to the site of injury is of higher attenuation (45-70 HU) than unclotted blood which flows away (Figs 3.2A and B). When source of intraperitoneal bleed is not evident, the location of highest attenuating blood clot is a clue to the most likely source.

Water Density Fluid Collection

Fluid collections of near water attenuation originate from rupture of gallbladder, urinary bladder, small bowel and cisterna chyli. When fluid of this density is encountered in the peritoneal cavity without an identifiable source, the safest assumption is that bowel injury is present.

Interloop Fluid

Triangular fluid collection(s) between the leaves of mesentery are important indicators of bowel or mesenteric injury. Hemoperitoneum from liver or spleen injury typically does not form such collections, but instead tracks from the upper abdomen along the paracolic gutters into the pelvis. When interloop fluid is of low attenuation (< 15 HU), bowel injury is suspected and when it is of high attenuation (> 30 HU), mesenteric hematoma is likely.

Hemodynamic Status

Size of the IVC in adults and size of aorta in children, give valuable morphological information that correlates with the intravascular volume and cardiac output.

Active Arterial Contrast Extravasation

It must be actively looked for as most oftenly it is an indicator for surgical/angiographic intervention. It must be distinguished from extravasated oral contrast material and from a vascular injury (pseudoaneurysm or arteriovenous fistula) within an injured organ. Vascular

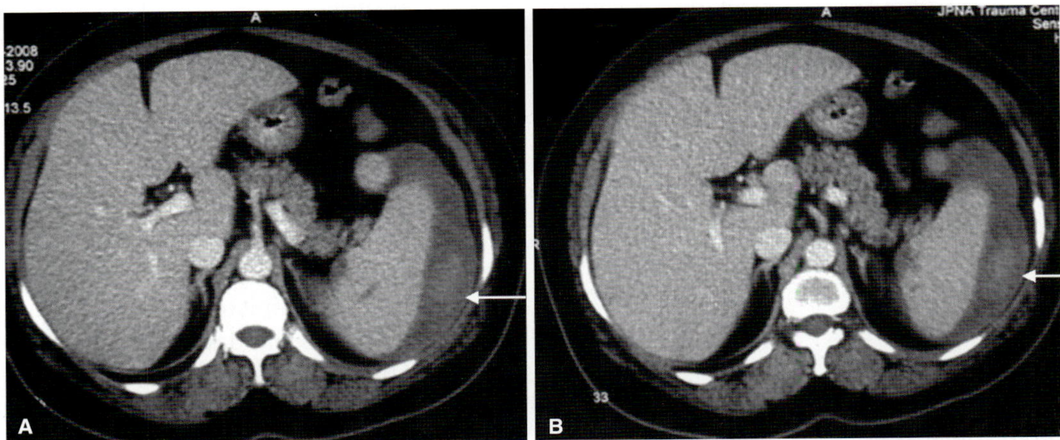

Figs 3.2A and B: Axial CECT scans show hemoperitoneum in perisplenic region. Note the presence of higher density clotted blood adjacent to the spleen (arrows)—the 'sentinel clot sign'

extravasation is typically poorly marginated, high attenuating collection, surrounded by a large hematoma. Extravasated gastrointestinal contrast is usually not surrounded by hematoma. Pseudoaneurysm usually has a well-defined margin. Vascular injuries show attenuation values paralleling the attenuation of adjacent vessel on delayed phase images while active bleeding shows attenuation values either increasing or remaining same.

CT Staging of Abdominal Injuries

Majority of the injuries to the liver, spleen and kidneys can be managed non-operatively. CT is required to evaluate the extent of injury and to exclude other intra and retroperitoneal injuries to determine the management approach. It is generally based on the premise that large and deep lacerations, large hematomas, and devitalised tissues are signs of more severe injuries and are more likely to require surgical management. Non-operative management is generally not appropriate in presence of active arterial hemorrhage, favouring urgent surgery or angiographic embolisation.

ORGAN TRAUMA

Peritoneal Cavity

Pneumoperitoneum

It is a sign of perforated hollow viscus, but may also occur following pneumothorax and mechanical ventilation.[11] Small amount of air is easily detectable under the right hemidiaphragm on erect chest radiograph. CT is the most sensitive investigation for detection for free peritoneal air. In order not to miss small amounts of free air the images should be viewed in the lung window settings. It may be detected on CT over the liver and anteriorly in the mid abdomen (Fig. 3.3). Bubbles of free air may be trapped between the leaves of the mesentery or in the peritoneal recesses.

Hemoperitoneum

Blood collects in the peritoneum following injury to the liver, spleen, bowel or mesentery. CT is sensitive in detecting intra-abdominal or pelvic hemorrhage. 'Sentinel clot' may be seen near the site of bleeding with lower attenuation blood elsewhere in the peritoneal cavity. In the supine position blood from the liver collects in the hepatorenal recess and travels down the right paracolic gutter into the pelvis. From the spleen the blood passes along the phrenico-colic ligament to the left paracolic gutter and pelvis. Hemoperitoneum typically has an attenuation value of 45 HU or greater, but a quarter of patients may have HU value less than 20 HU. Therefore hemoperitoneum may not be distinguishable from ascites, extravasated small intestinal fluid from bowel perforation or from intraperitoneal urine from ruptured urinary bladder.[12] In women of child bearing age small amounts of intraperitoneal fluid may be a normal finding. Detection of fluid in each paracolic gutter indicates that atleast 200 ml of blood must be present in each gutter. CT visualisation of blood in the abdomen and pelvis corresponds with the amounts of more than 500 ml.

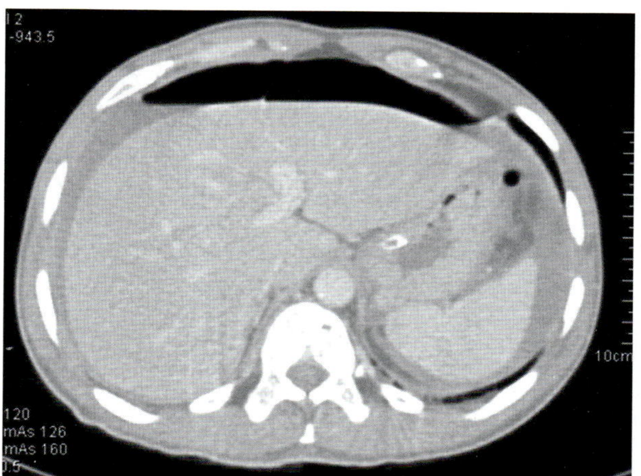

Fig. 3.3: Axial CECT scan through upper abdomen in lung window settings shows pneumoperitoneum anterior to liver

SPLEEN

Spleen is the most commonly injured organ following blunt abdominal trauma. The spleen is the most vascular organ of the body containing approximately 500-600 ml of blood. Although it may occur as an isolated injury, most patients with splenic trauma have associated intra-abdominal injuries. Over the last decade, there is increasing trend towards nonsurgical conservative management of splenic injuries. Imaging with multislice CT has greatly aided in evaluation of splenic trauma and contrast enhanced CT is the modality of choice for imaging of splenic injuries. The most widely used splenic injury grading system is the American Asssociation for the Surgery of Trauma (AAST) splenic injury scale.[13]

Grade I: Hematoma: subcapsular, < 10% surface area.

Laceration: capsular tear, < 1 cm in parenchymal depth.

Grade II: Hematoma: subcapsular, 10%-50% surface area; intraparenchymal, < 5 cm in diameter.

Laceration: 1-3 cm in parenchymal depth; does not involve a trabecular vessel.

Grade III: Hematoma: subcapsular, >50% surface area or expanding; ruptured subcapsular or parenchymal hematoma.

Laceration: >3 cm in parenchymal depth or involved trabecular vessels.

Grade IV: Laceration: Laceration involving segmental or hilar vessels and producing major devascularization (> 25% of spleen).

Grade V: Laceration: Completely shattered spleen.

Vascular: Hilar vascular injury that devascularizes spleen.

However, this AAST injury grading score is based on appearance of spleen on surgery. The CT may not be able to correctly show all the above features and hence may be a limitation in accurately grading the splenic injuries. Recently Marmery et al[14] have proposed a modified splenic injury grading system taking into account the findings of active splenic hemorrhage and vascular injuries on CT. According to their modified grading system, active intraparenchymal and subcapsular splenic bleeding, splenic vascular injury (pseudoaneurysm or arteriovenous fistula) and shattered spleen should be classified as grade IVa and active intraperitoneal bleeding as grade IVb. There is no grade V in their classification. It has now been well established that the presence of active hemorrhage and vascular injuries is predictive of the need for splenic artery transcatheter embolization or splenic surgery. The authors compared their modified grading with the AAST splenic injury grading scale and found it to be a better predictor for surgical or angiographic intervention in patients of splenic trauma (grade IV patients).

As already stated above, contrast enhanced CT is the preferred modality for imaging splenic trauma. The images should be obtained in portal venous phase as heterogenous enhancement of spleen in the arterial phase can simulate injury. In selective cases where there is dense contrast pooling seen within or around spleen, delayed CT images may be obtained to differentiate active bleeding from post traumatic vascular injuries. In delayed phase, the active bleeding would retain the same density or even may increase in attenuation but in case of vascular injuries including pseudoaneurysms and arteriovenous fistulas the attenuation would decrease in proportion to the attenuation of adjacent artery or aorta. Delayed phase may also be useful in differentiating a laceration from a splenic cleft.[14]

The various CT manifestation of splenic trauma are:

- Hematomas: Subcapsular or parenchymal. Subcapsular hematomas are characterized by their lenticular configuration and flattening of the adjacent splenic parenchyma. The compression of underlying parenchyma helps to differentiate subcapsular location of hematoma from free intraperitoneal fluid or blood. Uncomplicated subcapsular hematomas tend to resolve within 4-6 weeks. Parenchymal contusions/hematomas appear as focal, poorly marginated areas of low attenuation at contrast enhanced CT representing edema, hemorrhage and necrotic tissue (Fig. 3.4).
- Laceration of the spleen appears as non-enhancing linear or branching areas usually at the periphery of the parenchyma (Fig. 3.5). Lacerations decrease in size and number with time. When delayed phase images are taken, the lacerations appear to 'fill-in' from the periphery and become less visible. In contrast, splenic clefts remain unchanged in appearance on delayed phase images besides having smooth or rounded margins. Multiple lacerations can lead to shattered splenic parenchyma (Fig. 3.6).

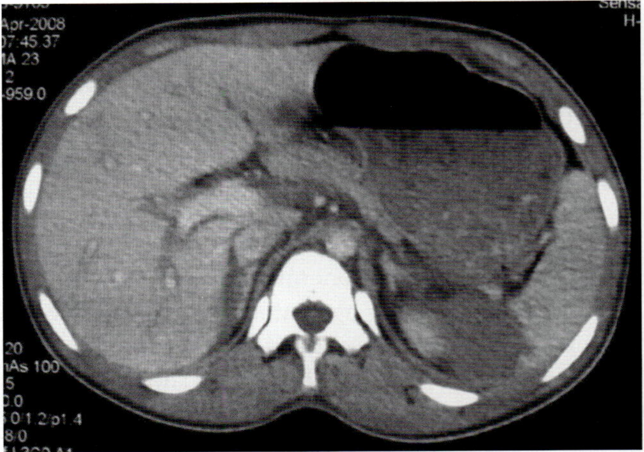

Fig. 3.4: Axial CECT scan through upper abdomen shows a splenic parenchymal hematoma

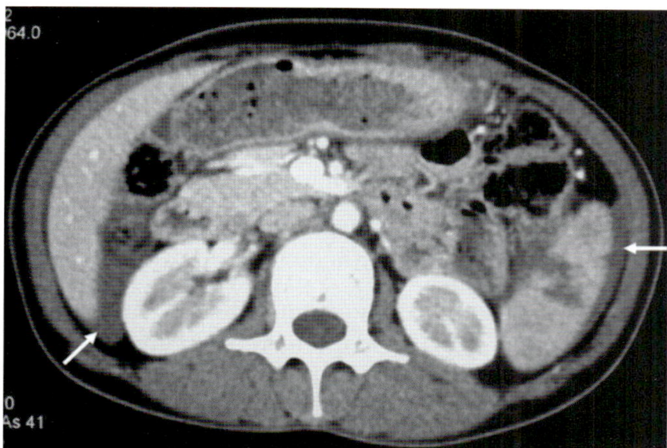

Fig. 3.5: Axial CECT scan at level of lower pole of spleen shows a splenic laceration. Note the presence of minimal fluid in perisplenic region and in hepatorenal pouch (arrows)

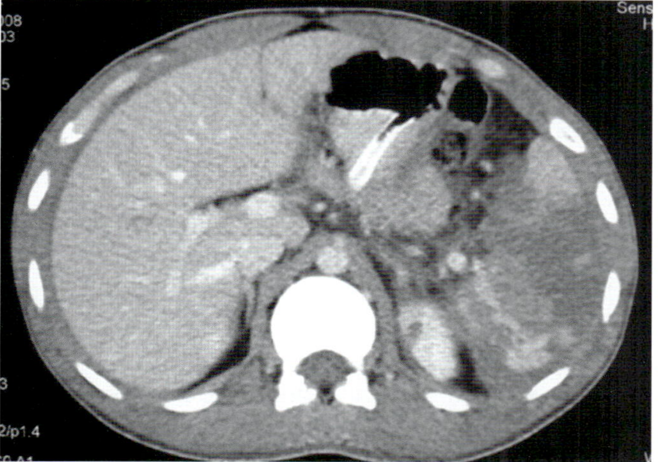

Fig. 3.6: Axial CECT scan through spleen shows shattered splenic parenchyma

- Active extravasation of contrast appears as linear or irregular hyperdensity (Figs 3.7A andB). The attenuation values ranges from 85-350 HU compared to that of clotted blood which lies between 40-70 HU. As described above, delayed phase imaging can help differentiate active bleeding from vascular injuries. Demonstration of active extravasation of contrast is a strong indicator of surgical or angiographic intervention.
- Vascular injuries including pseudoaneurysms and arteriovenous fistula appear as well circumscribed focal hyperattenuating areas on contrast enhanced CT with their attenuation value paralleling that of adjacent artery even on delayed images. Angiography is required to differentiate between pseudoaneurysm and arteriovenous fistula and possible embolization. Depiction of vascular injuries is also a strong marker for failure of non surgical management.
- Infarct appears as a well demarcated wedge shaped area of low attenuation which remains unchanged on delayed images. May decrease in size or remain unchanges on follow-up scans.
- Splenic vascular pedicle injury leads to splenic devascularization which appears as nonenhancing spleen (Fig. 3.8).

Some potential pitfalls in CT evaluation of splenic injury are: Motion artifacts simulating a subcapsular hematoma, volume averaging, splenic clefts or lobulation and peri-splenic fluid collection caused by ascites mistaken as hemoperitoneum, streak artifacts, premature scanning before the portal venous phase resulting in heterogeneous splenic enhancement etc. A sequel of splenic hematoma/laceration is the splenic pseudocyst,

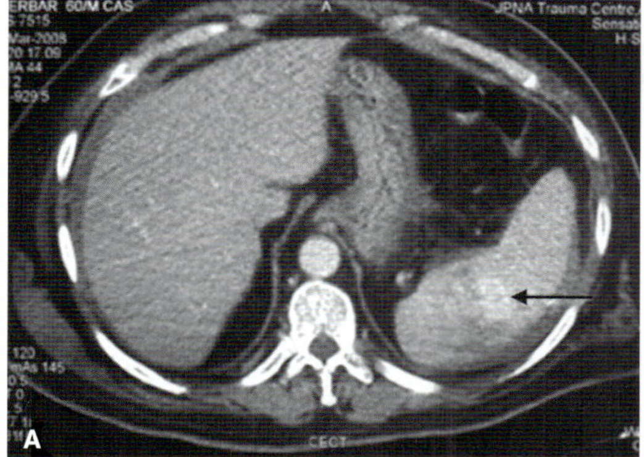

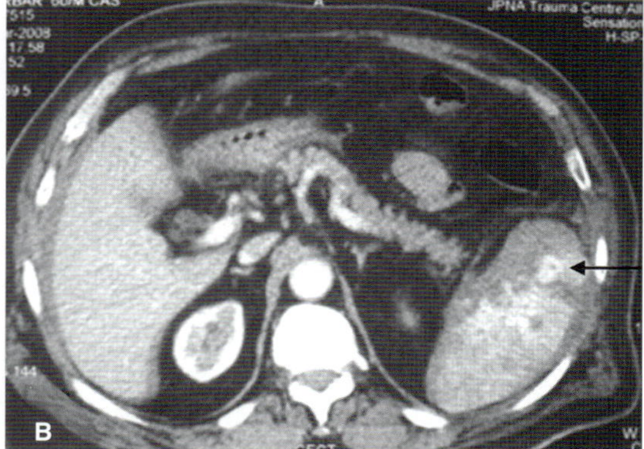

Figs 3.7A and B: Axial CECT scans through upper abdomen show active contrast extravasation (arrows) within the splenic parenchyma

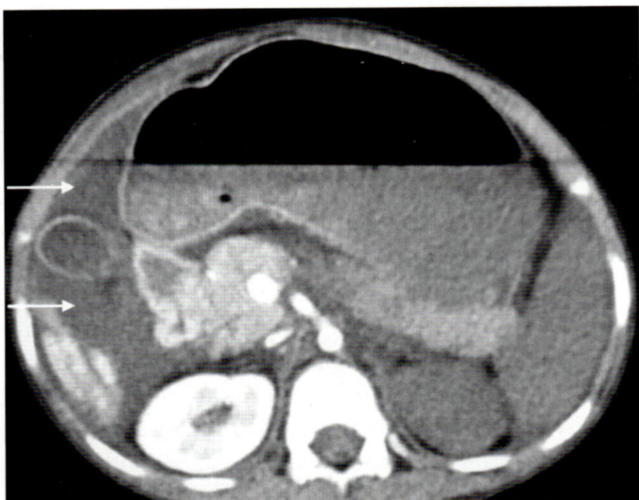

Fig. 3.8: Axial CECT scan shows nonenhancing spleen (devascularized). Also note the devascularization of left kidney and hemoperitoneum (arrows)

which appears as simple intra-splenic fluid collection of 20-30 HU and a fibrous capsule.

LIVER AND BILIARY TRACT

The liver is the second most frequently injured solid abdominal organ after spleen. The right lobe is injured more frequently and severely than the left and posterior segments are more frequently injured than anterior. As with spleen, CT is currently the diagnostic modality of choice for the evaluation of blunt liver trauma in hemodynamically stable patients. CT is the most accurate technique in detecting, defining and characterizing the hepatic injury, associated hemoperitoneum and other abdominal abnormalities. CT-based liver injury grading system established by the AAST is the most widely used grading system.[13]

AAST Liver Injury Grading System

Grade I: Hematoma: Subcapsular, < 10% surface area

Laceration: Capsular tear, < 1 cm in parenchymal depth

Grade II: Hematoma: Subcapsular, 10-50% surface area; intraparenchymal, < 10 cm in diameter.

Laceration: 1-3 cm in parenchymal depth, < 10 cm in length.

Grade III: Hematoma: subcapsular, > 50% surface area or expanding or ruptured subcapsular hematoma with active bleeding; intraparenchymal, > 10 cm or expanding or ruptured.

Laceration: > 3 cm in parenchymal depth.

Grade IV: Hematoma: Ruptured intraparenchymal hematoma with active bleeding.

Laceration: Parenchymal disruption involving 25-75% of a hepatic lobe or one to three Couinaud segments within a single lobe.

Grade V: Laceration: Parenchymal disruption involving >75% of a hepatic lobe or more than three Couinaud segments within a single lobe.

Vascular: Juxtahepatic venous injuries (i.e., retrohepatic vena cava or central major hepatic veins).

Grade VI: Vascular: Hepatic avulsion.

Majority (80%) of liver injuries cause hemoperitoneum. The finding of integrity of the liver capsule is important because it correlates with amount of blood loss. The various CT manifestations of liver trauma are:

- Subcapsular hematomas: The appearance is same as that described above in splenic trauma. They are located most commonly in antero-lateral aspect of right lobe of the liver (Figs 3. 9A and B).
- Parenchymal contusions and hematomas (Fig 3.10) have same appearance as described above in splenic trauma. Acute hematomas show increased density (40-60 HU) relative to adjacent normal liver parenchyma at unenhanced CT.
- Laceration is the most common type of liver injury. It appears as non-enhancing linear or branching areas usually at the periphery of the liver (Figs 3.11 and 3.12). Lacerations frequently travel along the vascular planes (portal vein branches and hepatic veins) and fissures (ligamentum teres and venosum), which are anatomic week zones. They can be classified as superficial (≤ 3 cm in depth) or deep (> 3 cm).
- Periportal tracking described by Foley et al.[15] is seen as low density areas along the portal vein branches. When accompanied by an adjacent parenchymal laceration, it indicates blood tracking along the periportal connective tissue (Fig. 3.12). It may also be secondary to distension of periportal lymphatic vessels due to increased central venous pressure of any cause

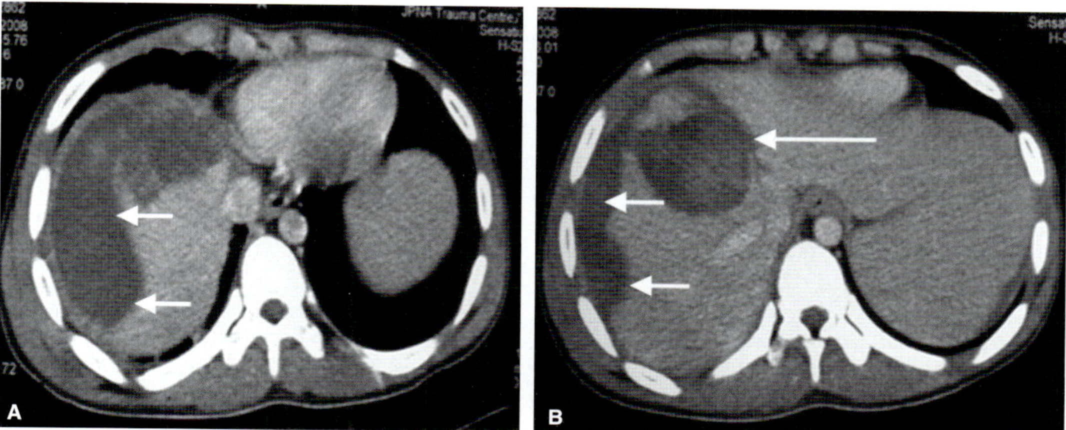

Figs 3.9A and B: Axial CECT scans show a large subcapsular liver hematoma (small arrows in A and B) caused due to rupture of a parenchymal hematoma (long arrow in B)

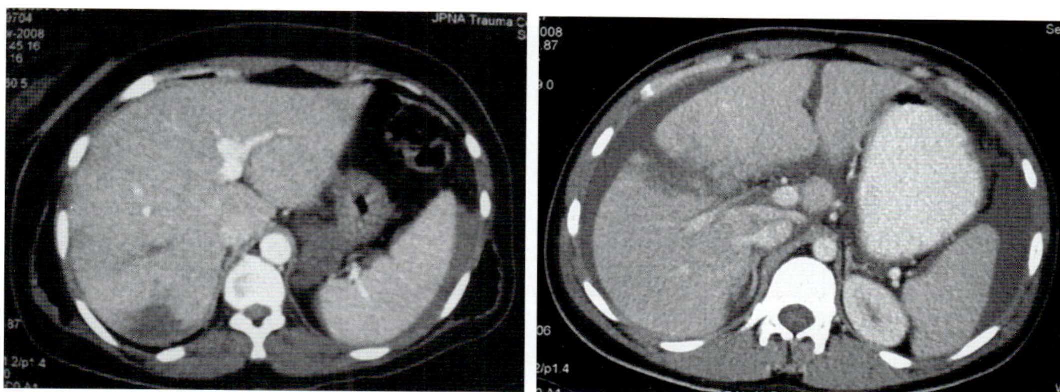

Fig. 3.10: Axial CECT scan shows a small liver parenchymal contusion

Fig. 3.11: Axial CECT scan shows a linear liver laceration

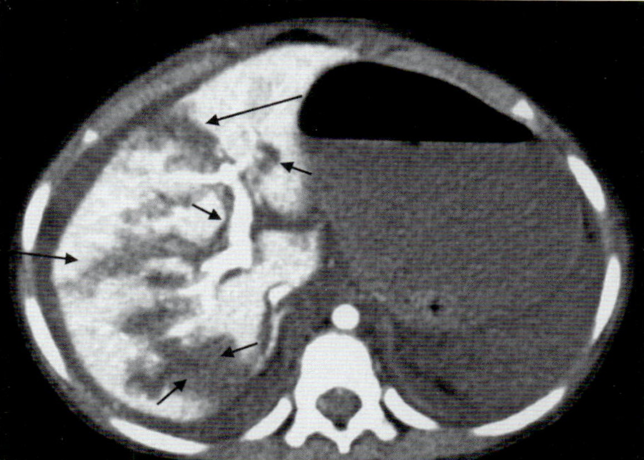

Fig. 3.12: Axial CECT scan though liver shows periportal fluid tracking (small arrows). The liver shows multiple lacerations (long arrows) and contusion (arrow heads)

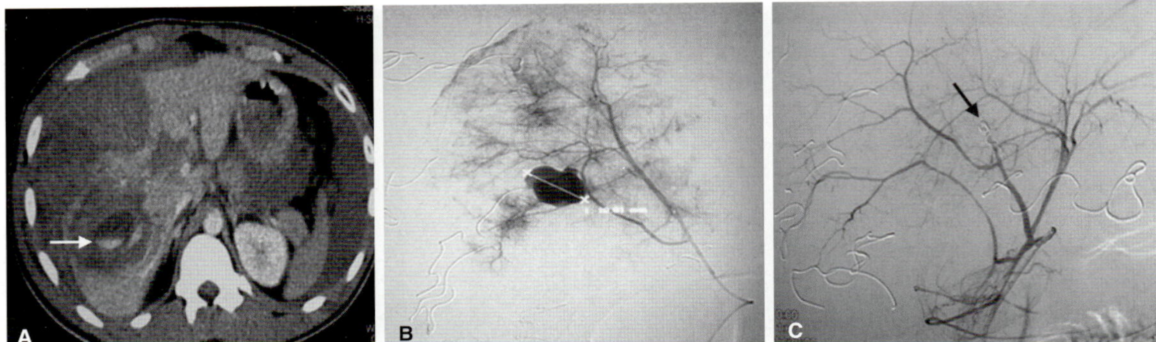

Figs 3.13A to C: Axial CECT scan (A) shows active contrast extravasation within liver parenchymal hematoma (arrow). The patient underwent DSA which showed a large pseudoaneurysm (B) filling from posterior branch of right hepatic artery.The patient underwent successful coil embolization (arrow in C)

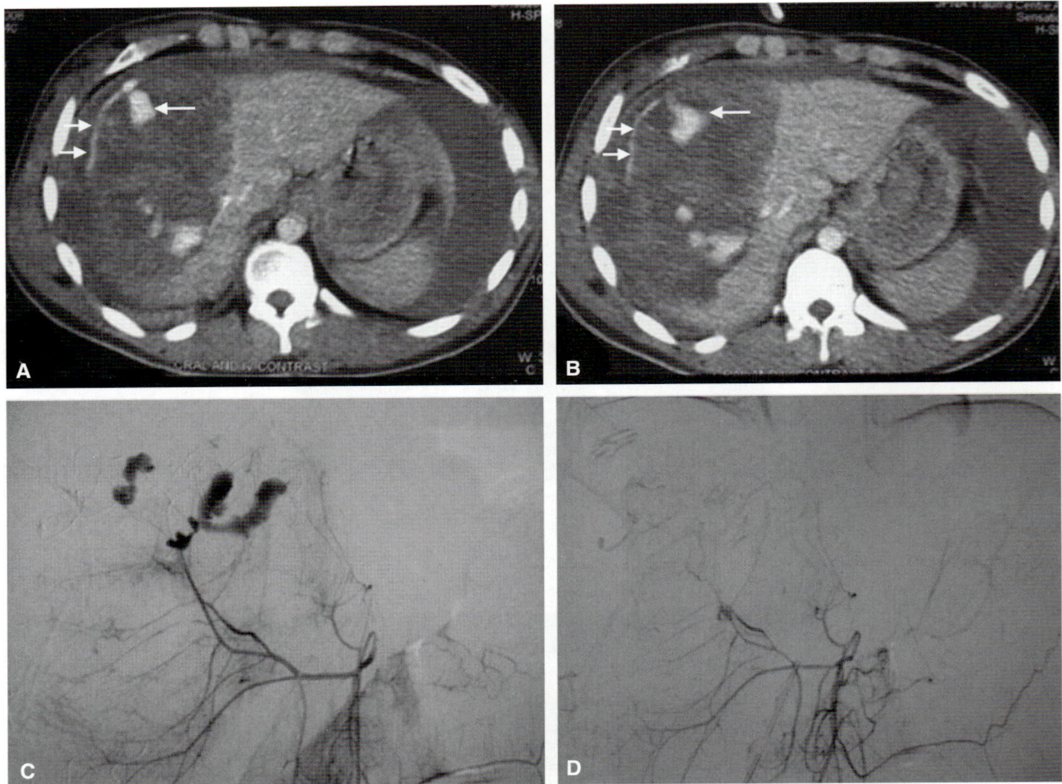

Figs 3.14A to D: Axial CECT scans (A and B) show active contrast extravasation within liver parenchyma (arrows) extending into peritoneal space (small arrows). DSA image (C) of selective hepatic artery injection shows active contrast extravasation. Post coil embolization (D) The extravasation has stopped

most commonly following vigorous intravenous fluid replacement.

- Active hemorrhage is best identified on early phase of contrast enhanced CT and is seen as focal high attenuation area representing extravasated contrast material secondary to arterial bleeding either within a parenchymal hematoma (Figs 3.13A to C) or freely into peritoneal space (Figs 3.14A to D). The attenuation value of extravasated blood measures within 10-20 HU of density of an adjacent major artery or aorta during the vascular phase of imaging and increases or pools on delayed phase of imaging[1]. The attenuation ranges from 91-274 HU in comparison to attenuation of clotted blood which ranges from 28-82 HU.[16]

- Major hepatic venous injury should be suspected if CT shows lacerations or hematomas extending into one or more major hepatic veins or IVC. If detected, it is an indicator for surgical treatment.
- Other uncommon manifestations include
  - Fragments of the liver may be completely avulsed from their dual blood supply, failing to enhance with the rest of the liver on CECT. Unavulsed infarcted segments appear as wedge shaped unenhanced areas extending upto the hepatic periphery.
  - Intrahepatic or subcapsular air may be seen usually for 2 days after the injury, and is attributed to necrosis rather than infection.
  - Hemobilia is seen as high attenuating material in the gallbladder or biliary channels (Figs 3.15A and B). It is caused when persistent arterial hemorrhage elevates intrahepatic pressure leading to parenchymal necrosis and blood spilling into the biliary tree and gut.
  - Intraperitoneal bile leak and peritonitis secondary to disruption of biliary system by trauma. Bile leaks are seen as relatively low attenuation fluid collections as compared to hemoperitoneum. These may be intrahepatic or extrahepatic, diffuse, focal or encapsulated (biloma).

The depiction of above mentioned findings on CT and the classification of the injury into grade based on AAST grading system has relevance in conjunction with the clinical status of the patient. However some of the findings in isolation also act as strong predictors for urgent surgical or angiographic intervention. It includes suspicion of major hepatic venous injury and detection of active contrast material extravasation on CT which indicates an ongoing, potentially life-threatening hemorrhage.

With the current concept of nonsurgical conservative management being employed in more and more patients of liver injury including those with severe grades, there is increased frequency of delayed complications visualized on follow-up CT. These include:[17]

- Delayed hemorrhage—Secondary to rupture of pseudoanuerysm formed by a biloma or secondary to an initially minimal but expanding injury.
- Hepatic artery pseudoaneurysm and hemobilia—A pseudoaneurysm is formed when the arterial continuity is disrupted and blood extravasates into a parenchymal hematoma with formation of a fibrous tissue capsule. They appear as focal rounded enhancing lesions paralleling the attenuation of the arterial blood in all phases. When the pseudo-aneurysm ruptures into biliary system it leads to hemobilia and subsequent drainage into duodenum can lead to hematemesis or melena. These pseudo-aneurysms should be treated early and angiographic embolization is the modality of choice.
- Abscess—Usually seen in follow-up of high grade liver injuries. It is visualized as fluid containing focal lesion with air bubbles or air-fluid levels. The treatment of choice is percutaneous catheter drainage.
- Biliary complications—Biliary leaks are usually self limiting with no definitive treatment required. Hepatic scintigraphy and MRCP may be helpful in detecting

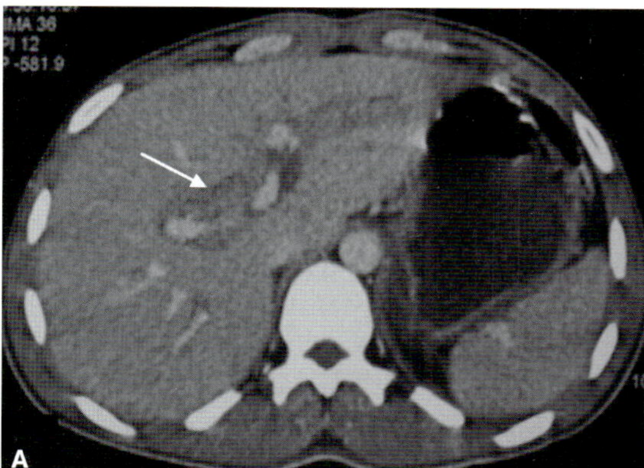

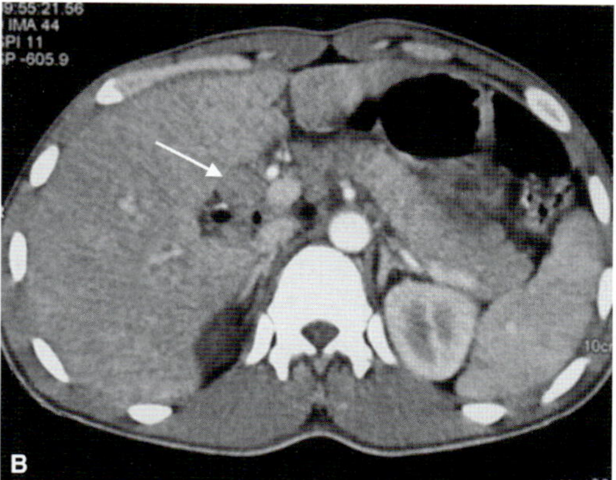

Figs 3.15A and B: Axial CECT scans through upper abdomen show hyperdensity within intrahepatic bile ducts (arrow in A) and within the CBD (arrow in B) suggesting hemobilia

bile leaks. Bile leak into a hematoma may cause necrosis of surrounding liver tissue leading to formation of biloma which on CT appears as low attenuation well circumscribed collection. Enlarging or symptomatic bilomas can be treated with percutaneous catheter drainage with or without ERCP guided endobiliary stent placement. Bile leak into peritoneal cavity leads to bile peritonitis which may be suspected on CT if peritoneal thickening and enhancement is seen with increasing amount of low attenuation fluid. It requires surgical intervention.

Follow-up CT is usually not required in low grade injuries unless patient's clinical status demands so. However in high grade injuries (grade IV or V), due to increased incidence of delayed complications a follow-up CT is usually required and should be done between 7-10 days after injury.

Evaluation of hepatic trauma can be associated with potential pitfalls on CT, viz., streak or beam hardening artifacts from the ribs, external tubes, patient's arms, air in the stomach, or unopacified hepatic veins. These may mimic lacerations. A false negative diagnosis can result in the setting of fatty liver when the enhanced fatty liver becomes isodense to a laceration or hematoma.

Gallbladder injuries are unusual. CT findings of ill defined contour of gallbladder, wall thickening, intraluminal hemorrhage, or collapsed lumen, especially in the presence of pericholecystic fluid suggests primary gallbladder injury in patients with abdominal trauma. Injuries to the extrahepatic bile ducts are uncommon and occur at the points of fixations, i.e. where the hepatic ducts enter the liver and where common bile duct enters the pancreas. The diagnosis is most often made at surgery.

PANCREAS

The pancreas is the least commonly injured solid organ, accounting for 3-12% of all abdominal injuries. This injury occurs after a sudden force that compresses the pancreatic neck against lumbar spine, e.g. in motor vehicle accidents in adults and bicycle accidents in children. Pancreatic injuries are difficult to diagnose. The presence of abdominal pain, leucocytosis and hyperamylasemia is nonspecific and frequently not present.

In contrast to liver and splenic injuries, CT is relatively insensitive to acute pancreatic injuries.[1] On CT, the findings may be subtle and must be actively sought.

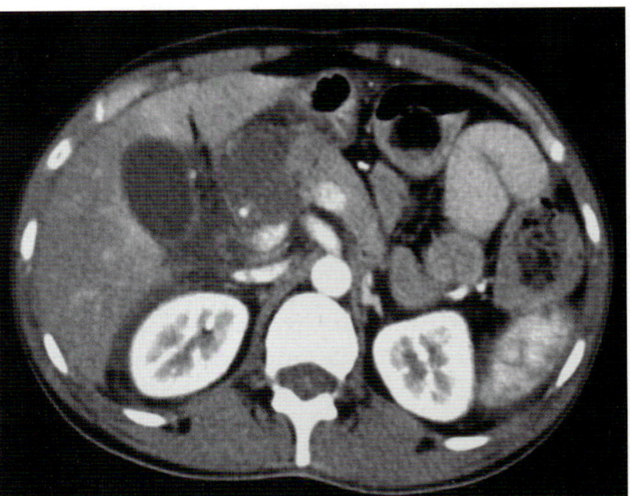

Fig. 3.16: Axial CECT scans show a contusion involving the head of pancreas

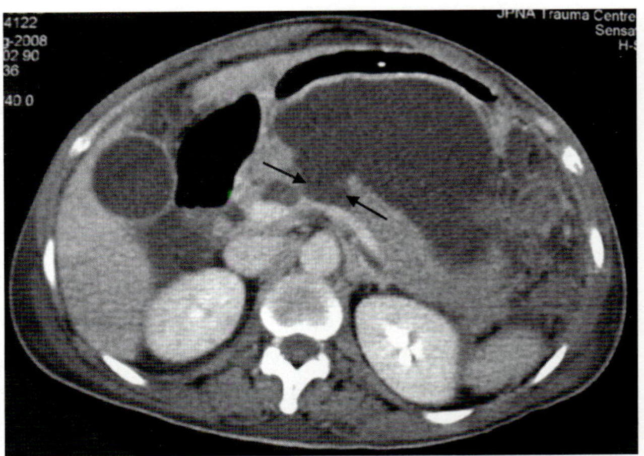

Fig. 3.17: Axial CECT scan through pancreas shows a laceration/ transection involving neck/proximal body of pancreas (arrows) with a large collection seen anterior to pancreas

Contusions, hematomas and superficial capsular lacerations are the most common findings (Fig. 3.16). Deeper lacerations may also occur with or without involvement of pancreatic duct. Direct signs include a fracture plane traversing the neck (most common), body or tail (Fig. 3.17). Lacerations of the pancreatic head are more likely to be complicated than are the more distal pancreatic injuries. These are usually associated with lacerations of the liver, spleen or duodenum. Transection of the pancreatic duct is an important source of morbidity and increased mortality. Indirect CT signs of pancreatic injury include focal or diffuse enlargement of the gland,

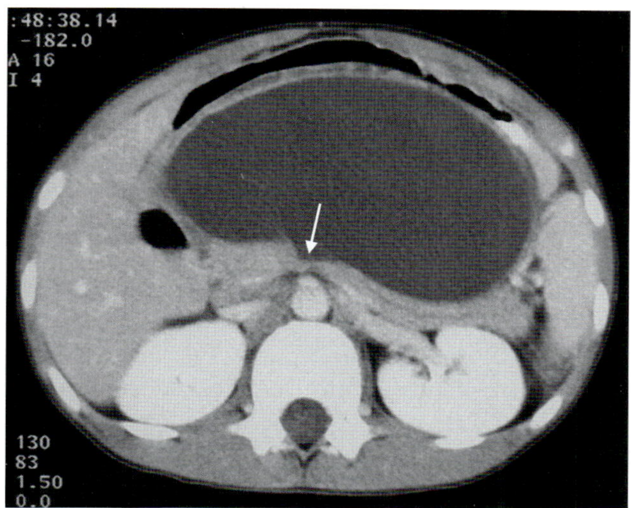

Fig. 3.18: Axial CECT scan at level of pancreas shows a large pseudocyst anterior to pancreas with a beak shape extension (arrow) in the neck of pancreas representing partial transection of pancreas

fluid in the peripancreatic fat, around the SMA, in the transverse mesocolon and lesser peritoneal sac, fluid separating pancreas from the splenic vein, and thickening of left anterior renal fascia. In a patient with suspected pancreatic injury in whom the initial CT scan shows a normal pancreas, a follow-up thin section CT scan within 24-48 hours of injury may show an injury not evident initially.

It is important to assess injury to main pancreatic duct because it usually requires surgical intervention or Endoscopic Retrograde cholangiopancreatography (ERCP) guided stent placement. CT is relatively insensitive in detecting this. In the clinical setting of a high index of suspicion of pancreatic ductal injury corroborated by elevated amylase and lipase, CT findings of a deep laceration or isolated peripancreatic fluid should suggest ductal injury and is an indication for surgical exploration. In doubtful cases, MRCP may be done to evaluate pancreatic ductal injury.[1,18] Endoscopic retrograde cholangiopancreatography (ERCP) may also be needed for confirmation purpose but its role is mainly limited for pancreatic ductal stenting for treatment of ductal injury.

Major complications can result following pancreatic trauma, e.g. pancreatic fistula, intra-abdominal abscess, pseudocyst formation (Fig. 3.18), hemorrhage, acute recurrent pancreatitis etc.

URINARY TRACT

Urinary tract injuries are outside the purview of this book and would be described in detail in a forthcoming book in this series on 'Urogenital Imaging'.

ADRENAL

With the advent of CT, adrenal injuries are now recognized as the most common retroperitoneal injury. It is usually associated with injury to other organs specially liver and kidneys. Adrenal hemorrhage due to trauma is unilateral in more than 90% of cases and usually the right adrenal gland is involved. The mechanism of injury may be compression of the adrenal gland between the liver and spine. On CT, adrenal hematoma appears as round to oval homogeneous density mass (40-75 HU) that replaces all or a portion of the normal adrenal gland (Figs 3.19A and B and 3.20). In addition there may be stranding of the

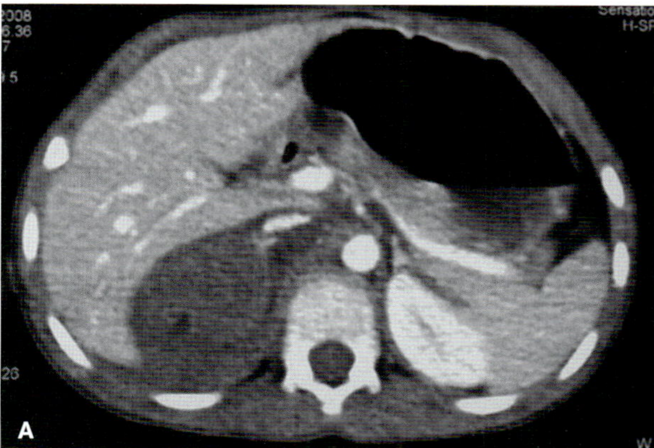

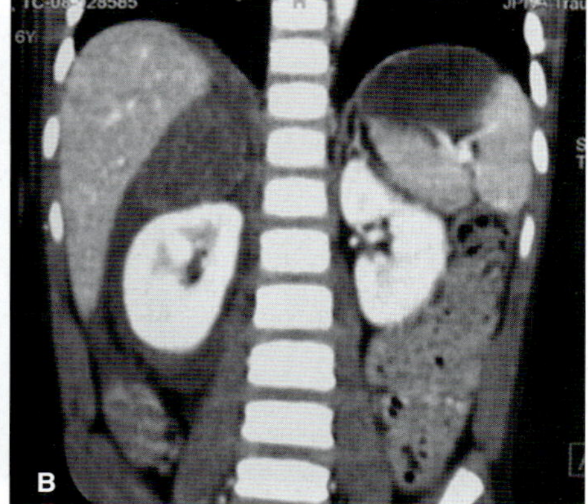

Figs. 3.19A and B: Axial (A) and coronal reformat (B) CECT scans show a right adrenal hematoma

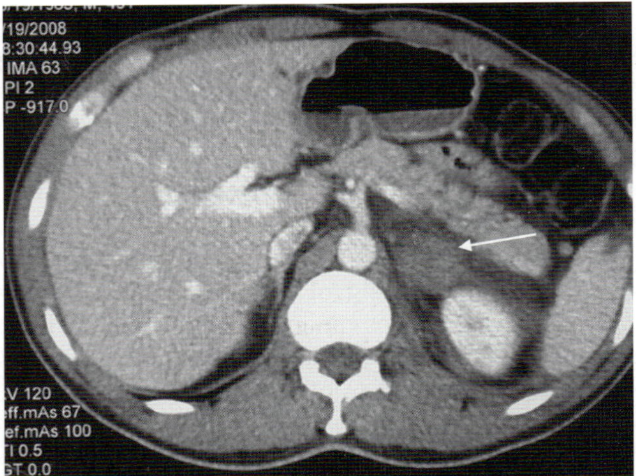

Fig. 3.20: Axial CECT scan shows a left adrenal hematoma (arrow)

peri-adrenal fat that extends to the upper pole of the kidney and apparent thickening of the ipsilateral diaphragmatic crus due to adjacent hemorrhage. A post-traumatic cyst or calcification may be seen as a sequel on long-term follow-up. Adrenal hemorrhage is of little clinical significance, particularly when it is unilateral.[19] Rarely bilateral adrenal hemorrhage has been shown to precipitate adrenal insufficiency.[20]

HOLLOW VISCUS, OMENTAL AND MESENTERIC INJURY

The diagnosis of intestinal injury is one of the most difficult and controversial aspects of trauma care. The symptoms may be delayed for many hours. If not surgically repaired it may lead to bleeding and leakage of gastrointestinal contents into the peritoneal cavity or retroperitoneum, leading to peritonitis or sepsis. The plain radiographs of the abdomen are relatively insensitive in detecting bowel injury. Rupture of a hollow viscus may produce free air either in the peritoneal cavity or retroperitoneum. Additional findings of free intraperitoneal fluid may be seen. Contrast studies employing water soluble contrast media are useful in detecting perforation and intraluminal obstruction in stable patients. MDCT is the diagnostic modality of choice for detection of bowel and mesenteric injuries and has been shown to be more sensitive and specific than clinical examination, diagnostic peritoneal lavage and abdominal ultrasound. The signs of bowel injury are frequently subtle. The most specific signs of bowel injury are:[21]

- Pneumoperitoneum or pneumo-retroperitoneum
- Extravasation of oral contrast material
- Low attenuation fluid between loops
- Bowel wall discontinuity (Figs 3.21A to C).

The presence of these signs usually mandate urgent laparotomy. All the above signs, though highly specific, are not as sensitive. Also care must be taken to exclude other causes of extraluminal contrast (bladder injury) and extraluminal air (mechanical ventilation, pneumothorax, chest injury, peritoneal lavage prior to CT, foley's catheter in a intraperitoneal bladder rupture). Retroperitoneal air tends to localize near the site of injury, often accompanied by fluid, either blood or intestinal.[22]

Less specific signs of bowel injury include:

- Peritoneal fluid without a known cause,
- Focal bowel wall thickening greater than 3 mm
- Mesenteric infiltration, thickening or hematoma abnormal bowel wall enhancement (Figs 3.22A and B)

Patients manifesting these signs may have bowel perforation requiring surgery, a less severe bowel contusion

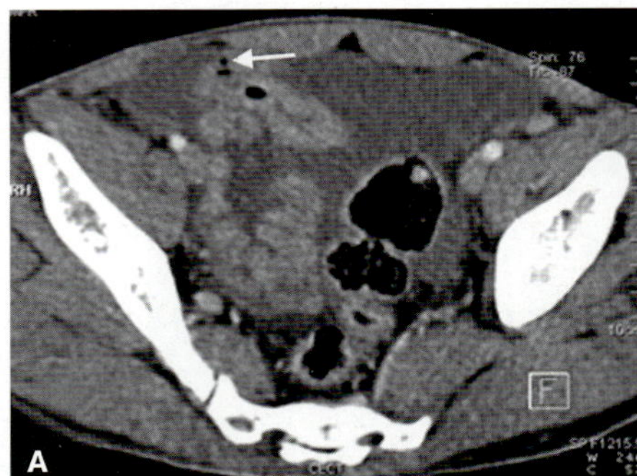

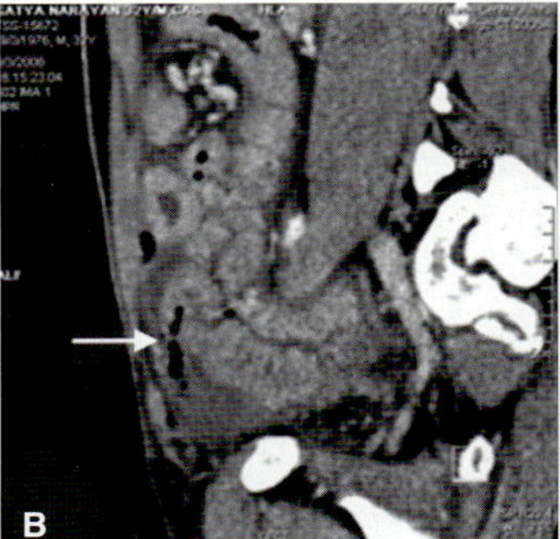

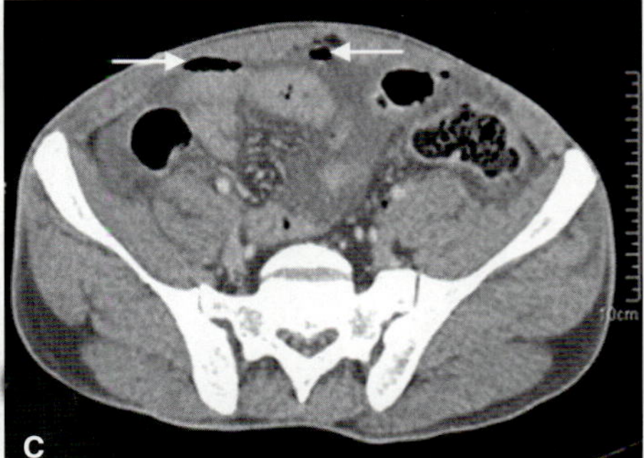

Figs 3.21A to C: Axial (A) and sagittal reformat (B) images of CECT shows a focal defect in wall of ileum (arrows) with air extending outside bowel lumen. An axial section at a different level with changed window settings shows the presence of pneumoperitoneum (arrows)

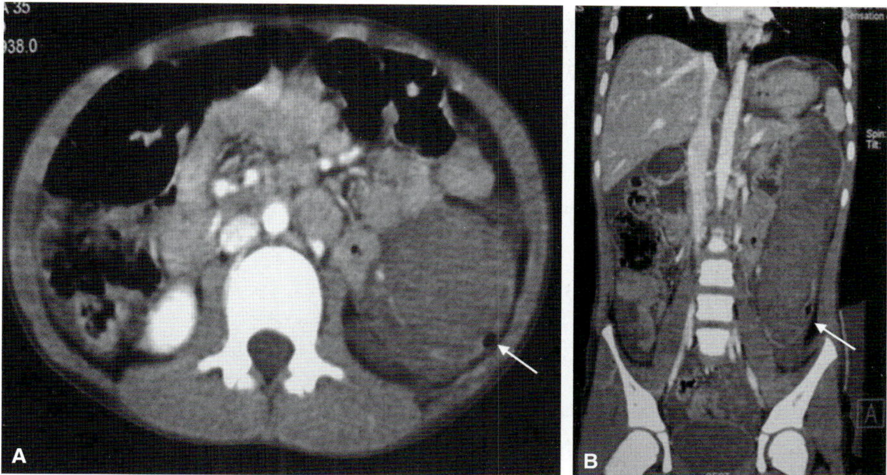

Figs 3.22A and B: Axial (A) and coronal reformat (B) CECT scans of abdomen show entire descending colon distended with hyperdense contents representing hematoma with thinned out abnormally enhancing walls and air within the wall (arrow in A,B) suggesting colonic injury

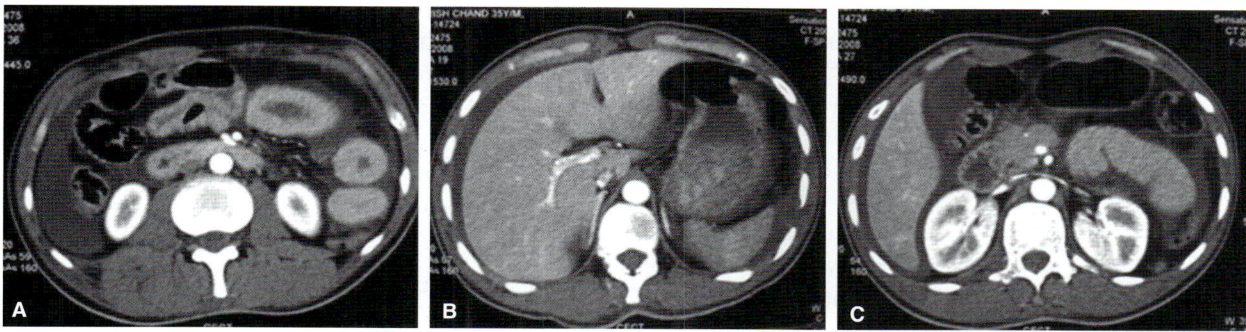

Figs 3.23A to C: Hypoperfusion state (shock bowel). Axial CECT scan through mid abdomen (A) shows diffuse thickening and hyperenhancement of jejunal loops. Note the presence of hemoperitoneum. Axial scan through adrenals (B) show hyperenhancing bilateral adrenal glands. Axial scan through kidneys (C) show flat IVC (arrow)

or hematoma that may be managed without surgery or no bowel injury at all. It must be remembered that diffuse bowel wall thickening may also be noted in fluid overload or in hypoperfusion state (shock bowel) (Figs 3.23A to C) wherein it would have accompanying features of increased wall enhancement, flat IVC, increased adrenal enhancement and pancreatic and retroperitoneal edema.[23] Abnormal pattern of bowel wall enhancement may be increased enhancement as in hypoperfusion state (due to increased vascular permeability with interstitial leakage of contrast), patchy and irregular enhancement due to wall injury or decreased or absent enhancement due to ischemia.

Blunt injuries to the stomach are uncommon. The second and third parts of duodenum are most frequently injured portion of small bowel. Duodenal hematoma has a characteristic appearance on CT scan. In the absence of duodenal perforation focal thickening or high attenuating mass in the duodenal wall, possibly associated with retroperitoneal fluid, is suggestive of intramural hematoma. With opacification of the bowel by oral contrast, the low density hematoma stands out clearly. Blunt injuries of the small intestine are most commonly seen at the points of fixation (ligament of Treitz and terminal ileum) but may occur anywhere along the length of the small intestine. Blunt colonic injuries are rare.

The mesentery and omentum are most often associated with injuries elsewhere in the abdomen and pelvis. Avulsion of the superior mesenteric artery and vein occurs most commonly near their origin, because of shearing effect. Massive hemorrhage can result from rupture or tear of these vessels. Vascular thrombosis and occlusion by an

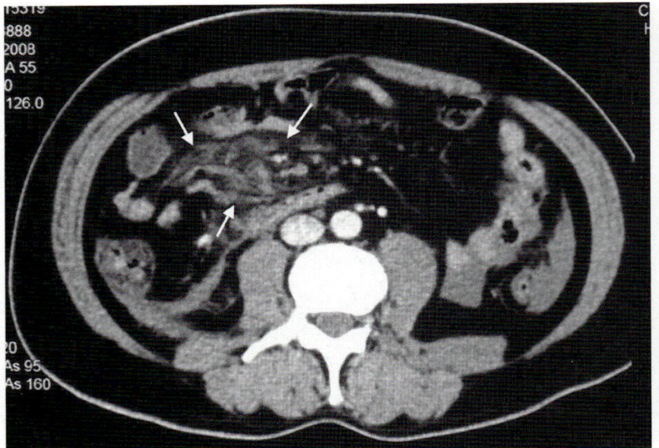

Fig. 3.24: Axial CECT scan through lower abdomen shows infiltration and hematoma (arrows) in mesentric root representing mesentric injury

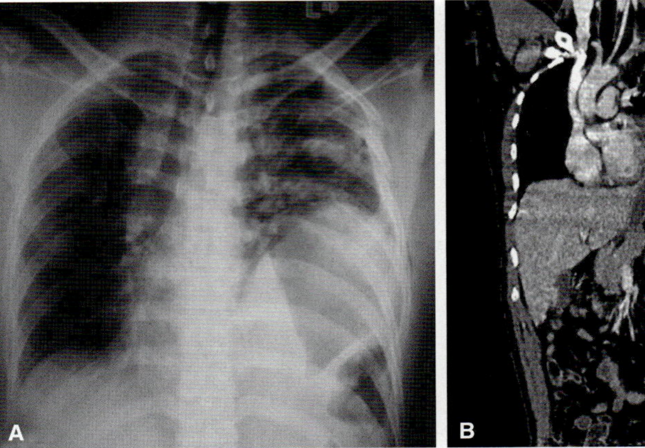

Figs 3.25A and B: Chest radiograph PA view (A) shows opacity in left lower zone with smooth convex upper margin and air lucencies within. Coronal reformatted CECT image (B) shows clearly the diaphragmatic defect (arrow) with stomach herniating through it into the thorax

intimal flap may also result from trauma. CT scan can be used to determine the extent and location of mesenteric injury. Specific CT features of mesenteric vascular injury include active contrast extravasation, beaded appearance of mesenteric vessels and abrupt termination of mesenteric vessels.[21] Other relatively non-specific findings include mesenteric hematoma (Fig. 3.24), mesenteric infiltration, bowel wall thickening and abnormal wall enhancement secondary to ischemia, increased fluid within the bowel lumen, intraperitoneal blood and pneumatosis intestinalis, etc. It must be remembered that some of these signs may also be seen in bowel injury alone without concomitant mesenteric injury.

DIAPHRAGM

Diaphragmatic rupture and subsequent herniation of abdominal contents into thorax is nine times more common on left side than right due to the protective effect of the liver.[24] On the right side most injuries to the diaphragm go unrecognized during the acute phase. In the interval phase, the abdominal viscus may not have herniated or the patient may have acclimatised to the presence of abdominal contents in the thorax. In the later phase, obstruction or strangulation presents with severe abdominal or chest pain. The injury may also be evident at a later stage in those patients who were earlier on positive pressure ventilation and have now been extubated. Chest radiograph may reveal non-specific findings that include an indistinct or elevated hemidiaphragm (Fig. 3.25A), pleural effusion, atelectasis with shift of the mediastinum to the contralateral side, hemothorax, pneumothorax or lower rib fractures. Specific findings are visualization of bowel loops or solid masses above the diaphragm and loss of the normal diaphragmatic contour. Detection of a nasogastric tube above the left hemidiaphragm is also a strong indicator. Contrast studies (barium meal or enema) can be used to clearly delineate the herniation.

The advent of MDCT with multiplanar reconstructions has significantly improved the sensitivity of CT in detecting diaphragmatic injuries. The various CT signs of diaphragmatic rupture include focal diaphragmatic discontinuity or elevation, focal diaphragmatic thickening (retraction), herniated abdominal contents into thorax, 'collar' sign – narrowed waist of a herniated intra-abdominal organ due to compression at the neck (diaphragm tear) and the 'dependent viscera' sign – herniated intrabdominal contents abutting the posterior thoracic wall (Fig. 3.25B). The 'dependent viscera' sign and the 'collar' signs are reported to be 100% specific.[1] CT is unreliable in diagnosing diaphragmatic tears before herniation. MRI also has been reported to be highly sensitive in detecting diaphragmatic rupture.[25]

RETROPERITONEUM

The most frequently injured retroperitoneal structures include the adrenals, pancreas, great vessels , gastro-intestinal tract, genitourinary tract and musculoskeletal system[26] Inability to account for blood loss either in the chest or abdomen in a patient with ongoing transfusion requirements should dictate angiographic investigation. The potential for simultaneous angiographic embolization of actively bleeding vessels is well documented and may be life saving since opening the retroperitoneum to control bleeding is associated with high mortality.

ABDOMINAL WALL INJURY

Abdominal wall injuries are easily overlooked if not specifically seen. Most common are bruises, which appear on CT as skin thickening and soft tissue infiltration of subcutaneous fat. Intramuscular hematomas may be seen (Fig. 3.26). Tearing of lateral abdominal wall or rectus abdominis is an unusual occurrence that results in subcutaneous hematoma and occasionally bowel herniation.[27]

PENETRATING ABDOMINAL TRAUMA

Traditionally, almost all stab and gun shot wounds to the abdomen have required surgical exploration. With increasing interest in non-operative management of penetrating injuries, CT has become important in evaluating extent of injury in selected hemodynamically stable patients to identify solid organ laceration, bowel perforation, retroperitoneal hematoma, and hemoperitoneum. It is often difficult to detect small perforations of the bowel that result in only small amounts of peritoneal fluid on CT. In contrast to stab wounds, gun shot wounds are potentially complex injuries and depend upon the type of weapon, distance between the weapon and victim amongst others. CT is directly able to demonstrate the path of the bullet.[28]

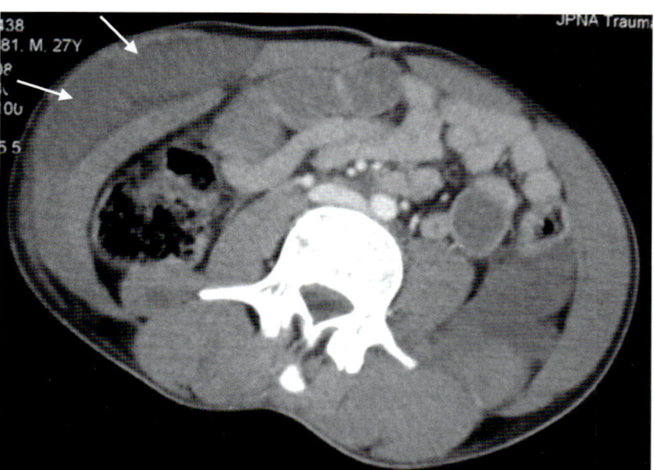

Fig. 3.26: Axial CECT scan through mid abdomen shows a large abdominal wall hematoma (arrows)

CONCLUSION

Diagnostic imaging technology has evolved considerably during the past decade and CT scanning in particular has increased the sensitivity and specificity of imaging in abdominal trauma. Currently, CT is universally accepted as a valuable tool for evaluating hemodynamically stable patients. The value of CT in diagnosis of abdominal injuries can be optimized by using the state of art MDCT scanners, maintaining adequate patient physiologic support and monitoring devices within the CT suite, using appropriate oral and intravenous contrast, paying careful attention to CT scanning technique and timely interpretation of CT images. However, CT must be considered as an adjunct to the clinical evaluation of the patient, which remains the most important criteria for guiding the management of the patient with abdominal trauma.

REFERENCES

1. Stanescu AL, Gross JA, Bittle M, Mann FA. Imaging of blunt abdominal trauma. Semin Roentgen 2006;41(3):196-204.
2. Anderson CB, Ballinger WF. Abdominal injuries. In Zuidema GD, Rutherford RB, Wallinger WF (Eds): The Management of trauma. Saunders, Philadelphia, 1985.
3. McClellan BA, Hanna SS, Montoya DR, et al. Analysis of peritoneal lavage parameters in blunt abdominal trauma. J Trauma 1985;25:393.
4. http://www.acr.org/SecondaryMainMenuCategories/quality_safety/app_criteria/pdf/Vascular/Blunt AbdominalTrauma.aspx.
5. Korner M, Krotz M, Degenhart C, Pfeifer KJ, Reiser MF, Linsenmaier U. Current role of emergency US in patients with major trauma. Radiographics 2008;28:225-44.
6. Alavi A. Detection of gastrointestinal bleeding with 99mTc sulphur colloid. Semin Nucl Med 1982;12:126-38.
7. Livingston DH, Lavery RF, Passannante MR, et al. Admission or observation is not necessary after a negative abdominal CT scan in patients with suspected blunt abdominal trauma: Result of prospective multi institutional trial. J Trauma 1998;44(2):273-82.
8. Stuhlfaut JW, Lucey BC, Varghese JC, Soto JA. Blunt abdominal trauma: Utility of 5-minute delayed CT with a reduced radiation dose. Radiology 2006;238(2):473-9.
9. Raptopoulos V. Abdominal trauma-emphasis on computed tomography. RCNA 1994;32:969-87.
10. Jeffrey RB Jr. Cross sectional imaging of the acute abdomen: Overview of philosophy and technique. In Jeffrey RB Jr, Ralls PW (Eds): CT and Sonography of Acute Abdomen. Lippincot-Raven, Philadelphia 1996;1-16.

11. Kane NM, Francis IR, Burney RE, et al. Traumatic pneumoperitoneum: Implications of CT diagnosis. Invest Radiol 1991;26(6):574-8.
12. Levine CD, Patel UJ, Silverman PM, et al. Low attenuation of acute traumatic haemoperitoneum on CT scans. AJR 1996;166(5):1089-93.
13. Moore EE, Cogbill TH, Jurkovich GJ, et al. Organ injury scaling: Spleen and liver (1994 revision). J Trauma 1995;38:323-4.
14. Marmery H, Shanmuganathan K, Alexander M, Mirvis S. Optimisation of selection for nonoperative management of blunt splenic injury: Comparison of MDCT grading systems. AJR 2007;189:1421-7.
15. Foley WSD, Cates JD, Kellman GM, et al. Treatment of blunt hepatic injuries: Role of CT. Radiology 1987;164: 635-8.
16. Willmann JK, Roos JE, Platz A, et al. Multidetector CT: detection of active hemorrhage in patients with blunt abdominal trauma. AJR 2006;179:437-44.
17. Yoon W, Jeong YY, Kim JK, Seo JJ, Lim HS, Shin SS, et al. CT in blunt liver trauma. Radiogrpahics 2005;25:87-104.
18. Stuhlfaut JW, Anderson SW, Soto JA. Blunt abdominal trauma: Current imaging techniques and CT findings in patients with solid organ, bowel, and mesenteric injury. Semin US, CT and MRI 2007;28:115-129.
19. Burks DW, Mirvis SE, Shanmuganathan K. Acute adrenal injury after blunt abdominal trauma: CT findings. AJR 1992;158(3):503-7.
20. Francque SM, Schwagten VM, Ysebaert DK, et al. Bilateral adrenal haemorrhage and acute adrenal insufficiency in a blunt abdominal trauma: A case-report and literature review. Eur J Emerg Med 2004;11:164-7
21. Brofman N, Atri M, Epid D, Hanson JM, Grinblat L, Chughtai T, Brenneman F. Evaluation of bowel and mesenteric blunt trauma with multidetector CT. Radiographics 2006;26:1119-26.
22. Rody JM, Leighton DB, Murphy BL, et al. CT of blunt trauma bowel and mesenteric injury: Hybrid findings and pitfalls. Radiographics 2000;20(6):1525-36.
23. Mirvis SE, Shanmuganathan K, Erb R. Diffuse small-bowel ischemia in hypotensive adults after blunt trauma (shock bowel): CT findings and clinical significance. AJR 1994;163:1375-79.
24. Heiberg E, Wolverson MK, Hud RN, et al. CT recognition of traumatic rupture of the diaphragm. AJR 1980;135:369-72.
25. Barbiera F, Nicastro N, Finazzo M, et al. The role of MRI in traumatic rupture of the diaphragm. Our experience in three cases and review of the literature. Radiol Med 2003;105(3):188-94.
26. Weil PH. Management of retroperitoneal trauma. Curr Prob Surg 1984;20:545.
27. Hill SA, Jackson MA, Fitz Gerald. Abdominal well haematoma mimicking visceral injury: The role of CT scanning. Injury 1995;26(9):605-7.
28. Easter DW, Shackford SR, Mattrey RF. A prospective randomized comparison of CT with conventional diagnostic methods in the evaluation of penetrating injuries to the back and flank. Arch Surg 1991;126(9): 1115-9.

Chapter Four

Imaging of the Esophagus

Sumedha Pawa

INTRODUCTION

A wide variety of disorders can affect the oesophagus. Difficulty in swallowing is a common manifestation of most of these disorders. Dysphagia is defined as the subjective awareness of swallowing difficulty during passage of a solid or liquid bolus from the mouth to the stomach.[1] It may be due to a motor disorder or to a lesion affecting the oropharynx or oesophageal lumen.[2]

In general, motor disturbances produce episodic dysphagia, which either does not progress or progresses slowly. Liquids are as difficult to swallow as solid foods. In contrast, structural lesions, which are more common than motor disturbances, produce relentless dysphagia that is initially worse with solid foods. As a lesion evolves, semisolids and liquids also become difficult to swallow.[2]

Pharyngeal and Esophageal Anatomy

The pharynx constitutes a musculomembranous tube approximately 12 cm long in adults. It is connected to the oral cavity by the pharyngeal inlet, which is open in the resting state, and to the oesophagus by the upper esophageal sphincter (UES) which is closed in the resting state.

The most cephalad segment is the nasopharynx, at and above the level of the soft palate. The most caudal segment is the laryngopharynx, or hypopharynx that extends from the level of the hyoid bone or pharyngo-epiglottic folds down to the cricopharyngeus muscle, the UES. Interposed between these two segments is the oropharynx.

The esophagus lies mainly in the posterior mediastinum and is 18-22 cm long in adults. It extends from the lower border of the horizontal fibers of cricopharyngeus at the level of C5-6 where the UES forms a 2.5 cm long high-pressure zone that separates the pharynx from the esophagus. The lowest 2-3 cm of the esophagus functions as the lower esophageal sphincter (LES).

The esophagus is composed of five layers: two muscle layers, submucosa, muscularis mucosae, and stratified squamous epithelium which changes abruptly at the cardia of the stomach into simple columnar epithelium. There is no serosal layer.[3]

The pharynx and the proximal 3-4 cm of esophageal body comprise of striated muscle. Distal to this, there is an intermingling of striated and smooth muscle and more distally, the esophageal body and the LES contain smooth muscle alone. Throughout its length, the esophagus has an outer longitudinal muscle layer and a thicker inner circular layer.

The abdominal esophagus is usually 3 cm or less in length and connects with the gastro-esophageal junction.

Physiology of Swallowing

Swallowing is a very complex activity that involves at least 37 paired striated muscles, six cranial nerves, C1,2 cervical nerves and supporting structures of the mandible, hyoid bone, cervical spine and skull. The cerebral cortex participates in the initiation of swallowing and it is a programmed medullary function.

The act of swallowing has been divided into four phases: (a) the preparatory phase of ingestion and bolus formation, (b) the oral phase, (c) the pharyngeal phase, and (d) the esophageal phase. In reality there is a continuous process which starts at the lips and tip of the tongue and ends at the gastric fundus.

a. Preparatory phase of swallowing includes the selection and placement of a bolus into the mouth. Solid or semisolid boluses are chewed and mixed with saliva while liquids are poured or sucked into the oral cavity and do not require much oral manipulation.
b. Oral phase of swallowing involves transfer of the bolus by the tongue to the oropharynx. Generally the bolus is held on the anterior tongue and pushed into the pharynx, a "tipper" type of swallow. The tongue holds the bolus in the anterior part of central groove and a combination of mandibular positioning and active tongue and soft palate contraction prevent anterior and lateral spill of the bolus. Spill from the back of the tongue is prevented by active contraction of the soft palate against the mid portion of the tongue.
c. During the pharyngeal phase of swallowing, the bolus passes through the pharynx without entering the nasopharynx or laryngeal vestibule. Pharyngeal and laryngeal elevation as a unit participates in laryngeal vestibule closure, epiglottic tilt, bolus transport, and UES opening. The bolus transport is accomplished by a combination of gravity, posterior push of the tongue, pharyngeal elevation over the bolus and sequential contraction of the constrictor muscles of the pharynx.
d. Primary esophageal peristalsis is induced by a swallow at the pharyngoesophageal junction. Caudad progression of a bolus is achieved by a wave of inhibition preceding the bolus and a wave of contraction behind it. This is seen radiographically as a V-shaped stripping wave. Normally, all of a liquid bolus is stripped, but some proximal escape may be seen at the level of the aortic arch even in normal individuals, which is then cleared by secondary peristalsis. The LES segment is 3-4 cm in length and is an area of high resting pressure which aids in the prevention of gastroesophageal reflux. The high resting pressure falls prior to the arrival of a bolus to allow its passage. Secondary peristalsis is induced by esophageal distension and initiates around the level of the aortic arch. It is a propulsive wave that occurs to clear the esophagus of any retained bolus.

Tertiary contractions are non-propulsive and cause a variable degree of narrowing of the lumen.

Between swallows, the esophagus is collapsed and the upper and lower esophageal sphincters are closed.

Clinical Perspective

Abnormality of the oral phase of swallowing results in food dribbling from the mouth, difficulty in drinking or chewing, or difficulty in initiating a swallow. Soft palate insufficiency results in a nasal quality of voice or nasal regurgitation. Coughing or choking during swallowing indicates laryngeal penetration.

Patients with pharyngeal dysphagia typically complain of a "lump in the throat" or of food "sticking in the throat" during swallowing. It may be caused by a functional abnormality such as cricopharyngeal dysmotility, amyotropic lateral sclerosis or by a morphologic abnormality such as Zenker diverticulum or pharyngeal tumor.

A sensation of blockage at the level of the suprasternal notch or thoracic inlet raises the possibility of a cervical esophageal web or tumor or of extrinsic compression of the cervical or upper thoracic esophagus by an enlarged thyroid, mediastinal lymphadenopathy, or other mass lesion.

Substernal localization of dysphagia is usually due to a structural disorder such as reflux esophagitis, peptic stricture or Schatzki ring or to a motility disorder of the esophagus such as achalasia. A distal lesion (even carcinoma of the gastric fundus) may refer dysphagia proximally as far as the pharynx.

The patient may complain of odynophagia (pain on swallowing) or chest pain. These symptoms may be due to esophageal spasm or other motor disorders but may also be caused by infectious esophagitis, gastroesophageal reflux disease and ulcerated pharyngeal or esophageal tumors.

Investigation of Dysphagia

A range of investigative modalities are available including radiology, pharyngolaryngoscopy, manometry, and scintigraphy.[4] Endoscopy and radiology are complimentary investigations but a contrast swallow is the investigation of first choice since it allows dynamic study of neuromuscular function, as well as the detection of structural abnormalities in the pharyngoesophageal segment. Barium studies may demonstrate lesions involving the valleculae, tongue base, lower hypopharynx and pharyngoesophageal segment that are difficult to visualize at endoscopy. Barium studies may also demonstrate diverticula that are difficult to circumvent safely at endoscopy. In addition, mild strictures and Schatzki ring can be overlooked by modern thin-calibre fiberscopes.[5,6] Radiographic studies are often able to define the length of an endoscopically impassable stenosing lesion and to provide information about extrinsic compression. Endoscopy is usually required for biopsy of radiologically demonstrated lesions and for radiologically negative dysphagia.[4]

Examination Technique

The patient is instructed to fast overnight before the examination. Although scout films are not obtained routinely, frontal and lateral plain films of the neck and chest may be helpful in cases of suspected foreign body, abscess, or fistula formation, and in the postoperative patient. The plain film may show fluid levels in the esophagus in a patient with achalasia. In major esophageal dilatation, the esophagus expands to the right, producing a mediastinal edge that runs from the neck to the diaphragm with a single indentation produced by the azygos vein (Fig. 4.1A).

Barium Studies

Examination of the pharynx and esophagus requires a dynamic evaluation of motility as well as double-contrast spot films to detect morphologic abnormalities. Cineradiography or videofluoroscopy should be used to study swallowing dynamics.

The purpose of the study is to define any structural abnormality, to demonstrate abnormal timing and abnormal structural movement, and to test the effect of maneuvers.

Videofluoroscopy allows an in depth examination of the cause of aspiration, and what remedial action, such as modification of posture or food consistency, will help. The recordings may be reviewed later to analyze tongue movement, soft palate elevation, epiglottic tilt, laryngeal closure, cricopharyngeal opening and pharyngeal peristalsis.[7,8]

Radiographically, hyoid elevation is best seen on the lateral view. Both frontal and lateral views demonstrate elevation, shortening and increased width of the pharynx. Epiglottic tilt is a very important component of laryngeal protection as the epiglottis diverts the bolus into the lateral swallowing channels of the hypopharynx. It is best seen on the lateral view while early tilt is seen as widening of the valleculae and broadening of the median glossoepiglottic fold.

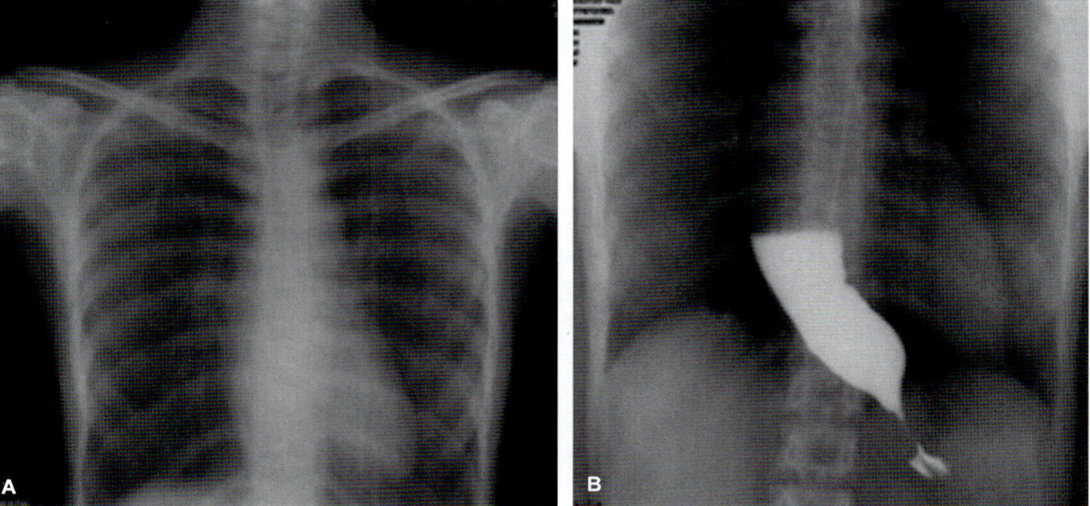

Figs 4.1A and B: (A) Chest PA showing right paracardiac shadow extending till the diaphragm due to dilated esophagus in a case of achalasia, (B) Barium swallow shows dilated esophagus with an air barium level, and a characteristic beak-like tapering of the distal esophagus—achalasia

Double-contrast spot films are then taken which extend from the superior surface of the soft palate at the top to the cricopharyngeus below in the lateral position. The pharynx is then examined in the frontal projection. This is the best view to show the surface of the tongue base enface and the contours of the tonsillar fossae, valleculae and lateral walls of the hypopharynx in profile. Oblique views are of value in assessing lesions of the aryepiglottic folds, valleculae, postcricoid region and upper cervical esophagus. An oblique view taken through the shoulders during swallowing may be necessary to visualize the region of cricopharyngeus.

The routine barium examination of the esophagus should be a biphasic study combining upright double contrast and prone single contrast techniques. In the double-contrast phase the aim is to achieve adequate gaseous distension of the lumen with a thin layer of high density barium coating the mucosa. Gaseous distension is improved by the patient swallowing effervescent agents. Rapid drinking causes air swallowing and thus esophageal distension. In addition it interrupts the esophageal peristalsis, thus resulting in esophageal hypotonia.

The effervescent agent may be omitted in patients with suspected esophageal infections or obstructing lesions (because it is painful and may cause artifacts).

All patients with a suspicion of esophageal dysfunction or defective transportation through the oesophagus should be examined in a recumbent position.[9]

Esophageal motility is evaluated with the patient swallowing a single mouthful of low density barium. Another swallow of barium should not be taken until after 20 seconds because this duration is the approximate refractory period of esophageal peristalsis. In suspected esophageal motility disorder, at least 5 swallows should be observed. This is followed by continuous drinking that optimally distends the esophagus. Prone views of the upper esophagus best show esophageal webs and aortic arch anomalies. Barium filled views of the distal oesophagus are important for the detection of hiatal hernias, strictures, webs or rings (Fig. 4.2) as these may not be visible in the erect double contrast phase.

Provocative testing in an attempt to reproduce symptoms may be useful in a patient with solid-food dysphagia who has a normal study with liquid barium. A barium-impregnated solid bolus may hold up at a subtle stricture or induce spasm not seen with liquid bolus.

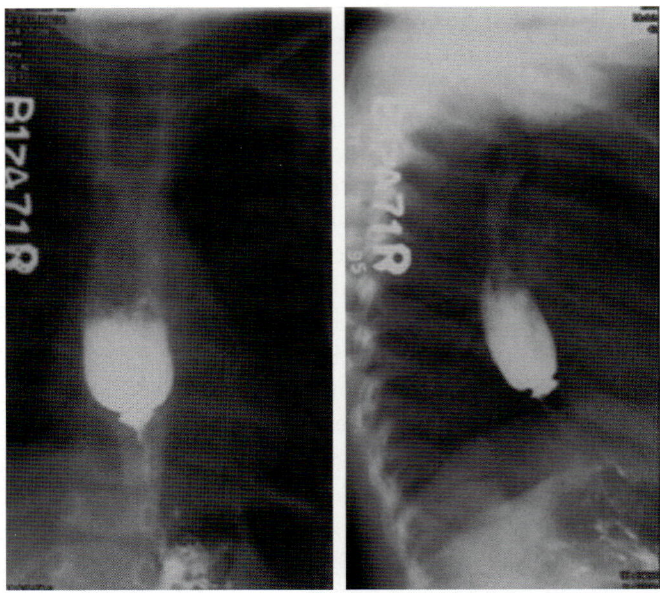

Fig. 4.2: Congenital ring in the distal esophagus causing hold up of barium, confirmed at endoscopy

Cross-sectional Studies

Imaging of the esophagus is challenging because the esophagus is a long tube, and poorly distansible, with a close relationship to many vital organs.[10]

Pharynx

Although the mucosal detail of the pharynx is studied best with barium contrast, the extraluminal anatomy is demonstrated in detail by CT, MRI and sonography. Axial techniques are therefore most useful as an adjunct to barium studies, particularly for tumor staging and the delineation of central and peripheral nervous system lesions producing pharyngeal dysfunction.

Esophagus

The apparent thickness of the esophageal wall at CT varies according to the degree of distension. A value of 5 mm, rather than 3 mm was found to be an appropriate maximum normal value for esophageal wall thickness.[11]

At T1–weighted imaging, the esophagus appears as a structure of low signal intensity, contrasted by fat of high signal intensity, while T2–weighted imaging indicates that its muscular wall, which shows moderate enhancement after the injection of intravenous Gd-DTPA, is of low intensity.[3]

CT provides considerable information on the intramural and extramural extent of esophageal malignancy and is also an indispensable part of the planning for radiation therapy. CT and MRI have been used to stage esophageal carcinoma, because these techniques can reveal extraesophageal extension into adjacent mediastinal structures, including the trachea, bronchi, aorta, and pericardium, and can detect lymphadenopathy in the mediastinum.[12] For assessing unresectability CT and MR have comparable accuracy when using criteria such as tracheobronchial invasion and aortic invasion, whereas CT appears more sensitive for detecting lymphadenopathy, particularly in the mediastinum. An advantage of MR is direct imaging in the coronal and sagittal planes which is useful for demonstrating the extent of disease.[13]

The ability of multi-detector computed tomography to cover a large volume in a very short scan time, and in a single breath hold with thin collimation and isotropic voxels, allows the imaging of the entire esophagus with high-quality multiplanar reformation and 3D reconstruction. Proper distension of the esophagus and stomach (by oral administration of effervescent granules and water) and optimally timed administration of intravenous contrast material are required to detect and characterize disease. Preoperative staging of oesophageal carcinoma appears to be the main indication for MDCT. In addition, MDCT allows detection of other esophageal malignancies and benign esophageal tumors. A diagnosis of rupture or fistula of the esophagus can be firmly established using MDCT. Other esophageal conditions such as achalasia, esophagitis, diverticula, and varices, can also be visualized with hydri-multi-detector CT. It is a valuable tool for esophageal wall disease and serves as an adjunct to endoscopy.[10]

Endoscopic Ultrasound

The prime purpose of imaging in cases of esophageal carcinoma is to stage the tumor by determining the depth and site of invasion, as well as longitudinal spread of tumor and to identify lymph node metastases. The depth of tumor infiltration into the esophageal wall can best be evaluated by EUS, which can directly visualize all layers of the esophageal wall.

On EUS, tumor is usually seen as poorly reflective tissue. Assessment of the extent to which this tissue is confined to an ultrasonographic layer is fairly reliable and in particular breaching of muscularis propria is well seen. The new TNM staging of esophageal tumor depends on the depth of invasion of local disease; this can only be performed with EUS.[14]

It has superior ability to determine the depth of tumor infiltration (T stage) and assess regional lymphadenopathy.[15] Small catheters containing 20 mHz transducers have recently become available for high resolution endoluminal ultrasound.[16] Miniprobe sonography has been found to be superior to spiral CT or MRI for T staging, especially in early esophageal cancer.[17] CT and MRI cannot definitively demonstrate the individual layers of the esophageal wall, therefore T1 and T2 tumors cannot be differentiated.[18]

In a prospective study in suspected early cancer in Barrett's esophagus, EUS was superior to CT for T staging and N staging. CT did not add any information relevant to the TNM classification that was in addition to that provided by EUS and abdominal ultrasonography in these patients.[19] By contrast, EUS is required in order to differentiate between patients with cancer in Barrett's esophagus in whom endoscopic therapy is suitable and those in whom surgical treatment is required.

Endoscopic ultrasound has also been shown to be helpful in diagnosing tumor recurrence at anastomoses in patients treated for esophageal carcinoma. Endoscopy in this situation is frequently negative as recurrence is submucosal or nodal. EUS has also been shown to be effective in staging tumors at the gastroesophageal junction.

Others Techniques for Evaluation of Esophagus

Videoendoscopic Swallowing Study

The key abnormalities best detected by endoscopic evaluation are of palatal function, vocal fold mobility and closure, degree and location of post-swallow residue, and pharyngeal and laryngeal sensation.[20]

Esophageal Scintigraphy

Radionuclide Esophageal transit studies allow safe, rapid, noninvasive and therefore, well-tolerated assessment of Esophageal transit time and function, using liquids and solids of a physiologic nature. It has well-established normal ranges and compares favorably with manometry in the investigation of dysmotility and other disease states. In addition it can provide quantifiable information that can be measured serially to assess response to treatment.[21]

In a study comparing esophagography and esophageal transit scintigraphy (ETS) in the evaluation of usefulness of Endoscopic Pneumatic Dilatation in Achalasia, the results showed, that even in patients with similar esophageal morphologies on esophagography, there was prominent variability in ETS. Therefore, barium esophagography was necessary for the evaluation of morphology, caliber of the esophagogastric channel, and post treatment complications, while ETS was necessary for the functional evaluation of esophageal emptying.[22]

Esophageal Manometry

Esophageal manometry remains the investigation of choice in suspected motility disorders.[23] Manometry can classify esophageal dysmotility into rare specific disorders such as achalasia and diffuse esophageal spasm or more common non-specific motility disorders.

Ambulatory pH Monitoring

Twenty four hour pH monitoring in the oesophagus remains the gold standard when reflux is a possible cause of dysphagia.[24] It is useful in patients with atypical symptoms or who have failed trials of antireflux treatment.[25]

Oropharyngeal Lesions

Neuromuscular Disease

Dysphagia may be the predominant symptom in a number of neuromuscular diseases. After a cerebrovascular accident, difficulty in feeding may result from peripheral weakness or paresis of the tongue, palate, or pharynx. A focal acute cerebrovascular accident in the brainstem may produce acute dysphagia with little or no other neurologic deficit.

It is seldom possible to diagnose specific diseases from the radiographically observed dysfunction, but we can often determine the pathophysiological mechanisms involved (Figs 4.3A and B). In motor neuron disease there is oropharyngeal muscle atrophy, pharyngeal paresis, nasopharyngeal regurgitation, airway penetration and compensatory extension of head and neck. In Parkinson's disease there is dysfunction of oral initiation, hesitancy and repetitive tongue movement, delayed swallow reflex, valleculae pooling and airway penetration. Aspiration may be silent. Pharyngeal muscle paresis and aspiration may occur in poliomyelitis (bulbar).

Myopathies may affect bulbar muscles. Striated muscles of cervical esophagus may also be affected with reduced peristalsis. Cricopharyngeal "chalasia" is seen in myotonic dystrophy.

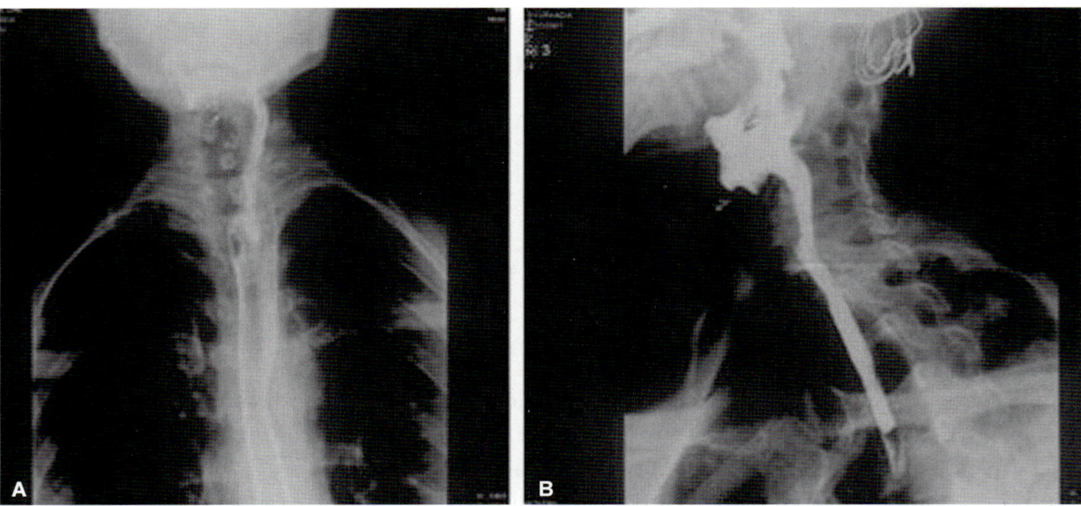

Figs 4.3A and B: Esophagogram shows barium outlining only the left side of the pharynx and cervical esophagus due to paralysis of left pharyngeal constrictor. The normal right pharyngeal constrictor is pushing the barium column to the left

Cricopharyngeal Prominence

The posterior indentation at approximately C5/6 level by cricopharyngeus muscle normally effaces as a bolus passes through. Mild persistent indentation may be normal but more obvious prominence may be seen in patients with gastroesophageal reflux or functional or mechanical esophageal obstruction. It is likely that acid reflux leads to edema, spasm and/or hypertrophy of cricopharyngeus.

Cricopharyngeal dysfunction or prominence may be seen as delayed opening, incomplete opening, or premature closure of the sphincter. Some of the barium is often trapped above the sphincter. This produces a "pseudodiverticulum" seen as a small barium collection in the lowermost hypopharynx just above the cricopharyngeal indentation. Extrinsic pharyngeal indentation caused by a cervical osteophyte may simulate cricopharyngeal prominence. Osteophytic impressions are fixed in position in relation to the spine, whereas cricopharyngeal indentations move with the pharynx and esophagus during swallowing.

Cricopharyngeal Webs

These mucosal folds occur on the anterior wall at the hypopharynx/esophagus junction. These are often thin and do not cause symptoms, but may be circumferential and cause luminal narrowing. (Figs 4.4A and B) Characteristic "jet effect" may be seen on contrast swallow when a large bolus passes through a web. Differentiation must be made between webs and the submucosal venous plexus which is a normal structure on anterior wall and causes an impression that is effaced as the bolus distends the lumen. At times webs are associated with iron-deficiency, glossitis and pharyngeal atrophy (Plummer-Vinson syndrome).

Pharyngeal Diverticula and Pouches

Zenker diverticulum is an acquired pulsion diverticulum herniating through Kilian dehiscence, an area of congenital weakness between the horizontal and oblique fibers of the cricopharyngeus muscle. It is seen on the lateral view as a bulge or true sac extending posteriorly from the posterior hypopharyngeal wall just above the cricopharyngeal impression. On the frontal view a Zenker diverticulum is seen as a barium-filled sac below the arcuate lines of the piriform sinuses. Dysphagia occurs as the diverticulum fills preferentially with food and obstructs the lumen of the esophagus. There is regurgitation of pouch contents and often, aspiration as it overflows. Zenker diverticulum is often associated with gastroesophageal reflux and hiatus hernia.

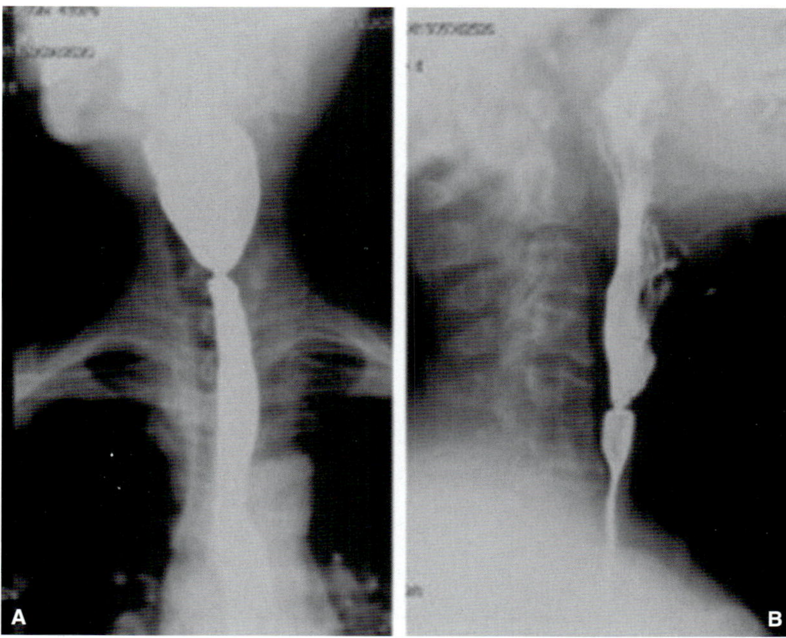

Figs 4.4A and B: Barium swallow shows well defined localized circumferential narrowing seen at the level of C5/C6 with minimal proximal dilatation – Cricopharyngeal web

Lateral pharyngeal pouches and diverticula are protrusions occurring through the thyrohyoid membrane between the hyoid bone and the thyroid cartilage. These are usually asymptomatic but may occasionally cause dysphagia or choking due to stasis and aspiration. Lateral pharyngeal pouches are seen as transient, wide-mouthed protrusions that fill during swallowing and empty during or after the swallow.

Lateral pharyngeal diverticula are persistent sacs with narrow necks and remain filled with barium after the swallow (Figs 4.5A and B). These pouches and diverticula are seen best on the frontal view because they protrude from the lateral pharyngeal walls. They may be seen on the lateral view, posterior to the valleculae along the anterior hypopharyngeal wall.

Killian-Jamieson diverticula or pouches are protrusions arising on the anterolateral wall of the proximal cervical oesophagus just below the level of the cricopharyngeus, arising in a region of anatomic weakness which is the site of passage of the inferior laryngeal nerve.

Pharyngeal Tumors

The majority of malignant pharyngeal tumors are squamous cell carcinomas. Small tumors may be seen as a nodular mucosal surface en face or as an irregular contour. Radiographic findings in large, advanced tumors include intraluminal mass, mucosal irregularity and asymmetric distensibility. An intra-luminal mass may be seen as an abnormal luminal contour, abnormally located extra barium-coated lines, a focal area of increased radiodensity, or a filling defect in the barium pool. Mucosal irregularity is recognized by abnormal barium collections due to ulceration or by a nonuniform nodular surface pattern. Asymmetric distensibility may be due to an infiltrating tumor or extrinsic mass.

The value of double-contrast pharyngography in patients with a known carcinoma is to determine the size, extent and inferior limit of the pharyngeal tumor and the degree of functional impairment. Pharyngoesophagograms are also useful for detecting separate co-existing carcinomas of the pharynx and esophagus. Extraluminal extent of the tumor (e.g. invasion of the preepiglottic space or cartilage destruction) and lymphadenopathy are best assessed by CT and MR imaging.

Pharyngeal Foreign Bodies

A lateral radiograph of the neck taken at soft tissue exposure may show a radioopaque foreign body, but many impacted fish or chicken bones are poorly opaque. Evidence of perforation should be sought, including

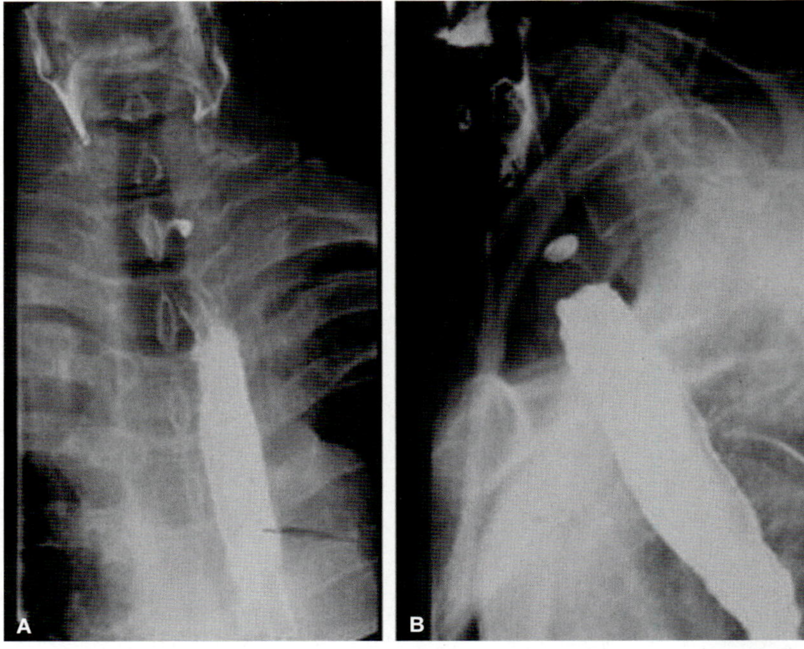

Figs 4.5A and B: Left sided lateral pharyngeal diverticulum – small, barium filled sac with narrow neck

extraluminal gas and widening of the prevertebral soft tissues. A contrast swallow is performed with a small volume of low density barium, or water-soluble non-ionic contrast if perforation is suspected.

Esophageal Motility Disorders

The oesophageal motor disorders have been classified as primary or secondary. In primary motor disorders the oesophagus is the site of major involvement. Achalasia, diffuse spasm and related disorders belong to this group. In secondary motor disorders the esophageal abnormalities are due to more generalized neural, muscular or systemic diseases, to metabolic disturbances or to inflammatory or tumoral lesions of the esophageal wall.

Primary

Nonspecific Esophageal Motility Disorder

Motility abnormalities that do not meet the criteria of specific motility disorders fall into this broad category. Manometrically, abnormal peristalsis is seen in 20% of such cases. Peristalsis may be intermittently absent or of low amplitude. Lower esophageal sphincter dysfunction (incomplete relaxation) and frequent spontaneous or repetitive contractions are also detected. Radiologically a nonspecific disturbance of primary peristalsis and tertiary contractions are seen in 40-50% of cases (Fig. 4.6).

Diffuse Esophageal Spasm

There is absence of primary peristalsis with simultaneous, spontaneous, repetitive, non-peristaltic contractions on manometry. The LES usually functions normally, although high resting pressures and incomplete relaxation may occur.

Radiographically, there is loss of primary peristalsis in the distal esophagus. Nonperistaltic contractions are usually repetitive and simultaneous and may produce a corkscrew or rosary bead appearance (Fig. 4.7). The findings are similar to those seen in nonspecific esophageal motility disorder. The clinical picture helps to distinguish the two conditions, because diffuse esophageal spasm is associated with chest pain. The esophagus is not usually dilated and the LES functions normally.

Achalasia

Achalasia is an uncommon motility disorder of the esophagus characterized by a loss of esophageal peristalsis, incomplete relaxation of the lower esophageal sphincter in response to deglutition, increased resting LES pressure, and increased intraesophageal pressure.[26,27]

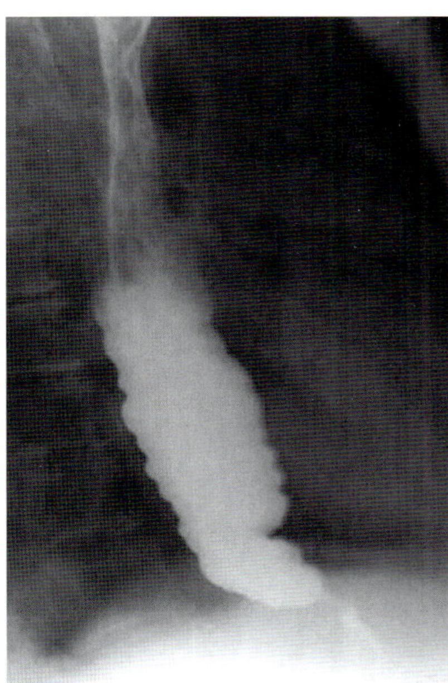

Fig. 4.6: Nonspecific esophageal motility disorder

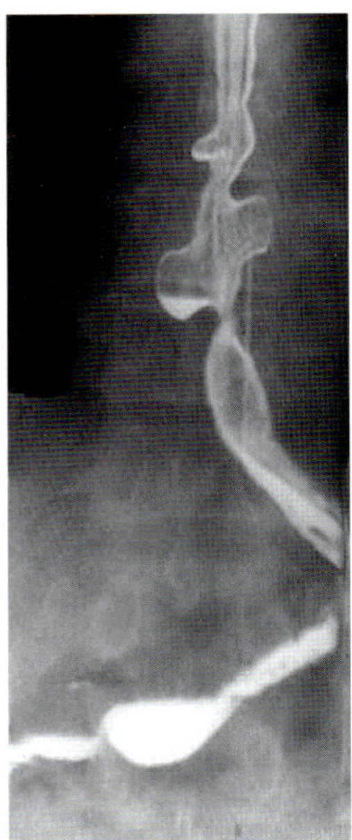

Fig. 4.7: 'Corkscrew' esophagus–non propulsive segmental contractions producing multiple areas of pronounced luminal narrowing with areas of sacculations

Achalasia can present at any age but is commonest in the 30-50 year age group. Dysphagia may initially be intermittent and eventually is persistent. It is diagnosed manometrically as esophageal aperistalsis and LES dysfunction, primary incomplete relaxation and elevated resting pressure. Esophageal dilatation is mild in the early stages, which may make radiographic diagnosis difficult, but is progressive. On plain radiography there may be an air-fluid level in the esophagus. The gastric air bubble is absent. Barium swallow with the patient erect demonstrates a variable degree of dilatation of the esophagus above a beak-like narrowing at the lower esophageal sphincter (Fig. 4.1B). The sphincter opens intermittently under the force of the hydrostatic pressure of the barium column above it to allow bolus passage. The distal two-thirds of the esophagus, which contains smooth muscle is aperistaltic. Secondary stasis esophagitis is common. Esophageal carcinoma may develop.

Secondary achalasia refers to carcinoma of the gastric cardia or metastases involving the gastroesophageal junction resulting in a radiographic picture simulating achalasia. It is related to destruction of the intramural myenteric plexus. Secondary achalasia should be considered in older patients if symptoms are acute or if the tapered gastroesophageal junction shows mucosal nodularity or mass effect. Repeating the esophagogram after patient inhales amylnitrate may help to distinguish this entity from achalasia. This smooth muscle relaxant relax the lower esophageal sphincter in achalasia while in secondary achalasia the LES remains rigid and unchanged.

Nutcracker Esophagus

Nutcracker esophagus is another possible cause of chest pain or dysphagia affecting predominantly older women. The diagnosis is made manometrically with normal peristalsis showing high amplitude. Radiologically, tertiary contractions are seen in half of the patients and the remainder appear normal. Esophageal transit is normal.

Secondary Motility Disorders

Many local and systemic disorders result in oesophageal dysmotility. Most of these are of a nonspecific nature and clinical correlation is needed to determine their significance and suggest etiology.

Scleroderma results in atrophy and fibrosis of connective tissues of the skin and various organs. Seventy five percent of these patients have involvement of the smooth muscle segment of the esophagus. Patients may present with dysphagia as a result of the functional disturbance or the commonly associated gastroesophageal reflux disease.

Radiographically there is a patulous, incompetent lower esophageal sphincter allowing marked gastroesophageal reflux in 40% cases. Distal esophageal peristalsis is absent or diminished and this contributes to the severity of reflux esophagitis (Fig. 4.8).

Other connective tissue diseases and collagen vascular disorders such as dermatomyositis, polymyositis, rheumatoid arthritis, systemic lupus erythematosus and polyarteritis nodosa can also involve the esophagus. Metabolic and endocrine disorders may affect esophageal function. The most common are diabetes and alcoholism, where the neuropathy results in decreased primary peristalsis, increased tertiary contractions and mild esophageal dilatation. Chagas' disease and

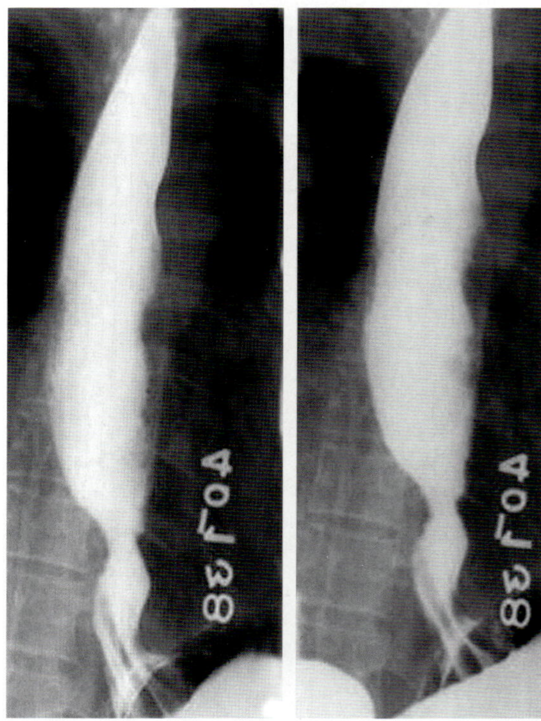

Fig. 4.8: Dilated esophagus with feeble peristalsis and patulous LES. Free gastroesophageal reflux was seen on fluoroscopy–Scleroderma

idiopathic intestinal pseudo-obstruction both mimic achalasia.

ESOPHAGITIS

Numerous etiologic factors may cause oesophagitis. The most common cause is gastroesophageal reflux.

Gastroesophageal Reflux Disease and Barrett's Esophagus

Patients with gastroesophageal reflux disease usually complain of a variety of symptoms like heartburn, regurgitation, substernal pain and also dysphagia in some cases.

On double-contrast esophagography, early changes of reflux esophagitis may be recognized as a fine mucosal nodularity or granular appearance of the mucosa in the distal third or half of the thoracic oesophagus, occurring due to the presence of mucosal oedema and inflammation during the early stages of reflux esophagitis (Fig. 4.9). As the disease progresses, double-contrast esophagography may demonstrate shallow ulcers and erosions, thickened longitudinal folds, inflammatory polyps and scarring.[28] Reflux esophagitis may be recognized also on mucosal relief views as lobulation or nodularity of slightly thickened longitudinal folds.

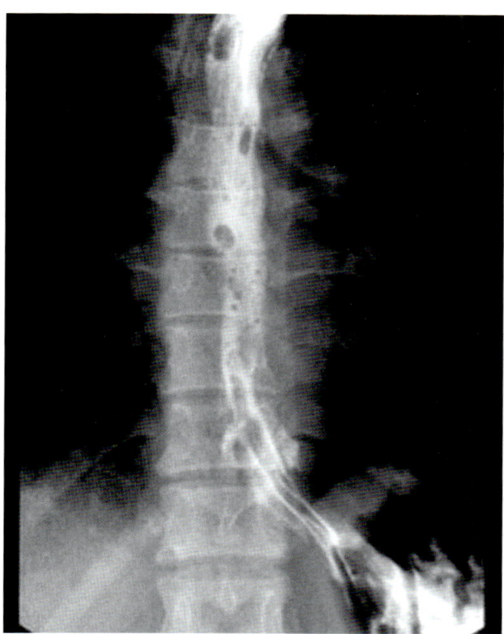

Fig. 4.9: Barium swallow shows minimal nodularity and thickening of mucosal folds in the distal esophagus in a case of peptic esophagitis

Superficial ulceration occurs with increasing severity, seen as tiny, punctate, linear or irregular collection of barium associated with mounds of edema and fold thickening and distortion. The changes of reflux esophagitis involve a continuous area in the distal esophagus extending proximally from the gastroesophageal junction. Sparing of distal esophagus indicates another cause for the radiographic abnormalities.

A stricture may develop with chronic gastroesophageal reflux disease, which is a smooth, tapered and concentric narrowing in the distal esophagus. Occasionally, the benign stricture is asymmetric due to scarring. Sacculations may form with severe scarring. A Schatzki ring is a thin, smooth, symmetric mucosal ring narrowing the gastroesophageal junction above a sliding hiatus hernia. It may be the result of gastroesophageal reflux disease. These usually cause dysphagia when less than 13 mm in diameter but are usually asymptomatic when greater than 20 mm in diameter. Esophageal dysmotility and dilatation of the esophagus due to atony may also be seen in gastroesophageal reflux disease.

Barrett's esophagus is progressive columnar metaplasia of the esophagus occurring in about 10 % of patients with long-standing gastroesophageal reflux and reflux esophagitis. There is 30-40 times greater risk of development of adenocarcinoma of the esophagus.[29] The characteristic radiologic feature of Barrett's esophagus is a midesophageal stricture or ulcer, often associated with a sliding hiatal hernia or gastroesophageal reflux.[28,30]

Infectious Esophagitis

Esophagitis may be caused by a variety of infectious agents which include monilia, herpes simplex, cytomegalic inclusion virus, tuberculosis, lactobacilli, cryptococcoses, blastomycosis, mixed bacterial infections and diphtheria. In most cases infectious esophagitis occurs in debilitated individuals; diabetics, immunosuppressed patients; or patients receiving steroids, antibiotics, radiotherapy or chemotherapy. It is seen with increasing frequency in immunosuppressed transplant patients and individuals with AIDS.

Candida Esophagitis

Candida albicans is the most common cause of infectious esophagitis. It usually occurs opportunistically in patients immunocompromised as a result of underlying malignancy; other debilitating illnesses; treatment with radiation, steroids, or cytotoxic agents; or most recently, AIDS. Candida esophagitis can also result from local oesophageal stasis caused by severe esophageal motility disorders such as achalasia and scleroderma. Symptoms range from asymptomatic to severe dysphagia. Since it is a mucosal disease, it can be identified on double-contrast barium examination. In the diagnosis of Candida esophagitis, double contrast esophagography shows a sensitivity of about 90%. The findings include discrete, linear, or irregular plaque like filling defects with intervening normal mucosa. (Fig. 4.10) The plaques may slough off resulting in ulcerations scattered on a background of plaques. In advanced disease, there may be coalescent plaques, which have been likened to a "cobblestone" or "snakeskin" appearance that correspond to the distinctive white plaques seen at endoscopy.[31] Patients with AIDS may get a severe form of this disease, resulting in a grossly irregular or shaggy appearance secondary to extensive plaques and pseudomembranes that trap barium between them.[32] A newly described sign associated with esophageal candidiasis is the "foamy" esophagus. This appears as innumerable tiny (1-3 mm), bubble-like lucencies producing a foamy appearance.[33]

The CT findings of Candida oesophagitis, though nonspecific and commonly seen in various kinds of esophagitis, are circumferential esophageal wall thickening of more than 5 mm, with relatively long segmental involvement. Enhanced scans may also depict the target sign (circumferential wall thickening and enhancing internal mucosa).[11]

Viral Esophagitis

Herpes esophagitis is manifest, usually as multiple discrete superficial ulcers separated by normal mucosa. The ulcers may be punctate, linear or stellate and are surrounded by radiolucent halos due to edema. In the appropriate clinical setting, the presence of small, discrete ulcers without plaques should be highly suggestive of herpes esophagitis, because ulceration in candidiasis almost always occurs against a background of diffuse plaque formation.[34]

When cytomegalovirus and HIV infect the esophagus, large, shallow ulcers up to several centimeters in size are seen in the mid- and sometimes the distal esophagus (Fig. 4.11). The ulcer is usually solitary, ovoid in shape and longitudinal in orientation with smooth

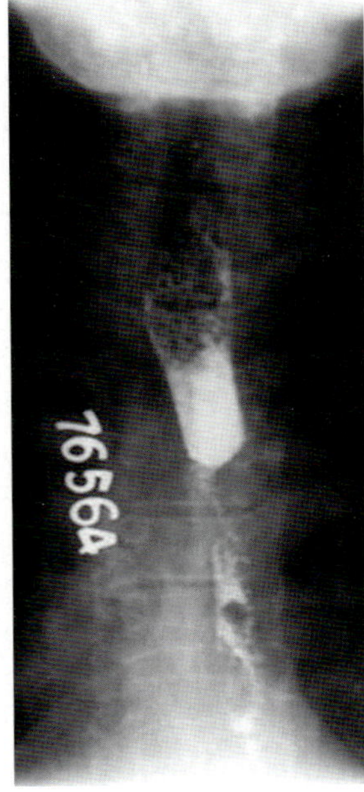

Fig. 4.10: Candida esophagitis: Esophagogram shows a shaggy contour with irregular plaque-like filling defects, seen above a stricture

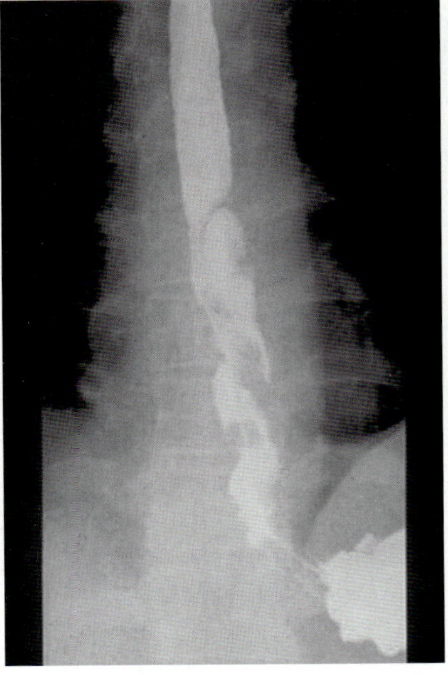

Fig. 4.11: Barium swallow in a case of CMV esophagitis shows irregular, shallow ulcers in the mid and distal esophagus

margins and often surrounded by a thin radiolucent rim of edematous mucosa.[35] Since the treatment of CMV and HIV esophagitis differs widely, endoscopy with biopsies and cultures is required to differentiate the two infections.

Tuberculosis

Tuberculous involvement of the esophagus is rare. When present, it is usually secondary to current or previous tuberculous infection in other sites. The esophagus may become infected as a result of direct extension from adjacent mediastinal or hilar lymph nodes, vertebral bodies, aortic aneurysms, tubeculous pharyngitis or laryngitis, or by inoculation of swallowed sputum, hematogenous or lymphatic spread.[36]

Tuberculous lesions can occur in any segment of the esophagus. However, they are most common in the middle third, just proximal to the tracheal bifurcation, because of its proximity to the mediastinal lymph nodes around the bifurcation of the trachea.[37] The changes in the esophagus may result from pressure, adhesions or actual involvement of mucosal surface.[36] The most common feature is extrinsic compression of the esophagus, usually by a mass of lymph nodes. Although the esophageal mucosa is often intact in such cases, the adventitia is usually implicated and this may produce classical traction diverticulam. When the disease process involves the esophageal mucosa, a tumoros lesion or an ulcer may result. Sinus or fistula as a result of rupture of caseous lymph nodes may also occur.[37] Amorphous gas collection at enlarged mediastinal lymph nodes in patients with tuberculous lymphadenitis suggests the presence of an esophagonodal fistula.[38] A constricting lesion or kinking of the esophagus may be seen as a result of fibrosis.[37]

Caustic Esophagitis

The severity and extent of esophageal injury depend on the type, concentration and volume of the caustic agent. Alkaline agents can produce deep coagulation necrosis in minutes. Necrosis from acids tends to be more superficial. In addition to esophageal injury, caustic agents may also produce burns of the pharynx and stomach. The initial clinical symptoms are the rapid onset of chest pain and dysphagia. Late complications are related primarily to fibrosis and stricture, which may cause dysphagia several weeks after the initial injury.

The radiographic findings vary, depending on the severity and extent. During the first 24 hours, the oesophagus may appear normal after a mild injury, or may show blurred margins, contour irregularity, ulceration or thickened folds when the changes are more severe. Generally, long segments of esophagus are involved. Moderate to severe injury usually abolishes peristalsis. In the acute stage the examination should be initiated with water-soluble contrast medium to exclude esophageal or gastric perforation; then barium may be used. During the first week an acute inflammatory response develops, and areas of significant injury show frank ulceration on esophagograms. A pseudomembrane may cause intramural trapping of barium (Fig. 4.12). The oesophageal wall is generally thickened with some luminal narrowing. By 2-6 weeks, healing progresses accompanied by severe fibrosis. Progressive narrowing of the esophageal lumen is heralded by the return or onset of dysphagia. The luminal contour may resume a smooth contour after epithelial regeneration, but focal areas of submucosal fibrosis cause nodular defects or scalloping (Figs 4.13A and B). Coexisting gastric involvement, primarily in the distal part of the stomach, may cause antral ulceration, pyloric stenosis, or frank gastric outlet obstruction (Fig. 4.14).

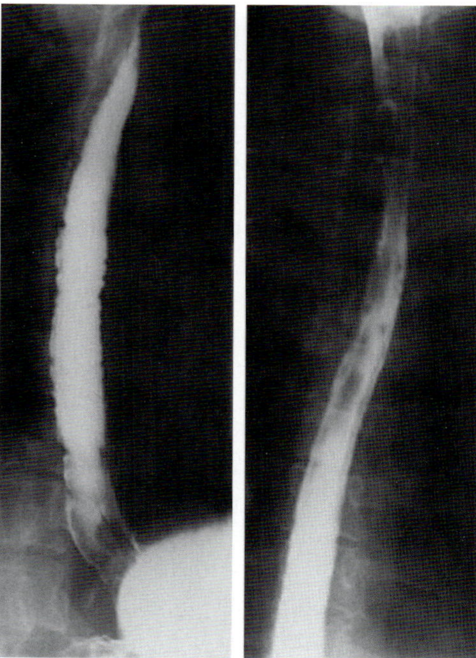

Fig. 4.12: Recent corrosive ingestion–esophagus showing frank ulcerations and pseudomembranes causing intramural trapping of barium

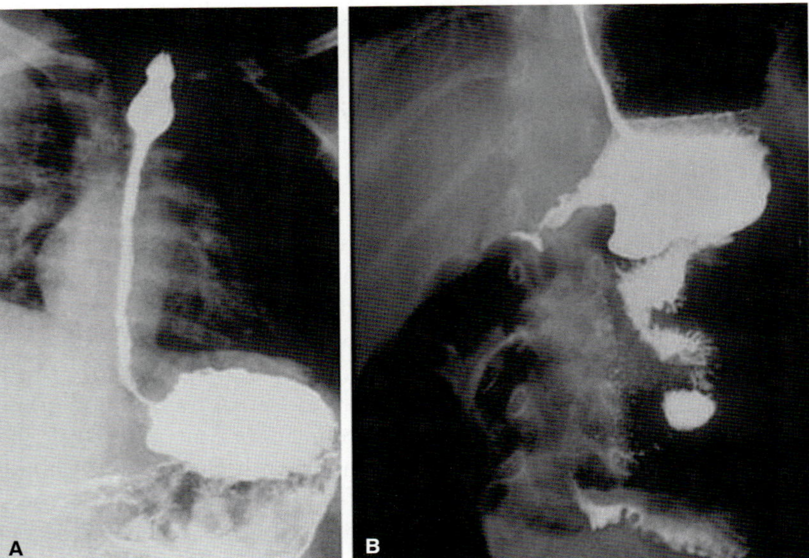

Figs 4.13A and B: (A) Barium swallow showing a long stricture with nodular defects due to focal areas of submucosal fibrosis in a case of Caustic esophagitis, (B) The stomach shows narrowing of distal body and antrum with mucosal irregularity

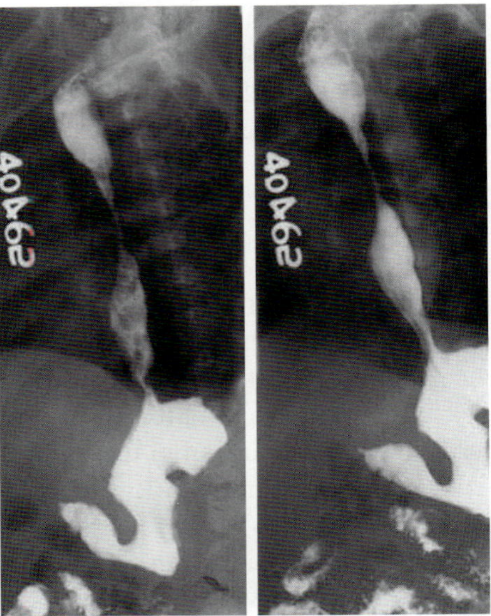

Fig. 4.14: Caustic ingestion in a child causing smooth long stricture in the mid esophagus with antral narrowing in the stomach

Drug-induced Esophagitis

Drug-induced esophagitis is caused most commonly by ingesting antibiotics, such as tetracycline and doxycycline. Other medications include potassium chloride, quinidine, ferrous sulphate and anti-inflammatory drugs. When such drugs dissolve in the esophagus, they cause mucosal injury by creating an acid pH or by a direct irritant effect in the epithelium. Hold up of tablets in the esophagus is favored by swallowing pills while lying down, taking them without water, abnormal esophageal motility, and cardiomegaly. Symptoms are usually sudden in onset and consist of chest pain, odynophagia or dysphagia. Drug-induced esophagitis usually involves the proximal or middle esophagus. A typical location is the aortic arch level, where tablets are delayed because of the aortic indentation on the esophagus and the low contractile force of peristalsis. The radiographic findings consist of luminal irregularity, frank ulceration and luminal narrowing. The ulcers are usually ovoid, occasionally linear and clustered circumferentially. A repeat study 7-10 days after withdrawal of the offending agent will show healing of ulcers.

Radiation-induced Esophagitis

Symptomatic radiation esophagitis may occur in a small percentage of patients receiving mediastinal radiation in doses of 50 Gy or more over a 6-8 week period. Mild heartburn or dysphagia develops several weeks after the onset of treatment. A mild superficial esophagitis is present during this period that heals rapidly. Late symptoms of dysphagia that develop weeks to months after the completion of therapy reflect deep injury to the esophageal muscle or nerves. Radiographically, the esophageal motor function is generally abnormal. Esophageal peristalsis commonly stops in the proximal esophagus at the upper margin of the radiation field and below this level repetitive, nonperistaltic contractions are seen. The LES may fail to relax. Occasionally diffuse ulceration that causes pain with swallowing may be seen and mimic moniliasis. Late findings consist of strictures which are smooth with tapering margin and rarely show irregularity or ulceration.

Miscellaneous Causes

These include bullous dermatoses, noninfectious granulomatous disease, Behçet's disease and ulcerative colitis. Allthough rare, Crohn's disease is probably the most common granulomatous esophagitis without an infectious cause.

ESOPHAGEAL DIVERTICULA

Most esophageal diverticula are acquired false diverticula and so comprise outpouchings of mucosa with or

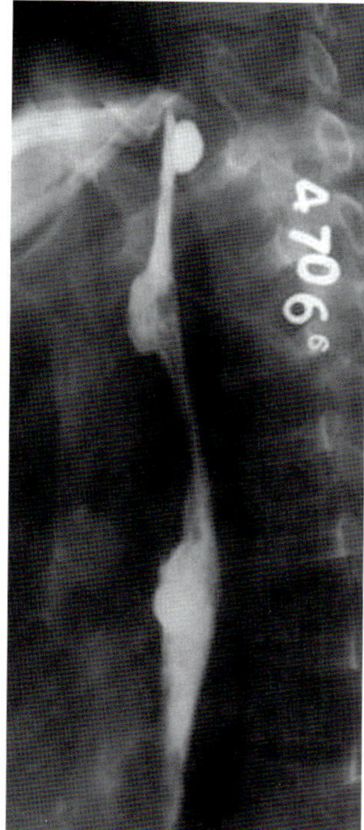

Fig. 4.15: Esophagogram showing multiple pulsion diverticula

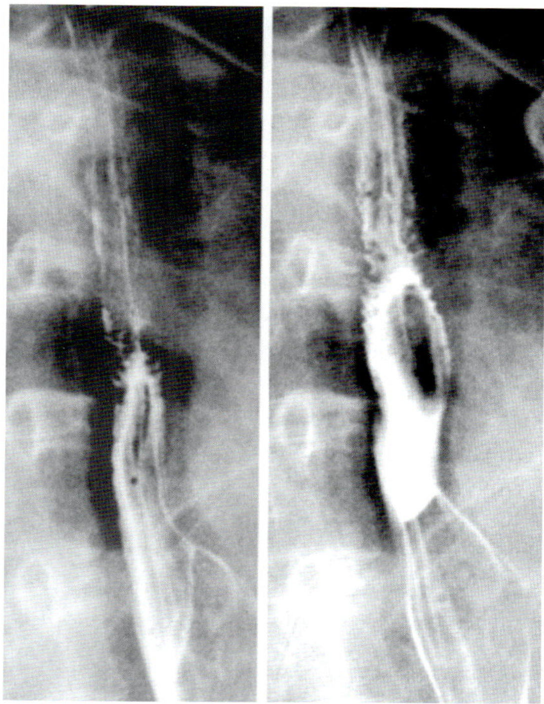

Fig. 4.16: Intramural Pseudodiverticulosis: Tiny, flask-shaped outpouchings arranged in longitudinal rows produced by barium entering dilated esophageal glands, seen in the thoracic esophagus

without submucosa (Fig. 4.15). They are most common in the middle and distal thirds of oesophagus. Nearly all of them are caused by pulsion forces as opposed to traction. A small percentage of diverticula in the midesophagus are conical in shape, have no neck and may be caused by traction. The causes of pulsion diverticula include esophageal motility disorders, mechanical obstruction and chronic wear-and-tear forces.

On barium swallow small esophageal diverticula, 0.5-2 cm in size are commonly observed as transient outpouchings that develop only during peristalsis. Large diverticula have a narrow neck, often retain fluid and gas and empty only by gravity. Epiphrenic diverticula located just above the LES, generally project to the right, whereas, elsewhere in the esophagus the diverticula project in any direction except posteriorly. In about 10- 20% of cases multiple diverticula are present.

Intramural Pseudodiverticulosis

It is an unusual condition in which inflammation leads to dilatation of the ducts of the deep mucous glands. Radiologically, they appear as tiny, flask-shaped outpouchings arranged in clusters or longitudinal rows (Fig. 4.16). Often the neck of the pseudodiverticula are not opacified and they appear to be separated from the esophageal lumen by 1 or 2 mm. The condition may be segmental or diffuse, and may be seen in association with a peptic stricture in the lower esophagus.

ESOPHAGEAL VARICES

Esophageal varices are dilated, subepithelial veins resulting from increased collateral blood flow via the azygos vein between the intra-abdominal portal venous system and the intrathoracic superior vena cava.

On mucosal spot films, esophageal varices seen enface appear as thickened longitudinal esophageal folds with fusiform separation. Beaded or serpiginous filling defects are more definite findings, that change in size during the examination. Varices are often effaced during esophageal distension. A thrombosed varix is extremely difficult to differentiate from a submucosal mass because the ability to efface the lesion is lost.

Uphill varices are usually caused by portal hypertension, with hepatofugal flow through dilated esophageal collateral vessels to the superior vena cava.

Uphill varices may cause marked upper gastrointestinal tract bleeding. Varices appear on barium studies as serpentine longitudinal filling defects in the distal half of the thoracic portion of the esophagus.[39] They are best seen on mucosal-relief views of the collapsed esophagus while the patient is in a prone RAO position, with use of a high-density barium suspension or barium paste to increase mucosal adherence.

Downhill varices are caused by superior vena cava obstruction with downward flow via dilated esophageal collateral vessels to the portal venous system and the inferior vena cava. Causes of downhill varices include central catheter-related thrombosis of the superior vena cava, bronchogenic carcinoma or other metastatic tumors involving the mediastinum, lymphoma, substernal goiter, mediastinal radiation, and sclerosing mediastinitis.[39] Such varices typically appear as serpentine longitudinal filling defects that, unlike uphill varices are confined to the upper or middle part of the esophagus.[35]

TRAUMATIC LESIONS

Esophageal injury may be caused by an ingested foreign body, endoscopy, dilatation procedures, penetrating wounds, blunt trauma, or surgical procedures.

Foreign Bodies

Smooth foreign bodies, such as coins, buttons, dental crowns generally pass through the esophagus but may lodge in areas of normal anatomic narrowing at the thoracic inlet, aortic arch, or diaphragmatic hiatus. Sharp objects may arrest at any esophageal level.

Metallic or dense foreign bodies are recognized on plain films of the neck or chest. Flat objects such as coins are oriented in the coronal plane of the esophagus in contrast to the sagittal plane orientation in the trachea. Obstructing foreign bodies may cause a gas-fluid level in the esophagus or tracheal displacement. Water-soluble contrast is indicated for the initial swallow to exclude perforation. Barium may be used for subsequent swallows. Cotton balls or marshmallows soaked in barium may be useful to demonstrate a small, hard-to-detect foreign body.

MISCELLANEOUS LESIONS

Esophageal hematomas are generally related to endoscopy, direct trauma, esophageal dilatations or truncal vagotomy but can occur spontaneously in patients on anticoagulants or with bleeding disorders. The hematoma causes acute lower chest pain and dysphagia. Radiologically, the oesophageal lumen is generally compressed by an elongated, eccentric intraluminal mass with smooth, lumpy, or sometimes irregular contour. In some cases, contrast medium fills a false channel.

ESOPHAGEAL TUMORS

Benign Tumors

Benign tumors of the esophagus are uncommon.

Benign mucosal tumors do not cause luminal narrowing. The commonest are squamous papillomas seen as small sessile polypoid lesions with a smooth or slightly lobulated contour on double contrast oesophagogram.[40]

Submucosal benign tumors are much more common; the vast majority of these are leiomyomas. Leiomyoma accounts for 60-70% of all benign esophageal neoplasms and is the most common benign tumour of the esophagus, while rare in the remaining gastrointestinal tract.[41,42] The tumor is present more often in male patients (2:1) at a median age of 30-35 years. Leiomyoma is discovered incidentally. When symptomatic, dysphagia for solids is the dominant symptom. Esophageal leiomyomas seldom ulcerate and are hardly ever malignant. Esophagograms demonstrate a smooth filling defect with the characteristic features of a submucosal lesion (Fig. 4.17A). On tangential views, a semilunar mass with intact mucosa narrows the barium column. Seen face on the lesion may cause splitting of the barium column, splaying of the longitudinal esophageal folds and segmental widening of the esophageal diameter. A soft tissue companion shadow may be observed, caused by the exophytic component of the lesion. Esophageal leiomyomas may occur as multiple lesions.

Enhanced CT scans reveal a smooth or lobulated tumor margin, with either iso or homogeneously low attenuation (Fig. 4.17B). Leiomyoma may appear as a well-circumscribed, intensely enhancing mass or may be a sessile, polypoidal, exophytic intraluminal solid mass, sometimes with seconday ulceration. Absence of infiltration of the esophageal wall or the absence of the typical circumferential growth pattern enables differentiation from esophageal cancer.[10]

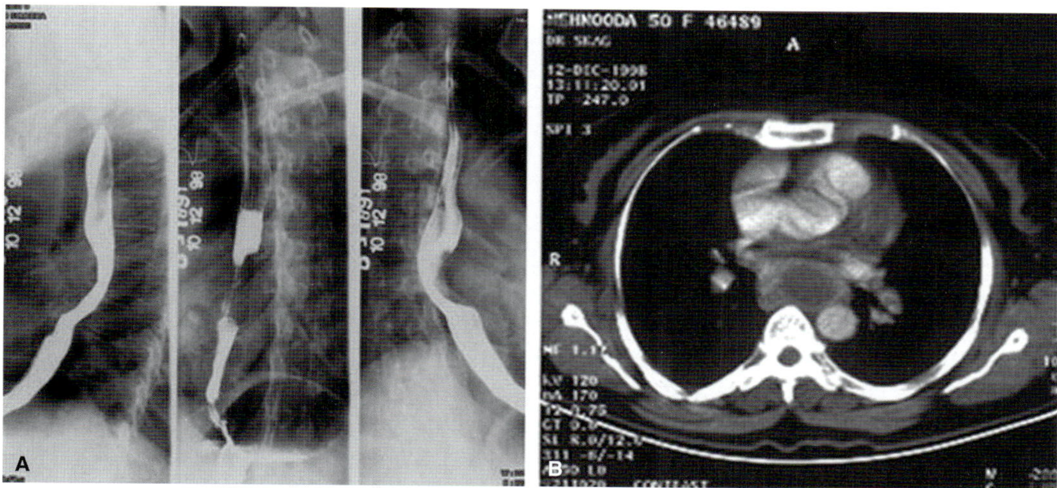

Figs 4.17A and B: (A) Leiomyoma in the distal thoracic esophagus seen as a semilunar mass with intact mucosa, narrowing the barium column and widening the esophageal diameter, (B) CECT shows smooth hypodense mass seen indenting the esophageal lumen with intact fat planes around esophagus–Leiomyoma

Other benign submucosal neoplasms include neurofibroma, fibroma, angioma, lipoma and granular cell tumor.

Malignant Tumors

In the esophagus, the majority of intrinsic tumors are primarily carcinomas.

Carcinoma

Esophageal carcinoma constitutes about 1% of all cancers in the United States and 7% of all gastrointestinal tumors.[43] Early dissemination of tumor occurs because the esophagus lacks a serosa, so there is no anatomic barrier to prevent these cancers from spreading rapidly into the mediastinum.

About 90% of esophageal carcinomas are of squamous cell origin. The remainder are adenocarcinomas that arise primarily in the distal esophagus. The predominant clinical complaint is dysphagia. Other symptoms include cough, hoarseness, weakness and weight loss.

Chest radiographs generally do not show any abnormalities but may reveal mediastinal widening, a soft tissue mass, an esophageal gas-fluid level, anterior tracheal bowing or a thickened retrotracheal stripe.

Early esophageal cancers are usually small protruded lesions less than 3.5 cm in size . On double-contrast studies moderate-sized lesions 1.5-3 cm in size, and generally occur as lobulated sessile lesions that are eccentric and may show evidence of ulceration. Some lesions are detected as an area of superficial irregularity or a flattened zone of decreased compliance (Fig. 4.18). Small lesions less than 1.5 cm in size may be seen as mound like sessile polyps, flattened sessile lesions, or a

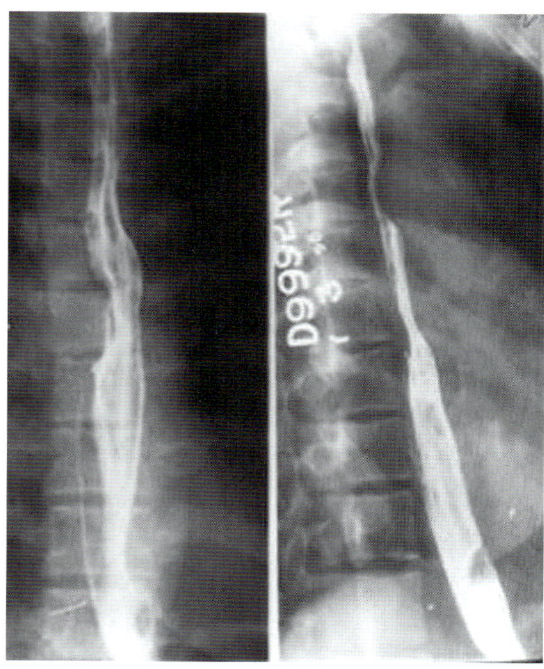

Fig. 4.18: A rigid plaque like area with flattened zone of decreased compliance in the right wall of mid esophagus – early malignancy

patch of mucosal irregularity. On esophagogram, advanced esophageal carcinoma presents a variety of morphologic abnormalities. Advanced tumors may appear as as annular apple-core lesion with overhanging margins (Fig. 4.19), irregular narrowed segment, smooth tapering stricture, bulky endophytic mass (Fig. 4.20), large ulceration, varicoid infiltrate (Fig. 4.21), or diffuse nodularity (Fig. 4.22). Varicoid carcinomas are those in which submucosal spread of tumor produces thickened, tortuous, longitudinal defects that mimic the appearance of varices. Varicoid tumors have a fixed configuration, however, whereas varices change in size and shape at fluoroscopy. In some cases esophageal carcinoma spreads submucosally via the lymphatics and reapperars at another site in the esophagus (Figs. 4.23A and B). These satellite metastases may appear as polypoid, plaque-like, or ulcerated lesions separated from the primary tumor by normal mucosa.[44] Tumor also spreads subdiaphragmatically to the proximal stomach via submucosal lymphatics. Fistulization may occur spontaneously, or after radiotherapy.[45]

Computed tomography and endoscopic ultrasound are the most accurate methods of staging esophageal carcinoma. Although many investigators have evaluated

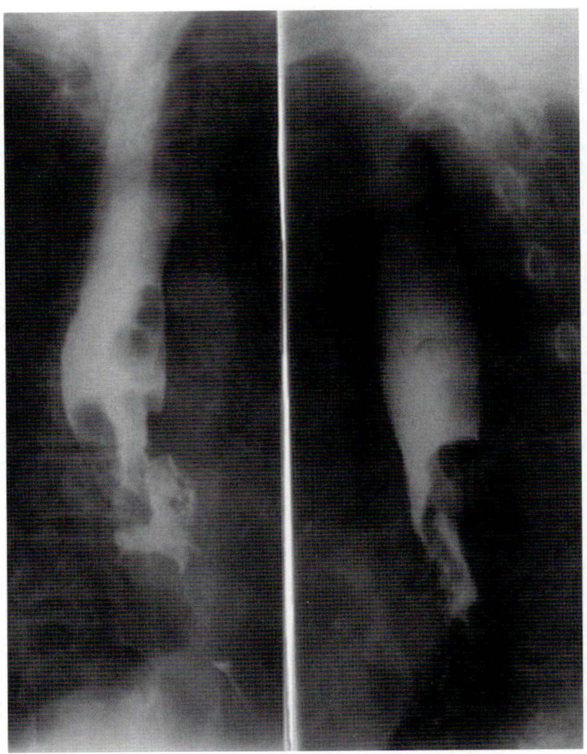

Fig. 4.20: Polypoidal filling defects with shouldering and irregular narrowing of lumen-carcinoma involving the mid and lower esophagus

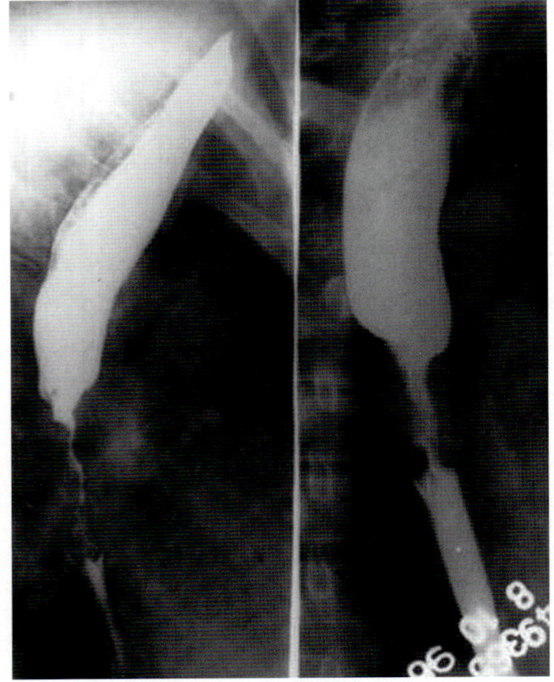

Fig. 4.19: Annular carcinoma in mid portion of esophagus with circumferential infiltration and overhanging margins

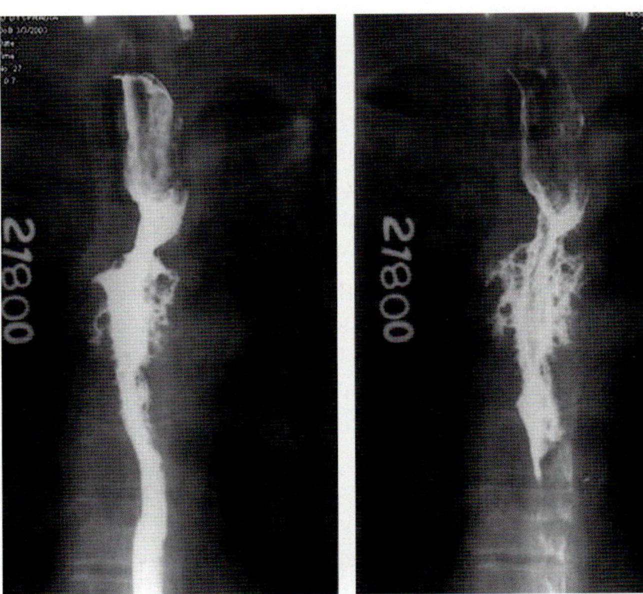

Fig. 4.21: Spot film of the esophagus at the level of aortic arch shows irregularity and nodularity of the mucosa with lymphatic infiltration-varicoid appearance in squamous cell carcinoma

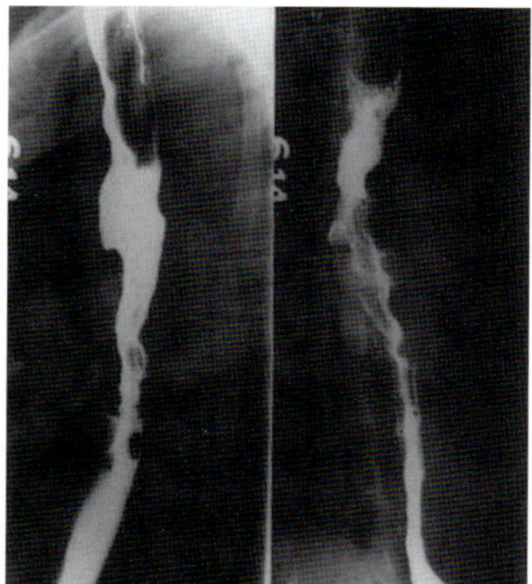

Fig. 4.22: Carcinoma involving mid esophagus with narrowing of lumen and diffuse nodular filling defects

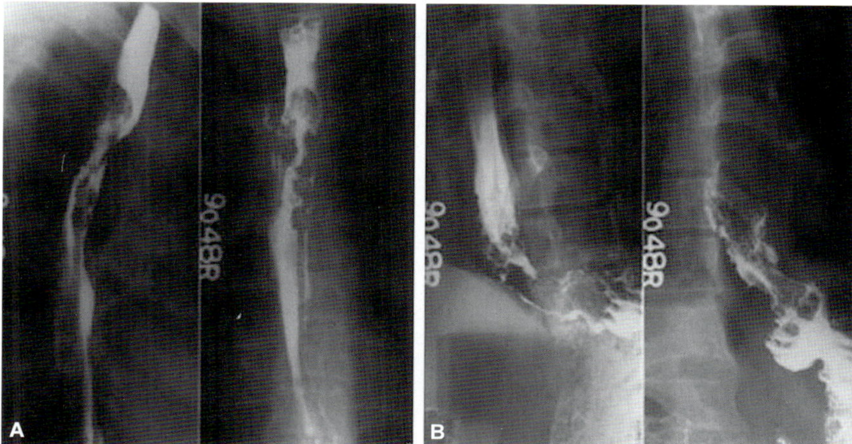

Figs 4.23A and B: Carcinoma involving upper and mid esophagus in a circumferential manner. Another lesion is seen just above the esophagogastric junction – Multicentric carcinoma

and compared the usefulness of CT and MRI in staging esophageal carcinoma, controversies remain about which imaging modality is superior. The extent of involvement of the esphageal wall by tumor, invasion of adjacent structures, and metastasis of disease to regional nodes or distant organs is the major issue for the radiologist.

On CT scans, esophageal carcinoma appears as mass or wall thickening with soft tissue attenuation (Figs 4.24 and 4.25). On MRI, esophageal carcinoma is seen as an area of isointensity relative to residual esophageal wall on T1W images and as an area of high signal intensity on T2W images (Fig. 4.26). The depth of tumor infiltration into the esophageal wall, one of the most important prognostic factors, can best by evaluated by EUS.

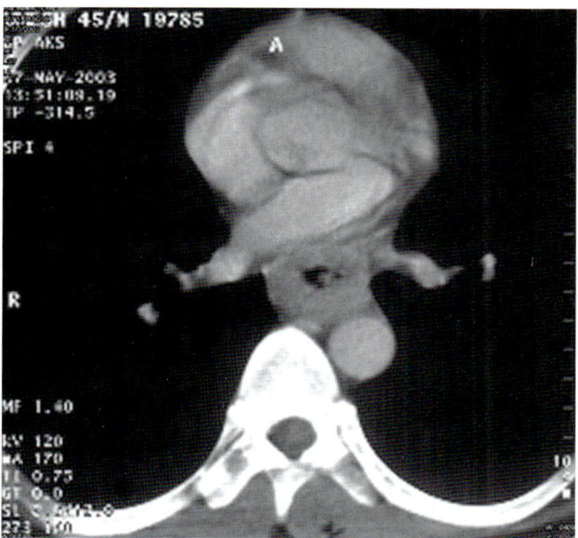

Fig. 4.24: CECT shows circumferential mural thickening in a case of carcinoma mid dorsal esophagus. There is indentation of left atrium anteriorly with less than 90° arc of contact with descending aorta

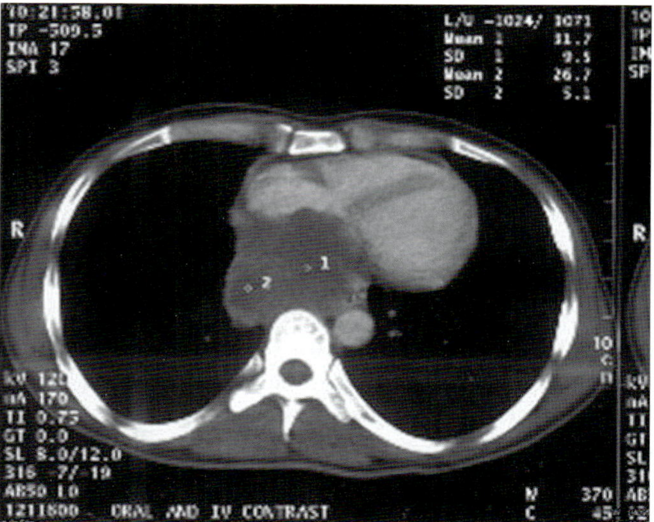

Fig. 4.25: CECT in a case of Ca Oesophagus shows a large hypodense mass invading the pericardium with extension into the adjacent left atrium. There is obliteration of fat planes around the aorta creating an arc of contact greater than 90°

Macroscopic periesphageal fat invasion by the tumour can be demonstrated with high accuracy on CT and MR images, although microscopic invasion to

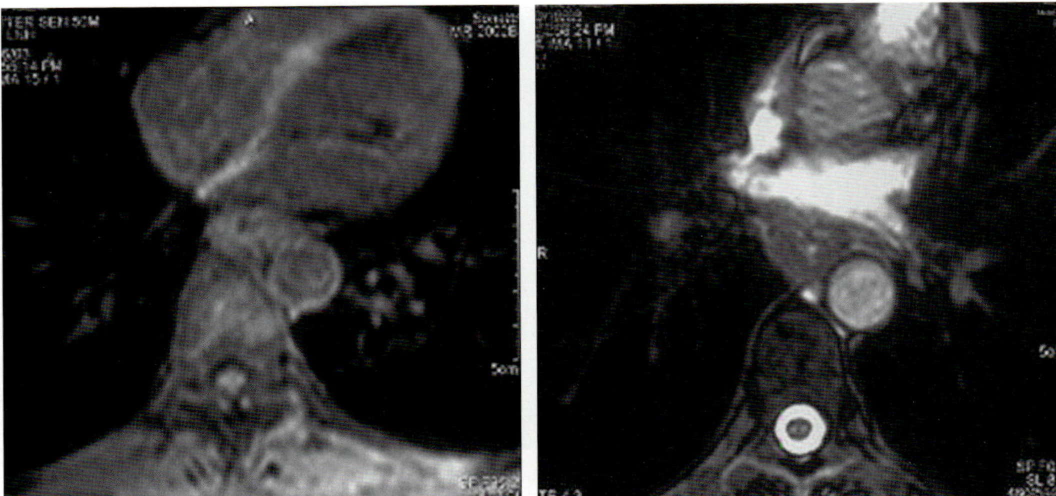

Fig. 4.26: MR images in case of carcinoma esophagus showing diffuse circumferential wall thickening with luminal narrowing in the dorsal esophagus. There is obliteration of fat plane between the mass and the left atrium, with angle of contact with aorta more than 90°

periesophageal fat is not revealed. On CT scans, periesophageal fat invasion is shown as strand like areas of soft tissue attenuation within the perioesophageal fat plane. On MRI, it is shown as having an illdefined, irregular margins, regional absence of a bright fat signal and tumor mass into the adjacent mediastinal fat.

Accurate evaluation of tracheobronchial, aortic, and bone invasion is important because these are contra-indications to surgical resection. CT or MRI appearance of trachobronchial invasion are displacement or indentation of the posterior wall of the trachea or the bronchus by the tumor mass as well as evidence of direct extension of the tumor into the lumen of the airway. The absence of an intervening fat plane alone however does not always suggest tumor invasion because this finding can be seen in normal patients. Moreover, an adjacent mass behind the trachea or main bronchus can produce concavity of the posterior portion without invasion because the cartilage rings are incomplete in the posterior portion of the trachea and main bronchi.[12]

According to Picus and co-workers,[46] aortic invasion can be diagnosed by CT if the area of contact between the oesophageal carcinoma and the aorta creates an arc of more than 90°. If the arc is less the 45°, aortic invasion is considered to be absent; an arc of 45-90° is considered indeterminate. The overall accuracy of MRI in evaluating aortic invasion is similar to that of CT.

Although the patient may be cachectic or may have undergone radiation, which can obliterate normal fat planes, tumour invasion should be suggested when a localized obliteration of fat plane is noted with preserved fat planes above and below the lesion.

Metastases

Secondary malignant involvement of the oesophagus may be of three types:

1. direct invasion
2. involvement from adjacent malignant nodes and
3. blood borne metastases, the least common form. Malignancy of the stomach, lung, thyroid, hypo-pharynx and larynx may extend directly into the oesophagus. Appearance of these lesions may simulate that of a primary carcinoma. Malignant mediastinal nodes may compress and constrict the oesophagus. The common origins are lung and breast carcinoma.

INDENTATIONS AND DISPLACEMENT

In healthy subjects, several normal structures commonly indent the barium-filled oesophagus. Mild indentations are caused commonly by the aortic knob, left mainstem bronchus and diaphragmatic hiatus. The dilated descending thoracic aorta indents the oesophagus just above the diaphragmatic hiatus, where the oesophagus passes immediately anterior to the aorta. Some reports suggest that ectasia of the descending aorta may rarely cause obstructive symptoms of "dysphagia aortica", especially when accompanied by cardiomegaly. Cervical or thoracic vertebral osteophytes may cause impression on the proximal esophagus and on rare occasions may also cause dysphagia. Symptomatic compression of the proximal esophagus has also been caused by scoliosis. A common cause of esophageal compression as well as displacement is cardiomegaly.

Esophageal impressions may also be caused by aberrant, anomalous or enlarged blood vessels. The majority of vascular impressions occur along the upper half of the thoracic esophagus. These rarely cause symptoms unless a complete ring exists around the esophagus and trachea. Symptoms in children are usually respiratory, whereas, adults have esophageal dysphagia. Although, an aberrant right subclavian artery may cause "dysphagia lusoria" obstructive symptoms are rare even when the vascular impression is pronounced on esophagograms.

Recent Advances and Future Directions

MR fluoroscopy of swallowing is feasible.[47] Real-time True FISP is well suited for this purpose because it is robust and provides good image contrast, as well as sufficient temporal and spatial resolution. Following the implementation of new strategies to further enhance spatial and temporal resolution, MR fluoroscopy may emerge as an additional tool for the assessment of the oropharynx.

To determine the diagnostic accuracy of high resolution MR imaging at 1.5T for evaluating the mural invasion of superficial esophageal carcinoma, an *in vitro* study[48] demonstrated that T2-weighted high resolution MR images clearly depict the normal esophageal wall as consisting of eight layers. MR imaging has a much higher soft-tissue contrast than do other imaging modalities and it does not cause the artifactual interface echoes in the esophageal wall that are seen in endoscopic US. Thus, high-resolution MR imaging can differentiate the normal layers of the esophageal wall more accurately than other imaging modalities. In a recent study it was demonstrated that high resolution 3D-CISS MRI *in vitro* clearly depicts the internal architecture of the esophageal wall and has a high diagnostic accuracy for evaluating mural invasion and macroscopic findings in esophageal carcinomas. Thus high-resolution 3D-CISS MRI may enable the preoperative histopathologic staging and morphologic evaluation of esophageal carcinomas.[49] Local staging of gastrointestinal tumors with the use of a nonferromagnetic endoscope with a radiofrequency coil embedded in its tip has been tried. High-resolution MR imaging of superficial esophageal carcinomas *in vivo* will be possible in the near future with the development of faster MR imaging techniques and with the use of an endoluminal surface-coil technique guided with endoscopy or a body-coil technique with a reduced or targeted field of view.[50] By means of high-resolution MR imaging which has a high diagnostic accuracy for the depth of carcinoma invasion, it may be possible to adopt either a smaller operation, laser treatment, or intracavitory irradiation for cases of superficial esophageal carcinomas without lymph node metastasis.

In another study,[51] Proton magnetic spectroscopy of esophageal biopsies combined with a statistical classification strategy data analysis provided a robust diagnosis with a high degree of accuracy for discriminating normal epithelium from esophageal adenocarcinoma and Barrett's esophagus. Different spectral categories of Barrett's epithelium were identified both by visual inspection and by statistical classification strategy, possibly reflecting the risk of future malignant transformation.

Functional MRI sequences acquired during the administration of oral contrast material can evaluate esophageal transit, providing information on motility and morphology. This modality can visualize the typical functional and morphological alterations of motility disorders.[52]

Position emission tomography ([18F] 2 flouro 2-deoxyglucose positron emission tomography [FDG]-PET) is gaining popularity in staging patients who have many types of malignant disease. Based on the finding that malignant cells possess higher rates of glucose uptake compared with normal cells, FDG-PET has been shown to detect occult distant metastatic disease in approximately 20% of patients who have esophageal cancer.[53,54] Drawbacks of FDG-PET are related to its lack of sensitivity for detecting small (< 1 cm) metastatic lesions and its relative lack of anatomic detail. The latter problem can be partially addressed by the advent of newer PET/CT fusion scanners. Until larger, confirmatory studies are performed examining the utility of

FDG-PET for detection of metastatic disease, the findings in patients who have esophageal cancer should be confirmed with a second imaging technique or a biopsy depending on the individual clinical scenario. This guideline is especially true in the assessment of potentially metastatic pulmonary lesions because although the FDG-PET scan is frequently positive in pulmonary metastases, a number of benign pulmonary lesions (mainly inflammatory) can also be glucose avid.[55]

PET/CT has important utility and limitations in the initial staging of esophageal cancer, evaluation of response to neoadjivant therapy, and detection of recurrent malignancy. Correct integration of PET/CT into the conventional work-up of esophageal cancer requires a multidisciplinary approach that combines the information from PET/CT with results of clinical assessment, diagnostic CT, endoscopic gastroduodenoscopy, and endoscopic ultrasonography.[56]

PET/CT has limited utility in T staging of esophageal cancer and relatively limited utility in detection of dissemination to locoregional lymph nodes. However, PET/CT allows detection of metastatic disease that may not be identifiable with other methods. PET/CT is not sufficiently reliable in the individual patient for determination of treatment response in the primary tumor.[56]

REFERENCES

1. Levine MS, Rubesin SE. Radiologic investigation of dysphagia. AJR 1990;154:1157-63.
2. Yang RD, Valenzuela JE: Dysphagia – A practical approach to diagnosis. Dysphagia 1992;92(7):129-46.
3. Jang KM, Lee KS, Lee SJ, et al. The spectrum of benign oesophageal Lesions: Imaging findings. Korean J Radiol 2002;3(3):199-210.
4. Cook IJ. Investigative techniques in the assessment of oral-pharyngeal dysphagia. Dig Dis 1998;16:125-33.
5. Mendelson RM. The gastrointestinal tract. In. Petterson H (Ed): A Global Textbook of Radiology. Vol II Series on diagnostic imaging, Oslo, the Nicer Institute 1995.
6. Levine MS, Rubesin SE, Ott DJ. Update on esophageal radiology. AJR 1990;155:933-41.
7. Leslie P, Carding PN, Wilson JA. Investigation and management of chronic dysphagia. BMJ 2003;326:433-6.
8. Kahrilas P. Esophageal motility disorders: Current concepts of pathogenesis and treatment. Can J Gastroenterol 2000;14:221-31.
9. Ekberg O, Olsson R. Dynamic radiology of swallowing disorders. Endoscopy 1997;29:439-46.
10. Ba- Ssalamah A, Zacheri J, Noebauer - Huhmann IM, et al. Dedicated multi-detector CT of the esophagus: Spectrum of diseases. Abdom Imaging 2007;26.
11. Berkovich GY, Levine MS, Miller WT. CT findings in patients with Oesophagitis. AJR 2000;175:1431-4.
12. Ha HK, Kim JK. The gastrointestinal tract. In Haaga JR, Lanzieri CF, Gilkeson RC (Eds)CT and MR Imaging of the Whole Body. 4th ed Mosby, 2003.
13. Paley MR, Ros PR. MRI of the gastrointestinal tract. Eur Radiol 1997;7:1387-97.
14. Shorvon PJ, Lees WR. The oesophagus, stomach and duodenum: In Cosgrove D, Meire H, Dewbury K (Eds): Abdominal and general ultrasound 2 (1st Edn). Churchill Livingstone, London, 1993.
15. Van Dam J. Endosonography of the oesophagus. Gastrointest Endosc Clin N Am 1994;4(4):803-26.
16. McLoughlin RF, Cooperberg PL, Malhieson JR, et al. High resolution endoluminal ultrasonography in the staging of oesophageal carcinoma. J Ultrasound Med 1995; 14(10):725-30.
17. Wu LF, Wang BZ, Feng JL, et al. Preoperative TN staging of oesophageal cancer: Comparison of miniprobe ultrasonography, spiral CT and MRI. World J Gastroenterol 2003;9(2):219-24.
18. Petrillo R, Balzarini L, Bidoli P, et al. Esophageal squamous cell carcinoma: MRI evaluation of mediastinum. Gastrointest Radiol 1990;15:275-8.
19. Pech O, May A, Gunter E, et al. The impact of endoscopic ultrasound and computed tomography on the TNM staging of early cancer in Barrett's oesophagus. AJR 2006;101:2223-9.
20. Batian RW. Contemporary diagnosis of the dysphagic patient. Otolaryngol Clin N Am 1998;31(3):489-506.
21. Stacey B, Patel P. Oesophageal scintigraphy for the investigation of dysphagia: In and out of favor – and underused when available. European Journal of Nuclear Medicine 2002;29(9):1216-20.
22. Chung JJ, Park HJ, Yu JS, et al. A comparison of oesophagography and oesophageal transit scintigraphy in the evaluation of usefulness of endoscopic pneumatic dilatation in achalasia. Acta Radiologica 2008;49:498-505.
23. Smount A. Manometry of the gastrointestinal tract: Toy or tool? Scand J Gastroenterol Suppl 2001;234:22-8.
24. Leite L, Castell O. Ambulatory oesophageal manometry in the evaluation of unexplained chest pain. Dig Dis 1995;13:145-52.
25. Dent J, Holloway R. Oesophageal motility and reflux testing: State-of-the-art and clinical role in the twenty first century. Gastroenterol Clin N Am 1996;25:51-73.
26. Reynold JC, Parkman HP. Achalasia. Gastroenterol Clin North Am 1989;18:223-257.
27. Gonlachanvit S, Fisher RS, Parkman HP. Diagnostic modalities for achalasia. Gastrointest Endosc Clin N Am 2001;11:293–310.
28. Laufer I. Radiology of Oesophagitis. Radiol Clin North Am 1982;20:687-99.

29. Reid BJ. Barrett's oesophagus and oesophageal adenocarcinoma. Gastroenterol Clin North Am 1991;20:817-34.
30. Levine MS. Barrett's oesophagus: A radiologic diagnosis ? AJR 1988;151:433–38.
31. Levine MS, Macones AJ Jr, Laufer I. Candida Oesophagitis: accuracy of radiographic diagnosis. Radiology 1985;154:581-87.
32. Mazzie DO, Wilson SR, Sadler MA, et al. Imaging of gastrointestinal tract infection. Seminars in Roentgenol 2007;42(2):102-116.
33. Sam JW, Levine MS, Rubesin SE, et al. The 'foamy' oesophagus: A radiographic sign of Candida Oesophagitis. AJR 2000;174:99-100.
34. Levine MS, Laufer I, Kressel HY, Friedman HM. Herpes Oesophagitis. AJR 1981;136:863-66.
35. Levine MS, Rubesin SE. Diseases of the Oesophagus: Diagnosis with esophagography. Radiology 2005; 237:414-27.
36. Rosario MT, Raso CL, Comer GM. Oesophageal tuberculosis. Dig Dis Sci 1989;34:1281.
37. Nagi B, Lal A, Kochhar R, et al. Imaging of oesophageal tuberculosis. Acta Radiologica 2003;44:329-33.
38. Im JG, Kim JH, Han MC, Kim CW. Computed tomography of oesophagomediastinal fistula in tuberculous mediastinal lymphadenitis. J Comput Assist Tomogr 1990;14:89-92.
39. Levine MS. Varices. In Gore RM, Levine MS, (Eds): Textbook of gastrointestinal radiology. (2nd Edn) Philadelphia. Pa: Saunders 2000;452-63.
40. Montesi A, Pesaresi A, Graziani L, et al. Small benign tumors of the oesophagus: Radiological diagnosis with double contrast examination. Gastrointest Radiol 1983;8:207-12.
41. Hatch GF 3rd, Wertheimer-Hatch L, Hatch KF, et al. Tumors of the oesophagus. World J Surg 2000;24:401-11.
42. Seremetis MG, Lyons WS, deGuzman VC, et al. Leiomyomata of the oesophagus. An analysis of 838 cases. Cancer 1976;38:2166-77.
43. Livstone EM, Skinner DB. Tumors of the oesophagus. In: Berk JE, (Ed): Bockus gastroenterology, (4th Edn) Philadelphia, Pa: Saunders 1985;818-40.
44. Levine MS, Halvorsen RA. Carcinoma of the oesophagus. In Gore RM, Levine MS, (Eds): Textbook of gastrointestinal radiology, (2nd Edn) Philadelphia, Pa: Saunders, 2000;403-33.
45. Stewart ET, Doods WJ. Radiology of the esophagus. In Freeny PC, Stevenson GW (Eds): Margulis and Burhenne's Alimentary Tract Radiology (5th Edn). St Louis, Mosby I: 1994.
46. Picus D, Balfe DM, Koehler RE, et al: Computed tomography in the staging of oesophageal carcinoma. Radiology 1983;146:433-8.
47. Barkhansen J, Goyen M, VonWinterfeld F, et al. Visualization of swallowing using real-time True FISP MR fluoroscopy. Eur Radiol 2002;12:129-33.
48. Yamada I, Izumi Y, Kawano T, et al. Superficial oesophageal carcinoma: An in vitro study of high resolution MR imaging at 1.5T. Journal of MRI 2001; 13:225-31.
49. Yamada I, Izumi Y, Kawano T, et al. Oesophageal carcinoma: Evaluation with high-resolution three-dimensional constructive interference in steady state MR imaging in vitro. Journal of Magnetic Resonance Imaging 2006;24:1326-32.
50. Cho ZH, Jo JM. Localized in vitro high resolution NMR imaging using gradient subencoding technique. Med Phys 1991;18(3):350-56.
51. Doran ST, Falk GL, Somorjai RL, et al. Pathology of Barrett's oesophagus by proton magnetic resonance spectroscopy and a statistical classification strategy. Am J Surg 2003;185(3):232-8.
52. Panebianco V, Tomei E, Anzidei M, et al. Functional MRI in the evaluation of oesophageal motility: Feasibility, MRI patterns of normality, and preliminary experience in subjects with motility disorders. La Radiologica Medica 2006;111:881-9.
53. Luketich JD, Friedman DM, Weigel TL, et al. Evaluation of distant metastases in oesophageal cancer: 100 consecutive positron emission tomography scans. Ann Thorac Surg 1999;68(4):1133-36.
54. Block MI, Patterson GA, Sundaresan RS, et al. Improvement in staging of oesophageal cancer with the addition of positron emission tomography. Ann Thorac Surg 1997;64(3):770-6.
55. Korst RJ, Altorki NK. Imaging for oesophageal tumors. Thorac Surg Clin 2004;14:61-9.
56. Bruzzi JF, Munden RF, Truong, MT, et al. PET/CT of oesophageal cancer: Its role in clinical management. Radiographics 2007;27:1635-52.

Chapter Five

Benign Lesions of Stomach and Small Intestine

Gaurav S Pradhan

INTRODUCTION

Stomach and duodenum can be involved by a wide variety of intrinsic diseases in isolation or as a part of systemic diseases or they can be involved by diseases involving adjacent structures. Common nonneoplastic processes affecting the stomach and duodenum include peptic ulcer disease, inflammatory and infective disorders, parasitic infestations, noxious agents or stimuli, congenital abnormalities, miscellaneous disorders and disease processes involving adjacent organs such as pancreatitis, hepatomegaly, etc.

While Hampton recognized the potential use of double contrast examination as an alternative to palpation method as early as 1937, it was in 1950 that after experimenting with double contrast examination of colon, a technique was developed to detect gastric lesions by Prof Hikoo Shirakabe. In 1952, Ruzicka and Rigler described a method for double contrast examination of stomach. This examination became standard in Japan in 1960's and spectacular results were achieved in both mass screening and evaluation of symptomatic patients of early gastric malignancy.

Although the double contrast examination of the stomach was developed primarily to enable the diagnosis of early gastric cancer, this technique has proved valuable in the depiction of gastric ulcers and their sequelae. Its accuracy in depiction of ulcers is substantially better than that of the single contrast method, which relies on the analysis of rugal folds. For double contrast barium meal, mucosal coating is critical, normal areae gastricae should be visualized and distensibility assessed for complete evaluation.

Techniques of Examination

In double contrast evaluation of the stomach and duodenum, an effervescent mixture is administered for gaseous distension of stomach along with 100-150 milliliters of high-density barium sulphate, which is 250% weight by volume. The patient lies on his left side to prevent barium reaching the duodenum quickly and obscuring the greater curvature. The patient then turns supine and on to the right side, to check for presence of gastroesophageal reflux.

Intravenous Buscopan, twenty milligram, is then given. The patient lies on the right side and then rolls over in a complete circle to right anterior oblique position so as to coat the gastric mucosa. Good coating is said to have been achieved if areae gastricae within the gastric antrum are visible. Normally, areae gastricae are round to oval, 1-2 millimeters in width and seen predominantly in body and antrum of stomach. They give a fine reticular to coarse nodular appearance (Fig. 5.1).

Gastric rugal folds can vary widely in dimensions. They are normally less than five millimeters in antrum and less than fifteen millimeters along greater curvature. *The views taken for stomach include*:

1. Right anterior oblique to demonstrate antrum and greater curvature.
2. Supine view to demonstrate antrum and body.

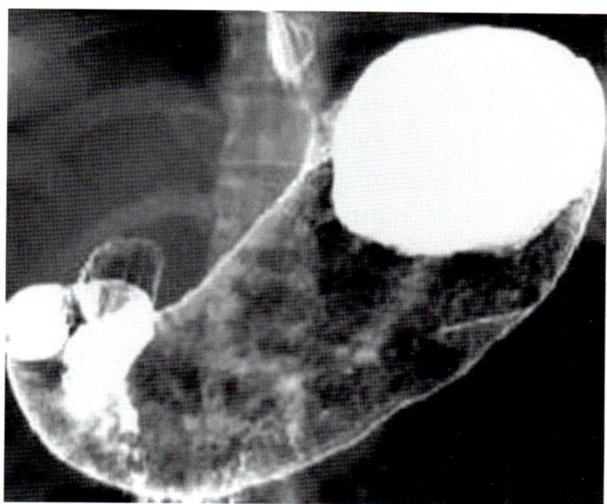

Fig. 5.1: Double contrast barium meal study showing normal areae gastricae [1-2 mm] in width and mucosal pattern in the region of body of stomach

3. Left anterior oblique to demonstrate lesser curvature en face.
4. Left lateral with table tilted forty-five degrees head up, to demonstrate the gastric fundus.

From left lateral position, the patient returns to supine position and then rolls onto left side into prone position to prevent flooding of 'C' loop of duodenum.

The views taken for duodenum include:

1. Spot films of the duodenal loop in prone position with compression pad and right anterior oblique views for anterior wall of the duodenal loop.
2. Spot films of the duodenal cap in prone, right oblique, supine and left anterior oblique positions for barium and gas filled phases.

Erect views of stomach and duodenum should also be taken to complete the examination.

In double contrast examination using barium and air contrast, a shallow barium pool outlines a protruding lesion on dependant surface as a radiolucent filling defect and a depressed lesion such as ulcer as a pool of barium.

Hypotonic Duodenography

A Bilbao-Dotter Teflon coated tube with guide wire is used for the examination. Twenty to thirty milliliters of high density barium sulphate is instilled through the tube into the duodenum, for mucosal coating. This is followed by pumping of air through the Bilbao-Dotter tube. Hyoscine-N-butyl bromide [Buscopan] is used as the hypotonic agent, as it has immediate onset of action and is preloaded into the intravenous tubing. Intravenous Buscopan, twenty milligram is given to paralyze peristalsis and immediately supine oblique and prone oblique views of the duodenum are obtained.

In double contrast examination, using the flow technique and distension with air, multiple projections as mentioned above are taken with varying degrees of patient rotation including profile views, showing projecting ulcer and enface views, showing pool of barium in ulcer crater. The flow technique is useful for ulcers on posterior wall and lesser curvature and prone compression views are useful for ulcers on anterior wall, in the region of antrum and body. The ulcers high on lesser curvature are difficult to see in profile views, so views in right posterior oblique position are required for their better delineation.

Other radiologic imaging modalities for evaluation of stomach and duodenum include gastrograffin studies in suspected perforation and in postoperative cases, angiography, ultrasound and computed tomography.

MDCT and 3D Imaging Techniques

With the advent of multidetector CT and 3D imaging techniques including volume rendering with interactive 3D and stereoscopic display, computed tomography is fast emerging as an important diagnostic tool in diagnosing diseases of stomach and duodenum.[1, 2] Dual phase scanning with rapid intravenous bolus of contrast is required. Dual phase scanning protocol allows acquisition of arterial phase images 25 seconds after and venous phase images 50 seconds after injection of contrast. MDCT with thin collimation (1.25 mm sections reformatted at 1 mm intervals) is performed using water as oral contrast agent. Water is preferred as an oral contrast agent over positive oral contrast medium, as enhancing gastric wall and subtle abnormalities can be well visualized and because it does not interfere with 3D imaging and CT angiography (Fig. 5.2). 750 ml of water should be given 15 minutes before scanning, with additional 250 ml when patient is on table. Intravenous Buscopan 10 mg is given for hypotonia. Effervescent granules can be given for distension. Supine, prone and decubitus scanning can be done for optimal distension and visualization of the region of interest. Some authors advocate use of left posterior oblique (LPO) position for maximum distensibility and minimal fluid retention in lower part of stomach, for producing excellent 3D CT

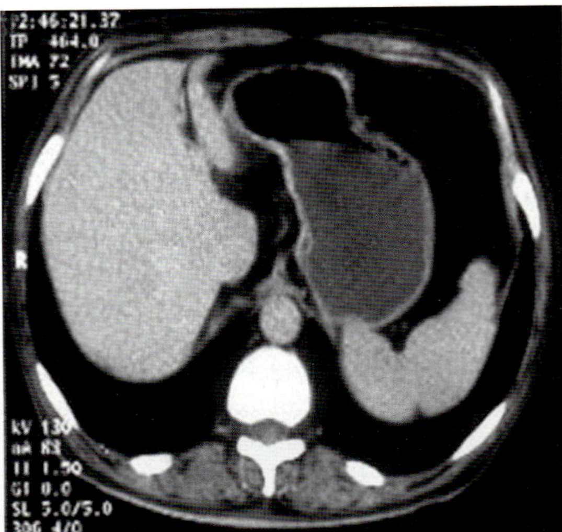

Fig. 5.2: Axial CT image with water as oral contrast showing enhancing gastric wall, well demarcated against negative intraluminal contrast and perigastric fat

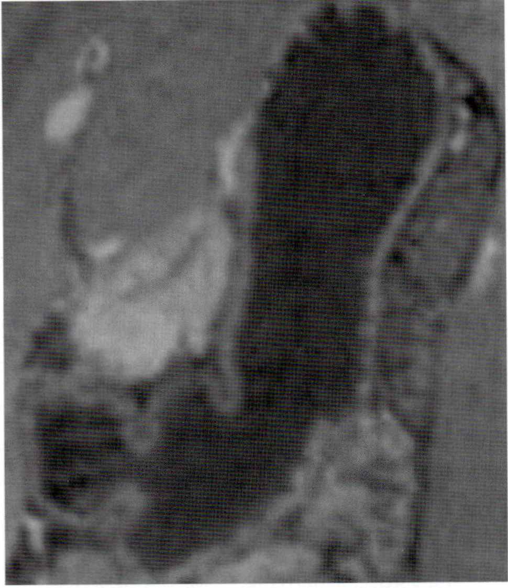

Fig. 5.3: 3D MPR CT image in coronal plane with water as oral contrast showing enhancing gastric wall and rugae

gastrographic images.[3] 3D MPR volume set in coronal, axial, and sagittal planes can be obtained which can be helpful in treatment planning (Fig. 5.3). Clinicians prefer coronal oblique projections, as the orientation is similar to routine upper GIT series. CT data can be processed to simulate endoscopic images (virtual gastroscopy).[4, 5] An added advantage is that transparency, brightness, window level and window width can be altered. Clip planes and different orientations can be used to visualize the entire stomach. This technique accentuates stomach rugal folds and wall. However, flat lesions are difficult to pick up by this technique.

CT is primarily required for detection and staging of malignancy. CT is not the modality of choice for benign conditions such as suspected peptic ulcer disease, but may have been requested for non-specific complaints. CT can diagnose free perforation when free intra-peritoneal air or gas is seen but cannot be used to determine the exact site of perforation. Enhancing mucosa and low attenuation submucosa due to edema can give rise to "halo" sign and help differentiate from neoplastic conditions.[5] The normal gastric wall measures 5-7 mm with optimal distension, with effacement of normal gastric folds. In gastritis, the thickness is usually less than 10 mm while in carcinoma it is usually more than 10 mm. In lymphoma, gastric wall thickness is usually more than 20 mm. Further, we should remember that focal thickening in adult hypertrophic pyloric stenosis and thickening involving antrum and greater curvature in *H. pylori* gastritis, can mimic gastric neoplasm. So, it is prudent to be careful while dealing with cases of focal thickening. Double contrast barium meal examination is the diagnostic modality of choice in such cases.

CT evaluation of duodenum requires dynamic administration of intravenous contrast with thin collimation, for identification of vascular structures and enhancement pattern of lesions affecting duodenum. Patient can be placed in the right posterior oblique position to maximize opacification of first and second parts of duodenum while left posterior oblique position is helpful when carbon dioxide is used for distension of duodenum.[6]

MR Imaging

With adequate distension of the gastric lumen, MR can provide adequate information regarding stomach wall and associated abnormality in perigastric region. MR requires rapid imaging to decrease the effect of respiratory motion and peristalsis. Negative intraluminal agents on fat suppressed gadolinium enhanced T1 weighted images are desirable, as dark lumen helps in highlighting the adjacent enhancing gastric wall (Fig. 5.4). The normal gastric wall enhances less than or equal to

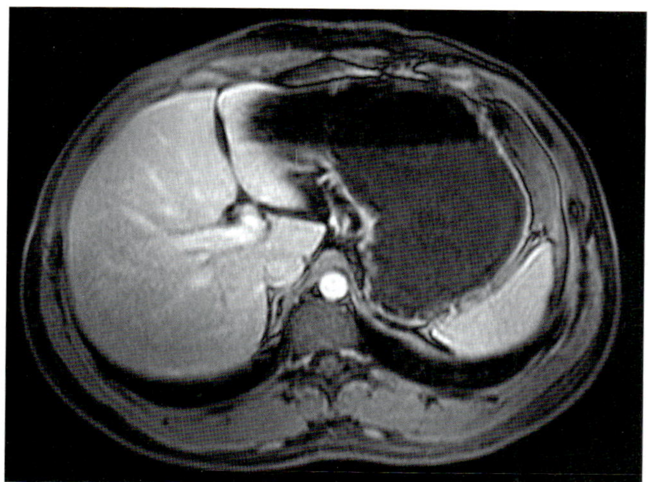

Fig. 5.4: MR T1 weighted gadolinium enhanced axial image, showing enhancing gastric wall, highlighted due to negative intraluminal contrast and perigastric fat

liver parenchyma. Multiplanar breath hold single shot rapid relaxation enhancement [SSRARE] for T2 weighted and breath hold fat suppressed spoiled gradient echo [SGE] imaging for T1 weighted acquisition, following gadolinium administration are required for evaluation of normal gastric mucosa and portion of stomach showing mural thickening with enhancement. Modifying SSRARE acquisition, by acquiring a thick slab coronal image with long TE [900 msec] can generate a MR hydrogram image similar to barium series. This acquisition shows high signal intensity of intraluminal contrast in stomach. Alternatively, volumetric imaging with 3D gradient echo pulse sequence like THRIVE, VIBE can be taken (Fig. 5.5A). Inversion recovery fat suppression can be added to 3D acquisition, to improve conspicuity of enhancing inflamed mucosa. True fast imaging with steady precession [FISP] can also be acquired for T2 weighted images[7] (Fig. 5.5B).

Double contrast barium upper gastrointestinal series are cost effective and have the advantage of speed, safety, patient comfort and do not require the administration of sedative drugs. Further, double contrast barium technique allows a detailed assessment of the mucosa of stomach and duodenum. Therefore, it is useful to consider a pattern approach for the radiologic diagnosis of benign lesions.

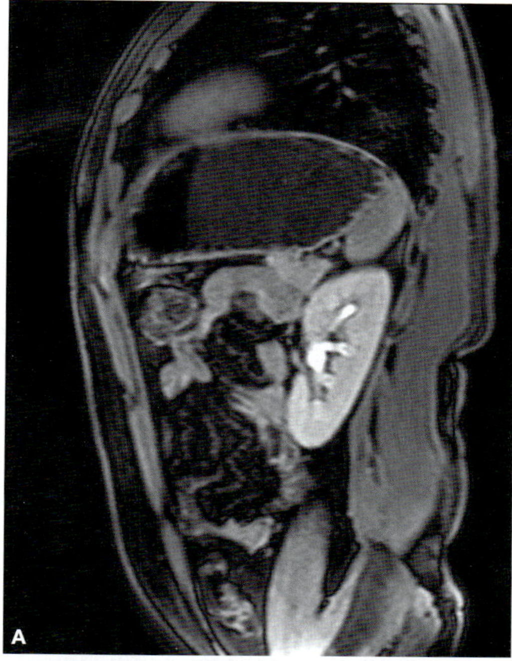

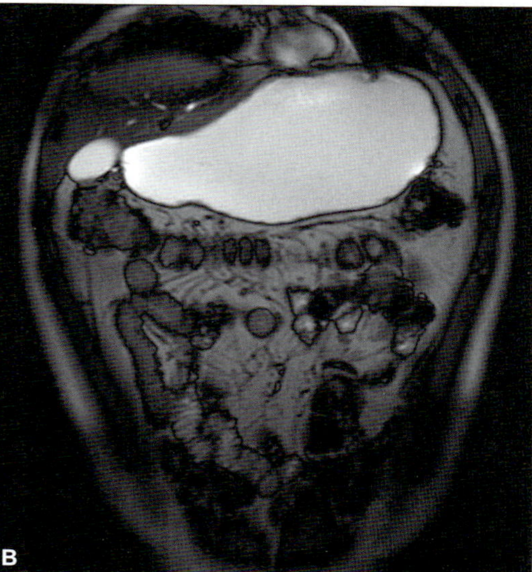

Figs 5.5A and B: (A) VIBE MR postgadolinium enhanced T1 weighted sagittal image showing enhancing wall of stomach, well demarcated against water and air distended stomach and perigastric fat, (B) True FISP MR coronal image in the same patient, for T2 weighted image

Erosive and Ulcerative Lesions of Stomach and Duodenum

Ulcer is a defect of full thickness of mucosa that may extend into deeper layers, while erosion is an epithelial defect not penetrating beyond muscularis mucosae.

Complete erosion also called varioliform erosion is associated with mucosal edema while incomplete erosion occurs without mucosal edema. The importance of identifying the ulcer lies not only because of its associated morbidity and mortality but also because of the risk of malignancy.

Approximately in half of the patients with erosive lesions the cause is not known. In the remainder, the cause may be traced to offending agents like aspirin, NSAID, corrosive substances, noxious stimuli, irradiation, and diseases such as Crohn's disease and sarcoidosis. The etiological agents may also include various infective agents like *H. pylori*, *cytomegalovirus* and parasitic infestation like *anisakiasis*.[8]

Most benign gastric ulcers occur on the lesser curvature while they can also occur in the antrum and body of the stomach. Fifteen percent of ulcers occur on anterior wall or greater curvature. In younger patients, ulcers occur in distal part of stomach while in older patients they occur high up on lesser curvature because junction of antral mucosa and corpus mucosa moves upwards with age. These ulcers in older patients are called "Geriatric ulcers". Benign ulcers on greater curvature occur in distal half and are associated with aspirin and NSAID use. All patients receiving aspirin develop erosions while 15-20% develop gastric ulcer.[9]

NSAID ulcer resembles gastric ulcer except that the surrounding mucosa shows less *H. pylori* associated gastritis. These ulcers appear intra luminal with presence of mass effect and thick mucosal folds. Biopsy may be required to differentiate from malignancy.

Duodenal ulcer is three times more common than gastric ulcer. Ninety-five percent of patients with duodenal ulcers have stomach infected with *H. pylori* . Patients with duodenal ulcers usually have antral predominant gastritis with gastric metaplasia of duodenal mucosa. Ninety-five percent of ulcers occur in bulb, with anterior and posterior wall involvement with equal frequency, while the remainder occur in postbulbar region and duodenal sweep.

Postbulbar ulceration commonly occurs on medial aspect of second part of duodenum with indentation on opposite wall due to spasm in early and fibrosis in late cases, which may lead to "ring stricture". Hypotonic duodenography may be required in cases where only eccentric indentation is seen without ulcer niche.

Common causes of postbulbar ulceration include peptic ulcer disease, Zollinger Ellison syndrome, Crohn's disease, and tuberculosis. In Zollinger Ellison syndrome there are ulcers in second, third and fourth part of duodenum besides gastric and jejunal ulcers. Ectopic pancreas can also simulate postbulbar ulceration.

The classic signs of a benign ulcer include projection beyond the contour, presence of Hampton line, smooth ulcer collar or mound, symmetrical radiating folds to edge of crater and penetration of ulcer on single and double contrast barium studies.[10]

The diagnostic features of an ulcer to be evaluated are its location, size, shape, multiplicity and healing which help distinguish between a benign and malignant ulcer.

Radiologic appearances of benign ulcer include:

a. *Ulcer crater or niche*

   Direct evidence of benign ulcer in the stomach is visualization of barium filled crater projecting beyond line of mucosal contour (Fig. 5.6). It should also be viewed enface to visualize surrounding mucosal folds reaching edge of ulcer crater or collar. Ring sign is seen when only margin of ulcer is coated with barium while double ring sign is seen when base of ulcer is broader than neck. Crescent sign results when barium is trapped in ulcer due to extensive edema. When barium collection has ellipsoid configuration, long

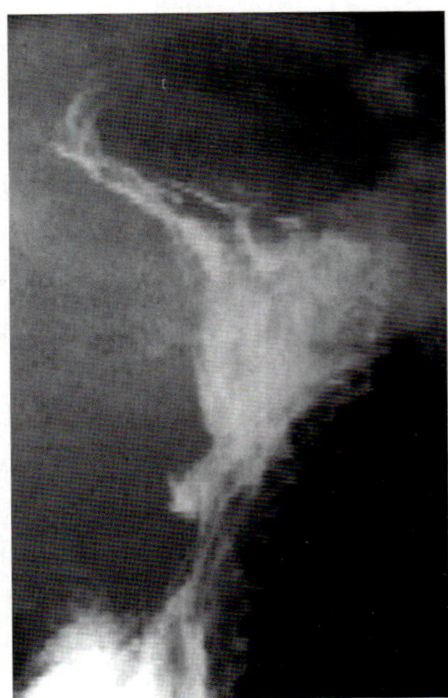

Fig. 5.6: Barium filled crater seen projecting beyond the line of gastric contour on profile view

axis being parallel to lumen it implies acute ulceration, while when it is perpendicular it represents deformity without ulceration. This is called ellipse sign. Both ulcer and deformity can coexist in the same area.

Majority of duodenal ulcers are round or oval although linear ulcers can also occur. Anterior wall ulcers are common and are seen as "ring" shadow since they are non-dependent. The mucosal folds are edematous and reach edge of the ulcer mound. Giant ulcers of more than two centimeters can occur and may mimic normal or scarred bulb, but they do not change size or shape.

Gadolinium enhanced spoiled gradient echo images can demonstrate mural thickening with central ulceration in peptic ulcer disease. Imaging in prone position can help in better gastric distension.

b. *Hampton's line, ulcer collar, and ulcer mound*

On profile view, overhanging edge of resistant mucosa produces a thin radiolucent line, which rims the mouth of ulcer crater, called the Hampton' s line (Fig. 5.7). Smooth translucent band or collar formation occurs when the overhanging mucosa is edematous. When there is marked edematous response ulcer mound results.

c. *Radiating folds*

In benign ulcer, the mucosal folds are smooth, symmetrical, and radiate from edge of ulcer crater, collar, or mound (Fig. 5.8).

d. *Incisura*

An incisura or indentation is seen on the wall opposite to ulcer due to edema or spasm of circular muscle.

e. *Hyperplastic polyps*

Hyperplastic polyps can occur because of inflammatory response of the gastric epithelium. They can be sessile or pedunculated, single or multiple and can occur anywhere in stomach. They do not grow or grow very slowly. Differentiation from malignancy is only possible histologically.

f. *Ulcer healing*

Complete healing is interpreted as a sign of benign ulcer, however, it is not 100% accurate, as a very small percentage of malignant ulcers may show healing similar to benign ulcer. H_2 antagonistic therapy of 6-8 weeks with concomitant withdrawal of causative agent like aspirin, NSAID results in decreasing size of ulcer and change in shape from round or oval to linear. With the usage of proton pump inhibitor like omeprazole, ulcers heal despite continuation of aspirin and NSAIDs. Splitting of ulcer can occur with healing. Two ulcer niches form at periphery because the rate of healing is more rapid at the center.

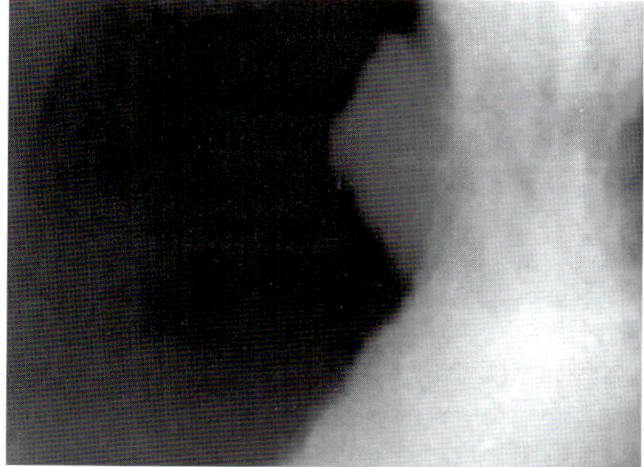

Fig. 5.7: Thin radiolucent line (Hampton's line) rimming the mouth of ulcer crater on profile view

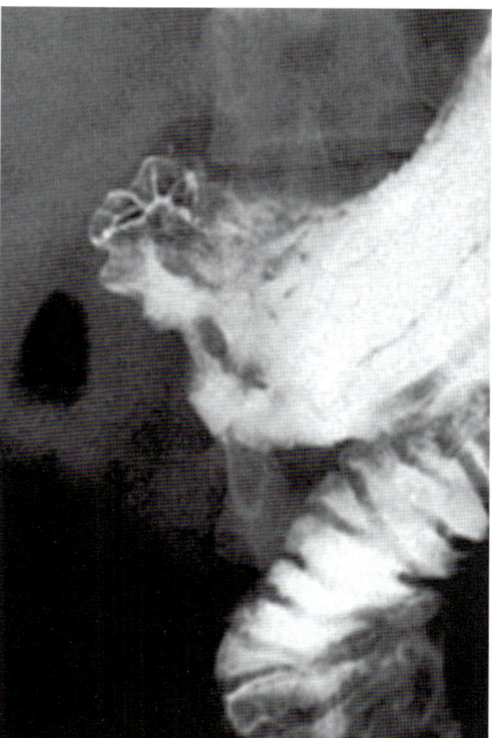

Fig. 5.8: Barium meal study showing barium filled ulcer crater with smooth, symmetrical radiating folds reaching edge of the ulcer crater

g. *Deformities and complications*
Pyloric spasm or scarring can result in gastric outlet obstruction (Fig. 5.9). Bizarre deformities can occur because of ulcer scarring. Some typical deformities like the *linitis plastica* pattern and the "Hour-Glass" deformity can also occur with gastric ulcer disease. Large ulcers with active bleeding can be seen on fluoroscopy, with barium displacing the non-opaque blood. Ulcers can perforate into abdominal cavity, which manifests as free air under dome of diaphragm along with signs of peritonitis. They can penetrate into pancreas, gastrohepatic omentum, biliary tract, liver, greater omentum, mesocolon and colon.[11] They can be walled off by neighboring structures and lead to perigastric pouch formation (Fig. 5.10). Seventy-five percent of duodenal ulcers perforating posteriorly into pancreas show evidence of extra-luminal air. CT can diagnose free perforation when free intra-peritoneal air or gas is seen but cannot be used to determine the exact site of perforation. Double pylorus, a form of gastroduodenal fistula, anterior to pyloric canal can develop with pyloric ulcer, with some reduction in symptoms of gastric outlet obstruction. Fistula formation can also occur as a complication of duodenal ulcer. Deformities that result in chronic duodenal ulcer include scarring and pseudodiverticula formation, which can be single or multiple. Multiple pseudodiverticulae can result in classical "Trifoliate" deformity (Fig. 5.11).

Radiological features that help in differentiating benign from malignant ulcers are that in malignant ulcer, the base is irregular and the ulcer does not project beyond contour as it is within a tumor mound. Further, there is obliteration of surrounding areae gastricae with involvement of radiating folds, which are thick, irregular, and amputated at tumor edge. Bull's eye lesion may be seen in metastatic deposits in patients of melanoma, carcinoma breast or carcinoma lung.

Pseudolymphoma is thought to be a response to chronic peptic ulcer disease manifesting as irregular large ulcer with thick enlarged folds. Linitis pattern in pseudolymphoma is associated with giant ulcers. Giant ulcers are more than three centimeters in diameter. These ulcers have also been associated with aspirin intake.

When gastric ulcer is intraluminal, has mass effect with shouldered edges with thick irregular folds and distorted areae gastricae, it is labeled as equivocal ulcer. Four to six biopsies are necessary to rule out malignancy.[11] With good enface views and three categories of diagnosis permitted, that is, benign, equivocal, and malignant, diagnosis of benign ulcer has high accuracy of 99%. Endoscopy is only indicated when radiologic findings are not typical of benign ulcer, when healing does not proceed at expected rate or when surrounding mucosa is nodular or irregular.[12,13]

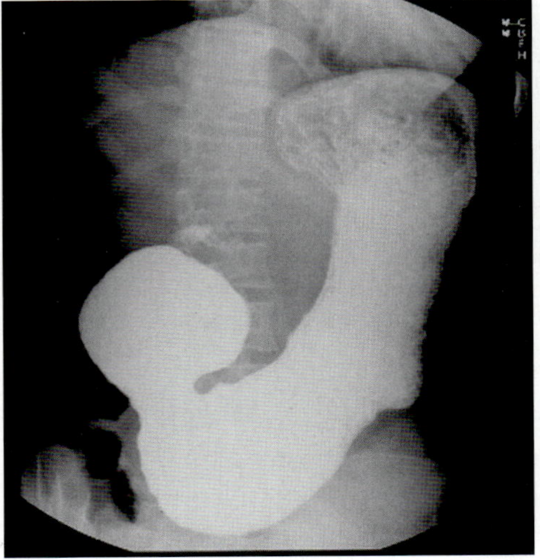

Fig. 5.9: A case of gastric outlet obstruction due to pyloric stenosis in which the stomach is enlarged and dilated with evidence of food mixed with barium

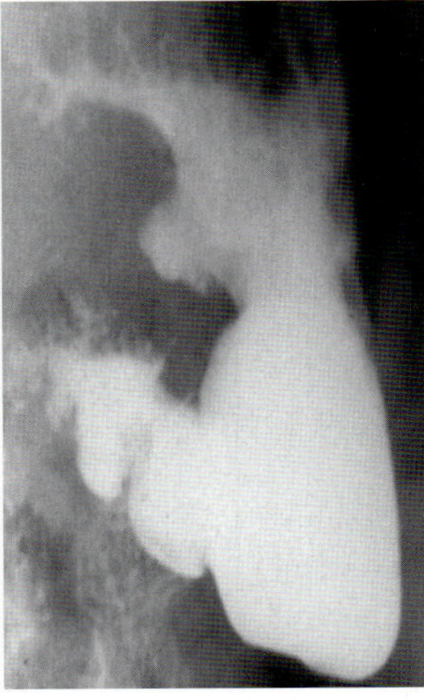

Fig. 5.10: Gastric ulcer in distal lesser curvature with perigastric pouch formation, due to localized leak

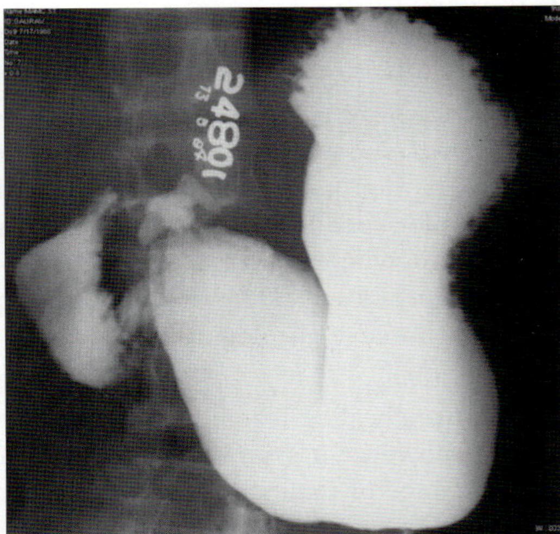

Fig. 5.11: Post-ulcer sequelae in a case of chronic duodenal ulcer, leading to pseudodiverticulum formation, with classical trifoliate deformity

NARROWING OF STOMACH

Several non-neoplastic diseases can cause narrowing of stomach. These include peptic ulcer disease, corrosives, iron intoxication, infiltrative disorders, and infective diseases, etc.

In peptic ulcer disease, there can be antral narrowing with rigidity. Acute ulcer may not be seen due to lack of distensibility.

In corrosive poisoning, there is antral stricturing due to coagulative necrosis, seen more with concentrated acids (Fig. 5.12). Acids produce more severe damage than alkali, though highly concentrated alkali in liquid form is capable of damaging the stomach wall as well. Gastric folds are thickened with mucosal ulceration, atony, or rigidity with fixed open pylorus. Differential diagnosis includes malignancy, if there is no history of corrosive intake. Associated changes in esophagus also help in differentiating from a malignant lesion.

Iron intoxication can occur in children due to ingestion of ferrous sulphate tablets. There is intense corrosive action on gastric mucosa with necrosis and hemorrhage, which is often fatal. Antral strictures develop in survivors, in ten days to six weeks. Freezing and radiation are associated with marked scarring and narrowing. There is high incidence of hemorrhage and perforation following gastric irradiation injury.

In Crohn's disease, there is narrowing of the antrum, widening of pylorus and narrowing of bulb with flared up tubular antrum opening into corpus of stomach giving the classical "ram's horn" appearance. Other findings include nodules, thickened folds, linear and transverse ulcers, and stricture formation. Gastric involvement occurs in two to twenty percent of cases of Crohn's disease elsewhere in gastrointestinal tract.[14]

Pseudolymphoma, amyloidosis, sarcoidosis, eosinophilc gastritis, syphilis, strongyloidosis can also cause narrowing of stomach.

Narrowing and elongation of pyloric canal of two to four centimeters, thick muscular wall of more than one centimeter, which can be easily diagnosed on ultrasound as sonolucent "doughnut" sign, characterize hypertrophic pyloric stenosis, both infantile and adult. Previously diagnosis was limited to barium study. Findings on barium study include narrow, elongated pyloric canal seen as "string sign", barium cleft in pyloric niche as "teat sign", mushroom shaped defect indenting base of bulb due to hypertrophic muscle and "double track sign" due to invagination into narrow pyloric canal.

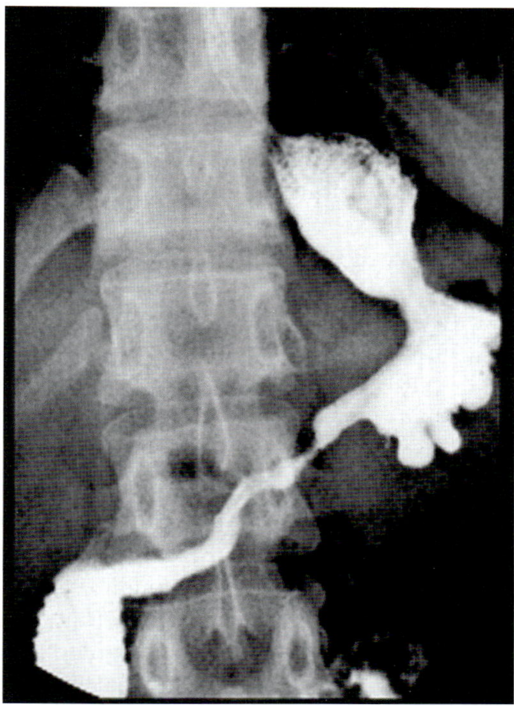

Fig. 5.12: Corrosive acid poisoning involving body of stomach with multiple pseudodiverticulae formation, with stricturing of antropyloric region

Gatroplasty, surgery done for weight reduction, results in localized narrowing.

Exogastric causes like hepatomegaly, pancreatic pseudocyst can cause extrinsic compression of stomach.

THICKENED GASTRIC FOLDS AND FILLING DEFECTS

Thickened gastric folds can be seen in gastritis, peptic ulcer disease, corrosives, irradiation, infections, Menetrier's disease, Crohn's disease and miscellaneous conditions like varices, etc. Gastric folds are usually thick and prominent in fundus and proximal body especially along greater curvature.

Alcohol intake can cause thickening of gastric folds, which subsides after withdrawal.

In hypertrophic gastritis there are thickened rugal folds of more than five millimeter in antral area and of more than one and a half centimeter along greater curvature. There are also prominent areae gastricae of four to five millimeters, which are polygonal or angular, throughout stomach. In antral gastritis, that is gastritis associated with *H.pylori*, there is mucosal fold thickening in antrum. We should remember that on computed tomography, focal thickening involving antrum and greater curvature in *H. pylori* gastritis can mimic gastric neoplasm. So, it is prudent to be careful while dealing with cases of focal thickening on computed tomography (Figs 5.13A and B). Adequate distension of region of interest, using decubitus scanning is essential.[15] Even then, double contrast barium examination remains the modality of choice to clinch the diagnosis.

Corrosive intake results in primarily distal involvement, as they travel along lesser curvature, with ulceration and fixed open pylorus. Irradiation results in ulceration with thick gastric folds, which heal with intense scarring.

Infections can result in thickening of gastric folds. Phelgmonous gastritis is an acute infective condition, with heightened risk of fatality, caused by various pathogenic organisms in which there is marked thickening of gastric walls with swollen rugae. At CT, the stomach is thickened and there is air within the layers of the stomach. In addition, there is a benign asymptomatic entity called gastric emphysema that may also lead to gas within the gastric wall. This condition resolves on its own, but the appearance of these two conditions is similar.

In peptic ulcer disease, ulceration with thick gastric folds is seen. Thick gastric and duodenal folds with multiple ulcerations in stomach, duodenum, and jejunum are seen in Zollinger Ellison syndrome.[16, 17] Hyperplastic polyps that constitute 90% of all gastric polyps are thought to be an unusual response of gastric epithelium to chronic peptic ulcer disease. They are small, multiple, smooth masses, distributed throughout the stomach, though may be clustered in fundus and body.

In Ménétrier's disease, there is massive enlargement of gastric rugae, folded on each other. There is also increased mucus secretion, with marked protein loss with decreased acid production with lesser curvature being infrequently involved. Thickened folds are soft and mobile and may simulate polypoidal-filling defects. The disease is associated with *H. pylori* in more than 90% cases and eradication of *H. pylori* with treatment results in return of giant folds to normal with normal mucosal histology and normal serum protein concentrations.[18-20]

Lymphocytic gastritis is also associated with giant gastric folds of about 13-20 millimeters. Giant gastric folds are also associated with inflammation due to *H.pylori* and in Ménétrier's disease. Echogenic thickening of mucosal layer, seen using endoscopic ultrasound may be a characteristic feature of protein losing gastropathy.[21] In acute phase of eosinophilic gastritis, there are enlarged rugae and polypoidal lesions.

In early phase of Crohn's disease, there is cobble stoning of antral folds, scalloping, fissuring, and aphthous ulcers. There is poorly distensile smooth tubular antrum in late stage.

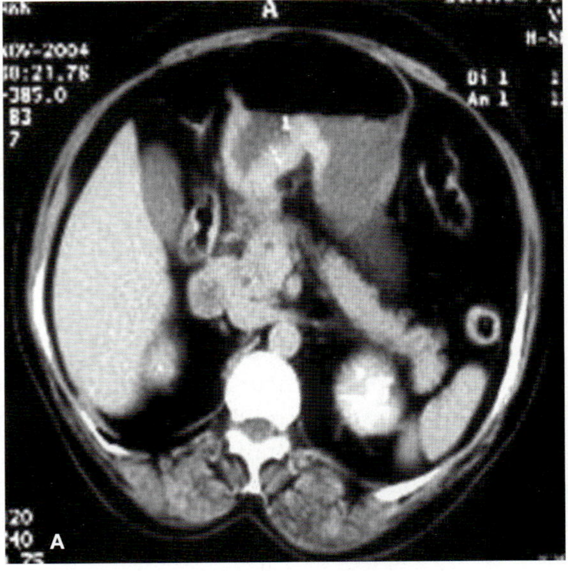

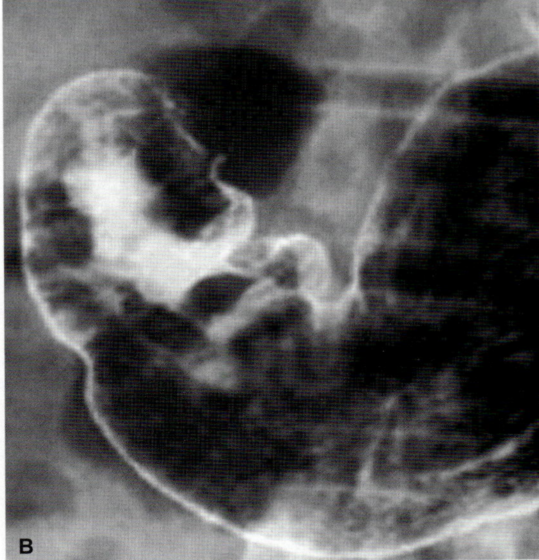

Figs 5.13A and B: (A) CECT abdomen in a patient, showing mural thickening [1.2 cm] of the gastric antrum with maintained perigastric planes. This case was misinterpreted as malignant on CT, (B) Double contrast barium meal study in the same patient showing abnormal areae gastricae in the gastric antrum with normal distensibility, suggestive of antral gastritis, thus ruling out malignancy

Thick rugal folds with superficial erosions, ulcerations, irregularly narrow rigid antrum can occur due to circumferential amyloid deposition in gastric amyloidosis.

Thickened gastric folds can be seen with gastric varices. Fundal varices are generally associated with esophageal varices, while isolated varices may occur with splenic vein occlusion. Gastric varices can also be seen as smooth lobulated defects in fundus and can extend along the lesser curvature. Gastric varices appear as enhancing vessels during the portal venous phase, along body and fundus of stomach (Fig. 5.14). Collateral vessels, in addition can be seen along gastrohepatic ligament. Varices typically will not enhance during arterial phase. CT angiography and 3D CT can help in identifying small perigastric vessels which are not picked up on routine computed tomography.

Fat suppressed gadolinium enhanced SGE MR images can also show enhancing tubular structures in gastric wall in portal venous phase, 45-90 seconds after injection of contrast. 3D gradient echo image can be post-processed, to create MR venogram image showing the extent of portal venous collaterals.

Gastric fold thickening may also be seen in tuberculosis.

Nodular, serpentine, mucosal folds are seen in posterior wall and along lesser curvature in pancreatitis.

Bezoars are intragastric masses composed of accumulated ingested material. These can be phytobezoars, composed of fruit and vegetable material, trichobezoars, made up of hairballs, which are seen more

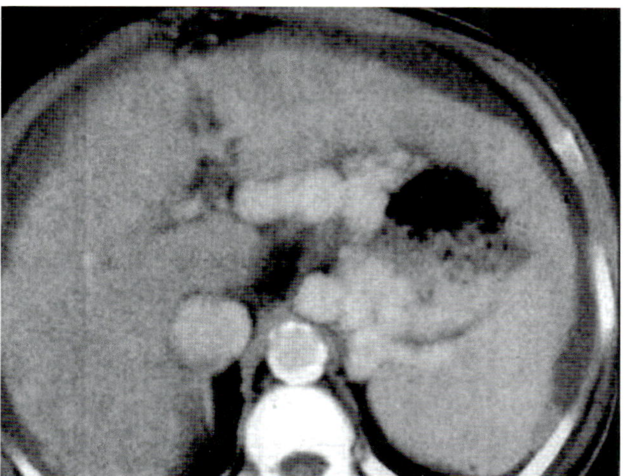

Fig. 5.14: Contrast enhanced axial CT image, in venous phase, showing enhancing gastric varices

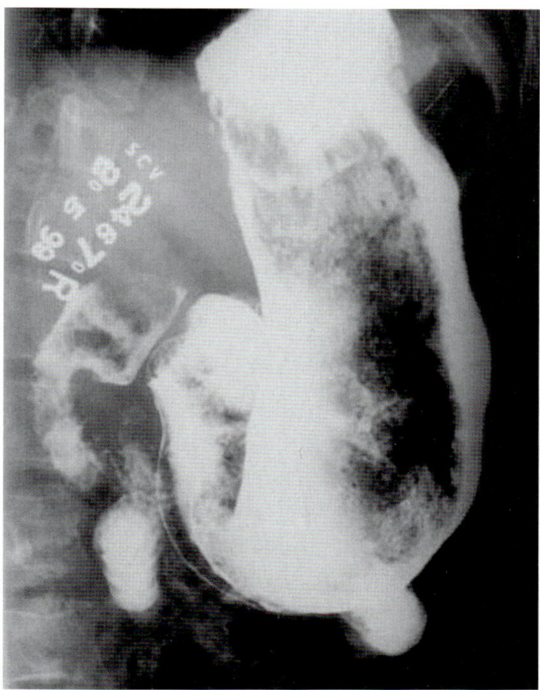

Fig. 5.15: A case of Trichobezoar showing hair balls constituting filling defect in the stomach, with extension into duodenum

in females and trichophytobezoars having features of both of the above, or rarely can be of other ingested material[22, 23] (Fig. 5.15). They are mobile masses, giving mottled appearance on barium, "compressed concentric ring" appearance free of gastric wall on CT and superficially located broadband of high amplitude echoes on ultrasound. Mechanical small bowel obstruction alone, or with perforation can result with distal extension of bezoar.[24]

Ectopic pancreas occur in greater curvature, within 3-6 centimeters of pylorus, presenting as sub-mucosal masses less than or equal to two centimeters with a central dimple or orifice, which may fill with barium and outline ductal structures.

Gastric duplication can be present as an extrinsic or intramural mass along greater curvature. If communicating with lumen, it can fill with barium. Computed tomography demonstrates relationship of mass to gastric wall as well as non-enhancing fluid content or debris in cyst. Gastric diverticulum is most commonly seen involving posterior gastric cardia. It can be seen on SSRARE MR images as air or fluid filled outpouching from adjacent stomach. Fat suppressed gadolinium enhanced SGE images show thin enhancing wall, similar to normal gastric mucosa.

REDUCED OR ABSENT RUGAL FOLDS

Absent or decreased rugal folds may be seen in atrophic gastritis. Type A atrophy gastritis is associated with pernicious anemia. There is decreased acid production, decreased intrinsic factor, and increased antibodies to parietal cells. There may be tubular stomach with lesser and greater curvature being parallel to each other.

There can be relative absence of folds in chronic alcoholic gastritis.

GAS IN WALL OF STOMACH

Gas bubbles in gastric wall with marked thickening of wall is seen in phelgmonous gastritis, which is an acute fulminant condition associated with necrosis caused by alpha hemolytic streptococci in more than 70% of the cases. Other agents include *Clostridium welchii, E. coli,* etc.

Gastric emphysema, that is air in the gastric wall, can also occur in the absence of infectious agents. Ingestion of corrosive agents is a common cause while gastric ulcers are a rare cause of this disease. It can also occur due to trauma, ischemia, and peptic ulcer with intramural perforation, gastric outlet obstruction, and following gastroscopy, and in a benign condition called "pneumatosis intestinalis".

GASTRIC OUTLET OBSTRUCTION

Gastric outlet obstruction can occur from peptic ulcer disease in about 60% of cases. Other non-neoplastic causes of obstruction include Crohn's disease, pancreatitis, volvulus, prior surgery, bezoar, corrosives, and prolapsed antral mucosa.

Certain congenital conditions like hypertrophic pyloric stenosis, antral diaphragm are also associated with outlet obstruction. Antral diaphragm is a membrane within three centimeters of pyloric canal. Gastric outlet obstruction does not occur if the diameter of the diaphragm is more than a centimeter.

Hypertrophic pyloric stenosis, both infantile and adult, are characterized by narrow and elongated pyloric canal and thick muscular wall, which can be confirmed by ultrasound.

GASTRIC DILATATION WITHOUT OBSTRUCTION

Acute gastric dilation is a serious condition and can occur with abdominal surgery, abdominal trauma, severe abdominal pain or renal colic, inflammatory conditions like peritonitis, pancreatitis, subphrenic abscess, septicemia, immobilization in case of a body plaster cast or in paraplegia because of difficulty in belching, or compression of third part of duodenum.

Chronic gastric dilatation can occur in diabetes mellitus, neuromuscular diseases like bulbar poliomyelitis, tabes dorsalis, vagotomy, scleroderma. It can also occur in electrolyte imbalance, emotional distress, porphyria and lead poisoning.

POSITIONAL ABNORMALITIES

Positional or configurational abnormalities include hiatus hernia, volvulus, and gastric hernias. The gastric hernias are rare occurring through incision or umbilicus. There is distorted appearance of stomach on anteroposterior view of barium study and the diagnosis is confirmed on lateral view.

In hiatus hernia, stomach is seen to herniate through the esophageal hiatus. The radiological features on barium study of hiatus hernia include:

a. A pouch of stomach above hiatus of size more than two centimeters.
b. Three or more gastric folds crossing hiatus.
c. Wide hiatus of more than three centimeters.
d. "Polyp and fold" complex.

Sliding hernia is more common than rolling hernia (Fig. 5.16). Gastroesophageal reflux and peptic esophagitis is often observed in sliding hiatus hernia. Para-

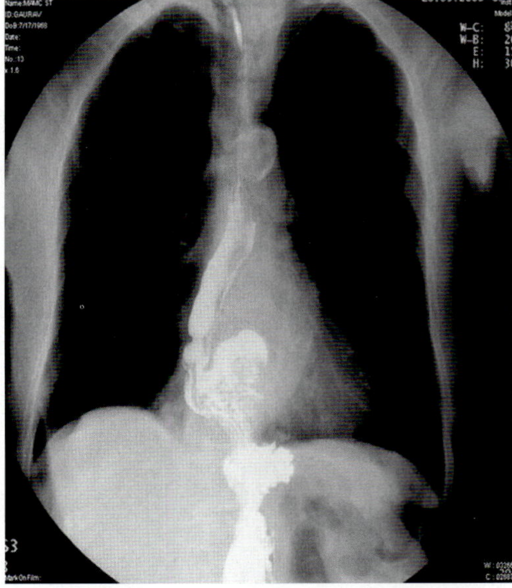

Fig. 5.16: Pouch of stomach seen above the diaphragmatic hiatus, with more than three gastric mucosal folds crossing the hiatus, in a case of sliding hiatus hernia

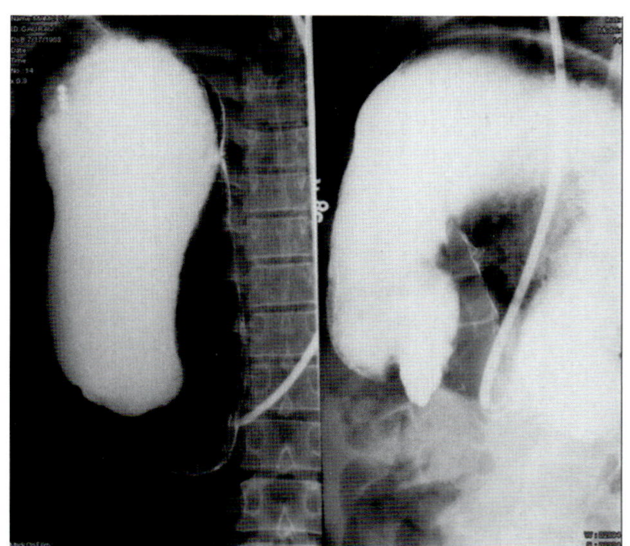

Fig. 5.17: Greater curvature seen lying above the level of lesser curvature, with down pointing of pylorus and duodenum, in a case of volvulus of stomach

esophageal or rolling hernia is less common, in which gastroesophageal junction position is maintained, and fundus of stomach herniates into thorax to lie in posterior mediastinum. It is more prone to ulceration, incarceration, and obstruction.

Herniation of stomach into thorax is also associated with traumatic rupture of left dome of diaphragm.

Volvulus of stomach can be organoaxial or mesentero-axial, depending on axis of rotation (Fig. 5.17). In organoaxial volvulus, stomach rotates upwards along long axis that is along cardia with pylorus, with antrum moving from inferior to superior position. It is commonly seen in elderly population and is usually asymptomatic.

In mesentero-axial volvulus, stomach rotates along axis of gastrohepatic omentum, that is, a line connecting middle of lesser and greater curvatures. There is inversion of stomach, that is greater curvature above level of lesser curvature with cardia and pylorus at same level and down pointing of pylorus and duodenum. It is associated with obstruction and common in children and following trauma.

Cascade stomach is a normal variant, in which fundal cup fills with barium and spills along lesser curvature and posterior wall.

THICKENING OF DUODENAL FOLDS

Thickening of duodenal folds can occur in peptic ulcer disease, Zollinger Ellison syndrome, pancreatitis uremia, Crohn's disease, eosinophilic gastroenteritis, amyloidosis, Whipple's disease, parasitic infestations like *Giardia* and strongyloidosis, in AIDS patients and miscellaneous conditions like vascular abnormalities, cystic fibrosis, etc.[25]

Fold thickening is the most common presentation of peptic ulcer disease. Cobble stone appearance results from Brunner gland hyperplasia, which occurs as response to peptic ulcer disease.[26] Fold thickening in duodenum and stomach with multiple ulcerations in duodenal bulb, stomach, and atypical sites like post-bulbar, second, third and fourth part of duodenum, jejunum is seen in Zollinger Ellison syndrome.

Thick folds may be seen in uremia involving bulb and second part of duodenum and in pancreatitis with mass impression on "C" loop.

Diffuse fold thickening, ulceration, luminal narrowing can be seen in Crohn's disease, Eosinophilic gastroenteritis, amyloidosis, and Whipple's disease. In Crohn's disease, there is tubular narrowing of antrum flaring into body of stomach with concomitant involvement of duodenal bulb and 'C' loop giving a pseudo post-Billroth I appearance. Eosinophilic gastroenteritis occurs after ingestion of specific foods like eggs and nuts and is associated with peripheral eosinophilia in sixty percent of cases. There is mucosal fold thickening and mural narrowing involving antropyloric region and duodenum.

Blurred thick folds due to increased secretion is seen in giardiasis, while ulceration with thick folds and stenosis is seen in strongyloidosis. In strongyloidosis, in addition, there are ulcerations and luminal narrowing involving antrum, bulbar and postbulbar regions.

Tubercular involvement is rare. When present, there are thick mucosal folds with ulcerative lesions with pyloro-duodenal nodularity.

In AIDS patients, nodular thickening of duodenal folds is seen in cytomegalovirus infection and in cryptosporidiosis, associated duodenal dilatation is seen. In *Mycobacterium avium* intercellulare infection, irregular coarsening giving "pseudowhipple" appearance is seen.[26-28]

Nodular and serpiginous thickening of duodenal folds is seen in duodenal varices and mesenteric arterial collaterals, secondary to celiac trunk or superior mesenteric artery occlusion (Figs 5.18A and B). Coarse thickening of folds can be seen in cystic fibrosis.

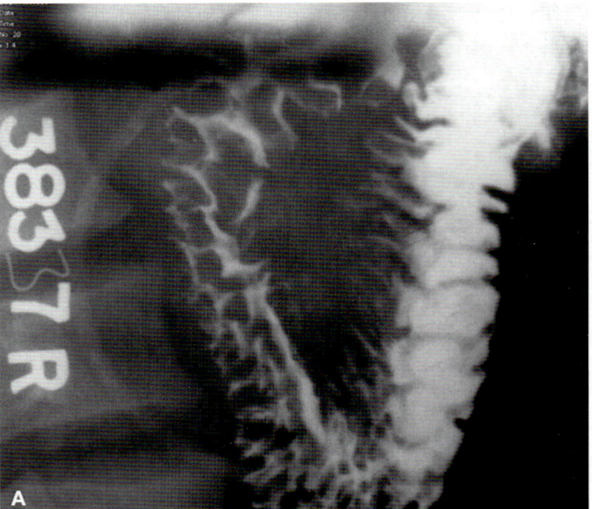

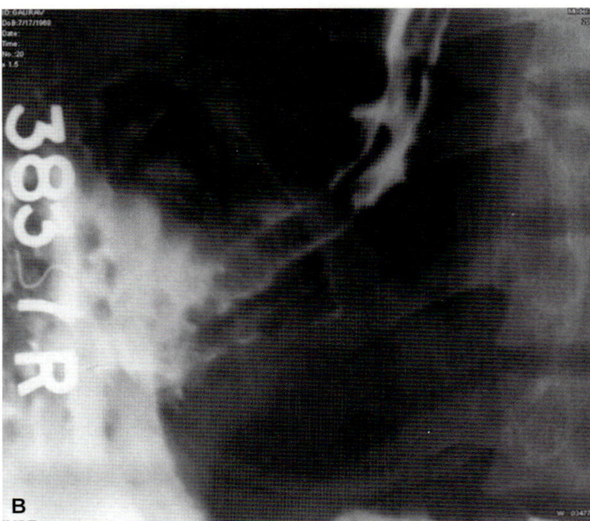

Figs 5.18A and B: Nodular and serpiginous thickening of duodenal mucosal folds involving: (A) Second part of duodenum in a case of alcoholic cirrhosis, (B) Esophageal varices are also present

DUODENAL FILLING DEFECTS

Filling defects in duodenum can occur due to pseudotumor, Brunner gland hyperplasia, benign lymphoid hyperplasia, heterotopic gastric mucosa, prolapsed antral mucosa, ectopic pancreas. It can also occur in non-erosive duodenitis, sprue, varices, mesenteric collaterals, intramural hematoma, and choledochocele.

Pseudotumor can occur due to flexure defect, blood clot, acute ulcer mound, intramural diverticulum, gallstone, and gallbladder impression (Fig. 5.19). Multiple nodular defects in bulb and second part of duodenum can occur in Brunner gland hyperplasia, which is thought to be a response to peptic ulcer disease. Tiny innumerable defects may occur in bulb with maintained normal distensibility in benign lymphoid hyperplasia. Multiple angular sharply marginated defects in bulb are seen in heterotopic gastric mucosa.

Mushroom-shaped filling defect at base of bulb may be seen due to prolapsed antral mucosa, which decreases with relaxation of peristaltic wave. Nodular folds more than five millimeters in size, simulating filling defects, may be seen in non-erosive duodenitis.[26] "Bubbly bulb" appearance due to hexagonal filling defects, of 1-4 millimeters in size, in bulb can be seen in sprue.[27]

Filling defects can occur with duodenal varices and mesenteric collaterals. Submucosal mass in second or third part of duodenum can be seen with intramural hematoma with irregular narrowing.

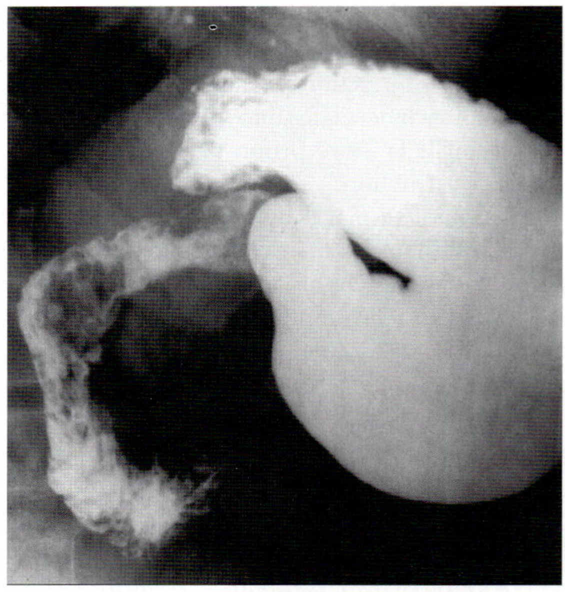

Fig. 5.19: Ulcer crater filled with barium with surrounding edema seen as a filling defect in the second part of duodenum

Filling defect can occur in medial wall of second part of duodenum due to a normal papilla of Vater or choledochocele. Filling defect can also occur due to enlargement of papilla of Vater. Enlargement of papilla of Vater can occur due to impacted CBD stone, in pancreatitis and in duodenal ulcer. Polypoidal enlargement of papilla can occur in papillits due to periductal inflammation and irregular enlargement with ulceration can occur in periampullary neoplasm. Smooth round defect with central dimple due to ductal structures in medial wall of second part of duodenum is seen in ectopic pancreas. Intraluminal diverticula are rare and usually limited to the second or third portion. At barium examination, such diverticula show the classic "windsock" deformity, with the contrast filled diverticulum seen to project into the true lumen. The diagnosis can also be made with CT, at which a collapsed or contrast filled diverticulum may be seen. Mass lesions due to benign and malignant tumors can also produce duodenal filling defects.

DUODENAL NARROWING OR OBSTRUCTION

Duodenal narrowing or obstruction can occur due to congenital, inflammatory, infiltrative, parasitic infestation, vascular, and miscellaneous conditions.

Congenital causes include duodenal atresia, duodenal stenosis, intramural diverticulum, annular pancreas, midgut volvulus, and Ladd's bands (Fig. 5.20). Complete obstruction with "Double bubble" appearance on plain radiographs occur in duodenal atresia, while "Double bubble" appearance with incomplete obstruction with presence of gas distally, occurs in duodenal stenosis. The "Double bubble" appearance is due to presence of gas in stomach and first part of duodenum. Duodenal obstruction can occur in second part of duodenum due to intraluminal diverticulum, which may balloon out producing comma shaped sac. Incomplete obstruction with notch like defect on lateral wall of second part of duodenum is seen in annular pancreas. The use of low attenuation oral contrast with imaging in arterial phase, may be helpful in detecting the enhancing pancreatic tissue. However, due to paucity of intra-abdominal fat, diagnosis of annular pancreas is difficult at CT and definitive diagnosis can be made at ERCP. Midgut volvulus is associated with incomplete rotation and abnormal position of cecum and it is associated with duodenal atresia, annular pancreas, and congenital duodenal diaphragm. Cecum is in mid abdomen or on left side. Duodeno-jejunal flexure is inferior and to right and there is spiral course of loops to right. Extrinsic obstruction in newborn can occur due to Ladd's bands. Dense fibrous bands extend from abnormally placed cecum or hepatic flexure over second and third part of duodenum, to inferior surface of liver. The obstruction is intermittent and partial. It increases on standing and decreases on lying down.

Eccentric narrowing initially due to spasm and later due to fibrosis, of opposite wall of second part of duodenum is seen in post-bulbar ulcer. "Ring Stricture" or concentric narrowing can also occur in post-bulbar ulcer (Fig. 5.21).

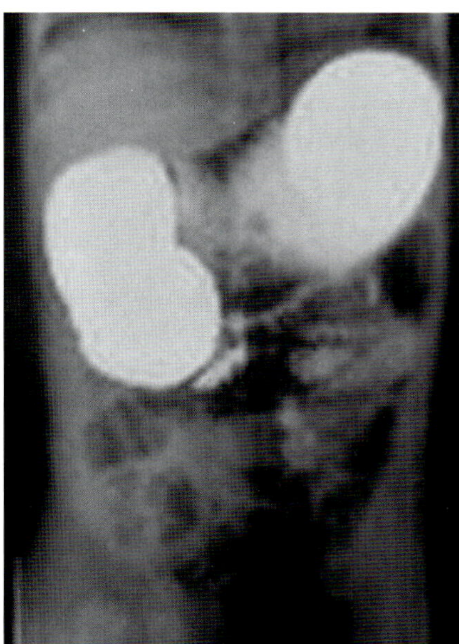

Fig. 5.20: Obstruction in second part of duodenum due to presence of duodenal web

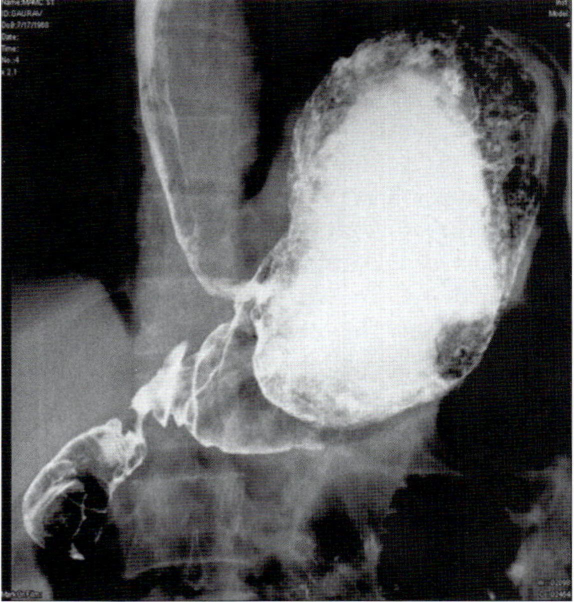

Fig. 5.21: Ring stricture formation, due to sequel of postbulbar ulcer, in second part of duodenum

Duodenal narrowing can occur in tuberculosis with antro-pyloric disease, with or without sinus or fistula formation.

Concentric tubular narrowing involving pyloroduodenal region with involvement of duodenal sweep in Crohn's disease results in pseudo-post Billroth-I appearance. Narrowing of duodenum can occur in nontropical sprue, which represents ulcer healing. Single or multiple areas of stenosis can occur in strongyloidosis.

Duodenal obstruction can also result from a gallstone that has perforated into the duodenum, which is referred to as Bouveret's syndrome. CT can detect the findings of pneumobilia, bowel obstruction, cholecysto or choledochoduodenal fistula and presence of thickened duodenal wall.[28]

Duodenal narrowing can occur due to extrinsic compression or involvement of duodenum by pancreatic disease with associated mucosal thickening in pancreatitis or destruction in pancreatic carcinoma.

Irregular tapered narrowing or "picket fence appearance" can be seen with intramural hematoma in the second or third part of duodenum. CT is an important modality in evaluation of duodenal injury. Duodenal injury can be suspected if air or fluid is present in the retroperitoneum or there is extravasation of oral contrast, along with edema of duodenal wall. Pancreatic transection and stranding of the peripancreatic fat are also important pointers to duodenal injury.[28] Extrinsic compression of third part of duodenum can occur as complication of abdominal aneurysm or due to placement of prosthetic graft due to resultant aortico-duodenal fistula.

Narrowing of third part of duodenum with proximal dilatation due to compression between superior mesenteric artery and aorta results in chronic intermittent obstruction that is known as the Superior Mesenteric Artery syndrome. This obstruction is relieved in left lateral decubitus, prone or knee chest position. Diagnosis is made by barium study of the upper gastrointestinal tract and hypotonic duodenography showing vertical cutoff in third part of duodenum (Figs 5.22A and B). There is delay of 4-6 hours in gastroduodenal transit. To-and-fro motion of barium in dilated proximal duodenum with anti-peristaltic waves can be seen on fluoroscopy with relief of obstruction by A-Hayes maneuver, that is, elevating the root of mesentery. There is decreased aorto-mesenteric angle of 6-25° as opposed to normal of 45° as seen by ultrasound and decreased aorto-mesenteric distance of 2-8 millimeters as opposed to normal of 8-10 millimeters by computed tomography.[29, 30]

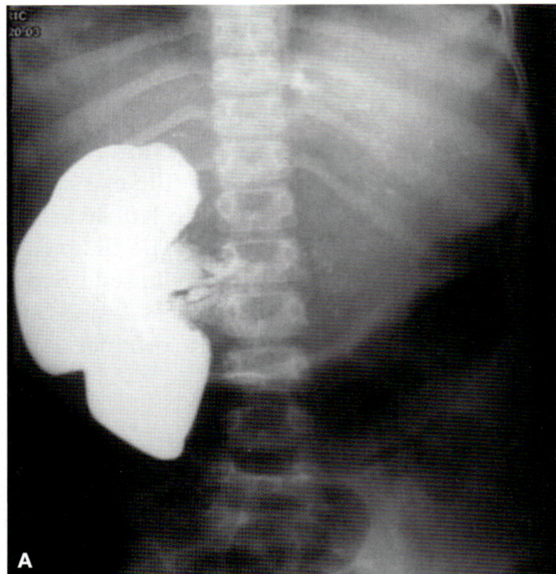

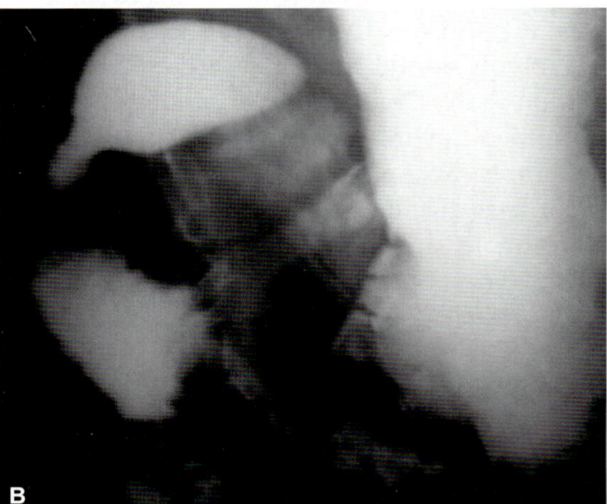

Figs 5.22A and B: Superior mesenteric artery syndrome (A) showing vertical cutoff at junction of second and third part of duodenum, (B) relieved in prone position

EXTRINSIC IMPRESSION ON BULB

Normal gallbladder or its enlargement can deform anterior aspect of bulb while enlargement of head of pancreas deforms bulb at its apex and along inferior wall. Massive dilatation of CBD can compress at apex or just beyond it.

Liver enlargement, lymph nodes, right adrenal or kidney enlargement, or masses, carcinoma hepatic flexure or colon can all cause extrinsic impression on duodenal bulb.

WIDENING OF DUODENAL SWEEP

Widening of duodenal sweep can occur as a normal variant, in pancreatic diseases, by lymphnodal or retroperitoneal masses, due to aortic-aneurysm and choledochal cyst (Fig. 5.23).

Widening of "C loop" of duodenum can occur, in obesity or due to high transverse stomach, as a normal variant.

Widening of duodenal sweep with thick duodenal folds can be seen in pancreatic disease with colon cutoff sign and sentinel loop in pancreatitis and mucosal ulceration and destruction in pancreatic malignancy. Lymphnode and retroperitonial masses can cause widening of duodenal sweep. Downward displacement of third part of duodenum can occur due to abdominal aortic aneurysm, which can be confirmed on ultrasound or Computed Tomography. Generalized widening of duodenal sweep, or local impression near papilla can occur with choledochal cyst.

MISCELLANEOUS ABNORMALITIES

Duodenum inversum is a developmental anomaly in which third part of duodenum passes across abdomen above cap. It is a variant of little clinical significance.

Duodenal duplication is rare and arise in medial wall of second or third portions of duodenum. They appear as cystic masses with fluid attenuation and typically do not communicate with the duodenal lumen. They are incidental finding at CT. Presence of mural nodules or vegetation in a duplication cyst should alert the radiologist to the possibility of carcinoma. Duodenal diverticula incidentally detected in 5% cases at barium meal, occur along inner border of "C loop", are often multiple and usually without clinical symptoms. They retain food residue or barium for weeks. Rarely, there can be biliary obstruction, perforation or bleeding. They can perforate and bleed following papillotomy if endoscopist is not aware of their presence (Fig. 5.24). Periampullary diverticulum can result in biliary obstruction. Diverticulum can be seen on SSRARE MR images as air or fluid filled outpouching from adjacent duodenum. Fat suppressed gadolinium enhanced SGE images show thin enhancing wall, similar to normal mucosa.

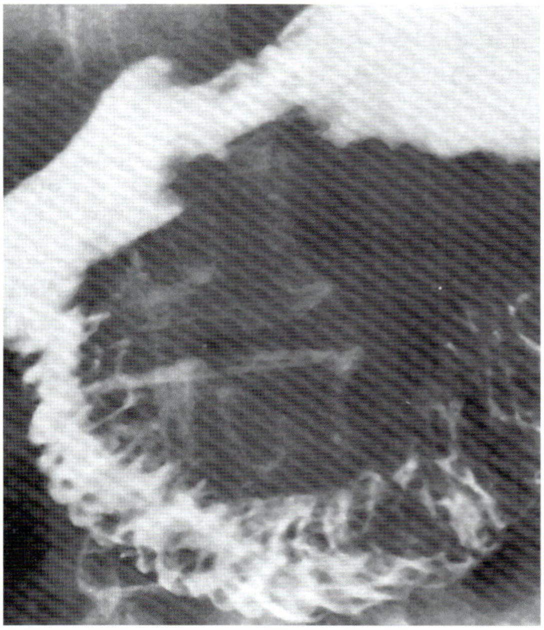

Fig. 5.23: Widening of 'C' loop of duodenum due to acute pancreatitis, with mass effect on second and third parts of duodenum

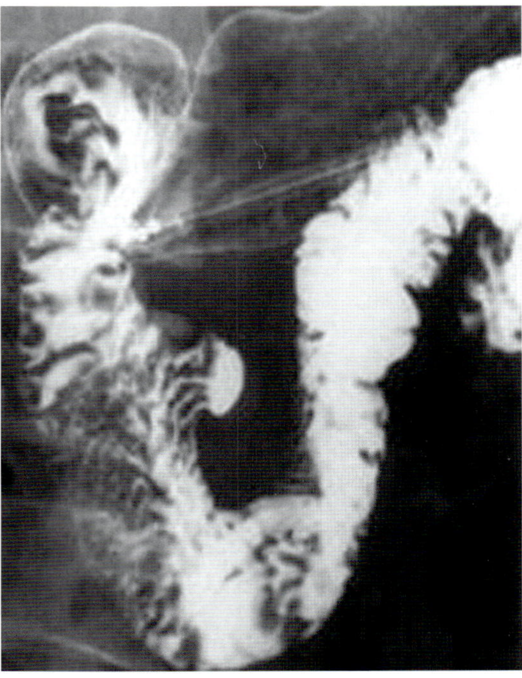

Fig. 5.24: Duodenal diverticula seen along mesenteric border of second part of duodenum, with mucosal folds seen in continuity with duodenum

CONCLUSION

A pattern recognition approach helps in recognizing various benign lesions of the stomach and duodenum, and differentiating them as mucosal fold abnormalities, ulcerative or erosive lesions, narrowing, filling defects and displacements due to various disease processes.

REFERENCES

1. Duan SY, Zhang DT, Lin QC, Wu YH. Clinical value of CT three-dimensional imaging in diagnosing gastrointestinal diseases. World J Gastroenterol 2006;12[18]: 2945-48.
2. Ogata I, Komohara Y, Mitsuzaki K, Takahashi M, Ogawa M. CT evaluation of gastric lesions with three-dimensional display and interactive virtual endoscopy: Comparison with conventional barium study and endoscopy. AJR Am J Roentgenol 1999;172:1263-70.
3. Kim SH, Lee JM, Han JK, Lee JY, Yang HK, Lee HJ Shin KS, Choi BI. Effect of adjusted positioning on gastric distension and fluid distribution during CT gastrography. AJR Am J Roentgenol 2005;185:1180-84.
4. Inamoto K, Kouzai K, Ueeda T, Marukawa T. CT virtual endoscopy of the stomach: comparison study with gastric fibrescopy. Abdom Imaging 2005;30:473-79.
5. Horton KM, Fishman EK. Current role of CT in imaging of the stomach. Radiographics 2003;23:75-87.
6. Jayaraman MV, Mayo-Smith WW, Movson JS, Wallach MT. CT of the duodenum—An overlooked segment gets its due. Radiographics 2001;21:S147-60.
7. Edelman Robert R, Hesselink John R, Zlatkin Michael B, Crees John S. Clinical Magnetic Resonance Imaging Vol-3, 3rd edition 2006;2684-2721.
8. Matsui T, Iida M, Murakami M, et al. Intestinal anisakiasis: Clinical and radiologic features. Radiology 1985;157:299.
9. Silverstein Fred E, Tytgat Guido NJ. Atlas of Gastrointestinal Endoscopy 1991, (2nd Edn). JB Lippincott, Philadelphia, Gower Medical Publishing; 5.2-5.21 and 7.2-7.19. ISBN–0-397-44616-0.
10. Sutton David. Text Book of Radiology and Imaging Vol-1 (7th Edn). 2003, ISBN- 0443071098.
11. Berry Manorama, Chowdhury Veena, Suri Sudha. Diagnostic Radiology (Hepatobiliary and Gastrointestinal Radiology) Jaypee Brothers 1997;246-54.
12. Levine MS, Rubesin SE, Herlinger H, Laufer I. Double contrast upper gastrointestinal examination—Technique and interpretation. Radiology1988;168:593-602.
13. Margulis AR, Burhenne HJ. Alimentary Tract Radiology 1994 5th edition.
14. Taveras Juan M, Ferrucci Joseph T. Radiology, Diagnosis-Imaging- Intervention 1986;4:ISBN–0-397-57115-1.
15. Jacobs JM, Hill MC, Steinberg WM. Peptic ulcer disease-CT evaluation. Radiology 1991;178:745-48.
16. Cotton PB, Shorvon PJ. Analysis of endoscopy and radiography in the diagnosis, follow up and treatment of peptic ulcer disease. Clin Gastroenterol 1994;13:383-403.
17. Dekker W, Opdenorth JO. Biphasic radiologic examination and endoscopy of the upper gastrointestinal tract-a comparative study: Journal of Clinical Gastroenterology 1988;10:461-65.
18. Eisenberg Ronald L. Clinical Imaging –An Atlas of Differential Diagnosis (4th edition 2003); Lippincott Williams and Wilkins.
19. Sleisenger Marvin H, Fordtran John S. Gastrointestinal Disease—Pathophysiology/Diagnosis/Management. Vol-I; Saunders 545-763,Year –2002, ISBN – 0-7216-8973-6.
20. Bayerdorffer E, Ritter MM, Hatz R, Brooks W, Ruckdeschel G, Stolte M. Healing of protein losing hypertrophic gastropathy by eradication of *Helicobacter pylori*-Is *Helicobacter pylori* a pathogenic factor in Menetrier's disease, Gut 1994;35(5):701-04.
21. Hizawa K, Kawasaki M, Yao T, Aoyagi K, Suekane H, Kawakubo K, Fujishima M. Endoscopic ultrasound features of protein losing gastropathy with hypertrophic gastric folds: Endoscopy 2000;32(5):394-97.
22. Newman B, Girdany BR. Gastric Trichobezoars- sonographic and computed tomographic appearance. Pediatric Radiology 1990;20:526-27.
23. Kaushik Narinder K, Sharma Yash P, Negi Asha, Jaswal Amal. Images-Gastric Trichobezoar, Ind J Radiol Imaging 1999;9:3:137-39.
24. Ko YT, Lim JH, and Lee DH et al. Small intestinal bezoar-Sonographic detection. Abdominal Imaging 1993;18: 271-72.
25. Federle MP, Megibow AJ, Naidich DP. Radiology of AIDS 1988:Raven Press, New York.
26. Langkamper R, et al. "Elevated lesions in the duodenal bulb caused by Heterotrophic Gastric mucosa" Radiology 1980;137:621-24.
27. Gelfand DW, Dale WJ, Ott DJ, et al. Duodenitis: Endoscopic-radiologic correlation in 272 patients, Radiology 1985;157:577-81.
28. Zissin R, Osadchy A, Gayer G, Shapiro-Feinberg. CT of duodenal pathology. British Journal of Radiology 2002;75:78-84.
29. Santer R, Young C, Rossi T. Computed Tomography in Superior Mesenteric Artery syndrome. Pediatric Radiology 1991;21(2):154-55.
30. Shetty Avinash, Hill Ivor D. Superior Mesenteric Artery syndrome – April 2003 http://www.emedicine.com/ped/byname/superior-mesenteric-artery-syndrome.htm.

Chapter Six

Malignant Lesions of the Stomach and Small Intestine

Sanjay Thulkar, Arun Kumar Gupta

INTRODUCTION

Malignant lesions of the stomach and small bowel include adenocarcinoma, lymphoma, carcinoids and gastrointestinal stromal tumors. Most common among these are carcinoma of the stomach and lymphoma, other tumors are comparatively uncommon. Lymphoma of the GIT is described elsewhere in this book. Stomach and small bowel can also be secondarily involved by other malignancies; either by contiguous extension of the tumors of the adjacent organs or by the hematogenous dissemination. Imaging is important not only for the diagnosis of these malignancies but it is also indispensable to assess the extent of the disease and staging, monitoring response to the treatment and to detect recurrence.

CARCINOMA OF THE STOMACH

Worldwide, carcinoma of the stomach is considered to be second only to lung cancer for cancer related deaths.[1] Incidence of gastric cancer varies in different parts of the world and it is most common in Japan, Eastern Europe and South America. It is the most common cancer in Japan with incidence of 160 cases per 100,000 persons per year. In India, the incidence of gastric cancer is about 10-13 cases per 100,000 persons per year and it is the most common cancer in males in Chennai.[2] Gastric cancer occurs above 40 years of age and the incidence rises with increasing age. Gastric cancer is twice more common in males than in females. Majority of gastric cancers are diagnosed at an advanced stage because of insidious onset of symptoms which are similar to benign dyspepsia.

Gastric cancer commonly affects body and antrum of the stomach, but over last two decades this has decreased and incidence of more aggressive carcinomas around gastroesophageal junction has increased at an alarming rate which is more than that of any other cancer.[3]

Risk Factors for Gastric Cancer

There are several risk factors for gastric cancer (Table 6.1); most important among them is chronic *Helicobacter pylori* infection. It increases the risk of gastric cancer by 3-6 fold.[4] The risk is considered to be related to development of chronic atrophic gastritis in people with this infection. Chronic atrophic gastritis resulting from other causes such as dietary factors, pernicious anemia and gastric

Table 6.1 Risk factor for gastric cancer

- *Helicobacter pylori* infection
- Chronic atrophic gastritis
- Pernicious anemia
- Salted, smoked or pickled food
- Diet with high nitrates
- Ménétrier's disease
- First degree relatives of gastric cancer patient
- Blood group A
- Gastric surgery for benign ulcers
- Gastroesophageal reflux
- Adenomatous polyp

surgery for benign ulcers also increase the risk of gastric cancer. Diet rich in salted, smoked or pickled food and diet with high nitrates increase the risk of gastric cancer.[5] High incidence of gastric cancer is found in patients with Ménétrier's disease.[1] More aggressive gastroesophageal region cancers however, are not related to *H. pylori* infection or chronic atrophic gastritis but genetic factors are important for their development. First degree relative of patients with gastric cancer and those with blood group A are genetically prone to develop gastric cancer.[3] Recurrent gastroesophageal reflux is also a risk factor. Adenomatous polyps increase the chances of gastric cancer, especially if more than 2 cm in size.[6] Hyperplastic gastric polyps and familial juvenile polyposis however, are at no increased risk.

Clinical Features

Early gastric cancers are asymptomatic. Abdominal pain and weight loss are the usual presenting symptoms and the disease is often advanced by this time.[7] Patients may also complain of abdominal lump. Tumors at GE junction cause dysphagia and those with antropyloric tumors present with recurrent vomiting. Occasionally, patients may present with early satiety (in linitis plastica). Massive GI bleeding is uncommon in gastric cancer. On examination, epigastric mass, ascites, left supraclavicular (Virchow's) or anterior axillary lymphadenopathy and hepatomegly may be found in patients with advanced gastric cancer. Serum CEA is elevated in about one-third of the patients. It is not sensitive for the diagnosis, however, it generally correlates well with the stage of the disease.[3]

Pathology

Gastric cancers can be classified according to cell types. More than 95% are adenocarcinoma and remaining are squamous or other varieties. However, this has little clinical usefulness. Division of gastric cancer into intestinal and diffuse types (Lauren's classification) provides better clinicopathological correlation and hence it is used most widely.[3,8,9] The intestinal type of gastric cancer resembles colon cancer and it has large glands lined by well differentiated columnar cells. It is also better circumscribed and usually ulcerated or polypoid on gross appearance. It is usually located in antrum and constitutes a predominant pathological type in areas with lower incidence of gastric cancer. Diffuse type of gastric cancer more commonly develop near cardia and produce wall thickening. These are ill-defined and well formed glands are usually absent. Diffuse submucosal spread and early metastases are common. It is the predominant variety in areas with high incidence of gastric cancer.[3]

Diagnosis

Upper GI endoscopy and biopsy is the most accurate way to diagnose the gastric cancer.[3] Direct vision of the mucosa and ability to take biopsy are the most important advantages of endoscopy. This combined with the natural bias of the gastroenterologist towards endoscopy has largely replaced the double contrast upper GI barium studies in the diagnosis of gastric pathologies. However, barium studies are not obsolete. They may still be performed in cases of failed endoscopy and are also better to demonstrate submucosal pathologies, subtle narrowing, motility and distensibility disorders.[10]

Barium UGI Series Features of Gastric Cancer

The technique of double contrast barium UGI series was perfected and popularized by Japanese for the screening of gastric cancer. The stomach is distended with effervescent agent and high density barium suspension (200% v/w, 100-150 ml) is used to coat the mucosal surface. IV glucagon or buscopan is also given to reduce peristalsis. Under fluoroscopy, various patient positions are then used to manoeuvre barium coating and air distension of different parts of the stomach and spot images are obtained.[11] With endoscopy becoming the mainstay of gastric mucosal evaluation, there is fast decline in the number of barium UGI examinations performed as well as the expertise to perform these satisfactorily.

Malignant ulcer is the most common feature of gastric cancer on barium UGI studies. Benign gastric ulcer, when seen enface, appears as round and smooth ulcer crater (Fig. 6.1). In profile, it extends beyond the gastric outline and has an overhanging mucosal edge, seen as a lucent line (Hampton's line) separating the ulcer from lumen of the stomach. With edema, this line may thicken to form a radiolucent band (ulcer collar). The edematous thickening of the stomach wall around the ulcer is seen as a smooth elevation (ulcer mound). Healing benign ulcer causes convergence of the mucosal folds which are smooth, tapered and extend to the edge of the ulcer.

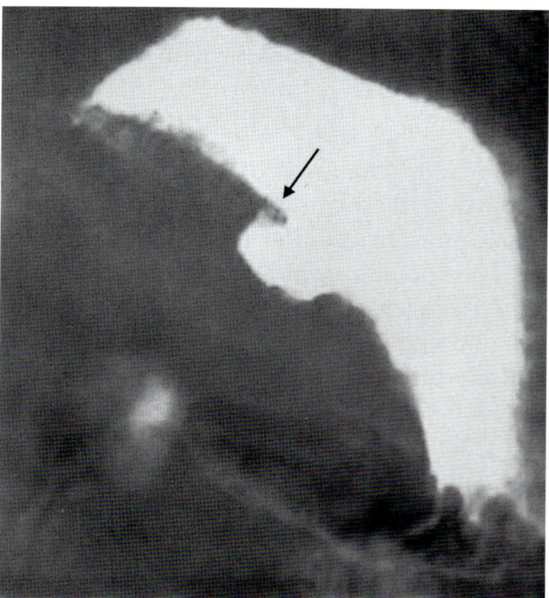

Fig. 6.1: Benign gastric ulcer: Barium UGI study shows a lesser curvature gastric ulcer which is projecting beyond the gastric outline. An ulcer collar (arrow) is seen separating the ulcer crater from gastric lumen

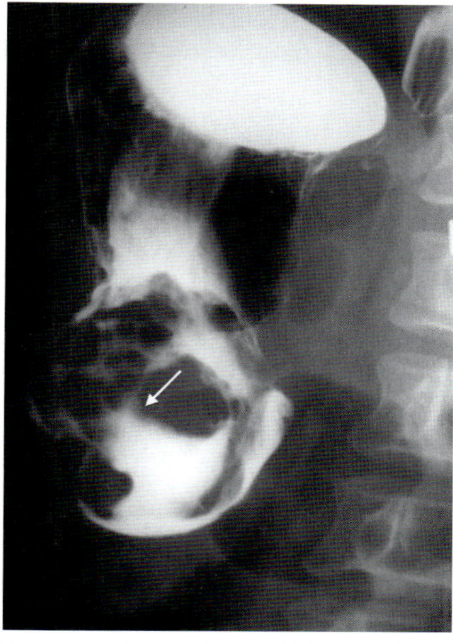

Fig. 6.2: Malignant gastric ulcer: Barium UGI study shows a mass with a large ulcer in lower stomach. Nodular thickening of adjacent mucosal folds is seen in the vicinity

Malignant gastric ulcer, when seen enface on double contrast barium study, appear as an irregular ulcer crater located eccentrically in a mass. Radiating folds do not reach up to the crater and these often have clubbed, fused or amputated tips. Viewed tangentially, the malignant ulcers do not project beyond the gastric outline as they essentially form within the gastric mass (Fig. 6.2). Gastric cancers of lesser curvature often produce a broad based lesion with central ulceration and elevated margins (Carman-Kirklin meniscus sign). It is convex towards the lumen. Size and location of the ulcer are not helpful in differentiation. Benign ulcers however, are rare at fundus and proximal greater curvature. Multiplicity is also known in both benign and malignant gastric ulcers.[11]

Early gastric cancer (EGC) is limited to mucosa and submucosa. These are generally small and asymptomatic. EGC are routinely detected in screening programs in Japan, however, these are rarely seen on barium studies or endoscopy in other parts of the world.[12] Japanese classification based on gross appearance divides EGC into three types.[13,14] Type I (elevated) EGC protrude into the lumen for more than 5 mm and seen on barium study as an elevation or polyp. Type II (superficial) EGC are further divided into elevated (IIa), flat (IIb) and depressed (IIc). These are seen as plaque like lesions, mucosal irregularity or shallow ulcers respectively (Fig. 6.3). Type III (excavated) EGC are malignant gastric ulcers.

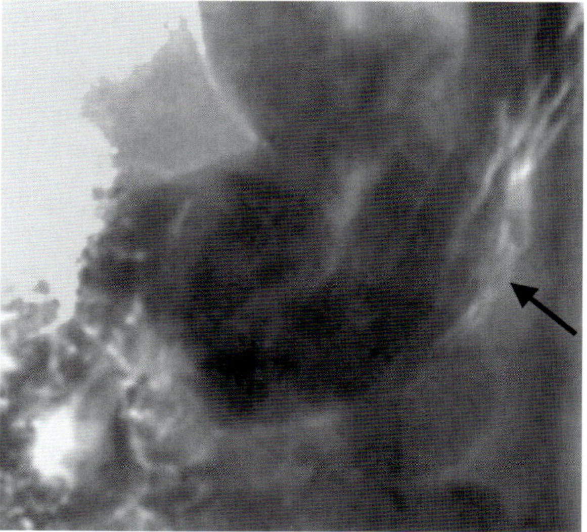

Fig. 6.3: Early gastric cancer: Double contrast barium UGI study shows mucosal irregularity with thickening and crowding of mucosal folds (arrow) at the greater curvature of the stomach

Advanced gastric cancers are usually larger than 3 cm.[1] Most symptomatic patients have advanced gastric cancer and hence, it is the type most commonly encountered on imaging or endoscopy. Advanced gastric cancers are morphologically described as per the Borrmann's classification[11] (Table 6.2). Bormann type 1

Table 6.2	Gastric cancer: Imaging findings

Barium studies (Bormann Classification)
- Type 1: Polypoid mass
- Type 2: Malignant ulcer
- Type 3: Ulcero-infiltrative wall thickening
- Type 4: Linitis plastica

CT
- Any of the above findings
- Invasion of perigastric tissues
- Invasion of adjacent organs
- Lymphadenopathy
- Liver metastases
- Peritoneal metastases
- Ascites

or polypoid cancers are masses protruding into the lumen (Figs 6.4A and B). Borrmann type 2 or ulcerative cancer is most common type which is seen as a large malignant ulcer (Fig. 6.2). Borrman type 3 or ulceroinfiltrative is a predominantly infiltrative lesion with ulcerations (Figs 6.5A and B). Borrmann type 4 or linitis plastica are scirrhous infiltrative tumors. These elicit desmoplastic reaction leading to thickening and rigidity of the stomach wall with luminal narrowing. Antrum is the most commonly affected part but in advanced cases, entire stomach is involved (Figs 6.6 and 6.7). Severe narrowing of the lumen however, is not a consistent feature of linitis plastica. Some lesions may cause only mild loss of distensiblity of the stomach along with fold thickening.[15]

Staging

Gastric cancer is diagnosed with endoscopy or barium study, however, these can assess the luminal component only. Assessment of local and distant extent can be made with CT and endoscopic ultrasound. The gold standard of staging is however, surgicopathological staging. Most patients undergo surgery for cure or palliation, unless distant metastases are demonstrated.[16]

AJCC-UICC staging based on TNM classification is used for staging of gastric cancer.[3] T staging is similar for most GIT cancers. T1 tumor involves lamina propria or submucosa, T2 is involvement of up to serosa (peritoneum), T3 is invasion outside the serosa (perigastric tissues, ligaments, omentum) and T4 is involvement of adjacent structures like liver, spleen, pancreas, colon or abdominal wall. N staging is based on number of positive lymph nodes on postoperative histopathology. N1 is up to six positive nodes, N2 is up to 15 positive nodes and N3 is more than 15 positive nodes. M1 is presence of distant metastases. This number based nodal staging correlates better with the prognosis than the earlier used location based nodal staging. However, preoperative identification of abnormal lymph nodes at various locations on CT is still important as it influences

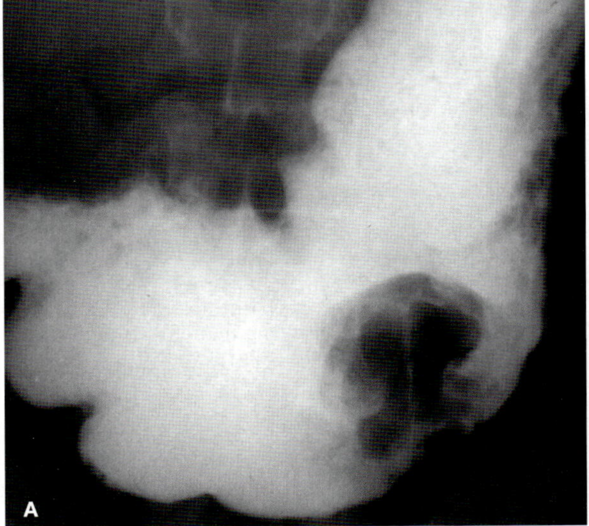

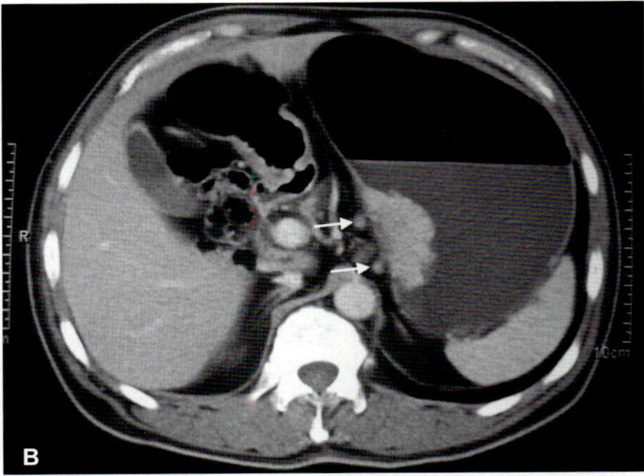

Figs 6.4A and B: Polypoid gastric cancer: (a) Barium meal UGI shows an irregular polypoid intraluminal growth arising from the greater curvature of the stomach, (b) CECT with water distension (hydro-CT) of another patient shows broad based enhancing polypoid mass along the lesser curvature of the stomach. Small but enhancing perigastric lymph nodes are also seen (arrows) which suggests their metastatic involvement

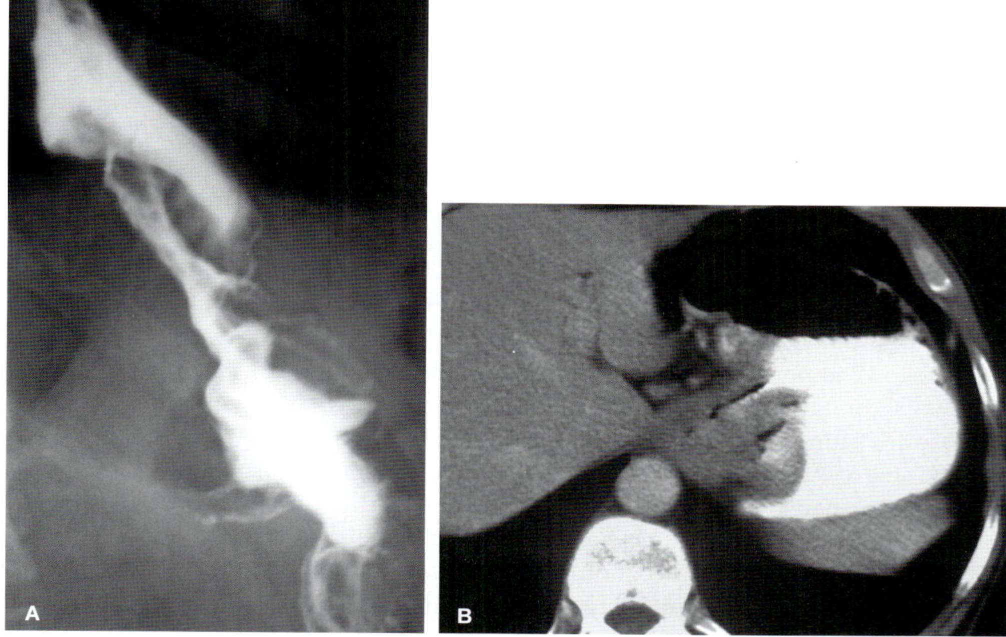

Figs 6.5A and B: Ulcero-infiltrative cancer at cardia of the stomach: (A) Barium study shows large ulceroproliferative mass involving gastroesophageal junction and the lesser curvature of the stomach, (B) CT scan shows infiltrative mass at the cardia with ulcerations

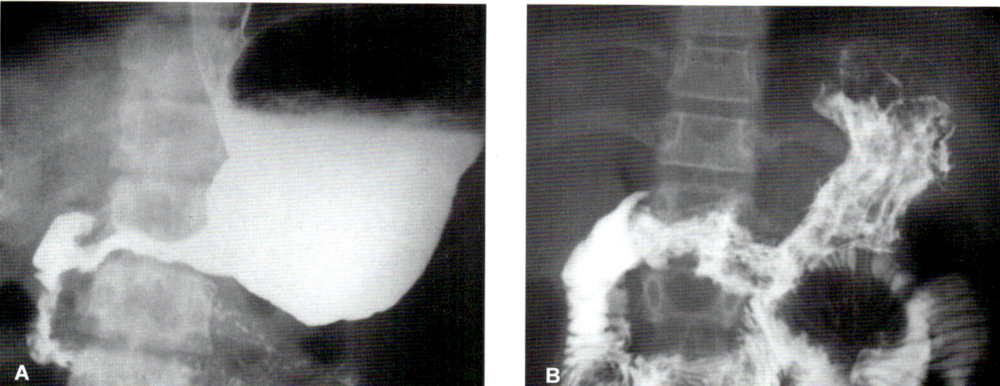

Figs 6.6A and B: Linitis plastica: (A) Barium UGI study shows diffuse narrowing of antrum with proximal dilatation of the stomach (B) Barium UGI of another patient with linitis plastica shows diffuse involvement and narrowing of the entire stomach

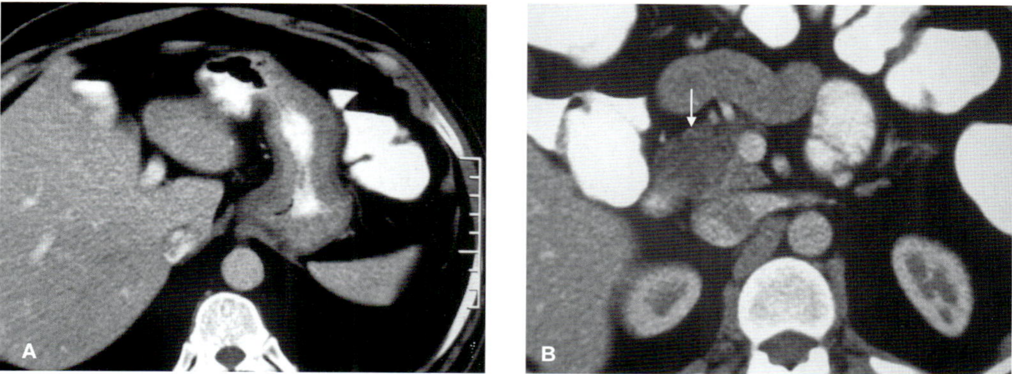

Figs 6.7A and B: Linitis plastica: (A) CT scan shows diffuse wall thickening and poor distensibility of the stomach, (B) CT section at the lower level shows an enlarged lymph node along the left gastric vessels (arrow)

the extent of nodal dissection that will be performed at surgery.[16,17] Perigastric nodes within 3 cm of the primary lesion are always removed during surgery and hence their radiological detection is not critical. Lymph nodes along the celiac artery or its branches are not always removed but are resectable. Enlarged lymph nodes at distant sites such as those at para-aortic, portal or retro-pancreatic locations cannot be removed on surgery and considered as distant metastases. Supraclavicular or any other extrabdominal lymph nodes are also distant metastases.[17]

Stage 1 disease is up to T2 tumor with no nodes. Stage 2 disease is up to either T3 or N2 disease. Stage 3 is with both T3 and N2 disease or T4 tumor without nodes. Stage 4 is N3 or M1 disease (Table 6.3). Japanese staging system for gastric cancer is more exhaustive. The T staging is more detailed and gross appearance of the tumor (Bormann's classification) is also taken into account. The nodal involvement is assessed as per 18 standard lymph node stations. Findings on laparoscopy and peritoneal cytology are also taken into account.[3]

CT Features of Gastric Cancer

On CT, normal gastric wall thickness is less than 5 mm in a well distended stomach. A wall thickness of more than 1 cm is considered abnormal. Stomach wall may appear thickened if it is poorly distended. GE junction and cardia are obliquely oriented to the scan plain and it normally shows increased wall thickness with variable appearances on CT, sometimes mimicking focal lesions.[18] For optimal evaluation, changing patient position so as to make the area of the lesion non-dependant and maximise its air distension is helpful. Thus, for proximal stomach lesions, right lateral decubitus and for antral lesions, left lateral decubitus positions of the patient are useful.[16] A modified technique (hydro-CT) can be used to increase the accuracy of CT in evaluation of gastric cancer (Fig. 6.4B). In this technique, large amount of water (approx 1 liter) is given orally followed by IV glucagon to increase the gastric distension and reduce peristalsis. Dual phase CT is then performed. With this technique, normal gastric wall is frequently seen in a multilayer pattern and any abnormal wall thickness or enhancement representing the tumor is accurately demonstrated[19](Fig. 6.4B). Combination of unenhanced MDCT with air distension of stomach (surface rendered 3D images or virtual endoscopy) and dual phase contrast enhanced MDCT with water distension also improves the detection and T staging of the primary lesion.[20-22] However, utility of such cumbersome procedures in routine clinical practice is not yet established.

On CT, the gastric cancer may is seen as focal wall thickening (Fig. 6.8), ulcerations (Fig. 6.5B), polypoid mass (Fig. 6.4B) or diffuse wall thickening (Fig. 6.7, Table 6.2). Transpyloric extension of antral carcinoma into the duodenum may sometimes be seen (Fig. 6.9). It is little more common in lymphoma, however, gastric carcinoma is statistically more common than lymphoma. Hence, extension into the duodenum is not a reliable finding to differentiate these two conditions.[23] Perigastric spread of gastric cancer (T3) is seen as blurred outer surface of the stomach wall or perigastric streakiness.[17] With further

Table 6.3 Gastric cancer: Staging overview

T1-invasion up to submucosa
T2-invasion up to serosa
T3-invasion of perigastric tissues/ligaments
T4-invasion of adjacent organs
N0 - no positive lymph nodes on HPE
N1 - up to 6 positive lymph nodes on HPE
N2 - up to 15 positive lymph nodes on HPE
N3 - more than 15 positive lymph nodes on HPE
M0 - no distant metastases
M1- distant metastases

- Stage 1 – up to T2, no nodes
- Stage 2 – up to T3 or N2
- Stage 3 – both T3 and N2 or T4 with no nodes
- Stage 4 – distant metastases with any T or N

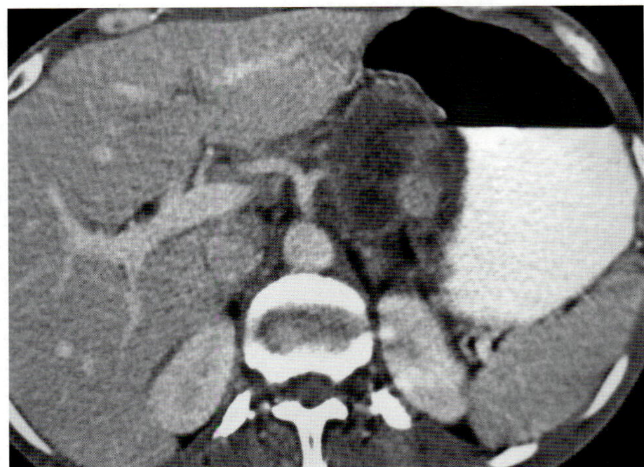

Fig. 6.8: Gastric cancer with coeliac lymphadenopathy: CT shows wall thickening at the lesser curvature of the stomach with necrotic conglomerate enlarged lymph nodes along the coeliac axis. The lymph node mass is not separately demarcated from the primary lesion

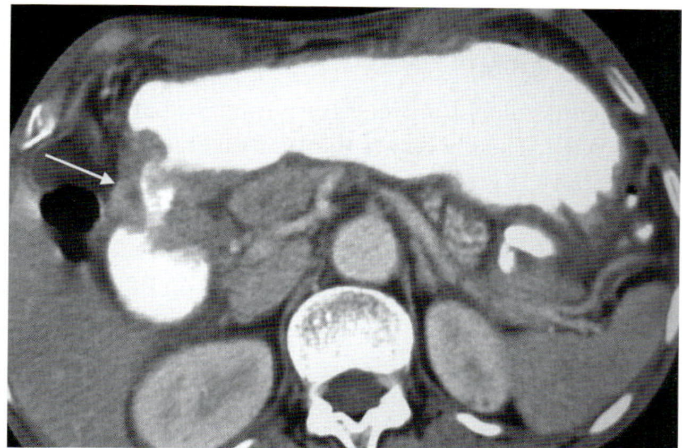

Fig. 6.9: Gastric cancer at the pylorus: CT shows an 'apple core' type of mass at the pylorus (arrow) which is extending into the duodenum

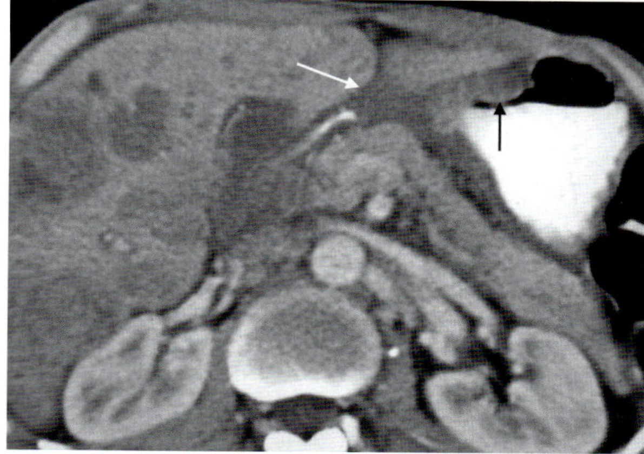

Fig. 6.10: Advanced gastric cancer: CT shows an infiltrative gastric cancer seen as the wall thickening of the antrum (black arrow). There is a contiguous extension of the soft tissue mass with loss of fat planes with the liver and the pancreas (white arrow). Multiple liver metastases are also seen

spread, adjacent structures are involved (T4). Gastric cancers located at cardia or lesser curvature tend to spread medially to involve lesser omentum (gastrohepatic and hepatoduodenal ligaments) and then porta hepatis or liver (Fig. 6.10). Proximal greater curvature tumors extend into gastrosplenic ligament and then to the spleen. Tumors of the distal greater curvature and antrum may invade pancreas via lesser sac and colon via greater omentum (gastrocolic ligament)[16,17] (Fig. 6.11). Diaphragm, adrenals or abdominal wall may also be involved by the advanced gastric cancer. Differentiation of T3 and T4 tumors on CT is important because that governs the feasibility of resection. Enlarged regional or distant lymph nodes are well demonstrated on CT. Lymphadenopathy is more common in diffuse variety of gastric cancer. Left gastric lymph nodes are consistently involved in most gastric cancers, regardless of its location in the stomach[3] (Fig. 6.7B). Patients with advanced gastric cancer may demonstrate liver deposits, ascites and peritoneal deposits. Liver metastases from gastric cancer are hypovascular and hence, best detected on portal venous phase CT (Fig. 6.10). Apart from liver; lungs, bones and adrenals are other common sites of hematogenous metastases from gastric cancer. Peritoneal deposits make the disease unresectable but these are often missed on CT and found only intraoperatively. On CT, these may be seen as nodules, plaque like thickening or enhancement of the peritoneum or small bowel wall thickening[1,16,17] (Figs 6.11 and 6.12). Drop metastases to ovaries produce bilateral, solid, heterogeneously enhancing masses which are known as Krukenberg's tumors (Fig. 6.11B).

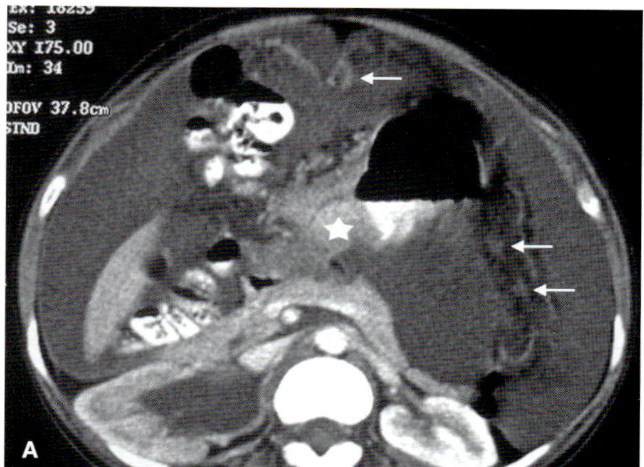

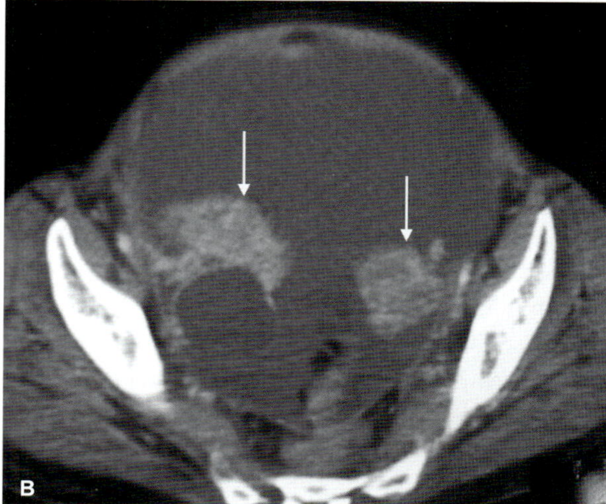

Figs 6.11A and B: Advanced gastric cancer: (A) CT shows wall thickening of the antrum (star) with multiple omental deposits (arrows). Ascites and right hydronephrosis is also seen, (B) CT section of the pelvis shows Krukenberg tumor as bilateral solid, heterogenously enhancing adnexal masses (arrows)

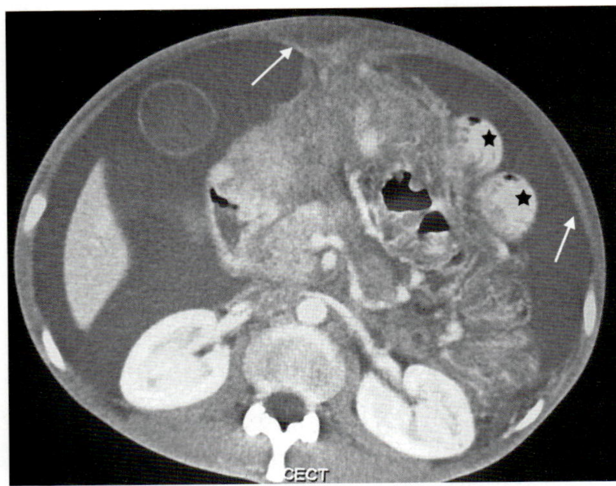

Fig. 6.12: Advanced gastric cancer: CT shows gastric cancer in the antrum of the stomach invading the transverse colon and the pancreas. Peritoneal deposits are seen as thickening of the small bowel wall (asterisks) and thickened and enhancing parietal peritoneum (arrows)

Limitations of CT

On CT, gastric cancers are seen as wall thickening or masses. However, CT cannot demonstrate all gastric cancers.[8] Also, wall thickening is not a specific finding. Hence, CT cannot be used as an alternative to barium study or endoscopy for the diagnosis of gastric cancer. CT should be performed for staging of the gastric cancer after histological diagnosis has been made.

For staging, major limitations of CT include its inability to determine the degree of gastric wall invasion. Accuracy in determination of perigastric spread is also variable. Small liver and peritoneal deposits are not identified on CT. Loss of fat plane between tumor and adjacent structures is only suggestive and not diagnostic of invasion. CT cannot differentiate metastatic and reactive lymph node enlargement. Sometimes, enlarged lymph nodes may be abutting the tumor and hence are not identified separately (Fig. 6.8). CT obviously cannot identify metastases in normal sized nodes. At CT, lymph nodes are considered positive if these show enlargement (short axis diameter 1cm or more), marked enhancement (Fig. 6.4B), rounded shape or central necrosis[17,19,24] (Fig. 6.8). Enlarged but uninvolved (reactive) nodes usually have low attenuation and retain their oval shape.[24]

Other Investigations for Preoperative Staging of Gastric Cancer

CT is the mainstay for preoperative staging of the gastric cancer. MRI is less accurate than CT for staging of gastric cancer. PET CT is not useful for staging work up as about one-third of the gastric cancers, mostly mucinous carcinomas, do not show significant FDG uptake. Peritoneal deposits are also often missed on PET.[17,25] PET is however useful to detect distant lymph nodes and metastases.

Endoscopic ultrasound (EUS) is complimentary to CT and it is performed if gross perigastric disease is absent on CT. EUS is more accurate than CT to assess the degree of stomach wall invasion.[17,26] On EUS, normal gastric wall shows five layers, three hyper-echoic layers separated by two hypo-echoic layers. Gastric carcinoma appears as a hypo-echoic mass reaching up to variable layers. Microscopic invasion is obviously not detected on EUS and hence its accuracy in T staging is about 85%.[1] EUS is also the most sensitive modality for detection of perigastric lymph node involvement. Criteria used on EUS to diagnose metastatic lymph nodes are enlargement, hypo-echogenicity or round shape. EUS guided FNAC can also be performed from abnormal lymph nodes, however, this is not a routine practice for staging of gastric cancer.[1] Preoperative staging laparoscopy may also be performed in some patients if the disease is localized on CT. It is especially useful to detect small (less than 5 mm) peritoneal and visceral surface deposits which are usually missed on CT. Laparoscopic ultrasonography, peritoneal biopsy or ascitic cytology may also be performed. If results of these investigations are positive, patients can be spared unnecessary surgery.[3]

Treatment and Prognosis

Complete resection of the tumors and adjacent lymph nodes is the only curative treatment of gastric cancer. Localized disease on CT may be found unresectable on surgery and hence, decision to proceed with radical resection is normally taken on laparotomy.[27] Gastric cancers within 5 cm of cardia are usually treated with distal esophagectomy and total or proximal gastrectomy. The esopahgo-gastric anastomosis is made in the thorax (with combined thoracic and abdominal surgery) or in lower cervical region (with trans-hiatal surgery). Distal tumors are treated with subtotal gastrectomy and gastrojejunostomy.[3] Lymph node dissection and sampling is a standard part of all surgical procedures. Small (less than 3 cm) early gastric cancers are successfully treated with endoscopic mucosal resection in Japan.[1] More extensive surgeries along with resection of spleen and distal pancreas may also be performed but this increases the morbidity and mortality.[1,3] Such procedures are successfully done and found effective to treat advanced cancers in Japan; however, similar results could not be reproduced in other parts of the world.

Many of the patients with localized disease undergo neo-adjuvant (preoperative) chemotherapy. It improves the chances of complete (R0) resection and also the overall survival.[3,9,28] CT is normally used to predict and assess the response to chemotherapy in these patients, but with limited success as most gastric cancers are not measurable on CT.[17,29,30] Although PET CT has a limited role in staging, it has been found useful to predict and assess the response to chemotherapy.[31] Adjuvant (post-operative) chemotherapy or radiotherapy offers no significant benefits.[3] Patients with locally advanced or metastatic disease may undergo palliative chemotherapy, radiotherapy or surgery (bypass gastrojejunostomy, feeding jejunostomy or palliative resection to relieve obstruction or bleeding).[1] Stents are also useful to palliate the obstructions at gastroesophageal junction or gastric outlet.[3,32]

Abscess, hematomas or pancreatitis may be seen on CT in postoperative setting. Anastomotic leaks are important cause of postoperative mortality and these can be accurately demonstrated on contrast radiography.[33] Patients with gastrojejunostomies may develop afferent loop syndrome. A fluid distended loop is seen on CT in this condition.

Tumor recurrence may be locoregional (local/ nodal) or at distant metastatic site. Both occur with similar frequency. Peritoneal recurrence is less common and usually seen with advanced T stage or diffuse variety of gastric cancer.[3] Recurrence of gastric cancer is difficult to detect on barium studies or endoscopy and CT is the modality of choice (Fig. 6.13). Local recurrence may be difficult to differentiate from postoperative thickening on CT and biopsy may be required. High attenuation of the wall thickening and perigastric infiltration favor recurrence over benign thickening.[34] PET-CT has also been found useful in patients who are clinically or radiologically suspected to have recurrence.[35,36] Patients

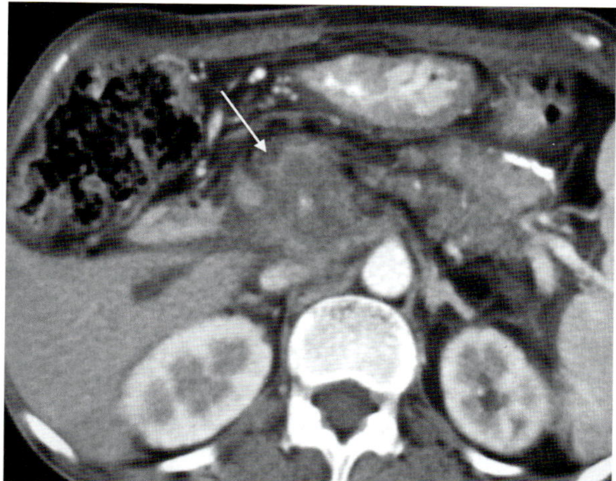

Fig. 6.13: Recurrent gastric cancer: CT shows a lymph nodal mass (arrow) with vascular encasement

treated with curative surgery have 40% five year survival. Those with proximal gastric cancer, Borrmann type 3 or 4 morphology, diffuse type of histology, presence of lymph node metastases or old age have worse prognosis.[1,3] Patients with unresectable disease usually die within six months.

CARCINOMA OF THE SMALL BOWEL

Although the small bowel constitutes the largest part of the GIT, it accounts for only 2% of GIT cancers.[37] Exact cause for this phenomenon is not known but several factors have been postulated. Rapid transit of contents reduces the duration of exposure of potential carcinogens. There is also a rapid turnover of intestinal mucosa and any premalignant transformation is rapidly shaded off. It is estimated that about 1 gm of mucosal cells are replaced every 20 minutes in small bowel.[38] Alkaline pH, few bacterial flora and mucosal enzymes are the other postulated factors.

Adenocarcinoma is considered as the most common primary malignancy of the small bowel.[39] Carcinoid, lymphoma and leiomyosarcoma are other tumors in that order. Incidence of adenocarcinoma is highest at the duodenum and it decreases gradually to have lowest incidence in terminal ileum. Incidence of carcinoid and lymphoma, on other hand, is highest in ileum and lowest in duodenum.

Adenocarcinoma of the Small Bowel

Adenocarcinoma of small bowel is a rare but aggressive tumor and it usually occurs after 50 years of age. In India,

Table 6.4	Small bowel carcinoma: risk factors

- Celiac disease
- Crohn's disease
- Familial adenomatous polyposis
- Lynch syndrome
- Peutz-Jegher's syndrome
- Neurofibromatosis

the incidence is 1-2 cases per 100,000 per year.[2] Celiac disease, Crohn's disease, familial adenomatous polyposis, Lynch syndrome, Peutz-Jeghers syndrome, neurofibromatosis are the risk factors[37,40] (Table 6.4). Small bowel adenocarcinoma shares the risk factors with colorectal cancer but not with gastric cancer. An adenomacarcinoma sequence, similar to colon, also occurs in the pathogenesis of small bowel adenocarcinoma.[41] However, no risk factor is evident in majority of the cases of small bowel adenocarcinoma.

Clinical Features

Most adenocarcinomas of small bowel arise in duodenum and periampullary region is the most favored site. Some of the patients with ampullary carcinoma present with obstructive jaundice early in the course of the disease. Patients with jejunal or ileal adenocarcinoma and those with ulceroinfiltrative duodenal adenocarcinoma usually have non-specific symptoms of nausea, vomiting, abdominal pain, weight loss or GI hemorrhage. Non-specific symptoms and rarity of the disease causes diagnostic delay and hence, most patients have advanced disease when diagnosed.[37] Radiological misinterpretation is also a major cause of diagnostic delay.[42] Many of the patients get treated like inflammatory bowel diseases for long before the correct diagnosis is made. About half of the patients present with acute events like obstruction, perforation or massive GI bleed.

Barium Studies of the Small Bowel

Endoscopy is now the most common modality to diagnose cancers in other parts of GIT, however, barium studies remain the primary modality for diagnosis of small bowel tumors. Distinctive morphological features as seen on barium studies of small bowel also allow specific diagnosis in majority of cases.[43] Barium evaluation of small bowel, however, is more difficult than the upper GIT or colon because of long segment of crowded and overlapping bowel loops and the rapid peristalsis. Many small bowel tumors are now diagnosed with wireless capsule endoscopy, push enteroscopy or double balloon enteroscopy.[37,44] However, these techniques are not common.

Barium meal follow through is the most commonly employed technique for small bowel evaluation. However, it is less sensitive (61%) than enteroclysis (95%) for the diagnosis of small bowel cancer.[45] Hence, enteroclysis should be preferred if small bowel cancer is suspected.[46] If this is not possible, then a carefully performed fluoroscopy and spot imaging during barium meal follow through may be helpful.

Biphasic enteroclysis is performed under mild sedation with catheter tip positioned at duodenojejunal junction. About 400 ml of 50% w/v barium suspension is slowly infused under intermittent fluoroscopy till pelvic ileal loops are opacified. This is followed by slow infusion of 1-2 liters of 0.5% methyl cellulose for double contrast effect. Quality of examination is highly dependent on infusion rate. A slow infusion of methyl cellulose is started and the rate is gradually increased so as to have moderate distension of the bowel without abolition of peristalsis. Higher infusion rate leads to overdistension and abolition of peristalsis. There may be poor mucosal coating and small lesions may be missed. Opacification of the distal ileal loops is especially affected with higher infusion rate. Examination is terminated when terminal ileum is seen transradiant. Intermittent fluoroscopy is performed with compression of the head of the barium column, if required and spot images are obtained during both single and double contrast phases. Some lesions may be less conspicuous on double contrast study and hence it should not be the only phase of evaluation.[47]

Barium Study Features of Carcinoma of the Small Bowel

About 70% of the duodenal adenocarcinomas are polypoidal.[47] Others are ulcerative or infiltrative. Jejunal and ileal adenocarcinoma are usually ulceroinfiltrative. Like most other GIT carcinomas, they present as an 'apple core' lesion on barium studies (Fig. 6.14) (Table 6.5). There is short segment annular narrowing with mucosal irregularity and ulcerations. The narrowing is abrupt and

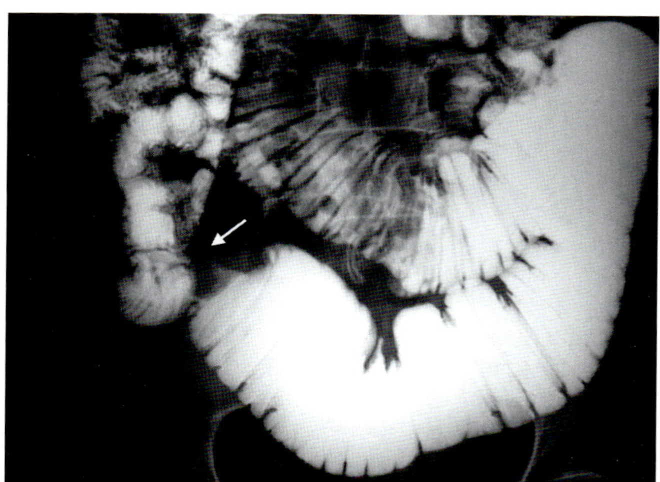

Fig. 6.14: Carcinoma of the jejunum: Barium follow through shows a tight abrupt short segment narrowing (arrow) with overhanging edges. Prestenotic segment of the bowel is dilated

Table 6.5	Small bowel carcinoma: Imaging findings

Barium studies
- Polypoid mass (proximal small bowel)
- Malignant apple core stricture (distal small bowel)
- Intestinal obstruction
- Intussusception

CT
- Above findings
- Lymphadenopathy
- Invasion of adjacent organs
- Invasion of mesentery, vessels
- Liver metastases
- Ascites

over hanging edges (shouldering) are usually present. Frequently, the stricture is tight and lumen barely seen on barium study.[40] There may be prestenotic dilatation of the small bowel. The stricture of the small bowel adenocarcinoma is rigid and does not change its shape on compression during barium studies. Strictures of lymphoma or GIST, on other hand, are softer. Other differential diagnoses of the small bowel strictures include metastases, Crohn's disease, tuberculosis and benign ulcers. When detected early, the jejuna-ileal adenocarcinoma may appear as a sessile polyp and cannot be differentiated from benign polyps. Unlike colorectal polyps, the malignancy cannot be predicted on the basis of size of the polyp in small bowel. Rarely, the polyp may produce intussusception.

CT of the Small Bowel

CT has traditionally been used to assess the extent of the disease, however, it can be used as a first investigation if patient presents with intestinal obstruction.[40] Newer MDCT techniques have been found useful both in the diagnosis as well as surgical planning of the small bowel tumors.[48] Advantages of the MDCT include acquisition in a single breath hold and high resolution axial, multiplanar or volume rendered images. Standard abdominal CT scans are normally performed with positive oral contrast and IV contrast. However, there is decreased contrast between lumen and bowel wall. Distension of the lumen may also be suboptimal. Hence, subtle bowel wall lesions may be missed. This can be improved using large amount of neutral luminal contrast agent (usually water) given orally (CT enterography) or using nasoduodenal tube (CT enteroclysis). Dual phase contrast enhanced MDCT is then performed. With CT enterography, luminal distension may be inadequate, especially in distal bowel loops. CT enteroclysis allows controlled and uniform distension of the bowel and it is more accurate (Fig. 6.15). However, it is more cumbersome to perform and also unpleasant for the patient.[49] Both these techniques combine the advantages of barium studies and standard abdominal CT. Mucosal details however, are better evaluated with barium enteroclysis.

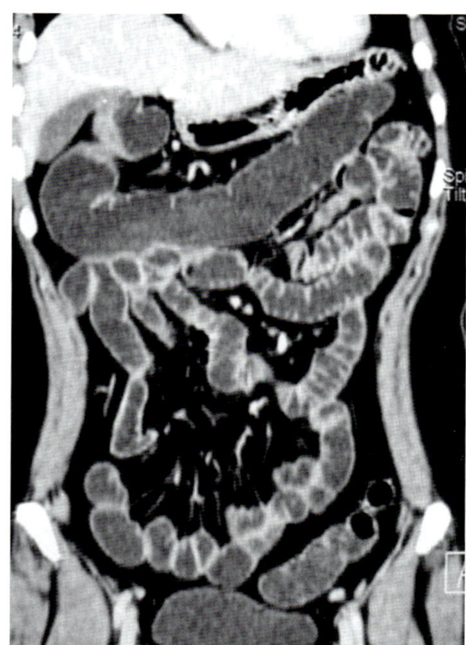

Fig. 6.15: CT enteroclysis

Overall, the CT enteroclysis has 85% sensitivity and 97% specificity in the diagnosis of small bowel tumors.[50] It also allows more accurate delineation of primary and metastatic lesions involving the small bowel when compared with standard abdominal CT.[51]

CT Features of Adenocarcinoma of the Small Bowel

On CT, small bowel adenocarcinoma is seen as ulcerative lesion, polypoidal mass or short segment stricture with wall thickening.[40,47,52] Small masses of adenocarcinoma cannot be differentiated from other polyps or benign tumors like leiomyoma (Fig. 6.16). Ulceration, proximal obstruction or intussusception may also be seen on CT[53]. Occasionally; the involved segment may be long and appear like a lymphoma. With further tumor growth, invasion of mesentery or adjacent organs is seen (Fig. 6.17). Other CT findings in advanced cases include ascites, retroperitoneal/mesenteric lymph node enlargement and liver and peritoneal metastases (Table 6.5). The enlarged lymph nodes may also invade mesenteric vessels.[40,47]

MRI of the Small Bowel

MRI and MR enteroclysis have been found useful for evaluation of the inflammatory small bowel diseases, however, it is less accurate than CT in the evaluation of small bowel tumors.[54-56] MRI and MR cholangiography may sometimes be useful to differentiate ampullary carcinoma of the duodenum from other periampullary carcinomas such as those arising from CBD or pancreas.[57]

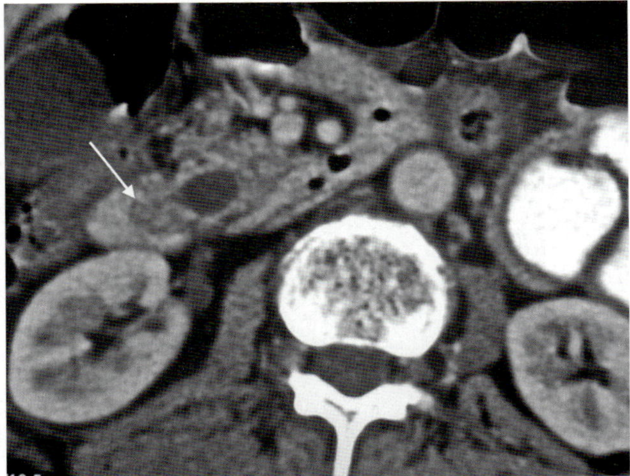

Fig. 6.16: Duodenal carcinoma: CT shows small rounded mass in the ampullary region of the duodenum (arrow). Obstruction and dilatation of the common bile duct is also seen

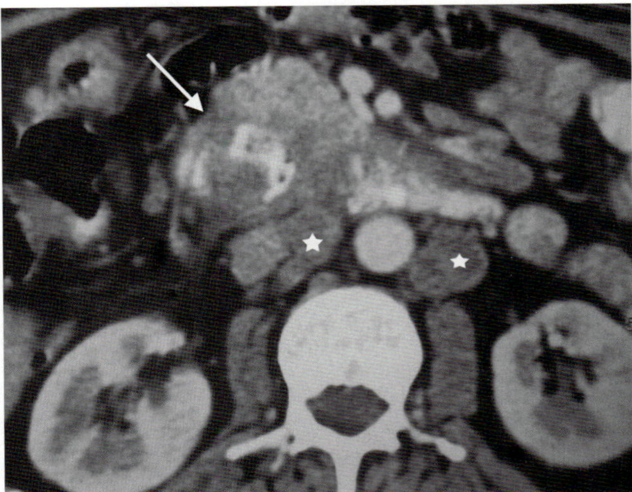

Fig. 6.17: Duodenal carcinoma: CT shows ulcerative and polypoidal duodenal mass with invasion of head of the pancreas (arrow). Enlarged para-aortic lymph nodes are also seen (asterisks)

Staging

AJCC-UICC staging is based on TNM classification (Table 6.6). It applies only to adenocarcinoma of the small bowel and not to GIST, lymphoma or carcinoids. T staging corresponds to the depth of invasion and it is similar to that of the gastric cancer. N and M are divided into only two groups (0 or 1) depending on whether lymphadenopathy or distant metastases are present or absent. Stage 1 disease is up to T2 and stage 2 disease is up to T4. Lymphadenopathy with any T makes it stage 3 while metastases make it stage 4.[40]

Treatment and Prognosis

Prognosis is generally poor. Small bowel adenocarcinomas are primarily treated with surgery. Few are

Table 6.6 Small bowel carcinoma: Staging overview

T1-invasion up to submucosa
T2-invasion up to serosa
T3-invasion beyond serosa
T4-invasion of adjacent organs
N0 - no lymphadenopathy
N1 - lymphadenopathy present
M0 - no distant metastases
M1 - distant metastases present

- Stage 1 - up to T2, no nodes
- Stage 2 - up to T4, no nodes
- Stage 3 - N1 with any T
- Stage 4 - M1 with any T or N

resectable when diagnosed and among them 5 years survival is only 20%. Periampullary carcinomas are usually diagnosed early and many of them are suitable for curative surgery (Whipple's procedure). In patients with advanced disease, chemotherapy, radiotherapy or surgery may be used for palliation with minimal benefits.[37]

Follow-up

CT is the modality of choice; however, there is no standard protocol. CT is performed six months after the curative resection of primary tumor and yearly thereafter. Postoperative changes and scar are sometimes difficult to differentiate from recurrent tumor and CT guided biopsy is required in these situations. More frequent CT may be required if chemo or radiotherapy is used, primarily to assess the response to the treatment.[40]

CARCINOID

Carcinoids are uncommon endocrine tumors of low malignant potential. They commonly occur in GIT followed by tracheobronchial system. Rare sites of origin include liver, gallbladder, gonads and thymus. Small bowel is the most common site of GIT carcinoids, followed by rectum, appendix and stomach.[58] Carcinoids are classified according their embryological origin into foregut carcinoids (tracheobronchial, stomach, duodenum and pancreas), midgut carcinoids (jejunum, ileum, appendix and ascending colon) and hindgut carcinoids (rest of the colon and rectum). Each of these groups has distinct clinical, pathological and imaging features.[59]

Carcinoids of the Stomach and Duodenum

Less than 10% of GIT carcinoids occur in stomach and the duodenum is a site for only 2% of GIT carcinoids.[58] Majority of gastric carcinoids are asymptomatic and incidentally detected on barium studies or endoscopy. Other patients present with abdominal pain and GI hemorrhage. Gastric carcinoids may or may not have endocrine functions. Very few of the gastric or duodenal carcinoids secret serotonin and hence carcinoid syndrome is uncommon with them when compared with the small bowel carcinoids.

Some of the gastric or duodenal carcinoids are associated with MEN 1. These are usually small, multiple and located in the antrum of the stomach or proximal duodenum. They secret gastrin (G-cell carcinoids) and patients present with Zollinger Ellison syndrome (ZES). It is characterized by abdominal pain, diarrhea, vomiting and gastroesphageal reflux. Recurrent gastric ulcers and bleeding from them is also common. Serum gastrin levels may be elevated. Sporadic gastrinomas are also carcinoids which produce ZES. These are located anywhere in gastrinoma triangle which is bounded by junction of cystic duct with CBD superiorly, third part of the duodenum inferiorly and body of the pancreas medially.[59] Other duodenal carcinoids are somatostatin producing tumors (D-cell carcinoids) associated with neurofibromatoisis-1. There are exclusively located around the ampulla and hence patients present with jaundice or pancreatitis.

Imaging Features of Gastric and Duodenal Carcinoids

On barium studies, most gastric carcinoids are seen as small mural masses located in fundus or the body of the stomach. These are usually single but may be multiple. They are often submucosal and hence endoscopic biopsy may be negative.[60] If central portion has ulcerated, it may have a 'bull's eye' appearance. These may also present as one or more sessile or pedunculated polyps. Large polypoid masses may simulate gastric carcinoma.[59] Carcinoids associated with MEN-1 and ZES also show diffuse mucosal fold thickening and ulcerations of the stomach (Table 6.7).

On CT, gastric or duodenal carcinoids are seen as single or multiple, well-defined, intramural or polypoid masses that may contain ulceration (Fig. 6.18). Larger and aggressive gastric carcinoids are seen as enhancing polypoid masses, frequently associated with lymphadenopathy and liver metastases.[59] Dual phase CECT

Table 6.7	Bowel carcinoid: Imaging findings

- Small rounded mural masses, with/without ulceration
- Sessile or pedunculated polyps
- Lobulated, polypoidal masses
- Strong contrast enhancement
- Mucosal fold thickening
- Bowel obstruction/ intussusception
- Rigidity, angulations and kinking of bowel
- Mesenteric fibrosis, masses, calcification
- Lymphadenopathy with calcification
- Hypervascular liver metastases

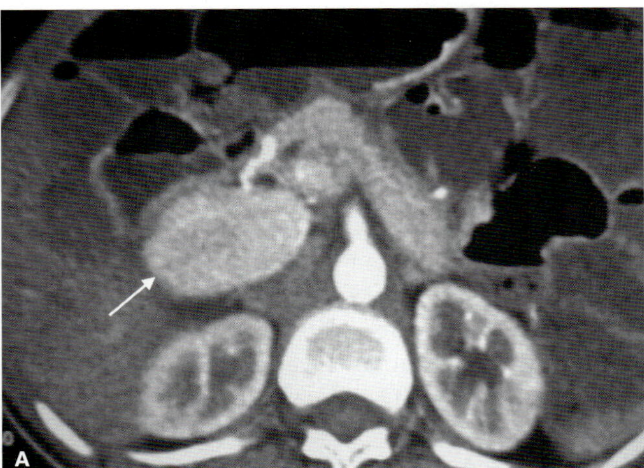

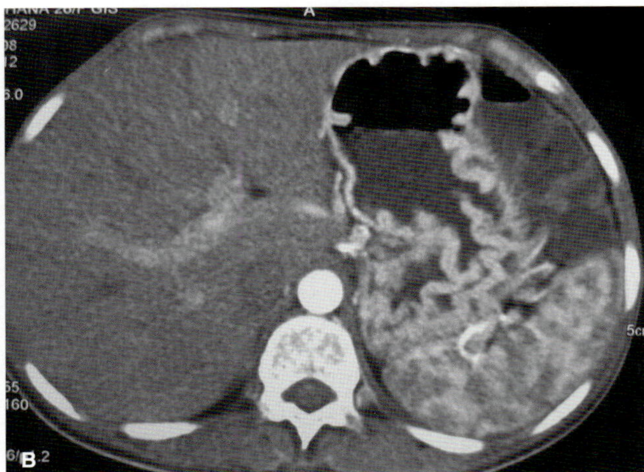

Figs 6.18A and B: Carcinoid: (A) CT shows a well, defined, oval, highly enhancing mass in the duodenum (arrow), (B) CT section at the higher level shows diffuse gastric mucosal fold thickening and enhancement

performed after adequate distension of the stomach with neutral oral contrast is especially useful to detect primary site and liver metastases from gastric carcinoids.[61] There is a strong enhancement on arterial phase and washout on delayed phase.[59] This feature helps to differentiate carcinoids from adenocarcinoma which may also be seen as masses.

Small Bowel Carcinoids

Carcinoid is the second most common malignant lesion of the small bowel. These are commonly located in the ileum, usually within two feet of ileocecal junction. These are multiple in about 30% patients and are associated with second malignancies (usually GIT adenocarcinoma) in up to 29% patients.[58] Most of the small bowel carcinoids are tiny and remain localized, however, up to 80% of small bowel carcinoids of more than 2 cm size have metastases.[62] Most small bowel carcinoids are asymptomatic and found incidentally. Symptomatic patients present with episodic abdominal pain of long duration or bowel obstruction.[63] Even though highly vascular, GI hemorrhage is an uncommon presentation of carcinoids.[40] Majority of the mesenteric small bowel carcinoids secrete serotonin. Up to 17% of patients with small bowel carcinoid present with carcinoid syndrome.[37] It occurs when tumor is large and liver metastases are present. Serotonin, bradykinin, prostaglandins and other pharmacologically active substances are secreted by carcinoids and these are deactivated in liver if tumor burden is small. However, with advanced disease, production of these substances exceeds the breakdown. Liver metastases may also release them directly into the hepatic veins. This produces various symptoms associated with carcinoid syndrome. It is characterized by episodic flushing, cyanosis, watery diarrhea, wheezing and right sided valvular heart disease. The flush is usually triggered by a physical or emotional stress, big meal or even by deep palpation of the abdominal mass. Elevated serum levels of chromogranin A and increased urinary secretion of 5-HIAA (a deaminated serotonin product) is diagnostic of midgut carcinoid tumor.[37]

Imaging Features of Small Bowel Carcinoids

On barium studies, small carcinoids are difficult to detect. Most are seen as smooth, rounded intramural mass lesion. They cannot be differentiated from other benign lesions. However, any distal ileal rounded lesion of more than 1 cm should be considered as carcinoid unless proved otherwise.[47] Presence of additional similar lesions further supports the diagnosis. Larger lesions are polypoidal and may cause intussusception. With further growth, it invades subserosa and adjacent mesentery. Mesenteric infiltration and local release of pharmacologically active substances produce extensive fibrosis in the mesentery and bowel wall. Initially tethering and crowding of adjacent mucosal folds are seen (Fig. 6.19). Chronic ischemia due to mesenteric fibrosis also causes mucosal fold thickening. Subsequently, bowel loops

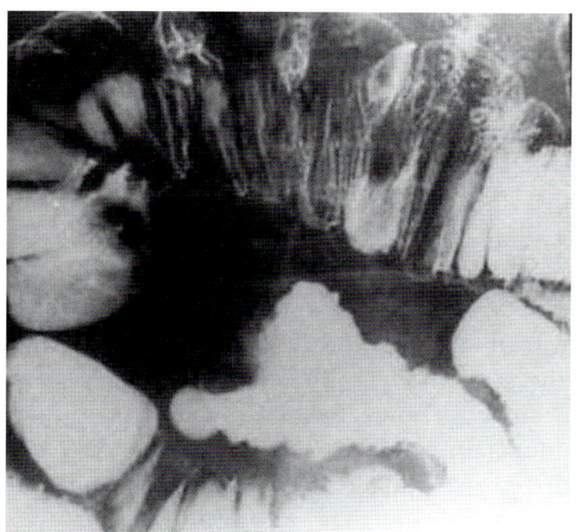

Fig. 6.19: Ileal carcinoid: Barium follow through shows irregularity and narrowing of the ileal loop. Adjacent bowel loops show kinking along with tethering and thickening of the mucosal folds

demonstrate rigidity, fixity, sharp angulations, kinking and narrowing.[40]

Extra-luminal extent of small bowel carcinoid is best demonstrated on CT (Table 6.7). Mesenteric fibrosis is seen as mesenteric streakiness, spiculated mesenteric mass formation and retraction of bowel loops.[64] Kinking, angulation, and narrowing of the small bowel loops are the characteristic features of carcinoid which are seen both on CT and barium studies (Figs 6.20A and B). Primary tumor of the small bowel carcinoid rarely exceed 3.5 cm. Hence, it is frequently overshadowed by extensive mesenteric fibrosis and not apparent on CT.[59] Mesenteric lymphadenopathy is common and calcification is seen in 70% of them.[65] Conglomerate bulky and enhancing mesenteric mass with calcifications is also a characteristic CT feature of carcinoid.[64] Vascular invasion by the mesenteric mass and liver metastases are also seen on CT in cases of advanced small bowel carcinoids. Liver metastases are hypervascular and show intense enhancement on arterial phase of a dual phase CT. Central necrosis with rim enhancement may also be seen.[66]

Differential Diagnosis of Carcinoids

Small, localized and rounded gastric or small bowel carcinoids cannot be differentiated from other similar lesions like leiomyoma, adenoma, lipoma or metastases. Larger polypoid lesions with ulcerations may mimic lymphoma, GIST, metastases or Kaposi's sarcoma. Advanced small bowel carcinoids with mesenteric fibrosis produce characteristic imaging appearances, however, similar features may rarely be seen with

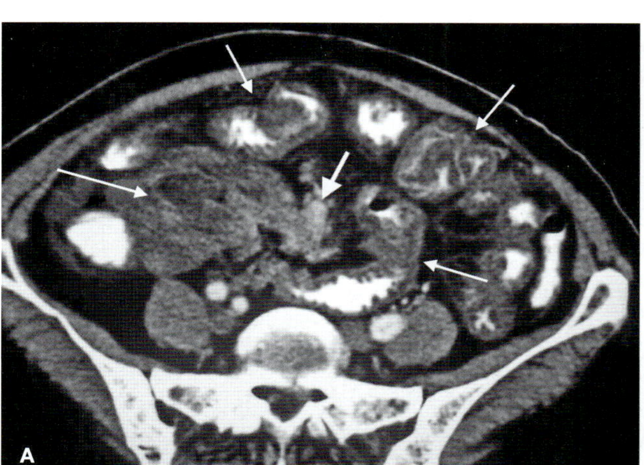

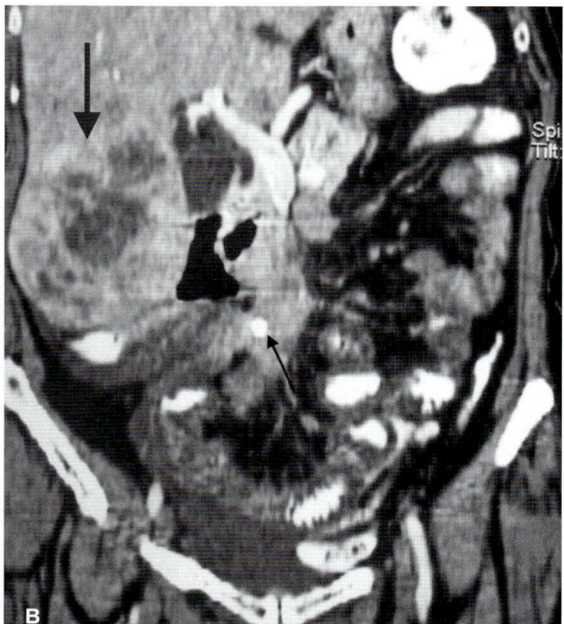

Figs 6.20A and B: Carcinoid of the ileum: (A) CT shows an ill-defined ileal mass with mesenteric extension (thick arrow). Adjacent bowel loops show mucosal wall thickening, kinking and sharp angulations (arrows), (B) Coronal reconstruction shows mesenteric fibrosis and spiculated mass with calcification (arrow). Thickening and kinking of adjacent small bowel loops as well as a large enhancing liver metastasis (thick arrow) are also seen

Crohn's disease, postoperative mesenteric fibrosis, radiation enteropathy and peritoneal metastases.[47] Scintigraphy or PET CT with somatostatin receptor analogue (Indium 111 octreotide) is useful in the diagnosis of primary as well as metastatic sites of carcinoids.[67]

Treatment and Prognosis

Overall, carcinoids have a better prognosis than adenocarcinoma. Small gastric carcinoids can be treated with endoscopic removal while larger require surgical resection.[1] Small bowel carcinoids are treated with bowel and regional lymph nodes resection. Patients with advanced and metastatic disease also benefit with debulking surgery and somatostatin medical therapy. Systemic chemotherapy is ineffective in the treatment of advanced carcinoids.[37] Hepatic artery chemoembolization is the mainstay of the treatment of carcinoid metastases in liver.[68] Radiofrequency ablation is also effective.[69] Overall five years survival after curative resection of carcinoid is 73%. Many patients survive longer, even with metastases.[37]

GASTROINTESTINAL STROMAL TUMORS (GIST)

These are the mesenchymal neoplasms of GIT with either smooth muscle or neural differentiation. Immunohistochemically they are C-KIT (CD 117) positive. This feature differentiates these tumors from rare true smooth muscle tumors (leiomyoma, leiomyosarcoma) and neurogenic tumors (schwannoma, neurofibroma).[70] Majority of GISTs are also CD 34 positive. Before the immunohistochemically distinct nature of GIST was recognized, these were classified as leiomyoma or leiomyosarcoma. True leiomyoma or leiomyosarcoma of the GIT are extremely rare, except in the esophagus.[37,71] These have identical imaging features as GISTs. Majority of GISTs arise in small bowel followed by the stomach. Rarely, they may originate in esophagus, colon, rectum, mesentery or omentum. Most GIST are benign, however, the malignant potential is variable. Malignant potential is assessed with size and mitotic figure rate on pathology.[37] Tumors smaller than 2 cm are usually benign while those larger than 5 cm behave aggressively.

Small GISTs are frequently detected incidentally. Patients with large and malignant GIST usually present with long duration of abdominal pain, abdominal mass or GI hemorrhage. They grow more slowly than adenocarcinoma.[70] In stomach, only 30% of GISTs are malignant and these are usually located in distal stomach. In small bowel, half of them are malignant and are usually located in distal small bowel.[72]

Imaging Features of GIST

GISTs may be submucosal, intramural or subserosal in location and small or large in size. Imaging cannot differentiate between benign and malignant GISTs.[73]

On barium studies, small submucosal GIST (or leiomyoma) appears as a smooth, round filling defect in stomach or small bowel (Fig. 6.21) (Table 6.8). Large subserosal tumors produce extrinsic impression or displacement of bowel loops[71] (Fig. 6.22). The growth of the tumor is predominantly in exophytic pattern and they produce large lobulated abdominal masses.[74] Because of this reason, the findings on barium studies are more subtle than seen on CT.

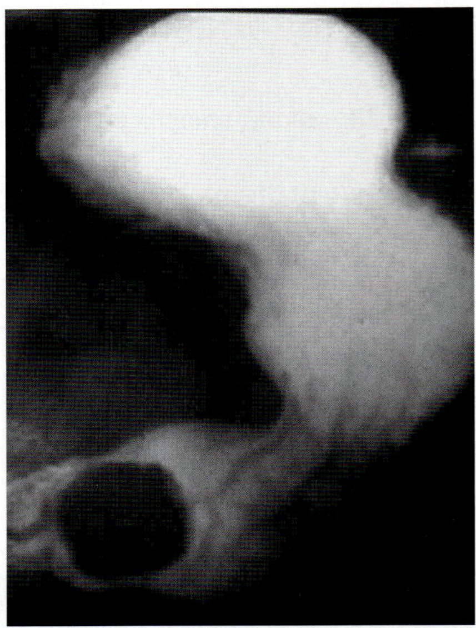

Fig. 6.21: GIST of the stomach: Barium UGI study shows it as a small, rounded, well-defined filling defect in the antrum

Table 6.8	GIST: Imaging findings
• Smooth rounded submucosal mass • Large exophytic mass • Heterogeneous contrast enhancement • Necrotic or cystic areas • Fistula with bowel • Invasion of other organs, mesentery • Liver metastases *Distinctly uncommon findings* • Bowel obstruction • Lymphadenopathy • Ascites	

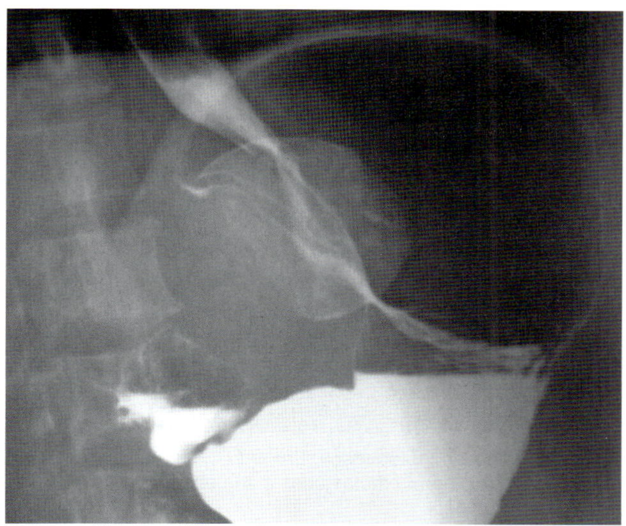

Fig. 6.22: GIST of the stomach: Barium UGI study shows a large mass with smooth mucosal surface and a mass effect along the lesser curvature of the stomach

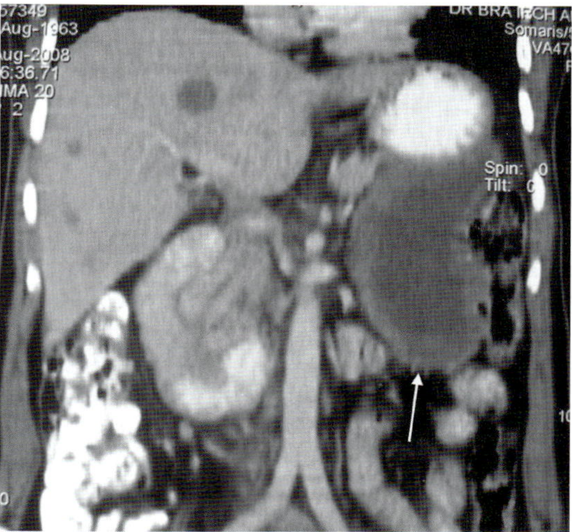

Fig. 6.23: Malignant GIST of the stomach: Coronal reconstruction of the CT shows a large, necrotic mass arising from the stomach (arrow). The mucosal folds are preserved as the growth is predominantly exophytic. Multiple liver metastases are also seen

On CT, small GISTs are seen as well-defined, solid stomach or small bowel masses with mild, homogenous contrast enhancement. Calcifications may be present.[52] Those protruding into the lumen form acute angle with adjacent mucosa. Predominantly exophytic lesions have obtuse angle with the lumen. Large tumors are seen as irregular, lobulated, exophytic masses (Fig. 6.23). The contrast enhancement is heterogeneous and large areas of necrosis are common. Rarely, the tumor may be entirely cystic.[75] Tumor margin is usually well-defined but may be ill-defined in large tumors. Mucosal ulceration and fistulous communication of necrotic cavity with the bowel lumen is common with large tumors[71] (Figs 6.24A and B). Ascites, lymphadenopathy and intestinal obstruction are uncommon in GIST (Table 6.8). Metastases are most common to liver, mesentery and peritoneum, however, unlike other sarcomas, are distinctly uncommon in lungs.[70,73] Peritoneal metastases are seen as solid peritoneal nodules with the morphology similar to the primary tumor. If extensive peritoneal dissemination is present, location of the primary tumors may be difficult to determine on CT. Direct invasion of adjacent bowel loops or vascular encasement may also be seen in advanced cases. MRI features of GISTs are similar to those seen on CT. They are seen as solid masses with variable signal intensity and intense, heterogeneous contrast enhancement.[74] MRI is especially useful to determine the organ of origin in difficult cases. Hemorrhages in the tumor can also be readily detected

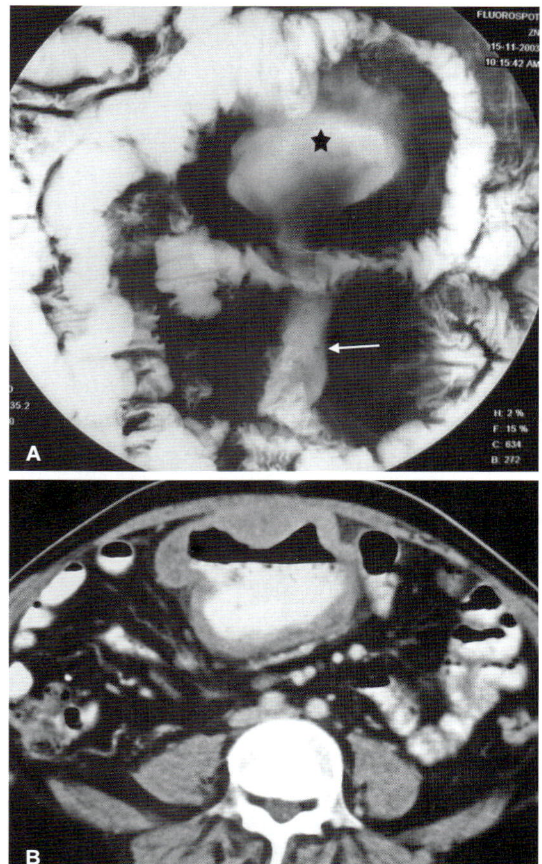

Figs 6.24A and B: GIST of the small bowel: (A) Barium follow through study shows narrowed segment of the ileum with mucosal irregularity (arrow) and mass effect seen as displacement of adjacent bowel loops. It is communicating with a large necrotic cavity (star), (B) CT shows the mass with necrotic cavity to a better extent

on MRI.[71] DSA may be performed in patients presenting with GI hemorrhage and it demonstrates a hypervascular mass.[75] PET imaging is useful to differentiate malignant from non-metastasizing GISTs.[70]

Treatment of GIST

Localized GISTs are treated effectively with surgical resection. Malignant GISTs have better prognosis than the adenocarcinoma of stomach or small bowel.[37] Tumors found incidentally are smaller and have better prognosis than the symptomatic patients. After surgical resection, 5 year recurrence free survival is 63%.[76] Malignant GISTs with high mitotic rate, size more than 10 cm and location in small bowel are more aggressive and have higher recurrence rates.[76] Chemotherapy with imatinib mesylate (Gleevec), a tyrosine kinase inhibitor, has been found effective in the treatment of metastatic GIST.[37] On imatinib treatment, tumor and liver metastases usually decrease in size and appear cystic on CT or MRI.[71] Rarely, the cystic lesions may remain stable in size or appear enlarged. This should not be confused with progressive disease.[77] PET imaging can assess the response to imatinib therapy much before the morphological changes are apparent.[78]

METASTASES TO THE STOMACH AND SMALL BOWEL

Metastases may spread to stomach or small bowel hematogenously (primaries from lung, breast, cervix, kidney or melanoma) or by intraperitoenal seedling (primaries from appendix, colon or ovary). Direct invasion of stomach or small bowel can also occur from adjacent tumors. Patients with stomach or small bowel metastases usually present with abdominal pain, GI hemorrhage or intestinal obstruction.[79] Clinical history is important in their diagnosis.

Metastases to stomach may appear as solitary or multiple nodules or diffuse wall thickening. Central 'bull's eye' ulceration may also be seen in nodules, especially in melanoma metastases[1] (Fig. 6.25). Rarely, large exophytic component is seen on CT. Infiltrative metastases, usually from breast, may produce linitis plastica type appearance in the antrum of the stomach. They also cause similar long segment narrowing with obstruction in small bowel.[40]

Intestinal metastases also manifest as single or multiple discrete intramural masses. These may be flat or polypoid. Ulceration may also be seen giving target appearance on barium studies. Intramural or intraluminal metastases may produce intussusceptions. Metastasis is the most common malignant cause of small bowel intussusceptions in adults.[79] Metastases in small bowel frequently produce annular constricting lesions which are difficult to differentiate from primary tumors on imaging. However, metastases tend to involve much longer segment of the bowel. They also cause desmoplastic reaction resulting in severe narrowing and angulations of the small bowel.[40] Desmoplastic reaction, however, does not occur with metastases from melanoma.[47] Annular malignant strictures in ileum usually represent metastases or lymphoma, rather than adenocarcinoma, which is rare in the ileum.[40] Other small bowel metastases, from lung cancer in particular, produce large mesenteric masses with infiltration and angulations of the small bowel wall.[40] Duodenal metastases may produce obstruction and dilatation of CBD and pancreatic duct.[80] Intraperitoneal seedlings are usually mucinous tumors. These produce multiple nodules or masses on the serosal surface of small bowel and in the mesentery and omentum. Ascites is usually present.

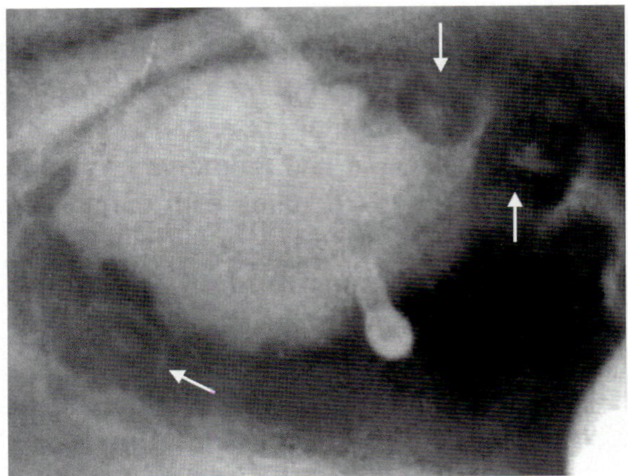

Fig. 6.25: Metastases to stomach: Barium UGI study shows multiple small, rounded melanoma metastases in the stomach with 'bull's eye' appearance (arrows)

MISCELLANEOUS MALIGNANT TUMORS OF STOMACH AND SMALL BOWEL

Lymphoma of the stomach and small bowel is described elsewhere in this book. Rarely, stomach may also be involved by leukemia or multiple myeloma.[1] Kaposi's sarcoma is a systemic multifocal malignancy characterized by visceral as well as pigmented skin lesions. It is rare in small bowel and always associated with AIDS. It is often multicentric. Most patients are asymptomatic and other may present with bowel obstruction or GI bleed. Imaging features are non-specific. It is usually seen as an elevated submucosal mass in small bowel. Multiple lesions may coalesce to form a mural mass with thickened mucosal fold and simulate lymphoma or GIST on imaging. Retroperitoneal and mesenteric lymphadenopathy is also commonly seen in Kaposi's sarcoma.[40] Angiosarcomas of the small bowel are extremely rare and patients may present with chronic anemia, massive GI bleed or intestinal obstruction. On imaging, they are seen as multiple filling defects or large annular lesions. Malignant liposarcomas are rare in small bowel, however, liposarcomas of retroperitoneum may secondarily involve it.

REFERENCES

1. Gore RM, Miller FH. Stomach cancer. In Brag DG, Rubin P, Hrickack H. (Ed) Oncologic imaging. Second edition. WB Saunders Co. Philadelphia, 2002;391-418.
2. National Cancer Registry Program: Two years report of population based cancer registries. Indian Council of Medical Research, New Delhi, 2005.
3. Pisters PWT, Keslen DP, Tepper JE. Cancer of the stomach. In: DeVita VT, Lawrence TS, Rosenberg SA (Ed). Cancer: principles and practice of oncology. Lippincott, Williams and Wilkins, 8th edition, 2008;1043-79.
4. Parsonnet J, Friedman GD, Vandersteen DP, et al. *Helicobacter pylori* infection and the risk of gastric carcinoma. N Engl J Med 1991;325;1127-31.
5. Ramon JM, Sera L, Cerdo C, et al. Dietary factors and gastric cancer risk: A case control study in Spain. Cancer 1993;71:1731-35.
6. Ginsberg GG, Al Kawas FH, Fleischer DE, et al. Gastric polyps: relationship of size and histology to cancer risk. Am J Gastroenterol 1996;91-714-17.
7. Crookes PF, Incarbone R, Peters JH, et al. A selective therapeutic approach to gastric cancer in a large public hospital. Am J Surg 1995;170:602-05.
8. Minami M, Kawauchi N, Itai Y. Gastric tumors: Radiologic-pathologic correlation and accuracy of T staging with dynamic CT. Radiology 1992;185:171-78.
9. Fuch CS, Meyer RJ. Gastric carcinoma. N Engl J Med 1995;333:32-41.
10. Levine MS, Laufer I. UGI series at crossroads. Am J Roentgenol 1993;161:1131-37.
11. Gore RM, Levine MS, Gahremani GG, et al. Gastric cancer: Radiologic diagnosis. Radiol Clin N Am 1997;35:311-29.
12. Farley DR, Donohue JH. Early gastric cancer. Surg Clin N Am 1992;72:401-21.
13. Gold RP, Green PH, O'Toole KM, et al. Early gastric cancer: Radiographic experience. Radiology 1984;152: 283-90.
14. Haruma K, Suzuki T, Tsuda T, et al. Evaluation of tumor growth rate in patients with early gastric carcinoma of elevated type. Gastrointest Radiology 1991;16:289-92.
15. Levine MS, Kong V, Rubesin SE, et al. Scirrhous carcinoma of the stomach: Radiologic and endoscopic diagnosis. Radiology 1990;175:151-54.
16. Miller FH, Kochman ML, Talamonti MS, et al. Gastric cancer: radiologic staging. Radiol Clin N Am 1997;35: 331-49.
17. Lim JS, Yun MJ, Kim MJ, et al. CT and PET in stomach cancer: preoperative staging and monitoring response to therapy. Radiographics 2006;26:143-56.
18. Marks WM, Callen PW, Moss AA. Gastroesophageal region: source of confusion on CT. Am J Roentgenol 1981;136:359-62.
19. D'Elia F, Zingarelli A, Palli D, et al. Hydrodynamic CT preoperative staging of gastric cancer: correlation with pathological findings. A prospective study of 107 cases. Eur Radiol 2000;10:1877-81.
20. Horton KM, Fishman EK. Current role of CT in imaging of the stomach. Radiographics 2003;23:75-87.
21. Kim HJ, Kim AY, Oh ST, et al. Gastric cancer staging at multidetector row CT gastrography: comparison of transverse and volumetric CT scanning. Radiology 2005;236:879-85.
22. Chen CY, Hsu JS, Wu DC, et al. Gastric cancer: preoperative local staging with 3D multidetector row CT – correlation with surgical and histopathological results. Radiology 2007;242:472-82.
23. Cho KC, Alterman DD, Fusco JM, et al. Transpyloric spread of gastric tumors: comparison of adenocarcinoma and lymphoma. Am J Roentgenol 1996;167:467-69.
24. Fukuya T, Honda H, Hayashi T, et al. Lymph node metastases: Efficacy for detection with helical CT in patients with gastric cancer. Radiology 1995;197:705-11.
25. Shah M, Yeung HW, Trocola D, et al. The characteristics and utility of FDG PET scans in patients with localized gastric cancer. Proc Am Soc Clin Oncol 2007;1:2.
26. Matsumato Y, Yanai H, Tokiyama H, et al. Endoscopic ultrasonography for diagnosis of submucosal invasion in early gastric cancer. J Gastroenterol 2000;35:326-30.
27. Moreaux J, Bougaran J. Early gastric cancer: A 25 years surgical experience. Ann Surg 1993;217:347-55.
28. Cunningham D, Allum WH, Stenning SP, et al. Perioperative chemotherapy versus surgery alone for resectable gastroesophageal cancers . N Engl J Med 2006; 355:11-17.
29. Beer AJ, Wieder HA, Lordick F, et al. Adenocarcinoma of esophagogastric junction: mutlidetector row CT to evaluate early response to neoadjuvant chemotherapy. Radiology 2006;239:471-80.
30. Park SR, Lee JS, Kim CG, et al. Endoscopic ultrasound and computed tomography in restaging and predicting

prognosis after neo-adjuvant chemotherapy in patients with locally advanced gastric cancer. Cancer 2008; 112:2368-76.

31. Weider HA, Peer AJ, Lordik F, et al. Comparison in tumor metabolic activity and tumor size during chemotherapy of adenocarcinomas of the esophago-gastric junction. J Nucl Med 2005;46:2029-32.
32. Binkert CA, Jost R, Steiner A, et al. Benign and malignant stenoses of stomach and duodenum: Treatment with self expanding metallic endoprostheses. Radiology 1996; 199:335-38.
33. Lamb PJ, Griffin SM, Chandrashekar MV, et al. Prospective study of routine contrast radiology after total gastrectomy. Br J Surg 2004;91:1015-19.
34. Kim JY, Kim SH, Lee JM, et al. Differentiating malignant from benign wall thickening in postoperative stomach using helical computed tomography: results of multivariate analysis. J Comput AssistTomogr 2007;31:455-62.
35. Sun L, Su XH, Guan YH, et al. Clinical role of 18 fluorodeoxyglucose positron emission tomography/ computed tomography in postoperative follow up of gastric cancer: initial results. World J Gastroenterol 2008;14:4627-32.
36. Park MJ, Lee WJ, Lim KH, et al. Detecting recurrence of gastric cancer: the value of FDG PET/CT. Abdom Imaging 2008;Epub.
37. Zeh HJ, Federle M. Cancer of the small intestine. In: DeVita VT, Lawrence TS, Rosenberg SA (Eds). Cancer: Principles and practice of oncology. Lippincott, Wiliams and Wilkins, 2008, 8th edition;1186-1204.
38. Calman KC. Why are small bowel tumors rare? An experimental model. Gut 1974;15-552-54.
39. Weis NS, Yang CP. Incidence of histologic types of cancer of the small intestine. J Natl Cancer Inst 1987;78:653-58.
40. Gourtosoyiannis NC, Odze RD, Ros PR. Malignant small bowel neoplasms. In: Gourtosoyiannis NC (Ed). Radiological imaging of the small bowel. Springer, Berlin, 2002; 398-428.
41. Selliner F. Investigations on significance of adenoma-carcinoma sequence in the small bowel. Cancer 1990; 66:702-06.
42. Maglinte DDT, O'Connor K, Bessette J, et al. The role of the physician in the late diagnosis of primary malignant tumors of the small intestine. Am J Gastroenterol 1991;86:304-08.
43. Nagi B, Verma V, Vaiphei K, et al. Primary small bowel tumors: a radiologic-pathologic correlation. Abdom Imaging 2001;26:474-80.
44. Kala Z, Valek V, Kysela P, et al. A shift in the diagnostics of small bowel tumors. Eur J Radiol 2007;62:160-66.
45. Bessette JR, Maglinte DDT, Kelvin FM, et al. Primary malignant tumors in small bowel: a comparison of small bowel enema and conventional follow through. Am J Roentgenol 1989;153:741-44.
46. Maglinte DDT, Kelvin FM, O'Connor K, et al. Current status of small bowel radiography. Abdom Imaging 1996;21:247-57.
47. Maglinte DDT, Reyes BL. Small bowel cancer: Radiologic diagnosis. Radiol Clin N Am 1997;35:361-80.
48. Horton KM, Fishman EK. Multidetector row computed tomography and 3-dimesional computed tomography imaging of small bowel neoplasms: current concept in diagnosis. J Comput Assist Tomogr 2004;28:106-16.
49. Patak MA, Mortele KJ, Ros PR. Mutlidetector row CT of the small bowel. Radiol Clin N Am 2005;43:1063-77.
50. Pilleul F, Penigaud M, Milt L, et al. Possible small bowel neoplasms: contrast enhanced and water enhanced multidetector CT enteroclysis. Radiology 2006;241: 796-801.
51. Maglinte DDT, Sandrasegaran K, Lappas JC, et al. CT enteroclysis. Radiology 2007;245:661-71.
52. Buckley JA, Fishman EK. CT evaluation of small bowel neoplasms: spectrum of disease. Radiographics 1998; 18:379-92.
53. Kazerooni EA, Quint LE, Francis IR. Duodenal neoplasms: Predictive value of CT for determining malignancy and tumor resectability. Am J Roentgenol 1992;159:303-09.
54. Schmidt S, Lepori D, Meuwly JY, et al. Prospective comparison of MR enteroclysis with multidetector spiral CT enteroclysis: interobserver agreement and sensitivity by means of 'sign-by-sign' correlation. Eur Radiol 2003;13:1303-11.
55. Fidlers J, MR imaging of small bowel. Radiol Clin N Am 2007;45:317-31.
56. Ryan ER, Heaslip IS. Magnetic resonance enteroclysis compared with conventional enteroclysis and computed tomography enteroclysis: a critically appraised topic. Abdom Imaging 2008;33:34-37.
57. Kim JH, Kim MJ, Chung J, et al. Differential diagnosis of periampullary carcinomas at MR imaging. Radiographics 2002;22:1335-52.
58. Modlin IM, Lye KD, Kidd M. A 5-decade analysis of 13,715 carcinoid tumors. Cancer 2003;97:934-59.
59. Levy AD, Sobin AH. Gastrointestinal carcinoids: imaging features with clinic-pathological correlation. Radiographics 2007;27:237-57.
60. Nakamura S, Lida M, Yao T, et al. Endoscopic features of gastric carcinoids. Gastrointest Endosc 1991;37:535-38.
61. Ba –Ssalamah A, Prokop M, Ufmann M, et al. Dedicated multidetector CT of the stomach: spectrum of diseases. Radiographics 2003;23:371-73.
62. Wallace S, Ajani JA, Charnasangavej C, et al. Carcinoid tumors: Imaging procedures and interventional radiology. World J Surg 1996;20:147-56.
63. McCleod Mk, Fig LM, et al. Clinical features, diagnosis and localization of carcinoid tumors and their management. Gastroenterol Clin N Am 1989;18:865-69.
64. Woodard PK, Feldman JM, Paine SS, et al. Midgut carcinoid tumors: CT findings and biochemical profiles. J Comput Assist Tomogr 1995;19:400-05.
65. Pantongrag-Brown L, Beutow PC, Carr NJ, et al. Calcification and fibrosis in mesenteric carcinoid tumor: CT findings and pathologic correlation. Am J Roentgenol 1995;164:387-91.

66. Pelage JP, Soyer P, Boudiaf M, et al. Carcinoid tumors of the abdomen: CT features. Abdom Imaging 1999;24: 240-45.
67. Nicou GC, Lygidakis NJ, Toubankis C, et al. Current diagnosis and treatment of gastrointestinal carcinoids in a series of 101 patient: the significance of serum chromogranin A, somatostatin receptor scintigraphy and somatostatin analogues. Hepatogastroenterology 2005;52:731-41.
68. Bloomston M, Al-Saif O, Klemanski D, et al. Hepatic artery chemoembolization in 122 patients with metastatic carcinoid tumor: lessons learned. J Gastrointest Surgery 2007;11:264-68.
69. Atwel TD, Charboneau JW, Que FG, et al. Treatment of neuroendocrine cancer metastatic to the liver: role of ablative techniques. Cardiovasc Intervent Radiol 2005;28:409-12.
70. Hersh MR, Choi J, Garrett C, et al. Imaging gastrointestinal stromal tumors. Cancer Control 2005;12: 111-15.
71. Levy AD, Remotti HE, Thompson WM, et al. Gastrointestinal stromal tumors: radiologic features with pathologic correlation. Radiographics 2003;23:283-304.
72. Horton KM, Juluru K Montgomery E, et al. Computed tomography imaging of gastrointestinal stromal tumors with pathologic correlation. J Comput Assist Tomogr 2004;28:811-17.
73. Gong JS, Zuo M, Yang P, et al. Value of CT in diagnosis and follow up of gastrointestinal stromal tumors. Clinical Imaging 2008;32:172-77.
74. Ranchod M, Kempson RL. Smooth muscle tumors of the gastrointestinal tract and retroperitoneum. A pathological analysis of 100 cases. Cancer 1977;39:255-58.
75. Darnell, A, Dalmau E, Pericay C, et al. Gastrointestinal stromal tumors. Abdom Imaging 2006;31:387-99.
76. Dematteo RP, Gold JS, Saran L, et al. Tumor mitotic rate, size, and location independently predict recurrence after resection of primary gastrointestinal stromal tumor (GIST). Cancer 2008;112:608-15.
77. Chen M, Bechtold R, Savage P, et al. Cystic changes in hepatic metastases from gastrointestinal stromal tumors (GISTs) treated with Gleevec (imatinib mesylate). Am J Roentgenol 2002;179:1059-62.
78. Choi H, Charnsangavej C, DeCastro FS, et al. CT evaluation of the response of gastrointestinal stromal tumors after imatinib mesylate treatment: a quantitative analysis correlated with FDG PET findings. Am J Roentgenol 2004;183:1619-28.
79. Subramanian S, Kumar M, Thulkar S, et al. Bowel metastases from primary leiyomyosarcoma of the gluteal region. Singapore Med J 2008;49:e68-70.
80. Farah MC, Jafri SZH, Schwab RE, et al. Duodenal neoplasms: role of CT. Radiology 1987;162:839-43.

Chapter Seven

Abdominal Tuberculosis

Anjali Prakash

Tuberculosis has been declared a global emergency by the world health organization and is the most important communicable disease worldwide. The prevalence of extra pulmonary tuberculosis seems to be rising, particularly due to the increasing incidence of acquired immunodeficiency syndrome (AIDS). Extrapulmonary form of TB which accounts for 10-15% of all cases may represent up to 50% of patients with AIDS. TB of the GIT is the sixth most common site of extrapulmonary TB, after lymphatic, genitourinary, bone and joint, miliary and meningeal TB.

The concept of abdominal tuberculosis refers to peritoneum and its reflections, gastrointestinal tract, abdominal lymphatic system and solid visceral organs, as they are subject to varying degrees of involvement, either alone or in combination.

The causative organisms include:

i. *Mycobacterium tuberculosis hominis*
ii. *Mycobacterium bovis*, and
iii. Atypical mycobacterium (*Mycobacterium avium* intracellulare)—associated with patients suffering from AIDS.

Most bacilli isolated in patients with abdominal tuberculosis are *Mycobacterium tuberculosis* and not *Mycobacterium bovis*. Suppression of host defenses by conditions such as malnutrition, weight loss, alcoholism, diabetes, chronic renal failure, immunosuppression, AIDS, etc, increases the risk of reactivation of an intestinal dormant focus.

Routes of GI infection include the following:

1. Spread by means of ingestion of infected sputum, in patients with active pulmonary TB and especially in patients with pulmonary cavitation and positive sputum smears.
2. Spread through a hematogenous route from a tuberculous focus in the lung to submucosal lymph nodes; and
3. Local spread from surrounding organs involved by primary tuberculous infection (e.g. renal TB causing fistulas into the duodenum or mediastinal TB lymphadenopathy involving the esophagus).

Although the presence of thoracic tuberculosis may be suggestive of associated abdominal tuberculosis, only 15% of patients with abdominal TB have evidence of pulmonary disease. The chest radiograph may be normal in 50-65% of these patients. [2, 3]

Pathological Findings

G.I TB is characterized by inflammation and fibrosis of the bowel wall and the regional lymph nodes, inflammation takes place in the submucosal lymphoid tissue of the intestine resulting in wall thickening due to formation of epitheliod tubercles, cellular infiltration and lymphatic hyperplasia. Within 2-4 weeks caseous necrosis of the tubercle begins which eventually leads to ulceration of the overlying mucosa. Further extension within the bowel wall and regional nodes occurs by lymphatic spead. Granuloma formation, fibrosis and scarring develop in a later stage. Regional lymphadenopathy may adhere to the diseased bowel wall, forming an inflammatory mass.The gross appearance of the intestinal tuberculous lesion has lead to its traditional categorization into three forms. The more common ulcerative form is characterized by the presence of multiple small ulcers, usually 3-6 mm in diameter, with an irregular margin; they usually present as transverse lesions located parallel to each other. This orientation is related to the arrangement of the submucosal lymphatic structures. In the less common hypertrophic form, extensive inflammatory response and reactive tissue produce a multinodular mucosal pattern resembling a neoplastic process. The ulcero-hypertrophic pattern consists of a combination of both types and may result in a cobble-stone appearance.

Clinical Spectrum

Abdominal tuberculosis is predominantly a disease of young adults. Two thirds of patients are 21-40 years old and sex incidence is equal, though some studies have shown a slight female preponderance. The spectrum of disease in children is different from adults[1,4] in whom adhesive peritoneal and lymph nodal involvement is more common than gastro-intestinal disease. The clinical presentation can be acute, chronic or acute on chronic. Most patients have constitutional symptoms. In addition they may present with diarrhea and malabsorption in ulcerative form or with recurrent sub acute intestinal obstruction in strictures type.

TUBERCULOUS PERITONITIS

Peritoneum and its reflections are common sites of tuberculous involvement of the abdomen. Most cases are as a result of reactivation of latent tuberculous foci in the peritoneum or due to tubercular salpingitis or discharge of caseous material from diseased lymph nodes.

Classically three forms of tuberculous peritonitis have been described[5-7]

i. Wet ascitic type-seen in 90% cases characterized by large amounts of free or loculated ascitic fluid (Fig. 7.1).
ii. Fibrotic fixed type-characterized by mesenteric and omental thickening and masses, matted bowel loops and occasionally loculated ascitis.
iii. Dry or 'plastic' type-unusual caseous nodules, fibrous peritoneal reaction and dense adhesions.

Ascitis: Free or loculated ascitis is seen in 30-100% of cases and is demonstrated by both ultrasound and CT.[8-10] Ultrasound is recommended as an initial investigation to image very small quantities of ascitis. Ultrasound reveals fine, multiple, complete or incomplete, mobile strands of fibrin and debris in the ascitis in 10-100% of patients (Fig. 7.2).

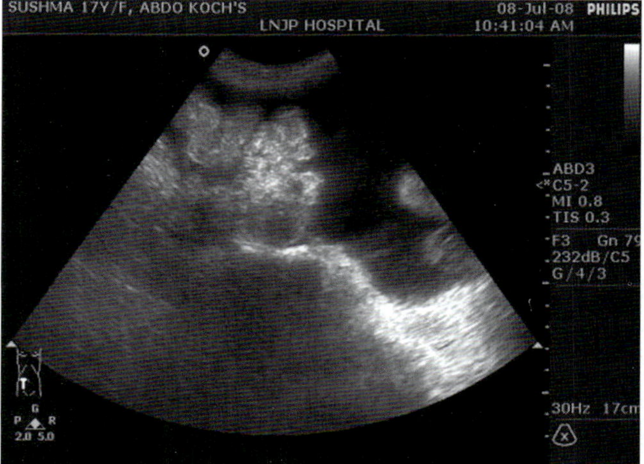

Fig. 7.1: USG:Voluminous free fluid with floating bowel loops in a case of peritonealTB

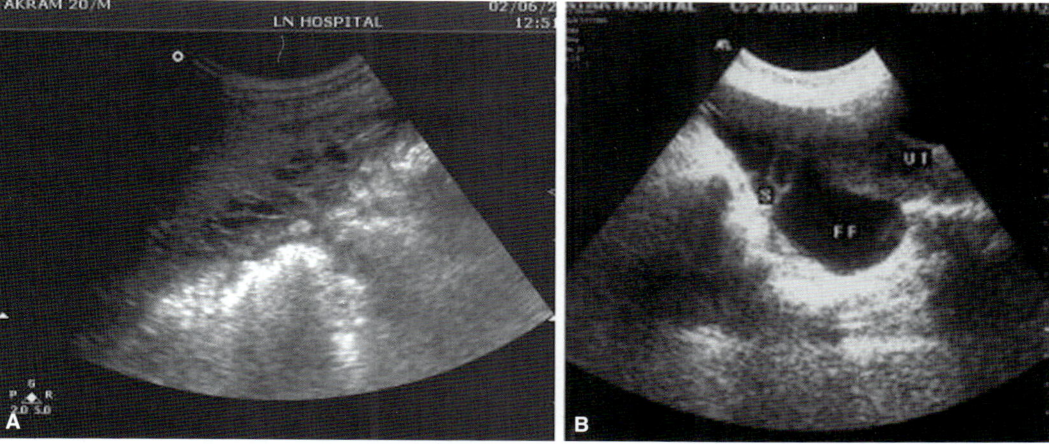

Figs. 7.2A and B: USG. Complex ascitis with loculations and septae seen in perihepatic (A) and rectovesical pouch (B)

On CT, high density (25-45 HU) of fluid due to high fibrin content and cellular debris is characteristic of TB.[6] However, ascitis may be near water density, representing an earlier transudative stage of immune reaction. Fat fluid level, a feature of chylous ascitis with supportive evidence of mesenteric adenopathy has been described in tuberculosis.[11] Computed tomography fails to show multiple, thin interlacing septa in most patients, especially in sub diaphragmatic and pelvic regions (Figs 7.3 and 7.4).[8-12]

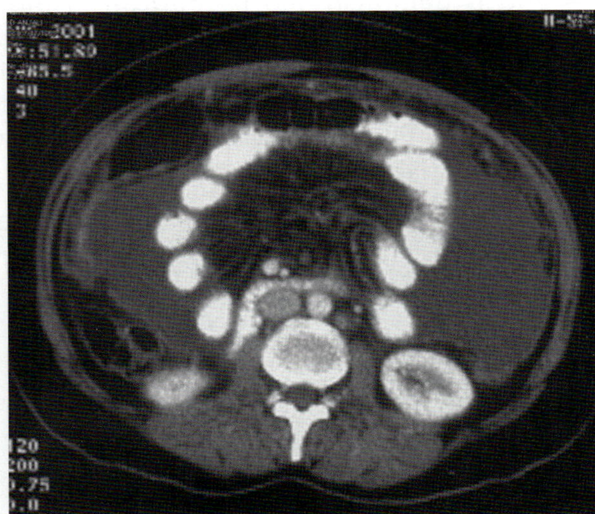

Fig. 7.3: CT: Ascitis with omental thickening and spread out bowel loops

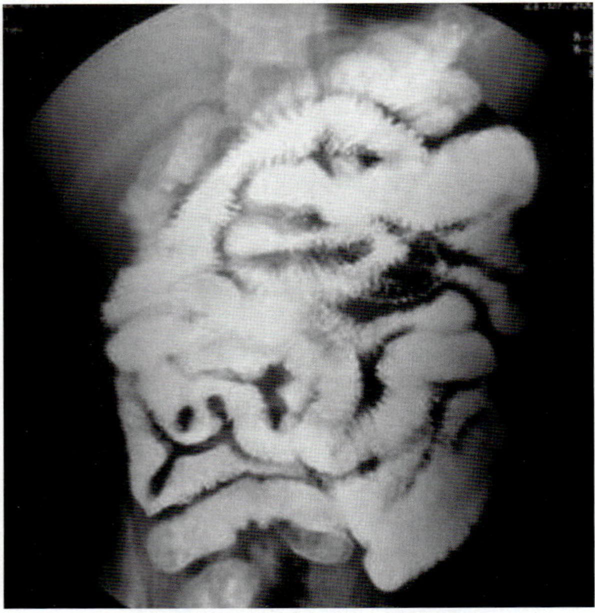

Fig. 7.4: Barium Meal FT-Mildly dilated small bowel loops with increased interloop distance in tubercular peritonitis

Enhancement of ascitis on MRI obtained 15-20 min after iv Gd-DTPA administration has been noted in tubercular peritonitis.[13]

Peritoneum

Peritoneal thickening and tiny nodules are better visualized in presence of ascitis on US. Smooth, slight peritoneal thickening and/or pronounced enhancement are seen in presence of ascitis on CT in almost all cases.

Omentum

Omental thickening is a feature of both TB and peritoneal carcinomatosis and many different appearances 'nodular' 'smudged' or 'caked' have been described. The nodular type has not been seen in any case of tuberculous peritonitis. Omental cake is seen in peritoneal carcinomatosis and tubercular peritonitis. Irregularly thickened outer contour of the infiltrated peritoneum favors malignancy, whereas a thin omental line, suggestive of a fibrous wall covering the infiltrated omentum is common in tubercular peritonitis. Computed tomography delineates omental changes better than other modalities (Fig. 7.5).[14, 15]

Small Bowel Mesentery

The mesentery is involved in most patients with tuberculous peritonitis. The most common changes are nodular lesions, mesenteric thickening and loss of normal mesenteric configuration. Mesenteric nodular lesions may present as micro (< 5 mm) or macro (>5 mm) nodules solid or cystic, lymph node or abscess.

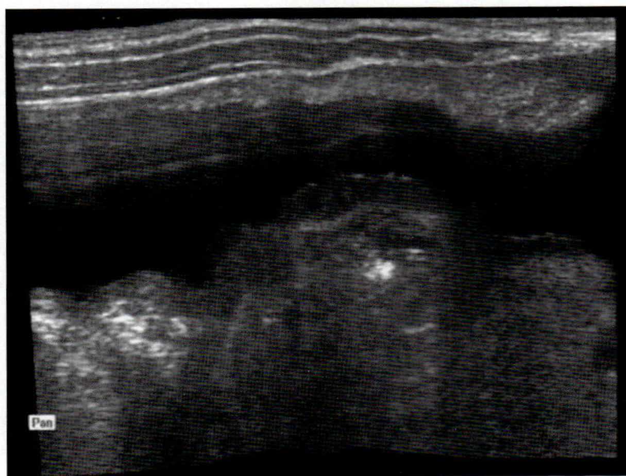

Fig. 7.5: Panoromic USG -smooth omental thickening and ascitis

Based on maximum observed thickness in healthy volunteers and patients at end of therapy, an arbitrary value of 15 mm is considered as a threshold for disease. Mesentery becomes echogenic as a result of increased fat deposition due to lymphatic obstruction (Fig. 7.6). Presence of enlarged lymph nodes adds to the diagnosis of early tuberculosis. Other conditions like portal hypertension and lymphoma can also give rise to mesenteric thickening.[16]

Fixed loops of bowel and mesentery standing out as spokes radiating out from the mesenteric root are described as US 'stellate' sign.

Computed tomography demonstrates thickened mesentery by its increased vascularity and thickened strands, tethering of bowel loops, forming an abdominal mass (Fig. 7.7)

'Club sandwich sign' or the 'sliced bread' appearance is due to localised or focal ascitis between radially oriented bowel loops due to local exudation from inflamed bowel or ruptured lymph nodes (Figs 7.8 and 7.9).[17] Differential diagnosis of tuberculous peritonitis constitutes peritoneal carcinomatosis, mesothelioma, peritonitis and rarely lymphoma.

The suggestive features in the peritoneal mesothelioma consist of multifocal peritoneal thickening of either sheet or nodular types up to 3cm, omental or mesenteric soft tissue masses, thick rigid septae between peritoneal leaves and fixed bowel loops and disproportionately small amount of ascitis to the degree of tumor dissemination, suggestive features of abdominal TB include smooth, minimal peritoneal thickening (< 5 mm), with pronounced smooth enhancement and multiple, fine, completeor incomplete mobile septae.[18]

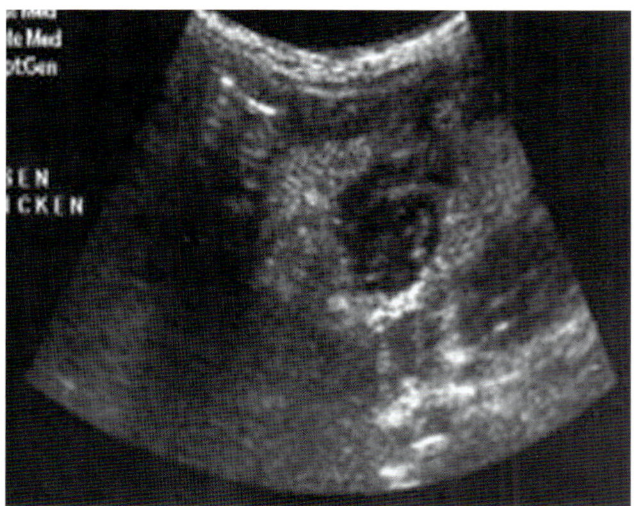

Fig. 7.6: USG-echogenic and thickened mesentry

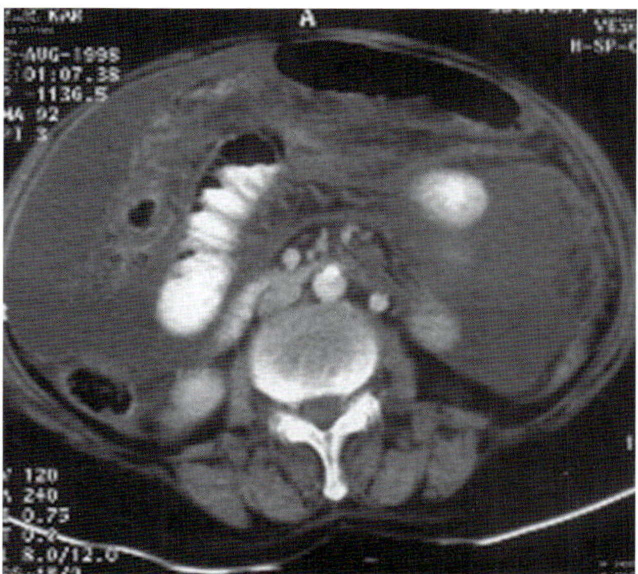

Fig. 7.7: CT-Ascitis with omental thickening

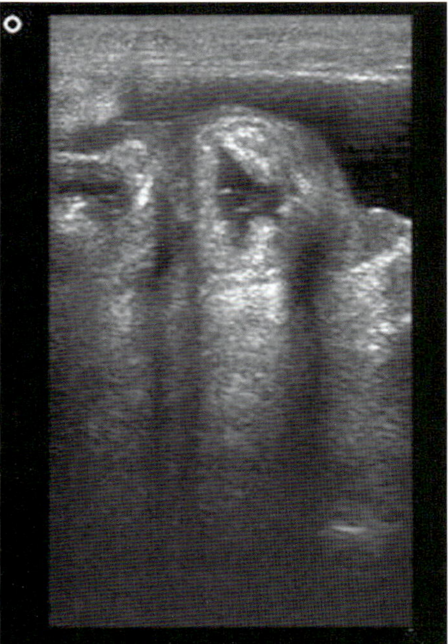

Fig. 7.8: USG- Mesenteric thickening seen between loops-"club sandwich"appearance

Tuberculosis has been implicated in the etiology of Sclerosing encapsulating peritonitis (abdominal cocoon). Ultrasound may shows a thick walled mass containing bowel loops, loculated ascitis and fibrous adhesions. CT shows small bowel loops congregated to the center of abdomen encased by a soft tissue density mantle.[19, 20]

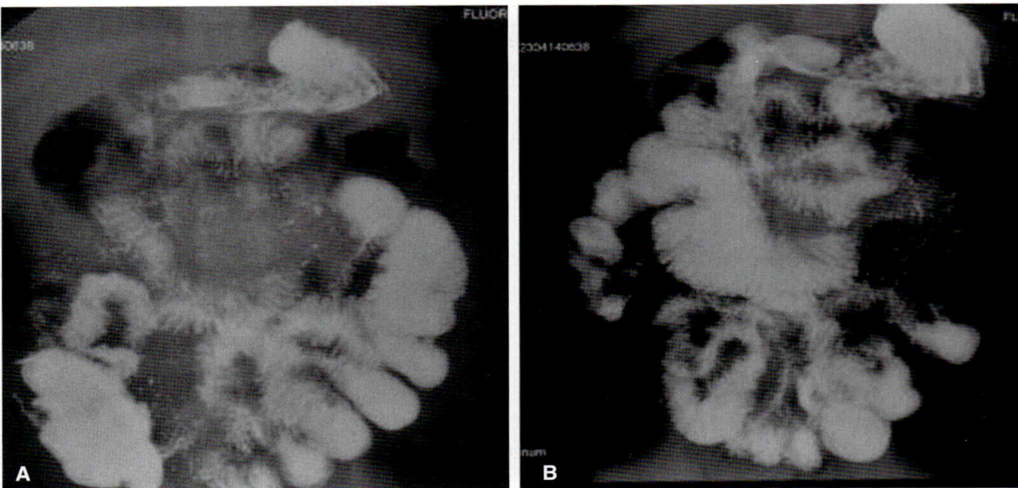

Figs. 7.9A and B: BaMFT-Fixity of loops with mucosal thickening-TB

Tubercular peritonitis should be considered when ultrasound shows ascitis, complex, loculated or accompanied by hepatosplenomegaly, omental cake, bowel wall thickening and an appropriate history and clinical presentation.

TUBERCULAR LYMPHADENITIS

Lymphadenopathy is the commonest manifestation of abdominal tuberculosis and may occur without any other evidence of abdominal involvement. However, it may be associated with gastrointestinal tuberculosis and less commonly peritoneal or solid organ involvement. The rates of lymphadenopathy in patients with abdominal tuberculosis vary widely between 25-93% of cases.[3, 8, 16, 17] Tubercular adenitis, alone may be confused with nodes of lymphoma and clinical and radiological differentiation may be difficult.

Although tuberculosis can involve every lymphatic region in the abdomen, the distribution of enlarged nodes reflects the lymphatic drainage of the involved organs. Lymphatic drainage from bowel explains the involvement of mesenteric periportal, anterior pararenal, upper para-aortic and lesser omental lymph nodes with exclusion of lower para-aortic lymph node (Fig. 7.6). Hematogeneous spread to nodes can involve mesenteric, lesser omentum, anterior pararenal and upper and lower para-aortic lymph nodes. Direct spread of infection from adjacent infected glands or organs is possible.

The nodes may vary from increased number of normal sized nodes to massive conglomerates with matting, the latter resulting from adhesions due to periadenitis.

On ultrasonography, the lymph nodes are either discrete or conglomerate masses Enlarged nodes contain central hypoechoic area with a mixed heterogeneous echo texture, in contrast to homogeneously hypoechoic nodes seen in lymphoma. Heterogeneity of echo patterns, in nodes of a single anatomic subgroup, prior to treatment, is strongly suggestive of tuberculosis, rather than lymphoma. Larger areas of caseation may coalesce with adjacent nodes, resulting in larger collections. Lymph nodes may be adherent to intra-abdominal vasculature and a fibrous reaction surrounding clusters of nodes, may be seen as increase in background echogenicity. With the institution of appropriate treatment, nodal masses tend to show a transient increase in size for 3-4 weeks followed by a gradual reduction in overall dimensions. Focal macro calcification may occur in nodal and omental masses and collections, which may be clustered along the periphery or may be central in location (Figs. 7.10 and 7.11). Both

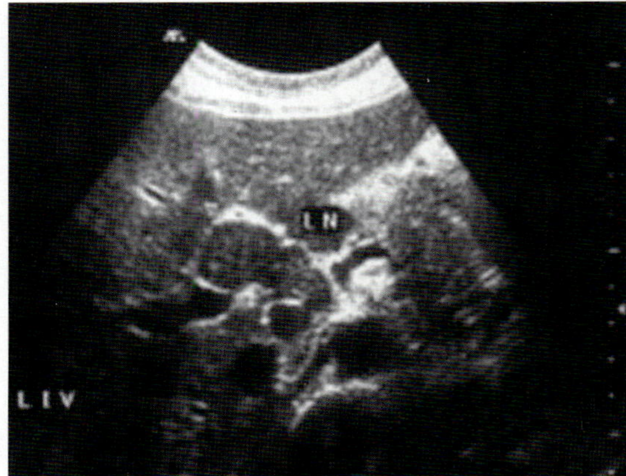

Fig. 7.10: Multiple hypoechoic enlarged discrete nodes in periportal and peripancreatic region

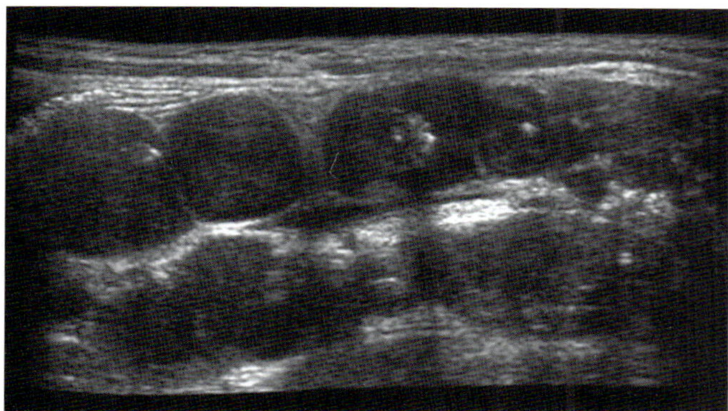

Fig. 7.11: USG-Multiple enlarged hypoechoic mesenteric nodes, with foci of calcification

caseation and calcification are features, highly suggestive of tubercular etiology, being uncommon in malignant lymphoma.[16, 21]

Despite considerable bulk of adenopathy, significant GI or urinary obstruction has not been reported. Biliary obstruction may be occurring secondary to direct ductal compression by infected nodes in association with periductal inflammation and stricture. Portal vein thrombosis and portal hypertension may rarely occur as a complication of abdominal tuberculosis involving hepatic hilar lymph nodes.[22] A case of vascular compression by nodes leading to renovascular hypertension has been reported.[23]

Abdominal lymphadenopathy is well evaluated on CT. Its multi-compartmental localization with relative sparing of the retroperitoneal compartment is the most characteristic feature of tuberculosis.

On unenhanced scans, the nodes may display low attenuation values <30 HU or soft tissue attenuation values similar to muscle. Four different patterns of nodal enhancement are noted after contrast administration in patients with tuberculosis.[24, 25]

Peripheral enhancement, the most frequent pattern, is characterised by peripheral rim enhancement, with or without low attenuation centre. This pattern seen in younger patients reflects significant central liquefactive or caseous necrosis and a highly vascular perinodal inflammatory reaction which is relatively diagnostic for tuberculosis.[11] However, it is not pathgnomonic, as has been noted in some malignant and benign conditions such as metastasis from testicular tumours, head and neck squamous carcinomas, lymphoma, Whipple's and Crohn's disease (Figs 7.12 and 7.13).

Inhomogeneous enhancement is also a frequent manifestation of tubercular adenitis, revealing intra-nodal granulomas and relatively less necrosis than in nodes that show peripheral enhancement.

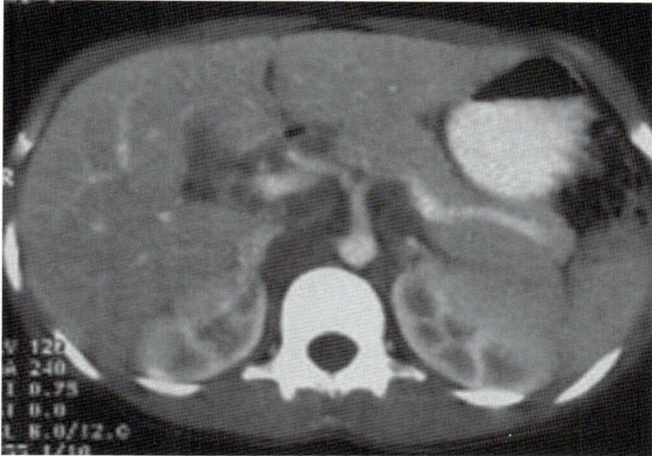

Fig. 7.12: CT -Hypodense nodes with peripheral rim enhancement in periportal region

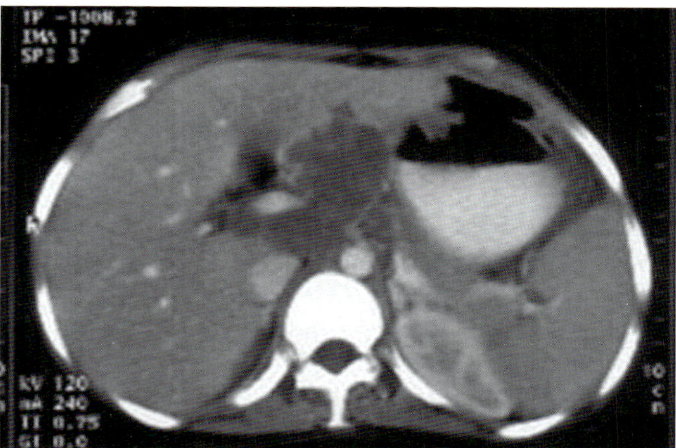

Fig. 7.13: CT- Large conglomerate hypodense nodal mass in periportal and peripancreatic region

Nodes showing homogeneous contrast enhancement represent a less frequent manifestation of infection by mycobacterium tuberculosis. These are indistinguishable from untreated lymphomatous nodes and are seen in patients with infection with mycobacterium avium intracellular and AIDS.Lymphatic involvement is the commonest feature in patients with AIDS. The nodes in these are usually located in mesenteric and retroperitoneal region. Non-enhanced low attenuation nodes may be seen in AIDS.

A variety of patterns of contrast enhancement on CT even within the same nodal group may be seen in tubercular adenitis, probably relating to the different stages of pathological process. However, this feature cannot be considered characteristic of the disease.

MR imaging of abdominal tubercular lymphadenopathy shows that majority of nodes are hypointense on T1 and hyperintense on T2 weighted images, compared to abdominal wall muscle, with a few demonstrating a rim, hypo on T1 and hyperintense on T2. Minority of nodes are hypo to isointense on both T1 and T2 weighted images. Nodes especially when large may show intranodal areas of high signal intensity on T2-weighted images corresponding to nonenhancing portions on CT (Figs 7.14A to C). This finding corresponds to caseation or liquefaction necrosis at the center of the enlarged nodes. Obliteration of the perinodal fat, characterized by increased signal on T2 weighted images, is also seen and probably reflects capsular disruption. On contrast enhanced images, different enhancement patterns, including peripheral, heterogeneous and less frequently homogeneous enhancement may be seen.[26-28]

A promising role of MRI, in the evaluation of tubercular adenopathy is to differentiate enlarged nodes that are abutting the pancreas, from a cystic neoplasm of the pancreas.

GASTROINTESTINAL TUBERCULOSIS

It is a common form of abdominal tuberculosis. Any segment of the gastrointestinal tract can be involved, but the ileocecal region is the most commonly affected, involved in up to 90% of cases with intestinal tuberculosis.

Patients with gastrointestinal tuberculosis present with diarrhea, abdominal pain and distension, anorexia, wt. loss, gola formation and doughy feel of the abdomen. Complications include obstruction, perforation, perianal fistula, enterolithiasis formation proximal to the stricture, hemorrhage. Traditionally the diagnosis has been based on barium studies with a reported sensitivity of 70-100%.

Cross sectional imaging modalities like USG, CT and MRI offer a comprehensive overview of abdominal structure with direct imaging of bowel, mesentry and lymph nodes, but does not replace the demonstration of mucosal detail by barium techniques. Small bowel enteroscopy can be used for proximal small bowel. Capsule endoscopy has added another dimension to small bowel evaluation.

OESOPHAGEAL TUBERCULOSIS

Oesophageal tuberculosis is a rare condition and is usually secondary to advanced pulmonary or mediastinal disease. Spread occurs from tubercular laryngitis, adjacent caseating lymph nodes, vertebral body, lymphatics or the hematogeneous route. Primary esophageal tuberculosis involves, most commonly the tracheal bifurcation. Patients usually presents with dysphagia, odynophagia, chest pain or cough.

Barium studies show evidence of extrinsic compression by the enlarged nodes, smooth strictures, ulceration, mucosal irregularity, and traction diverticuli. Sinus tracts and fistulous communication may develop with the mediastinum or tracheobronchial tree. Computed tomography is a more reliable method to determine full extent of the disease in the mediastinum. Oesophageal tuberculosis in AIDS patients manifests as deep ulcerations, transmural inflammation with fistula and sinus

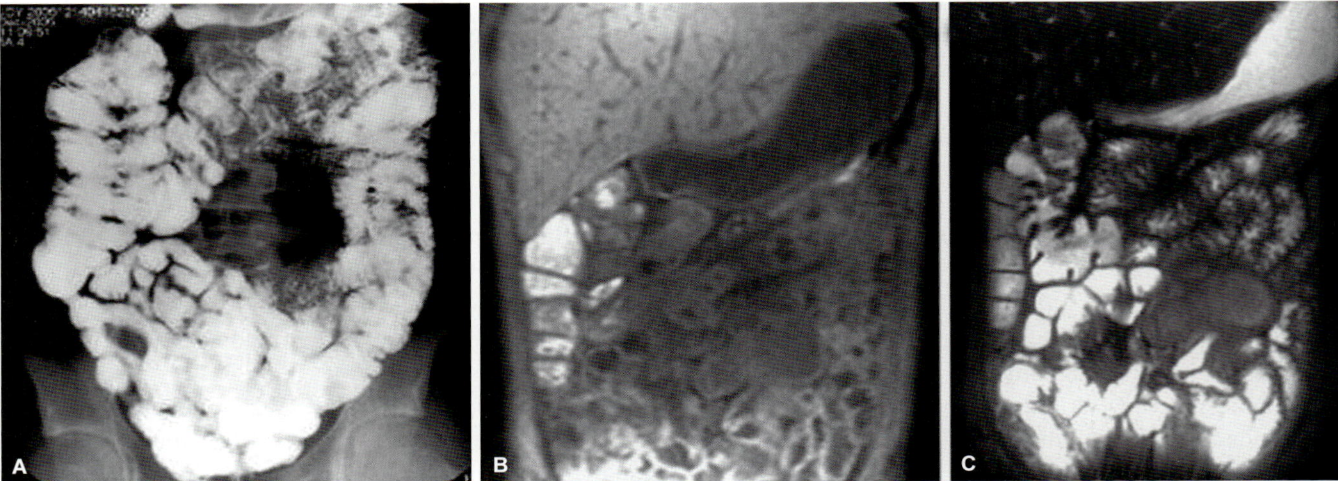

Figs 7.14A to C: (A) BariumFT - displaced bowel loops with paucity in central abdomen (B) T1 FLASH-coronal multiple enlarged mesenteric lymphnodes isointenseon T1WI (C) T2 TRUE FISP coronal shows iso to mildly hyperintense lymph nodes

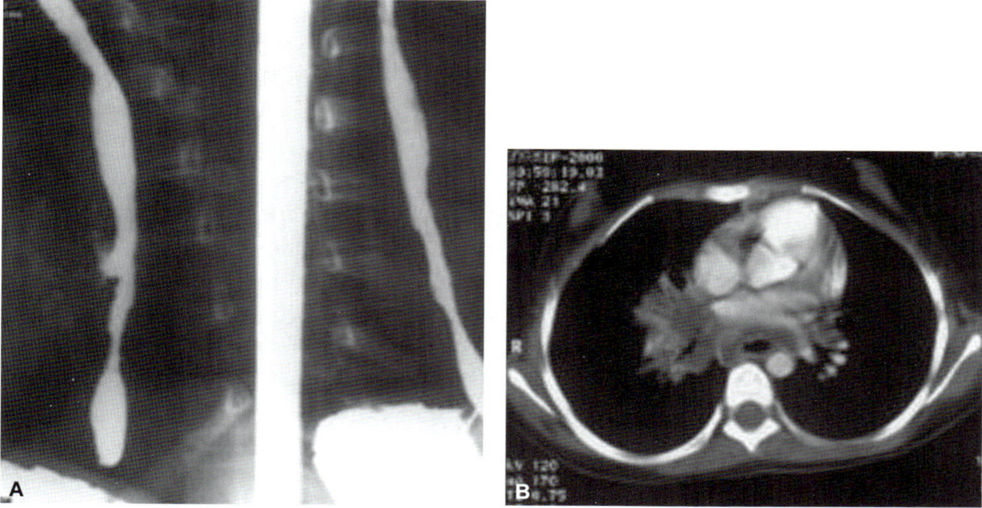

Figs 7.15A and B: (A) Barium Swallow- esophageal stricture with ulceration and periesophageal leak - tubercular (B) CT Concentric mural, esophageal wall thickening with periesophageal leak with mediastinal adenopalthy

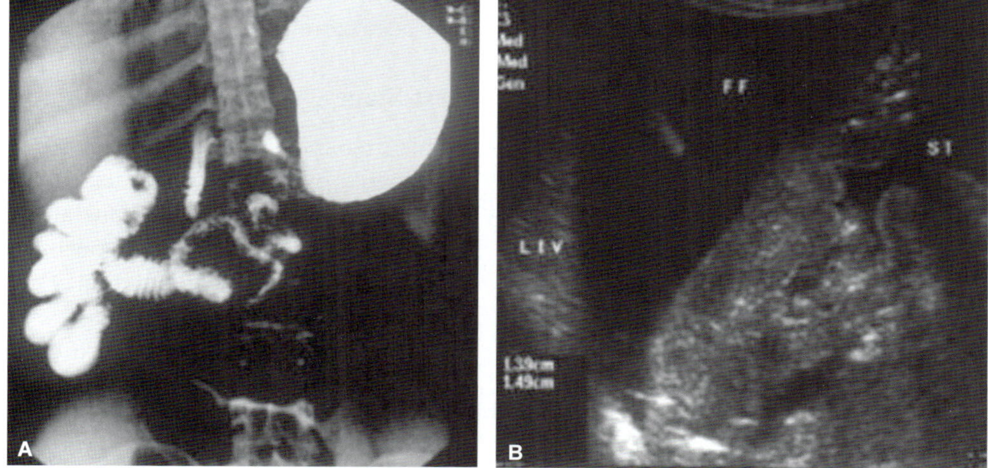

Fig. 7.16A and B: (A) Ba Meal gastric outlet obstruction with antropyloric narrowing with mildly dilated jejunal loops and enterolith. (B) USG shows wall thickening of antrophyloric region with free fluid

formation and adjacent lymphadenopathy. The differential diagnosis of oesophageal tuberculosis includes other benign and malignant strictures (Figs 7.15A and B).[6, 18]

GASTRIC TUBERCULOSIS

Gastric tuberculosis is very rare, reported to occur in 0.36-2.3% of patients with pulmonary TB, in an autopsy series. It usually occurs with secondary spread from adjacent lymph nodes or via the hematogeneous route. The most common symptoms are epigastric discomfort, vomiting, weight loss, fever and hemorrhage. A palpable abdominal lump may be present.

Pathologically gastric tuberculosis is of the following types:

a. Ulcerative commonest, usually along the lesser curve and pylorus
b. Hypertrophic
c. Miliary tubercles
d. Tubercular pyloric stenosis
e. Solitary tuberculoma, and
f. Tubercular lymphadenitis

Radiological features are nonspecific, mimicking a benign ulcer in ulcerative and that of a malignant ulcer in the hypertrophic form. Outlet obstruction may be seen due to inflammatory changes, fibrosis or enlarged lymph nodes. Gastric tuberculosis must be differentiated radiologically from gastric carcinoma, lymphoma and syphilis (Figs 7.16A and B).[6, 18, 29]

DUODENAL TUBERCULOSIS

Two percent of all intestinal TB is duodenal. An extrinsic or intrinsic process, extrinsic involvement being more common due to lymphadenopathy or adhesions, may affect the duodenum.[9] On barium studies, lymphadenopathy leads to widening or impressions on the medial aspect of the C loop and can simulate superior mesenteric artery syndrome whereas intrinsic involvement may be ulcerative or hyperplastic. Incompetence of sphincter of oddi often leads to reflux of air into biliary tree.[29] Perforation with fistula formation can occur. Healing may cause contraction and stenosis leading to duodenal obstruction. Endoscopic biopsies are often negative because of the submucosal nature of the disease. The differential diagnosis of duodenal tuberculosis includes lymphoma, malignancy, carcinoma pancreas, atypical peptic ulcer disease (Figs 7.17A and B).

TUBERCULOSIS ENTERITIS

In India, tuberculosis is a common cause of small bowel obstruction. The radiographic features of small bowel tuberculosis closely reflect the underlying pathological changes. The ulcerative form is most common, .the ulcers have stellate or linear shape. Stellate ulcers are characterized by a barium speck with converging mucosal folds. Linear ulcers are perpendicular to the long axis, resulting in spasm and circumferential strictures. Strictures are usually multiple and short. The hypertrophic form is less common, usually seen in ileocecal area. The bowel loops are matted and fixed by adhesion and fibrosis.

Plain X-ray abdomen may show enteroliths with features of obstruction, i.e. dilated bowel loops with multiple air-fluid levels, evidence of ascitis, perforation or intussusceptions. In addition, there may be calcified lymph nodes, calcified granulomas and hepatosplenomegaly.

In all patients suspected of bowel tuberculosis, barium studies should include the barium meal follow through/ enteroclysis followed by a barium enema, if there is a colonic involvement. The barium meal evaluates the motility and organic lesions in the terminal ileum and other parts of small bowel, while the per oral pneumocolon and enema, best evaluate the caecum and ileocecal valve. Small bowel enteroclysis scores over cross sectional imaging and conventional intestinal studies in providing mucosal details and since this investigation requires adequate distension of intestine, early and incomplete strictures are better detected, as prestenotic dilatation develops at sites of minimal strictures.[30]

The radiographic features of intestinal tuberculosis have been correlated with the pathological state of disease.

First Stage

In this first stage of superficial invasion of the mucosa, radiological examination reveals:

a. An accelerated intestinal transit (Fig. 7.18)
b. Disturbances in tone and peristaltic contractions resulting in hypersegmentation of the barium column, the so-called 'chicken intestine'.
c. Disturbances in secretion, resulting in precipitation, flocculation or dilution of the barium suspension.

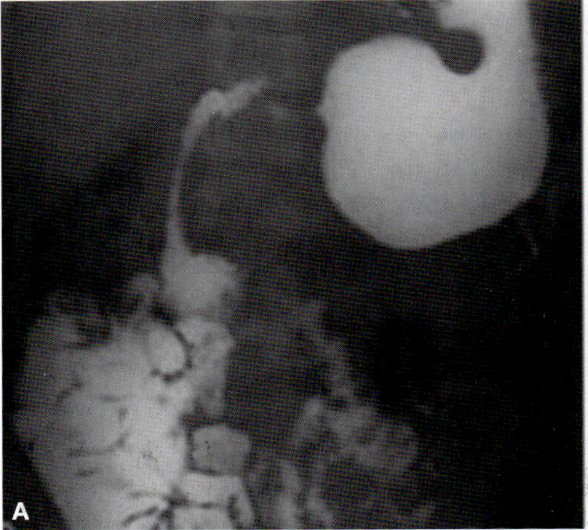

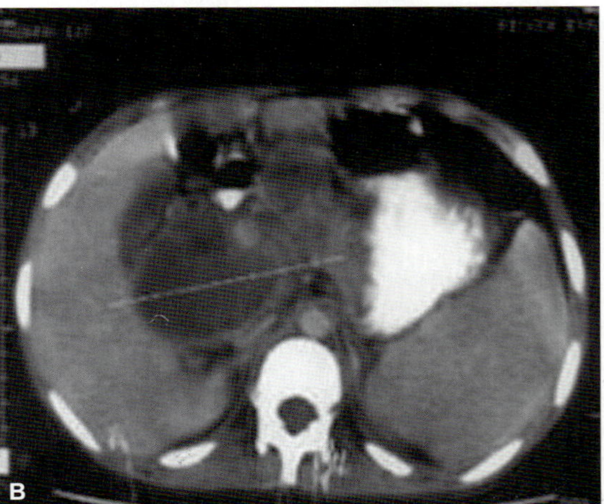

Figs 7.17A and B: Ba MUGIT in a case of duodenal tuberculosis with both extrinsic and intrinsic involvement (B) CT large peripancreatic lymphnodal mass

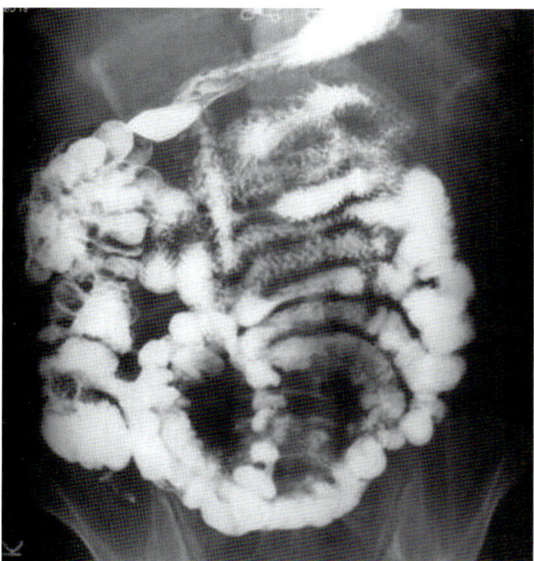

Fig. 7.18: Ba MFT: Accelerated transit time is seen with barium reaching large bowel in Ist film

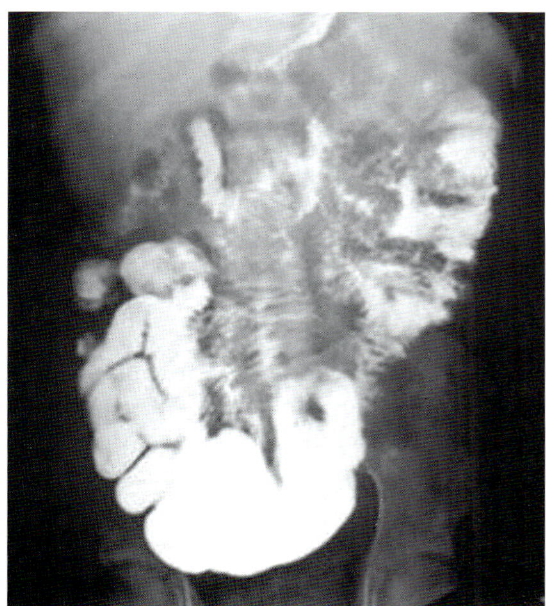

Fig. 7.19: Ba MFT. Early TB with mucosal irregularity and spiculation

d. Changes in intestinal contours, which are irregular, crenated and interrupted by spicule.
e. Changes in the mucosal pattern manifested by softened and thickened folds (Figs 7.14 and 7.19).

Second Stage

The second stage, in addition to above comprise of ulcerations, characterized by a barium fleck surrounded by either a thickened wall or by converging folds.

Third Stage

The third stage is of sclerosis, hypertrophy and stenosis. In the small intestine penetrating ulcers cause very short 'hour glass' stenosis, that have smooth, but stiff contours and in which the mucosal relief has disappeared. Multiple strictures with segmental dilatation of bowel loops may occur. Other features include fixity of loops, spiculation, matting and signs of malabsorption (Figs 7.20 and 7.21).

Mucosal changes that occur in early stages of tuberculous enteritis are not usually sonographically visible. However, deep ulcerations can be detected and appear as radial extensions of the echogenic luminal contents into the surrounding thickened wall. With disease progression, wall thickening and short segment strictures develop in the intestine, resulting in partial intestinal obstruction and occasionally in intestinal perforations. On transverse sonograms, areas of narrowing representing strictures appear as segments of circumferential mural thickening and reduced luminal content. Real time sonography can assess hyperperistalsis proximal to the obstruction.[5]

ILEOCAECAL TUBERCULOSIS

The ileocaecal region is most commonly affected in small bowel TB, because of physiological stasis, abundant lymphoid tissue, increased rate of absorption in the region and closer contact of the bacilli with the mucosa of the region.[6] The lesion may be:

i. Hyperplastic with long segments of narrowing, rigidity and loss of distensibility, i.e., the 'pipe stem colon', which is the commonest,

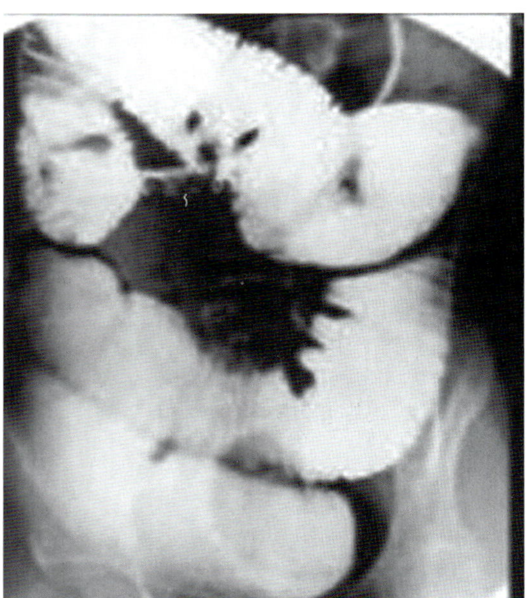

Fig. 7.20: Enteroclysis - Multiple stricture segments with dilated small bowel loops

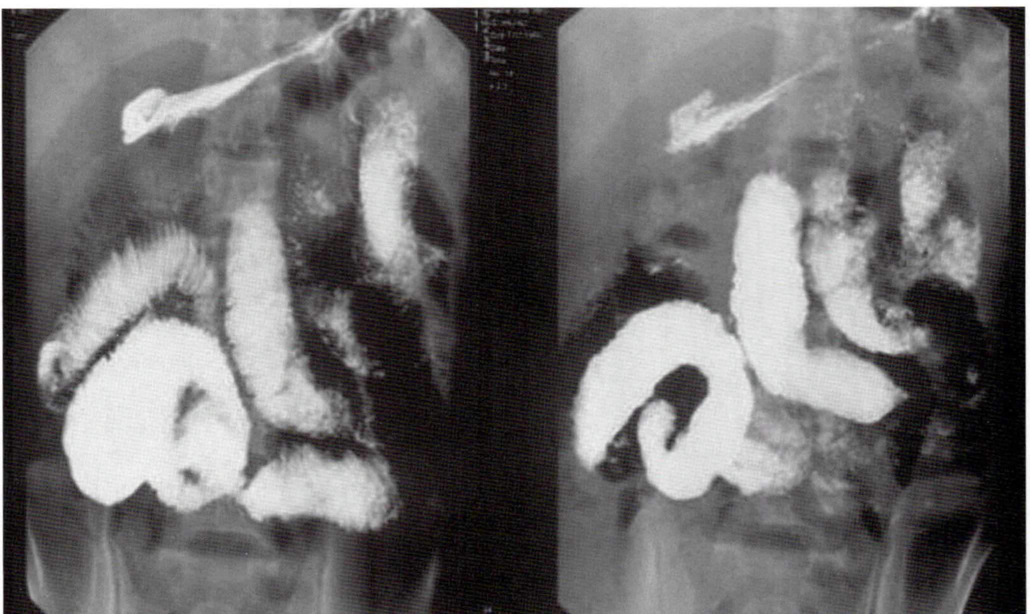

Fig. 7.21: BaMFT - Fixed matted and dilated small bowel loops with mucosal thickening

ii. Ulcerative
iii. Ulcerohyperplastic, and
iv. Carcinoma type with a short annular defect and overhanging edges.

Early involvement of the ileocaecal region is manifest as spasm and hypermotility with edema of the valve. Thickening of the ileocaecal valve lips and/or wide gaping of the valve, with narrowing of the terminal ileum (the 'Fleischner or inverted umbrella' sign)[31] are considered characteristic of tuberculosis (Figs 7.22A and B).

In advanced disease, the characteristic deformity includes symmetric, annular, 'napkin ring' stenosis and obstruction or shortening, retraction and pouch formation. The caecum classically becomes conical, shrunken and retracted out of the iliac fossa due to contraction of the mesocolon. Hepatic flexure may also be pulled down. There may be loss of the normal ileocecal angle and the dilated terminal ileum may appear suspended and hanging from a retracted, shortened cecum (goose neck deformity) (Fig. 7.18). Localised partial stenosis opposite the ileocecal value with a rounded off smooth cecum and a dilated terminal ileum resembles a purse string stenosis. The ileocaecal value becomes fixed, irregular, gaping and incompetent. The terminal ileum may be fixed and narrowed due to stricture formation. Narrowing of the terminal ileum may occur due to irritability with rapid

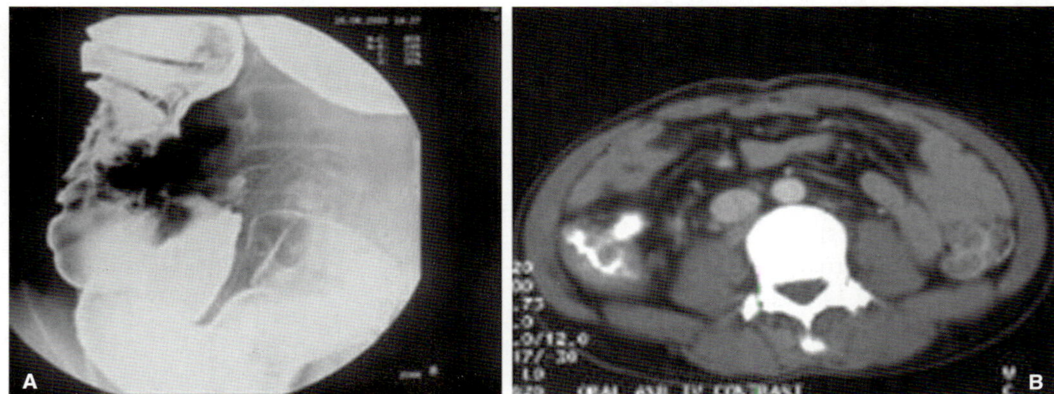

Figs 7.22A and B: (A) Ba MFT - Fleischner sign - Thickening of ileocecal valve with narrowing of terminal ileum (B) CT narrowing of terminal ileum with thickening in region of I.C Valve

emptying through a gaping ileocecal value with a shortened, rigid or obliterated caecum "Stierlin's sign". This represents acute inflammation superimposed on a chronically involved segment of the ileum, cecum or ascending colon with a normal configured column of barium on either side. A persistent narrow stream of barium in the bowel indicates stenosis and is known as the 'string sign' (Figs 7. 23 to 7.25). Both Stierlin's sign and string sign are also noted in Crohn's disease and cannot be considered specific for tuberculosis. Hyperplastic tuberculosis mimics carcinoma and histological diagnosis is mandatory.

The findings on barium studies have been separated into the following groups.[32]

Group 1

Highly suggestive, if one or more of the following features are present.

a. Deformed ileocaecal valve with dilatation of the terminal ileum.
b. Contracted caecum with an abnormal ileocecal valve and/or terminal ileum (Fig. 7.19).
c. Stricture of the ascending colon with shortening and involvement of the ileocaecal region.

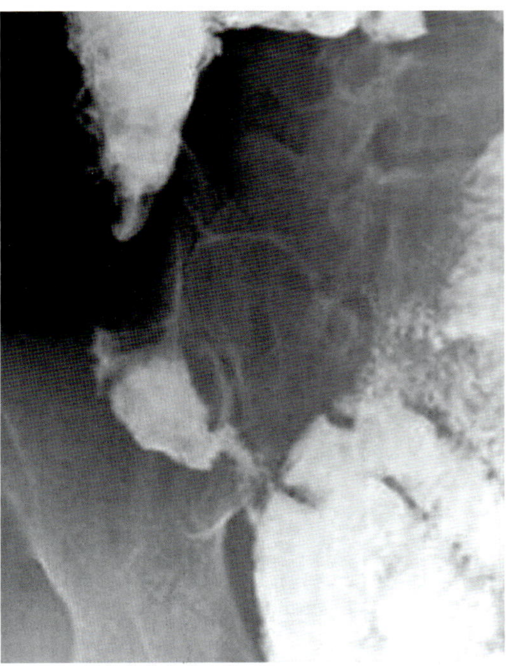

Fig. 7.23: BaMFT string sign: Persistent narrow stream of barium in bowel indicating stenosis

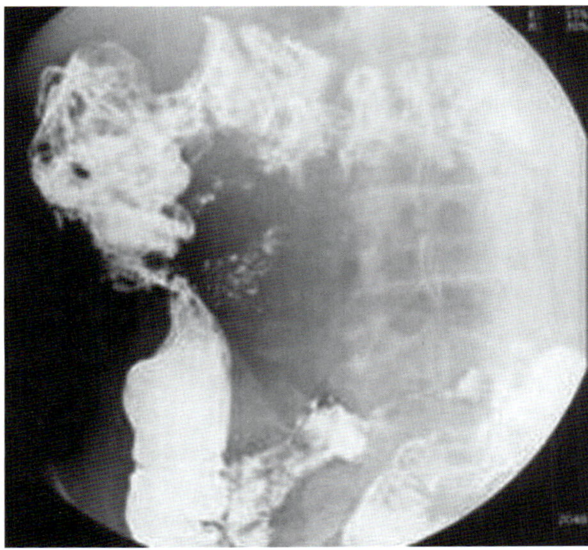

Fig. 7.24: BaMFT-Retracted and contracted caecum with terminal ileum appearing suspended with loss of I-C angle-goose neck deformity

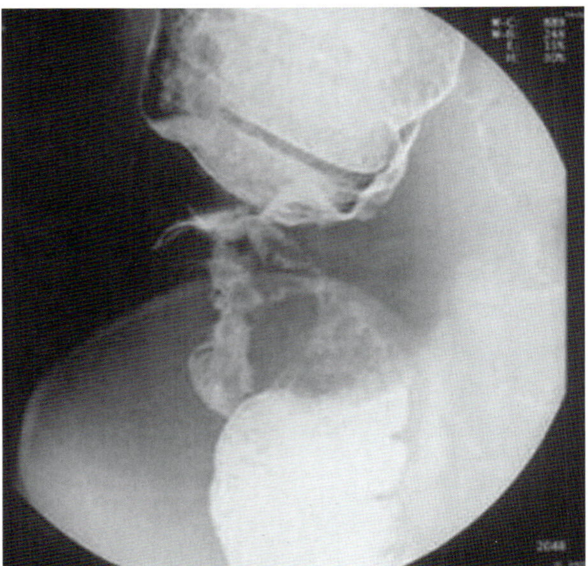

Fig. 7.25: BaMFT - Advanced IC Koch's with symmetric annular napkin ring stenosis with conical shrunken and caecum

Group 2

Suggestive-if any of the following features are present:

a. Contracted caecum
b. Ulcerations or narrowing of the terminal ileum
c. Stricture of the ascending colon
d. Multiple areas of dilatation, narrowing and matting of small bowel loops.

Group 3

Nonspecific-includes features of matting, dilatation or mucosal thickening of small bowel loops.

Group 4

Normal study.

Sonography shows extramucosal changes and can occasionally detect mucosal changes. In early stages of ileocecal tuberculosis, a few regional nodes and circumferential thickening of the wall of the cecum and terminal ileum may be visualised. The bowel wall is considered thickened when it measures > 5 mm in the small bowel when non-distended, and > 3 mm when distended. In later stages of disease, the ileocaecal value and adjacent medial wall of the cecum are predominantly and asymmetrically thickened. These changes are nonspecific and may be seen in other conditions such as carcinoma, Crohn's disease, lymphoma and amoebiasis. However, in Crohn's disease eccentric thickening may be noted at mesenteric border and a variegated appearance is seen in malignancy. Due to the predilection of TB for the ileocecal region and the tendency of the ileocaecal region to be pulled upto a subhepatic position, a pseudo-kidney sign seen in this location is highly suggestive of a tuberculous pathology. In advanced ileocaecal tuberculosis, gross wall thickening, adherent loops, large regional nodes and mesenteric thickening may together form a complex mass of varied echogenicity centered on the ileocaecal region (Figs 7.26 and 7.27). These changes are highly suggestive of tuberculosis in the appropriate clinical setting. Ultrasound can detect ulcerations, however due to associated spasm, there is low sensitivity of the same. Lesions in jejunum or proximal ileum can be missed due to difficulty in scanning the entire length of the intestines, and is also limited by presence of overlying bowel gas.[5, 6, 17]

CT scans of the ileocaecal region, may show circumferential bowel wall thickening up to 3.0 cm in diameter in terminal ileum and caecum with enlargement of ileocaecal valve and adjacent mesenteric adenopathy (Fig. 7.28). The bowel wall thickening may be mild and symmetric or severe and asymmetric with a homogeneous density and areas of slight heterogeneous appearance. A CT appearance more characteristic of TB is asymmetric thickening of the ileocecal valve and medial wall of the caecum with an exophytic extension engulfing the terminal ileum and massive lymphadenopathy with central low attenuation area. Pericaecal or mesenteric fat shows either absence or only minimal haziness. CT may also show distal small bowel obstruction.[6, 32-34]

CT enteroclysis has a greater sensitivity and specificity than nonhelical CT in patients suspected of having low grade small bowel obstruction, a feature commonly seen

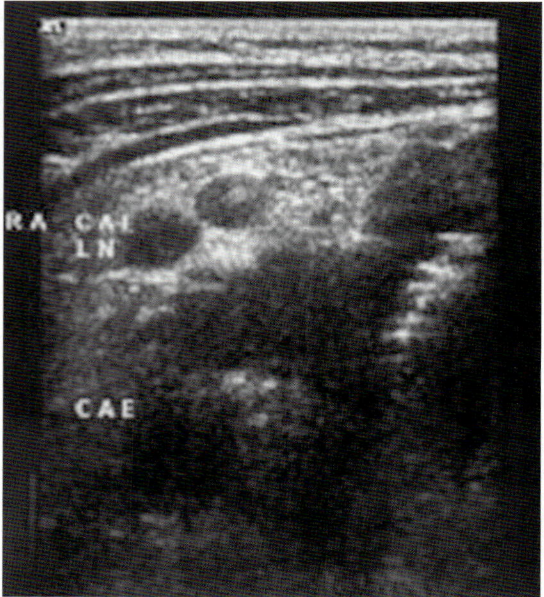

Fig. 7.26: USG- Hypoechoic mural thickening of the ileum and cecum with paracaecal lymphadenopathy

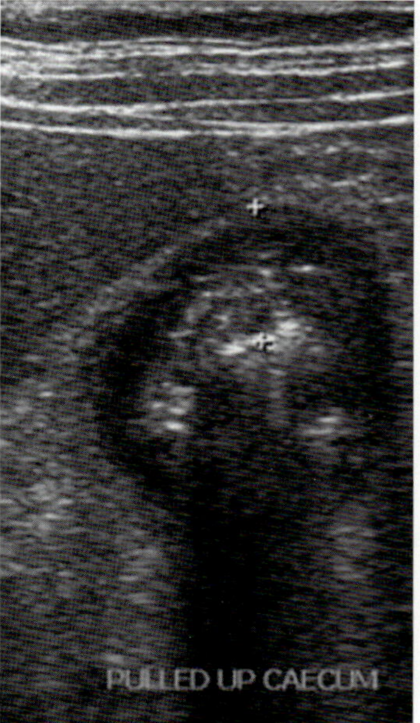

Fig. 7.27: USG-Retracted and pulled up caecum wall with thickening in the subhepatic region

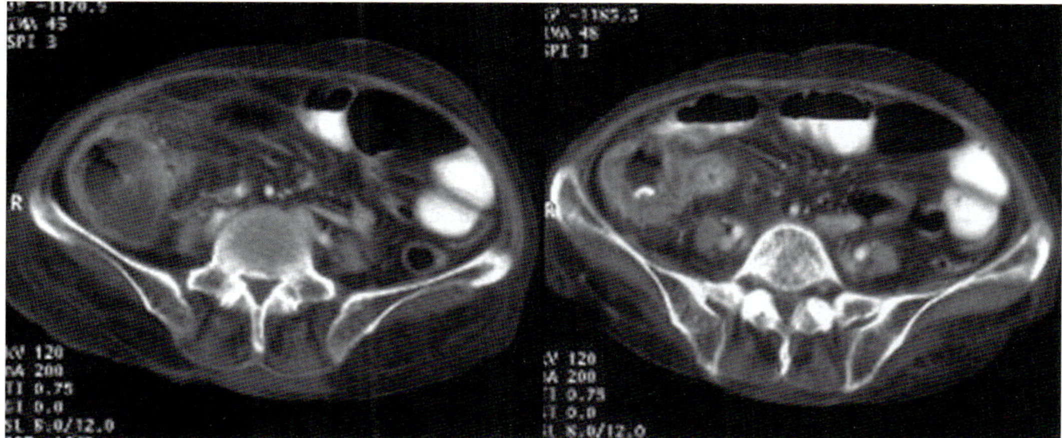

Fig. 7.28: CT-Shows mural thickening of terminal ileum and caecum with enterolith

in small bowel TB. CT enteroclysis allows detection of luminal and extraluminal disease.[35]

On MRI, bowel wall changes in tuberculosis are varied and reflect the various stages of disease. They range from exophytic soft tissue masses surrounding a constricted and ulcerated lumen, minimal but asymmetric wall thickening with spiky or tethered mucosal outline, minimal symmetric wall thickening or normal wall thickness. The tuberculous lesion may show decreased signal intensity and increased, slight heterogeneous signal intensities on T_1W and T_2W images respectively.The inflammatory mass may have a heterogeneous appearance on contrast-enhanced images (Figs 7.29 and 7.30). Bowel wall thickness larger than 3 mm must be considered abnormal. In the acute stage of intestinal tuberculosis, ulcerations can be seen; in the sub acute stage, scarring effects on the bowel wall can be identified. Mucosal abnormalities are less well demonstrated on MRI, due to lower spatial resolution of MRI as compared to barium studies for demonstration of subtle mucosal abnormalities.[36-38]

Radiological differentiation of early stage ileocecal tuberculosis from Crohn's disease and lymphoma is usually impossible. CT is capable of identifying changes in bowel wall and mesentery to provide differentiating factors between advanced intestinal tuberculosis and Crohn's disease. In tuberculosis, bowel wall changes are varied and reflect the various stages of the disease. These are exophytic soft tissue masses surrounding a constricted and ulcerated lumen, minimal but asymmetrical bowel wall thickening with spiky or tethered mucosal outline, minimal symmetrical wall thickening and absence of wall thickening. Mucosal stratification does not occur. In

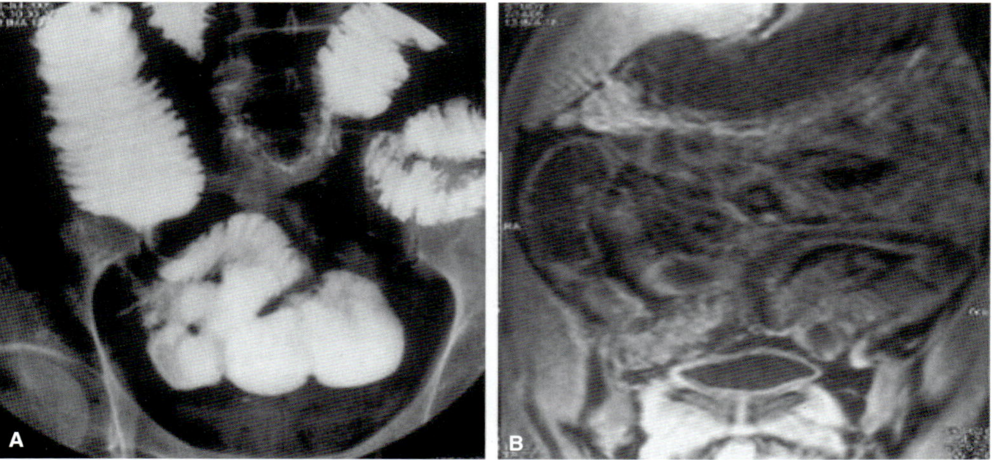

Figs 7.29A and B: Ba enteroclysis (A) MRI enteroclysis (B) Stricture segment in ileum seen in both with proximal dilation

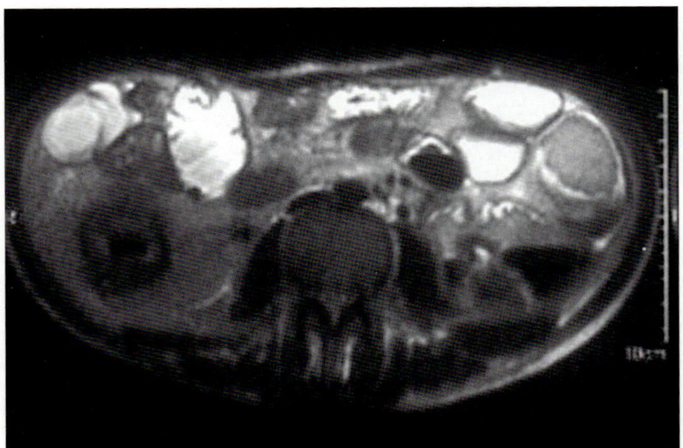

Fig. 7.30: TRUE FISP axial-cecal wall thickening with pericolonic inflammatory changes

comparison, Crohn's disease has a uniform pattern of wall thickening, which is concentric or largely symmetrical, ranging from 0.6 to 1.7 cm, few showing mural stratification.[39] Although amebiasis may produce the typical shrunken caecum seen in TB, associated small bowel involvement is rare. Caecal malignancy is always limited by the ileocaecal valve (Figs 7.20 and 7.21).

The differentiating imaging features of ileocecal involvement can be summarized as:[40]

Tuberculosis	Crohn's Disease
1. Asymmetric wall thickening, irregular	Circumferential bowel wall thickening ulceration on mesenteric surface
2. Fleischner sign on barium studies	Cobblestone appearance on barium
3. No creeping fat	Creeping fat (abnormal quantity of mesenteric fat) present
4. Positive chest film (50%)	Negative chest film
5. Omental and peritoneal thickening	Normal omentum and peritoneum
6. Enlarged lymph nodes with low-density centers	Enlarged soft-tissue density lymph nodes

APPENDICEAL TUBERCULOSIS[41]

Isolated appendiceal tuberculosis is very rare and usually presents as chronic appendicitis due to intrinsic disease of the appendix, involvement by surrounding nodes and/or occlusion of the lumen by a caecal mass.

COLONIC TUBERCULOSIS

The large bowel is involved in 9% of cases without small bowel involvement.[42] Colonic disease may present as a segmental involvement (long or short) with spiculation, spasm, rigidity and ulceration. Occasionally, inflammatory polyps, perforations and fistulae may occur with pericolic abscesses. The differential diagnosis of extensive colonic tuberculosis include ulcerative colitis, Crohn's disease, amoebic colitis, ischemic and pseudomembranous colitis, as well as malignancy. Anal involvement and internal fistulae are more common in Crohn's disease while free perforation is more common in TB. The ulceration in TB is circumferential while that in Crohn's disease is along the mesenteric border (Fig. 7.31).

ANORECTAL TUBERCULOSIS[29]

Tubercular infection may rarely present as ulcerating proctitis. Fistulae, strictures and chronic ischiorectal abscesses may occur. In the anal canal, it may present as ulcers fissures, fistulae, abscesses and as warty growths. The differential diagnosis include LGV, amoebiasis, actinomycosis and schistosomiasis.Anal tuberculosis is also seen in peadiatric patients (Fig. 7.32).

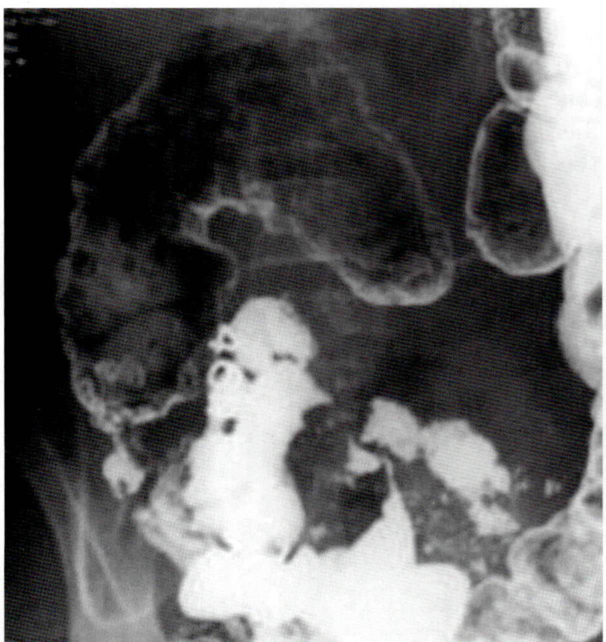

Fig. 7.31: Double contrast barium enema showing a stricture in mid transverse colon- tubercular

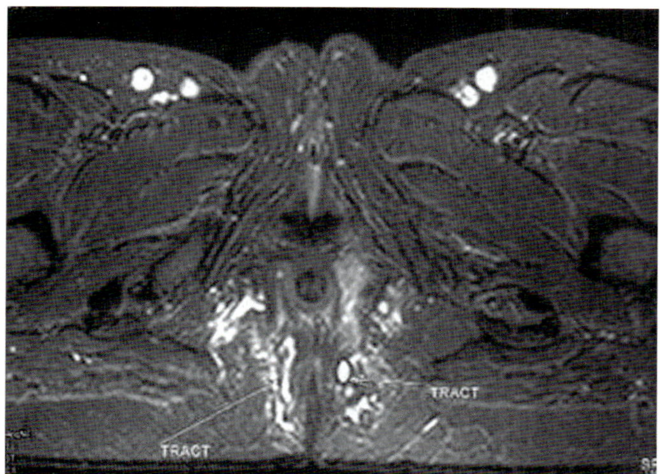

Fig. 7.32: MRI STIR axial - Multiple small tracts seen in perianal region. Fistula in ano- anal tuberculosis

Enterolithiasis

Intestinal calculi may form above any bowel stricture. When the stricture is high in the small bowel, the enteroliths are usually nonopaque, being composed of choleic acid. In the lower small bowel, due to a more alkaline medium and a higher concentration of calcium salts, enteroliths are often opaque. They may be completely opacified or have translucent centres with a ring of calcification. They vary from being multiple, small stones to a large lamellated calculus and must be differentiated from renal stones, gallstones, vesical stones and calcified granulomas (Figs 7.33A and B).

VISCERAL TUBERCULOSIS

Involvement of solid organs (liver, spleen, pancreas).

Liver and Spleen

Hepatosplenic tuberculosis is common in miliary tuberculosis and is found in 80-100%[43] of autopsied patients with disseminated pulmonary tuberculosis. Hepatosplenic tuberculosis may occur secondary to pulmonary or miliary tuberculosis or through portal vein from GI lesions.

The micro nodular form is observed in miliary form of pulmonary tuberculosis. On Ultrasound, micro nodular form of hepatosplenic involvement presents as diffuse hyperechogenicity, the 'bright liver or spleen' pattern. On CT, miliary nodules measuring from 0.5 to 2 mm in diameter are not appreciated, but the liver or spleen may be enlarged and appear homogeneous or heterogeneous (Fig. 7. 34).[18, 31] These features are non-specific and are seen in several benign or malignant lesions.

Macronodular form is a rare manifestation of hepato-splenic tuberculosis. Infection probably spreads via the portal vein or hepatic artery from the para-aortic or portal nodes. The lesion may be multiple or single. Multiple lesions in the liver and spleen are often hypo echoic on ultrasound (Fig. 7.35) and hypodense on CT, as well as marginated small masses scattered throughout the organ. In a few cases, lesions are hyperechoic with or without calcification (Fig. 7. 36). The differential diagnosis includes

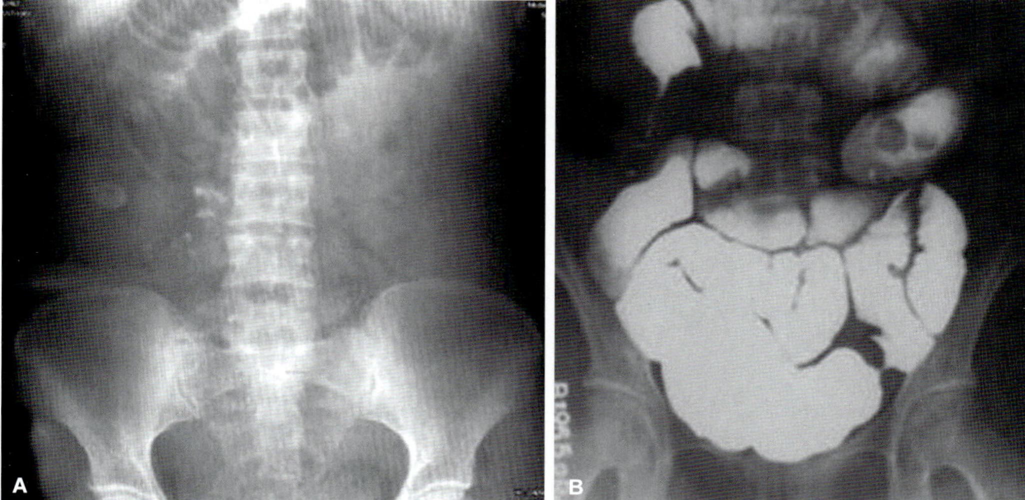

Figs 7.33A and B: (A) Plain Film showing a large lamellated enterolith with evidence of dilated small bowl loops and calcified nodes in a case of abdominal tuberculosis (B) BaMFT: multiple strictures in small bowel, shrunken, pulled up caecum and filling defects suggestion of enteroliths

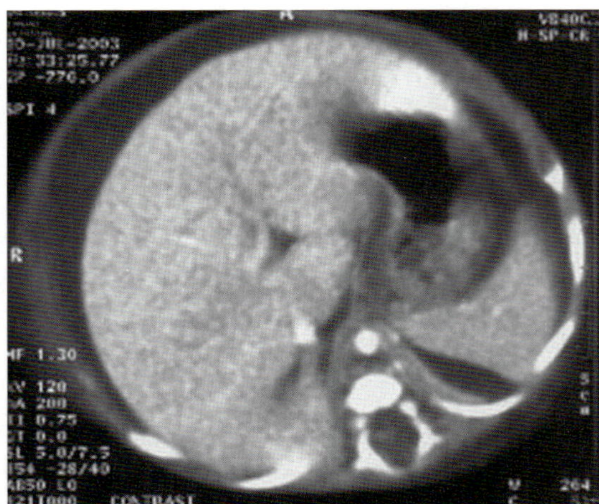

Fig. 7.34: CT-Liver and spleen shows multiple small pinpoint hypodense lesion with ascitis - Miliary TB

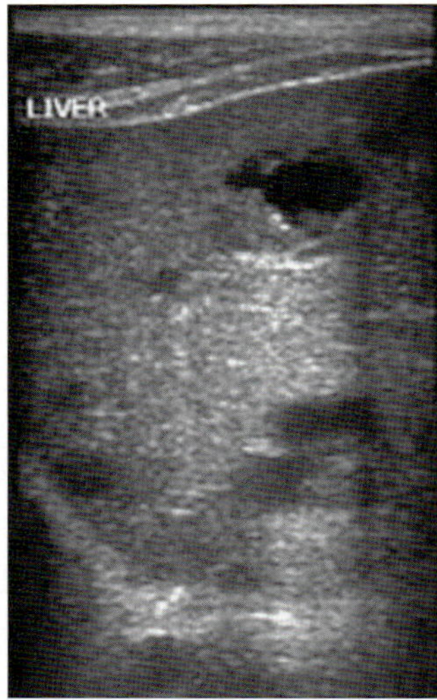

Fig. 7.35: USG-Small irregular hypoechoic nodules in liver—a case of disseminated Kochs

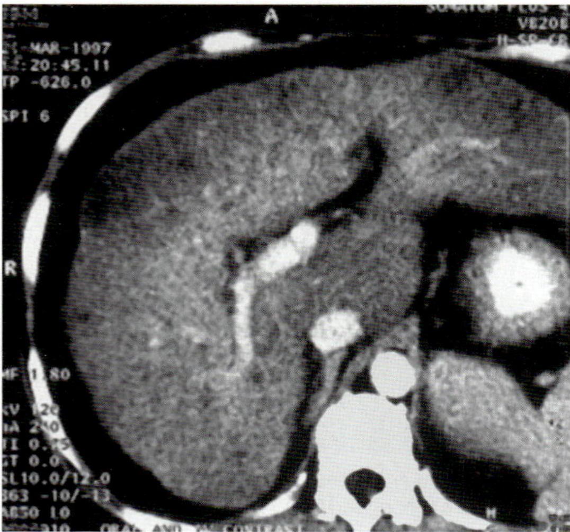

Fig. 7.36: CT-Multiple hypodense nodules in the liver

fungal infections, pyogenic or ameobic abcessess, Hodgkins disease and metastatic carcinoma.

A single visceral lesion in liver and spleen is often seen as hypoechoic, heterogeneous or calcified mass on sonography. Uncommon appearance of hepatosplenic TB, included a septated honeycomb and a hyperechoic, uncalcified tuberculoma. Both echogenic and echo poor tuberculomas have been reported. These probably represent different phases of the disease; the echogenic lesions are seen in the early phase while the echopoor lesions seen later represent the phase of caseation and necrosis. On CT, the solitary tuberculoma appears as solid, hypodense and heterogeneous mass with low attenuation ranging from 14 to 45 HU. After administration of iv contrast, the lesion shows minimal uptake centrally, with moderate peripheral enhancement.[43-45]

MRI of the liver demonstrates a hypointense nodule with a hypo intense rim on T_1 weighted images and a isointense or hyper intense nodule with a less intense rim on T_2 weighted images.[48]

Splenic TB is generally found in patients with severe, disseminated disease, splenic lesions present as single or multiple focal hypoechoic lesions on ultrasound (Fig. 7.37). These may be hemorrhagic or necrotic. Irregular hypoechoic lesions typically represent splenic abscesses, an important manifestation of splenic TB, specially in HIV disease. Splenic involvement is common in HIV positive patients with TB, with macronodular involvement seen in 15% of HIV+ patients.[37]

The differential diagnosis of hepatic and splenic tuberculosis includes sarcoidosis, histoplasmosis, metastasis, hepatocellular carcinoma and parasitic

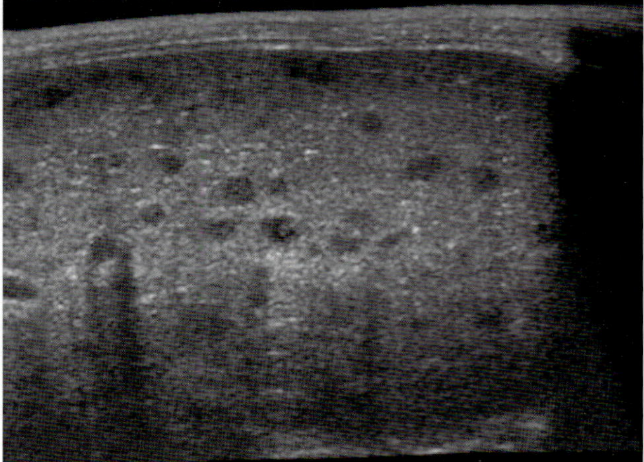

Fig. 7.37: USG - spleen is studded with small hypoechoic nodules

diseases. These may be distinguished from each other by history, laboratory tests and liver biopsy. Associated intestinal, peritoneal and nodal involvement may suggest tuberculosis despite the nonspecific radiological appearances.

Pancreas

Tuberculosis of the pancreas is rare and only a few cases have been reported. Pancreas is involved in the miliary form of tuberculosis, but may be the only site of reactivation in later years. Tuberculous lesions in the pancreas are usually located in the head and less commonly in the body or tail. Solitary lesions are seen as well-defined hypoechoic mass on US and as hypodense mass with irregular margin, with or without pancreatic enlargement on CT. Peripancreatic nodes may be present. Endoscopic retrograde cholangiopancreatography may show displacement and stenosis of the pancreatic duct, which is usually mistaken for a tumour.[49] Calcification has been observed in tubercular pancreas.

Radiological appearance might be similar to a mucinous cystic neoplasm or shows a pancreatic mass with involvement of peripancreatic lymph node. Pancreatic biopsy and culture is indicated, endoscopic ultrasound with fine needle aspiration cytology is the preferred technique. Diagnosis is made by percutaneous biopsy as malignancies; abscesses and chronic pancreatitis are included in the differential diagnosis (Fig. 7.38).

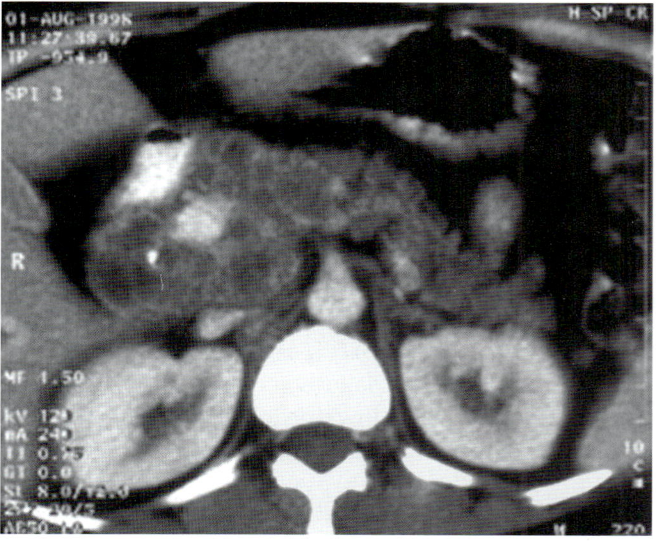

Fig. 7.38: CT- Small hypodense nodules, one showing a speck of calcification in region of head and proximal body of pancreas-TB

Vascular Involvement in Gastrointestinal Tuberculosis

Vascular involvement constitutes an important aspect of gastrointestinal tuberculosis. During the ulcerative phase, the superior mesenteric angiography shows hypervascularity in the affected region, hence selective embolisation or vasopressin infusion are important in patients with patients presenting with massive gastrointestinal bleed. Occlusive arterial changes are most marked in the vasa recta and develop in later stages, in the region of the strictures. Encasement and narrowing of vessels in the primary and secondary order branches occur secondary to tubercular peritonitis.[50]

Submucosal and subserosal vessels can be involved with caseating granulomas with occlusion resulting in localised infarction followed by fibrosis, stricture formation or obstruction. These lesions are rare and occur most commonly in the colon. The differential diagnosis on angiography includes Crohn's disease.

M tuberculosis may affect the vascular wall, resulting in pseudo aneurysm formation - mycotic aneurysm of the aorta. Local extension of a tuberculous mass may result in involvement of adjacent vascular structures. Involvement of the adjacent mesentery and major mesenteric vessels has been described with abdominal TB associated with perforation and intestinal obstruction. [51]

On colour Doppler imaging, characteristic changes take place in the SMA waveform in the presence of small bowel disease. Intestinal perfusion is increased with an associated decrease in vascular resistance resulting in an increase in volume and velocities (PSV, EDV and Vmean) of blood flow to the small bowel (Fig. 7.39). There is a consequent decrease in RI.[52]

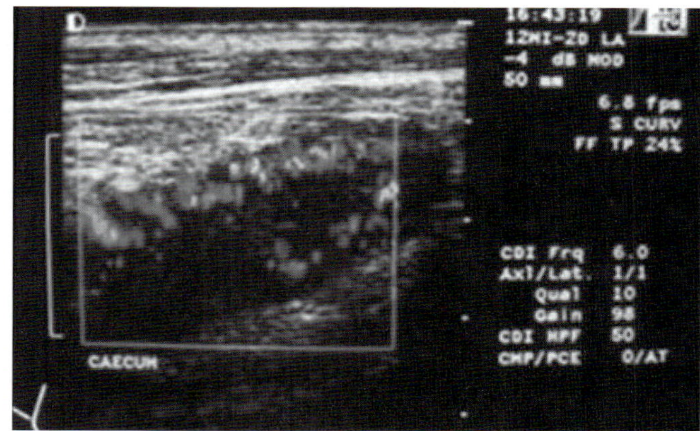

Fig. 7.39: CDFI. Shows a thick walled caecum with increased submuscosal vascularity *(For color version see plate 1)*

In a study conducted in the Dept. of Radio-diagnosis MAMC, 40% of cases with tubercular enteritis showed hypervascularity on CDFI. Preferentially the vascularity was seen in the mucosal and submucosal layers indicating acute stage of the disease. The intramural arterial signals in almost all cases showed a PSV <20 cm per sec and an RI of<0.6 suggesting low resistance waveform within the inflamed bowel segment. As the lesion progresses towards chronicity and with the setting in of fibrosis in the inflamed bowel segment, the vascularity decreases with a reduction in the PSV.

AIDS AND TUBERCULOSIS

There is a high incidence of tuberculosis in patients with HIV infection. Tuberculosis adopts atypical forms in HIV + patients. The extrapulmonary dissemination of the disease is very common (in 50-70% of cases)[41] and has been adopted by Centre for Disease Control as criterion for diagnosis of AIDS.

Mycobacterium tuberculosis infection in AIDS patients tends to be disseminated and may involve mesenteric lymph nodes, the peritoneum, solid visceral organs and virtually any part of the gastrointestinal tract. Infection with atypical mycobacterium (mycobacterium avium and mycobacterium intracellulare MAC), although rarely encountered in non-immunocompromised patients, is frequently noted in AIDS.

Significant abdominal lymphadenopathy is noted, with the radiographic appearance of tuberculous lymphadenitis in AIDS and non AIDS patients being similar. The majority have multiple enlarged nodes with peripheral enhancement and low attenuation centres. However in 25% of AIDS cases, nodes may be large, show low attenuation with no significant enhancement, a pattern not seen in non-AIDS patients. This is possibly due to lack of inflammatory response due to impaired immunity. A typical mycobacterial involvement produces a more impressive bulky retroperitoneal and mesenteric lymphadenopathy, which is similar to that in lymphoma and metastatic Kaposi's sarcoma. In contrast to mycobacterium tuberculosis, infection, most (55%) of the cases demonstrate homogeneous soft tissue attenuation with moderate homogeneous enhancement.[8, 24]

Splenic involvement is common among HIV positive patients with disseminated tuberculosis, the involvement being of the miliary type. Macro-nodular/focal splenic involvement occurs in about 15% of cases with HIV, and is considered of greater diagnostic value.[54] MAC infection in AIDS produces marked enlargement of liver in 20% and of spleen in 14% of patients. MAC may also cause focal abscesses within liver or spleen. Cholangitis in AIDS patients due to MAC produces intrahepatic and extrahepatic ductal stenosis and dilatation similar to that seen in primary sclerosing cholangitis.[55] These may be indistinguishable from more common infections such as cytomegalovirus or cryptosporidium.

Enteritis in AIDS patient is usually due to MAC on barium studies, this appears as diffuse small bowel dilatation and irregular fold thickening, simulating Whipple's disease. Barium dilution may be noted. Diffuse jejunal wall thickening visible on CT has been described in 18% of patients with MAC infection.[56] Ileocaecal involvement is usually by M. tuberculosis and produces similar radiographic changes as non-AIDS patients, except when the disease is advanced. In this stage with a primary ileocecal involvement, colonic abnormalities are more extensive, greater circumferential inflammatory involvement of the surrounding mesentery is seen, and bulky lymphadenopathy occurs. Unusual sites of involvement, such as the duodenum are also noted.[57]

Percutaneous Biopsy in the Diagnosis of Abdominal Tuberculosis

The diagnosis of abdominal tuberculosis, is difficult to establish. For a definitive diagnosis, microbiological or histological proof is mandatory. Percutaneous aspiration or biopsy, under CT or US guidance provides an excellent opportunity for the same by microscopic visualisation or culture of acid fast bacilli or histological identification of caseating granulomas. It is important to obtain the aspirate from the low attenuation area as the tubercle bacilli are less likely to be found in adjacent solid tissue. Direct visualisation of acid fast bacilli is rarely noted, ranging between 0-45% among patients with miliary TB. Positive culture is obtained in 10%, increasing in patients of miliary TB to 60%. Fine needle aspiration cytology from splenic and lymph node involvement has a high sensitivity (87.5-78.6% respectively) in the diagnosis of tuberculosis.[58] Peritoneal biopsies by laparoscopy detect caseating granulomas in 85-90% of cases with tuberculous peritonitis.

US guided FNAC is recommended over non-guided FNAC, even in palpable lesions, as the operator can actually visualise the needle tip. Diagnostic yield from bowel lesions has been reported to be low due to desmoplastic reaction secondary to chronic hypertrophic lesions.[58]

NUCLEAR IMAGING

Gallium-67 citrate, indium-111-labeled autologous leukocyte (white blood cell) scintigraphy, are useful in the setting of pyrexia of unknown origin, in which tuberculosis is implicated and no definitive source has been identified with other imaging techniques. In one study, Ga-67 scintigraphy has a sensitivity of 78% in identifying extrapulmonary tuberculosis. Nuclear imaging techniques do not help distinguish between the different causes of sepsis, but they do help identify a focus of interest. Further imaging of the area in question, along with additional tissue sampling, can then be performed to aid in diagnosis.Tc 99^{m} Ciprofloxacin (infecton) has shown a promising role in the diagnosis of abdominal tuberculosis. FDG-PET is an evolving diagnostic modality. Initial reports suggest that a diffuse peritoneal uptake may be indicative of peritoneal tuberculosis, rather than peritoneal carcinomatosa.[59, 60]Active tubercular lesions, often exhibit a high degree of FDG uptake. Though not specific for TB, PET-CT can demonstrate activity of lesions, guide biopsy from active sites, assess disease extent, detect occult distant foci and evaluate response to therapy.[61]

Table 7.1 Specificity of various imaging modalities in detecting specific changes encountered in abdominal tuberculosis [18]

Involved organ	*Findings*	*GI series*	*US*	*CT*
Peritoneum and its reflection	Ascitis	-	++	++
	Septa	-	++	-/+
	Slight peritoneal thickening	-	++ (if ascitis)	++
	Tiny nodules	-	++	++
	Peritoneal enhancement	-	-	++
	Omental changes	-	+	++
	Mesenteric changes	-	+	++
Lymph nodes	Enlargement	-	+	++
	Node characteristics	-	+	++
Solid organs	Hepato-splenomegaly	-	++	++
	Bright liver spleen	-	++	-
	Macronodules (liver-spleen)	-	++	++
	Pancreatic lesions	-	+	++
GI tract	Ulcers	++	-/+	+
	Irregular narrowed segment	++	+	++
	Wall thickening	-/+	+	++
	Regional lymph nodes	-	+	++
	Regional fat involvement	-	-	++

CONCLUSION

Diagnosis of abdominal TB is difficult because of vague and nonspecific clinical features and low yield of mycobacterium culture. Further invasive and costly procedures are requires for obtaining tissue for histopathological examination. Diagnosis based on radiology is rapid and less expensive, but is presumptive and cannot completely exclude other pathologies such as Crohn's. A high index of suspicion is required to make an early diagnosis.

Judicious and appropriate use of the various imaging modality will avoid laparotomies for the diagnosis of abdominal tuberculosis.

REFERENCES

1. Sharma MP, Vikram Bhatia. Abdominal Tuberculosis. Indian J Med Res 2004;120:305-15.
2. Manohar A, Simjee AE, Haffejee AA, et al. Symptoms and investigative findings in 145 patients with tuberculous peritonitis diagnosed by peritoneoscopy and biopsy over a 5 year period. Gut 1990;31:1130-32.
3. Bhansali SK. Abdominal Tuberculosis, experiences with 300 cases. Am J Gastroenterol 1977;67:324-37.
4. Sharma AK, Agarwal LD, Sharma CS et al. Abdominal tuberculosis in children. Experience over a decade. Indian Paediatr 1993;30:1149-53.
5. Batra A, Gulati MS, Sarma D, Paul SB. Sonographic appearances in abdominal tuberculosis. J Clin Ultrasound 2000;28:233-45.
6. Leder RA, Low VHS. Tuberculosis of the abdomen. Radiol Clin North Am 1995;33:691-705.
7. Burrill J, Williams CJ, Bain G et al. Tuberculosis : A Radiologic Review Radiographics 2007; 27:1255-73.
8. Hulnick DH, Megibow AJ, Nadiach DP, et al. Abdominal tuberculosis: CT evaluation. Radiology 1985;157:199-204.
9. Lundstedt C, Nymon R, Brimsar J, Hugosson C, Kagevi I. Imaging of abdominal tuberculosis, Abdominal manifestations in 112 patients. Acta Radiol 1996;37:489-95.
10. Mali A, Saxena NC. Ultrasound in abdominal tuberculosis. Abdom Imaging 2003.
11. Anbarasu A, Upadhyay A, Merchant SA, Amonkar P, et al. Tuberculous chylous ascitis: pathognomonic CT findings. Abdom Imaging 1997;22:50-51.
12. Demirkazik FB, Akhan O, Ozmn MN, Akata D. US and CT findings in the diagnosis of tuberculous peritonitis. Acta Radiol 1996;36:1-4.
13. Arai K, Makino H, Morioka T, et al. Enhancement of ascitis on MRI following intravenous administration of Gd-DTPA. J Comput Asst Tomogr 1993;17:617-22 .
14. Ha HK, Jung JM, Lee MS, et al. CT differentiation of Tuberculous peritonitis and Peritoneal carcinomatosis. AJR 1996;167:743-48.
15. Rodriquez E and Pombo F. Peritoneal Tuberculosis versus peritoneal carcinomatosis:Distinction based on CT findings. J Comput Asst Tomogr 1996;20(2).

16. Jain R, Sawhney S, Bhargava DK, et al. Diagnosis of Abdominal Tuberculosis: sonographic findings in patients with early disease. AJR 1995;165:1391-95.
17. Kedar RP, Shah PP, Shirde RS, et al. Sonographic findings in gastrointestinal and Peritoneal Tuberculosis. Clinical Radiology 1994;49:24-29.
18. Akhan O, Pringot J. Imaging of abdominal Tuberculosis Eur. Radiol 2002;12:312-23.
19. Kaushik R, Punia R, Mohan H et al. Tuberculous abdominal cocoon - a report of 6 cases and review of the literature. World J Emerg - Surg 2006;1:18.
20. Ping Xu, Li Hua Chen, You Ming Li. Idiopathic sclerosing encapsulating peritonitis (or abdominal cocoon) A report of 5 cases. World J Gastroenterol 2007; 13(26):3649-365.
21. Ganeshan S, Indrajit IK. US in Abdominal lymph node Tuberculosis-A review of 42 cases. Ind J Radiol Imag 1993;3: 231-36.
22. Caroli - Bosc FX, Conio M, Maes B, et al. Abdominal tuberculosis involving hepatic hilar lymph nodes. J Clin Gastroenterol 1997;25:541-43.
23. Puri S, Khurana SB, Malhotra S. Tuberculous abdominal lymphadenopathy causing reversible renovascular hypertension. J Assoc Physicians India 2000;48(5):530-32.
24. Pombo F, Rodriquez E, Mato J, Perez-Fontan, et al. Patterns of contrast enhancement of tuberculous lymph nodes demonstrated by computed tomography. Clin Radiol 1992;46:13-17.
25. Yang ZG, Min P, Sone S, He Z, et al. Tuberculosis versus lymphomas in the abdominal lymph nodes. Evaluation with contrast enhanced CT. AJR 1999;172:619-23.
26. Kim S-Y, Kim M-J, Chung J-J, Le et al. Abdominal tuberculous lymphadenopathy: MR imaging findings. Abdom Imaging 2000;25:627-32.
27. Moon W, Im J, Yu I, et al. Mediastinal tuberculous lymphadenitis: MR imaging appearance with clinicopathological correlation. AJR 1996;166:21-25.
28. Backer Dc A.1, Mortete KJ, Deeren D et al. Abdominal Tuberculour lymphadenopathy : MRI features. Eur Radiol 2005 DOI: 10 : 1007/S 00330 - 005-2745-6.
29. Shah P: Gastrointestinal, Tuberculosis-A review Ind. J Radiol Imag 1993;3:243-51.
30. Nagi B., Sodhi KS, Kochhar R, et al. Small bowel tuberculosis : enteroclysis findings. Abdom Imaging 2004;29:335-40.
31. Carrera GF, Young S, Lewincki AM. Intestinal tuberculosis. Gastrointest Radiol 1976;1:147-55.
32. Suri S, Kaur H, Wig JD, Singh K. CT in Abdominal Tuberculosis-Comparison with barium studies. Ind. J Radiol Imag 1993;3:237-42.
33. Suri S, Gupta S, Suri R. Pictoral review-Computed tomography in abdominal tuberculosis. The British Journal of Radiology 1999;72:92-98.
34. Balthazar EJ, Cordon R, Hulnick D. Ileocecal tuberculosis : CT and Radiological evaluation. AJR 1990;154:499-503.
35. Boudiaf M, jaff A, Soyer Petal. Small bowel diseases, Prospective evaluation of Multidetector Row Helical CT enteroclysis in 107 Consecutive patients. Radiology 2004;233:338-44.
36. Backer De A.1, Mortele K.J., Keulenaer De. CT and MR imaging of gastrointestinal Tuberculosis. JBR-BTR 2006; 89:190-95.
37. Schunk K. Small Bowel magnetic resonance imaging for inflammatory bowel disease. Topics in magnetic resonance imaging 2002;13(6):409-25.
38. Masserli G, Brisi GM, Parelle et al. Crohn's disease Magnetic Resonance enteroclysis. Abdominal Imaging 2004;29:326-34.
39. Makajuola D. Is it Crohn's disease or intestinal tuberculosis? CT Analysis Eur J Radiol 1998;28:55-61.
40. Jose M Pereira, Antonio J Madurerira Alberto Vieira et al. Abdominal Tuberculosis: Imaging features. European Journal of Radiology EJR 2005;55:173-80.
41. Morrison H, Mixter CG, Schlesinger MJ, et al. Tuberculosis localised in the vermiform appendix. N Engl J Med 1952;246:329-31.
42. Theoni RF, Margullis AR. Gastrointestinal Tuberculosis. Semin Roentgenol 1979;14:283-94.
43. Brauner M, Buuffard MD, Jeantils V, et al. Sonography and computed tomography of macroscopic tuberculosis of the liver. J Clin Ultrasound 1989;17:563-68.
44. Topal U, Savci G, Sadikoglu MY, et al. Splenic involvement of tuberculosis: US and CT findings. Eur Radiol 1994;43:128-29.
45. Levine C. Primary macronodular hepatic tuberculosis : US and CT appearances. Gastrointest Radiol 1990;15:307-09.
46. Kawamori Y, Matsui O, Kitagawa K, et al. Macronodular tuberculoma of the liver: CT and MR findings. AJR 1992;158:311-13.
47. Sharma SK, Duncan Smith - Rohrberg, Mohammad Tahir et al. Radiological manifestations of splenic tuberculosis : A 23 patient case series from India. Indian J Med Res 2007;125:669-78.
48. Monilla-Serra JM, Martinez-Noguera A, Montserrat E, et al. Abdominal ultrasound findings of disseminated tuberculosis in AIDS. J Clin Ultrasound 1997;25:1-6.
49. Fischer G, Splengler U, Neubrand M, Kodoya M, et al. Isolated tuberculosis of the pancreas masquerading as a pancreatic mass. Am J Gastroenterol 1995;90:2227-29.
50. Shah P, Ravi R. Role of vasculitis in the natural history of abdominal TB-evaluation by mesenteric angiography. Indian J Gastroenterol 1991;10:127-30.
51. De Backer A.I., Mortele KJ, De Keulenaer B.L. et al. Vascular involvement secondary to tuberculosis of the abdomen. Abdom Imaging 2005;30:714-18.
52. Erden Ayse, Cumhur T, Olcer T: Superior mesenteric artery blood flow in patients with small bowel diseases: Evaluation with Duplex Doppler Sonography. JCU 1998;26(1):37-41.

53. Shafer RW, Kim DS, Weiss JP, et al. Extrapulmonary tuberculosis in patients with human immunovirus deficiency virus infection. Medicine 1991;70:384-96.
54. Monilla-Serra JM, Martinez Noguera A, Montserral E, et al. Abdominal ultrasound findings of disseminated tuberculosis in AIDS. J Clin Ultrasound 1997;25: 1-6.
55. Farman J, Brunetti J, Baer JW, et al. AIDS related cholangiopancreatographic changes. Abdominal Imaging 1994;19:417.
56. Radin DR. Intraabdominal Mycobacterium tuberculosis vs Mycobacterium avium intracellulare infections in patients with AIDS. AJR Am J Roentgenol 1991;156:487.
57. Bargallo N, Nicolau C, Luburich P, et al. Intestinal tuberculosis in AIDS. Gastrointest Radiol 1992:17;115.
58. Suri R, Gupta S, Gupta SK, et al. Ultrasound guided fine needle aspiration cytology in abdominal tuberculosis. Br J Radiol 1998:71;723-27.
59. Adams Bruce K, Youssef Inas, Parker et al. Tc 99m Ciprofloxacin (Infecton) in Abdominal Tuberculosis. Clinical Nuclear Medicine 2006;31(3):157-58.
60. Shimmota H, Hamada K, Higuch I et al. Abdominal Tuberculosis : Peritoneal Involvement shown by F-18 FDG PET ; Clin Nucl Med 2007;32:716-18.
61. Harkirat S, Anand SS, Indrajit IK, Dash AK.Pictoral essay. PET-CT in tuberculosis. Indian J Radiol Imaging 2008;18:141-7.

Chapter Eight

Non-tubercular Inflammatory Bowel Diseases

Birinder Nagi, Anupam Lal, Manphool Singhal

INFLAMMATORY BOWEL DISEASES

Inflammatory bowel disease (IBD) refers to a group of disorders characterized by intestinal inflammation, extra intestinal manifestations and a relapsing course. Ulcerative colitis (UC) and Crohn's disease (CD) are the two distinct idiopathic inflammatory diseases accounting for the majority of cases of IBD.

UC is a superficial inflammatory disease characterized by symmetric, uniform and contiguous process that usually involves the rectum, extending proximally until the entire colon is affected, producing a pancolitis. The disease is confined to colon spreading in a contiguous manner from the rectum proximally, and terminal ileum may be affected only when ascending colon and cecum are involved (backwash ileitis).

Crohn's disease is a granulomatous process characterized by transmural and discontinuous inflammation of the bowel, often complicated by fistulae and abscesses. It can affect any part of the gastrointestinal (GI) tract, from the mouth to the anus, often involving multiple discontinuous segments. The small intestine is involved in 80% of cases, most commonly at the terminal ileum. The colon is affected either with (50%) or without (15-20%) involvement of the small intestine. [1]

RADIOLOGY

Various imaging modalities used in the evaluation of IBD include barium studies, ultrasonography (US), computed tomography (CT), magnetic resonance imaging (MRI) and positron emission tomography (PET-CT). In the appropriate clinical settings, these modalities help confirm the diagnosis, localize lesions, assess their extent, severity and activity, identify the presence of extra intestinal complications and monitor the response to therapy. [2-6]

Double contrast barium enema (DCBE), barium meal follow through and enteroclysis are the primary radiological tools for confirming the presence of IBD and to determine the extent of disease. Barium studies though provide superb visualization of mucosa, are limited in their capacity to demonstrate the transmural and extramural extent of disease and extra intestinal complications.

Computed tomography is the cross-sectional imaging modality of choice for detection and characterization of inflammatory conditions of bowel and evaluating the mural and extra intestinal manifestations of IBD.[7] The advent of multi-detector CT (MDCT) and use of high quality 3D and virtual images have opened up the opportunity to evaluate these patients with non-invasive technique. CT perfusion studies can demonstrate actively inflamed segments of bowel.

Virtual colonoscopy or CT colonography is a novel and rapidly evolving technique for colon imaging. It can depict early and advanced changes in both UC and CD bearing a strong resemblance to those of conventional colonoscopy. [8] Colon distension should be carried out carefully in these patients as there are reports of colonic perforation because of inflamed colonic wall. [9]

MDCT is associated with considerable dose of ionizing radiation and could be an issue in patients with IBD, who need frequent follow up examinations. MRI is having an increasing diagnostic impact on patients with IBD. Its attributes include high soft tissue contrast, multiplaner capabilities and the use of non-ionizing radiation. MRI is safe in pregnancy and renal failure. The greatest advantage is its ability to differentiate active inflammation from fibrosis. Fibrotic wall thickening demonstrates low signal intensity both on T1WI and T2WI sequences.

MR colonography is a new technique applied to evaluate IBD of colon. For colonic evaluations, T1 weighted positive signal is referred to as "Bright lumen" imaging which can be performed using mixture of water and gadolinium per rectally. The "Dark lumen" technique produces a dark intraluminal contrast on T1W1 after application of rectal water enema to contrast with a bright bowel wall which is achieved by intravenous contrast agent. A good correlation has been seen between colonoscopy and MR colonography using "Dark lumen" technique. This has opened a new promising role in monitoring IBD activity. [10] The presence of bowel wall thickening with mural enhancement after administration of IV contrast allows assessing disease activity. Abnormally high bowel wall signal intensity on T2W1, caused by edema and inflammation, associated with high signal intensity after contrast enhancement on T1WI indicates active disease. Mural thickening without high T2WI signal and enhancement after contrast is correlated with clinical remission and decreased disease activity.

MR colonography is still considered inadequate to diagnose colonic inflammation. New techniques such as color coding of bowel wall thickness and new generation of inflammation sensitive contrast media in MRI may improve the diagnostic accuracy of MR colonography and need to be evaluated intensively in the future.

Ultrasound is a simple, non-invasive, easily available modality without ionizing radiation. It is able to detect bowel wall abnormalities and complications such as fistulae and abscesses in most of IBD patients. High resolution sonography has a good sensitivity in detecting bowel inflammation. Inflamed bowel often shows hypervascularization, which can be assessed by using Doppler ultrasound, thus providing additional information on the degree of disease activity. [11] Hydrocolonic sonography allows detailed evaluation of the bowel lumen and all the five anatomic layers of colonic wall. [12]

PET/CT scanners provide accurately fused morphological and functional imaging within a single examination. PET-CT colonography offers a simple non-invasive study to identify and localize active intestinal inflammation. [13] Detection of disease activity in IBD is of crucial importance for the purpose of management 18F - FDG accumulates at sites of infection, inflammation and in granulomatous diseases by the over expression of glucose transporter isotypes (GLUT) mainly GLUT-1 and GLUT-3 and by an overproduction of glycolytic enzymes in inflammatory cells. PET activity correlates well with active inflammation in both UC and CD, suggesting that this is a non-invasive method of identifying disease activity in patients with IBD. It simultaneously detects inflammation and disease activity in large and small bowel.

ULCERATIVE COLITIS

In UC the earliest finding on DCBE is characterized by fine granular appearance of mucosa, usually involving the recto sigmoid junction caused by edema and hyperemia of mucosa. Abscesses of the crypts of lieberkuhn may erode into the lumen, producing a stippled appearance as a result of superimposition of multiple erosions on a background of mucosal granularity (Fig. 8.1). With further progression, deeper ulcers may erode into the submucosa, resulting in characteristics 'collar-button' ulcers that undermine the mucosa (Fig. 8.2). These ulcers can be seen in various other inflammatory conditions also (Table 8.1). In advanced disease, ulcerative colitis is characterized by pancolitis with diffuse ulcerations, absence of haustral folds and narrowing of the colon, with the possible development of inflammatory pseudopolyps, representing mounds of inflamed tissue

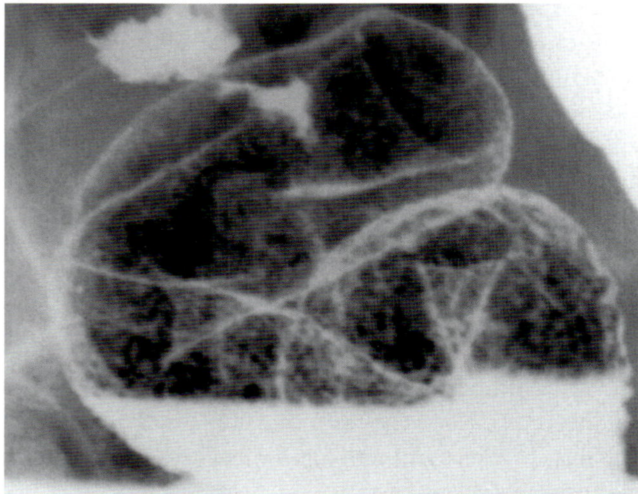

Fig. 8.1: DCBE showing granular mucosal pattern in sigmoid colon

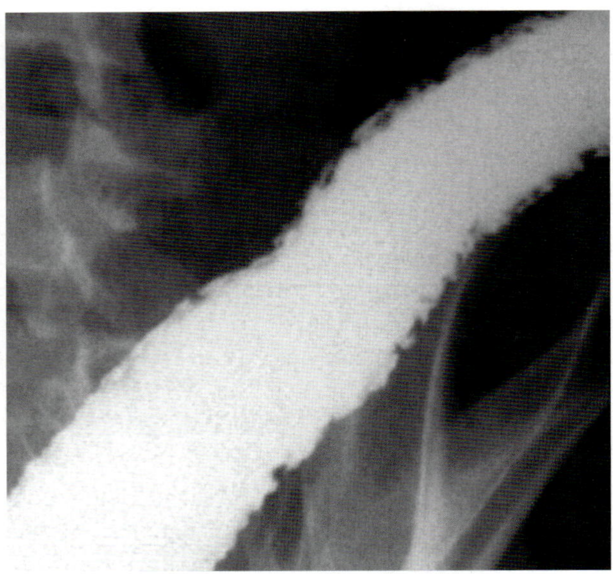

Fig. 8.2: Collar button ulcers seen in descending colon

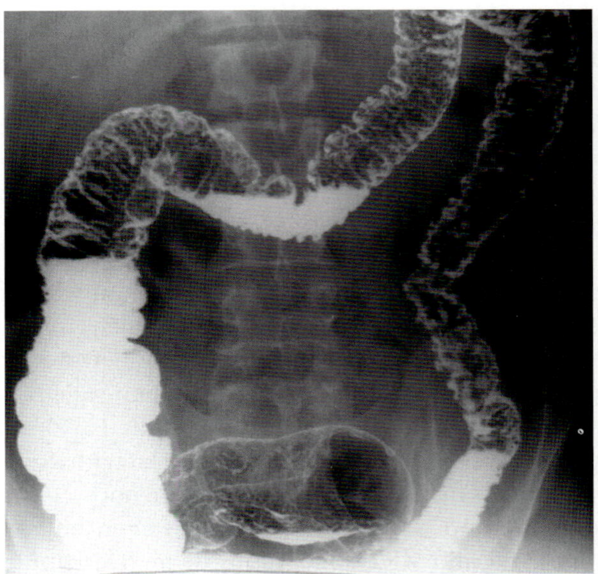

Fig. 8.3: Diffuse involvement of colon with ulcers, pseudo polyps and loss of haustrations

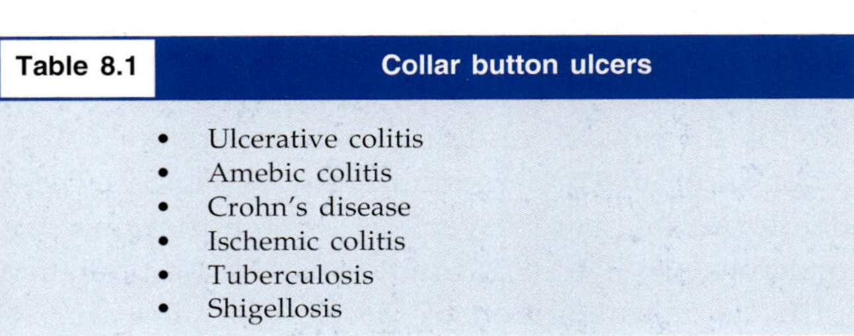

Table 8.1	Collar button ulcers
	• Ulcerative colitis • Amebic colitis • Crohn's disease • Ischemic colitis • Tuberculosis • Shigellosis

between areas of denuded mucosa (Fig. 8.3). About 15 - 20% of patients with severe UC can show associated backwash ileitis characterized by a fixed, patulous ileocecal valve and a dilated granular terminal ileum.

In chronic disease, DCBE reveals marked colonic shortening, tubular narrowing, loss of haustration and widening of presacral space (Fig. 8.4). Colonic shortening is caused by thickening and contraction of muscularis mucosae without actual fibrosis. These findings may be reversible after treatment. As healing occurs, patients may develop post inflammatory polyps, representing areas of residual granulation tissue after the acute inflammatory process (Fig. 8.5).[2, 6]

CT is not a useful technique in early UC for detecting mucosal abnormalities. Abnormal findings are seen in advanced disease in the form of colonic wall thickening which is diffuse, symmetric and measures 7-8 mm with inhomogeneous enhancement and preservation of mural stratification (Fig. 8.6).[14] The "target sign", a low attenuation ring in the bowel wall due to deposition of sub-mucosal fat is characterized by an inner soft tissue density ring comprising (mucosa, lamina propria and muscularis mucosae), a central low density ring (sub-mucosa) and an outer soft tissue density ring (muscularis propria and serosa) is seen more commonly in UC than CD. [15] In chronic UC rectal narrowing with widening of retrorectal space is commonly seen. There is also proliferation of peri-rectal fat which is non-specific and can be present in UC, CD, pseudo membranous colitis or radiation colitis. CT colonography clearly depicts early and advanced changes of UC bearing a strong resemblance to that of conventional colonoscopy.

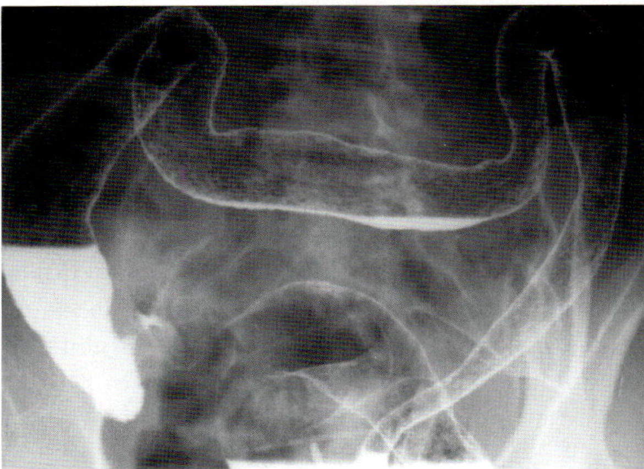

Fig. 8.4: Total colitis with narrowing and shortening of colon

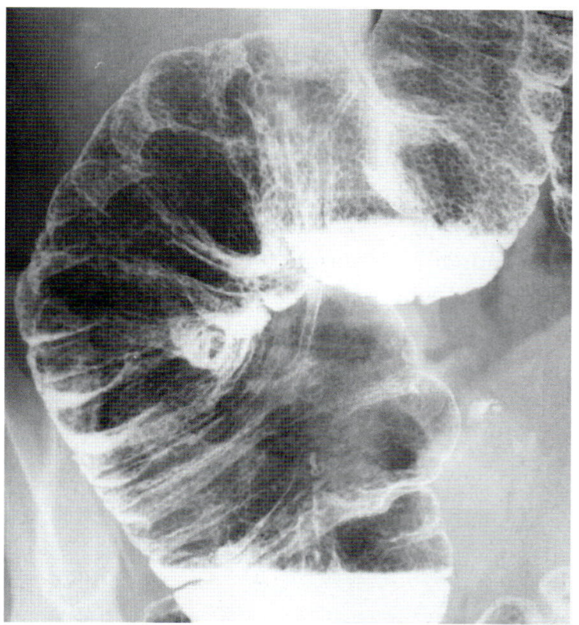

Fig. 8.5: Multiple post-inflammatory polyps

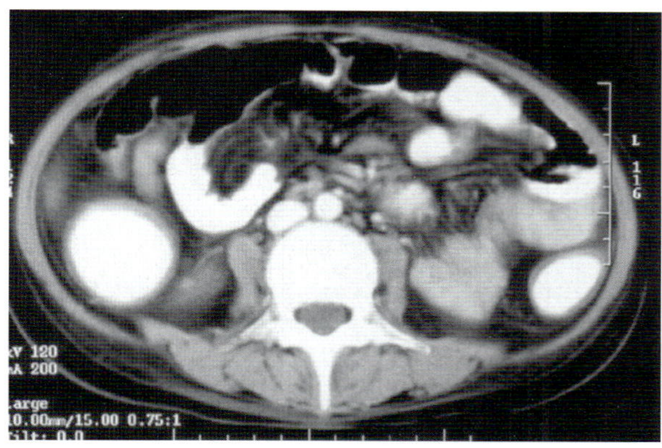

Fig. 8.6: CECT showing symmetrical mild thickening of ascending and descending colon

With PET-CT colonography, there is excellent correlation between PET activity and disease activity as determined by colonoscopy (Fig. 8.7).

On ultrasound, there is intermediate thickening of colonic wall (5-10 mm) with preservation of mural stratification both in active and chronic phases.[2-5]

CROHN'S DISEASE

Crohn's disease of small bowel has been categorized into subtypes based upon imaging studies so as to help clinicians to plan appropriate therapy.

Radiological classification of small bowel Crohn's disease is as follows:[16]

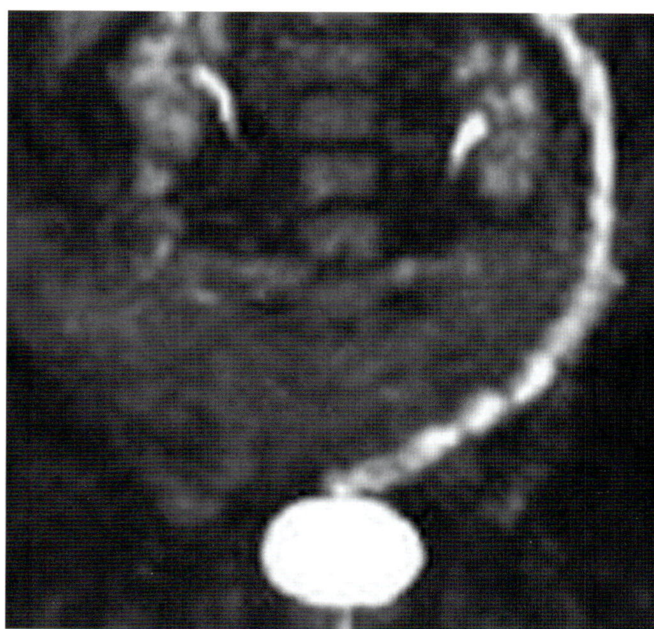

Fig. 8.7: PET activity seen in rectosigmoid and descending colon in active ulcerative colitis

Active Inflammatory Subtype

Minimal Changes

1. Superficial ulcers (Aphthae)
2. Fold thickening

Severe Changes

1. Deep ulcers, cobblestone mucosa
2. Wall thickening

"Comb sign"

Fibrostenotic Subtype

Minimal stenosis
Severe stenosis

Fistulizing/Perforating Subtype

Deep fissuring ulcers, sinus tracts
Fistulae to adjacent organs
Associated inflammatory mass

Reparative or Regenerative Subtype

Mucosa atrophy
Regenerative polyps

Barium examination is traditionally considered the cornerstone of the radiologic evaluation of CD. Barium enteroclysis particularly double contrast (barium and air) enteroclysis is superior for evaluation of early lesion. The diagnosis of CD should include assessment of (a) Presence, severity and extent of disease (b) Inflammatory lesion activity and (c) The presence of extra intestinal complications.

The earliest pathological changes are in the form of hyperplasia of the lymphoid tissue and obstructive lymphedema in the submucosa which may not be manifested as on barium studies. The earliest appreciable radiological finding is the presence of aphthous ulcers, which typically appear as punctate collections (1 to 3 mm in size) of barium surrounded by radiolucent halos. These ulcers can only be well-appreciated on double contrast (barium and air) enteroclysis. Pathologically these represent shallow mucosal erosions on the surface of hyperplastic lymphoid follicles in the lamina propria surrounded by a small halo of edema. In appropriate clinical setting this finding is considered highly specific for Crohn's disease. As the disease progresses, aphthous ulcers enlarge to form satellite, serpiginous or linear areas of ulceration (Fig. 8.8). Contiguous progression of the disease leads to development of deep fissuring ulcers (Fig. 8.9) and cobblestone appearance as a result of deep transverse and longitudinal ulcers separated by residual areas of edematous mucosa (Fig. 8.10). In the fibrostenotic subtype, there is stenosis of bowel with or without

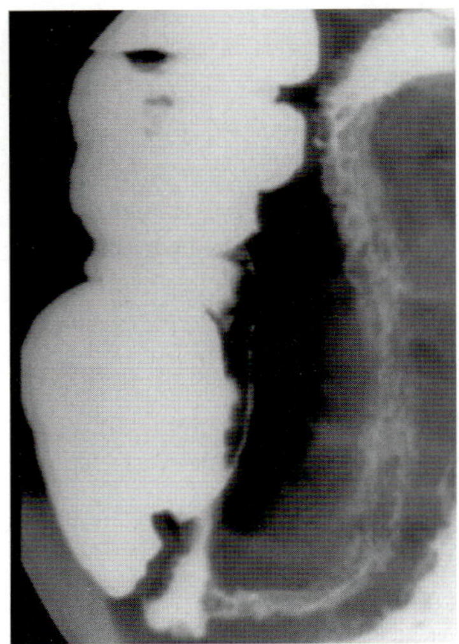

Fig. 8.8: Barium enteroclysis showing serpiginous ulcers in ileum

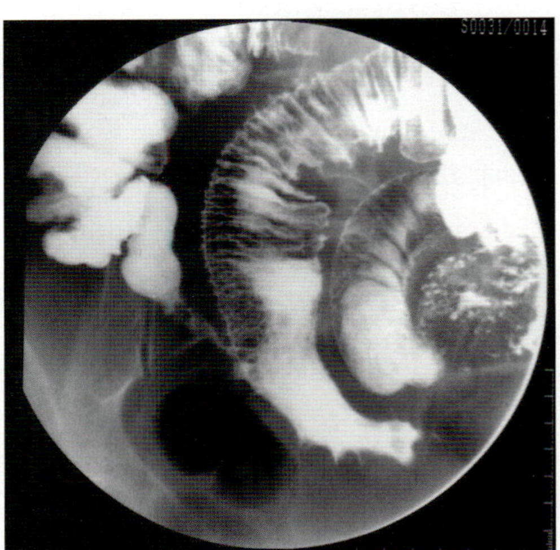

Fig. 8.9: Fissuring ulcers seen in ileum

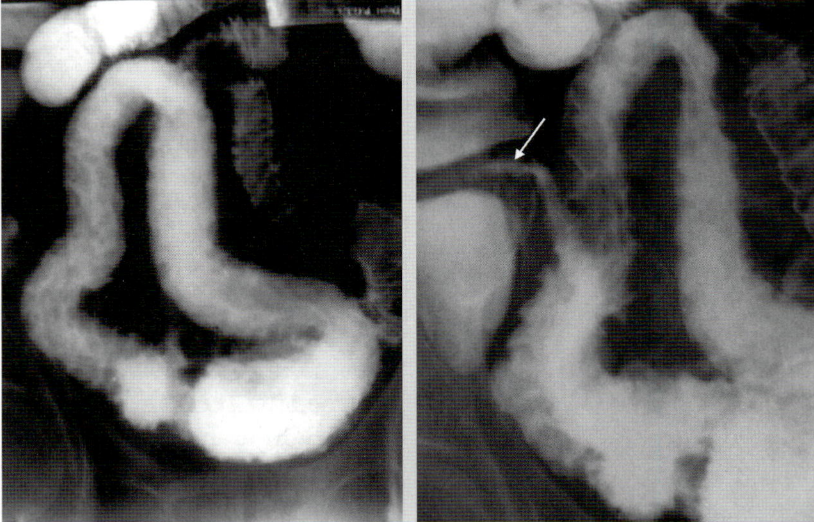

Fig. 8.10: Barium enteroclysis showing cobblestone pattern involving long segment of ileum. Note sparing of ileo-cecal junction (arrow)

significant prestenotic dilatation (Fig. 8.11). The narrowing is usually eccentric along the mesenteric border which is associated with thickening, sclerosis, and retraction of the adjacent mesentery. The unaffected antimesentric border assumes appearance of pleating or sacculation (Fig. 8.12). A persistent stream of barium in the bowel is termed as "string sign" indicating long segment of stenosis and is more often seen in Crohn's disease. Sinus tracts, fistulae and perforations are predominant findings in fistulizing/perforating subtype (Fig. 8.13).[16]

The changes of only severe inflammatory disease activity are detectable by CT enteroclysis. Aphthoid ulcers are not shown by CT. Various constellations of findings on CT are moderate to marked thickening of bowel wall (1-2 cms.) with stratification indicative of edema from active inflammation of bowel wall (Figs 8.14 and 8.15). This correlates very well with the disease activity and subsides with treatment. This is useful for monitoring the response to medical treatment. [16-20] Other findings seen are deep ulcers presenting as contrast protrusion into the bowel wall and cobble stone mucosa. "Comb sign" is seen

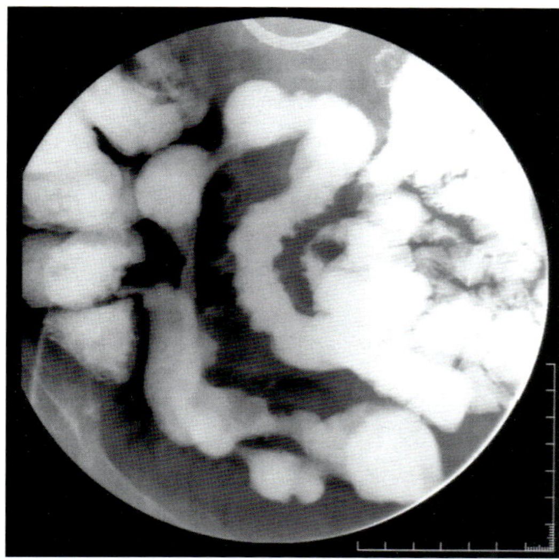

Fig. 8.11: Multiple eccentric strictures with intervening areas of dilatation

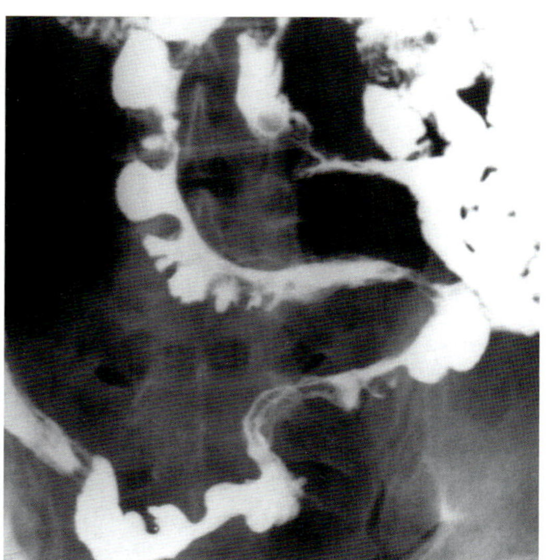

Fig. 8.12: Barium examination showing asymmetric narrowing and pseudosacculations at anti-mesenteric border

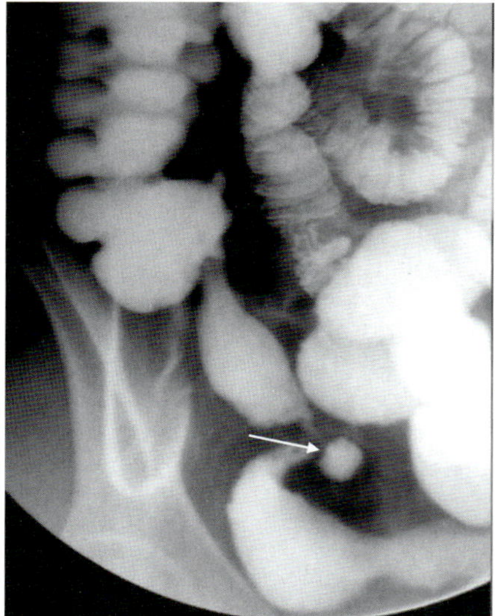

Fig. 8.13: Localized perforation of ileum (arrow)

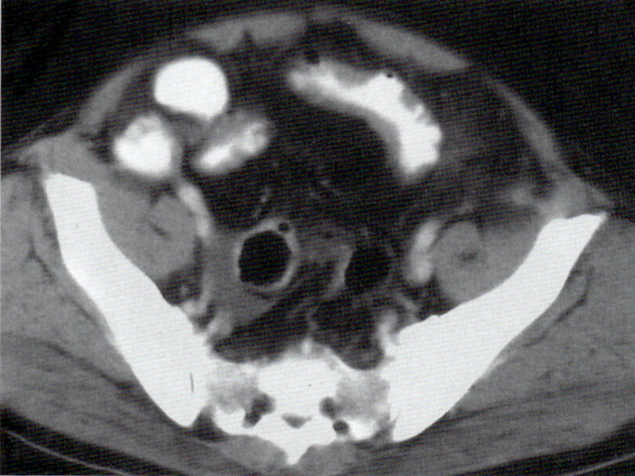

Fig. 8.14: CECT showing asymmetric mural thickening of ileum with pseudosacculations

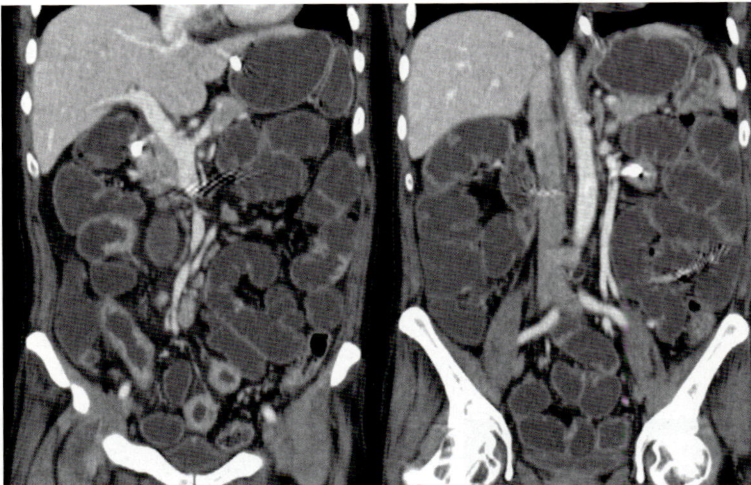

Fig. 8.15: CT enteroclysis showing skip lesions in ileum in the form of mural thickening with enhancement and sparing of ileocecal junction

as prominent vasa recta of mesenteric vessels representing perienteric inflammation and bowel wall inflammation. [21] Fibrofatty proliferation of mesentery is a predominant finding seen in CD. Mesenteric lymphadenopathy is seen as hypodense enlarged nodes without any central necrosis (Fig. 8.16). In the fibrostenotic subtype transmural fibrosis manifests as homogeneous attenuation of bowel wall. Entero-cutaneous and entero-vesical fistulae are best demonstrated on CT (Figs 8.17A to C). Intraabdominal abscesses can also be detected and CT can guide percutaneous drainage procedures. The sequential CT enterography examination has excellent potential for reliably monitoring Crohn's disease progression and regression.[22] Virtual ileoscopy, which is an extension of virtual colonoscopy can show thickening of folds and nodularity in the ileum (Figs 8.18A to C).

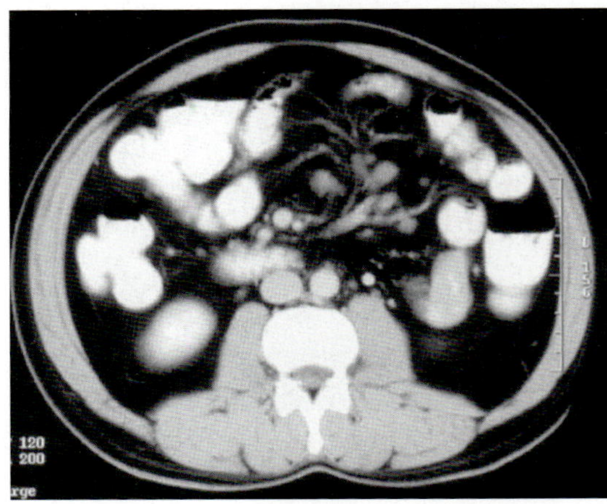

Fig. 8.16: CECT showing mesenteric vascular engorgement with fibrofatty proliferation of mesentery and lymphadenopathy

MR enteroclysis shows multiple strictures with thickened bowel wall. Bowel wall thickening appears as increased signal on T2-weighted images which on contrast enhanced T1-weighted sequences shows enhancement. [20,23]

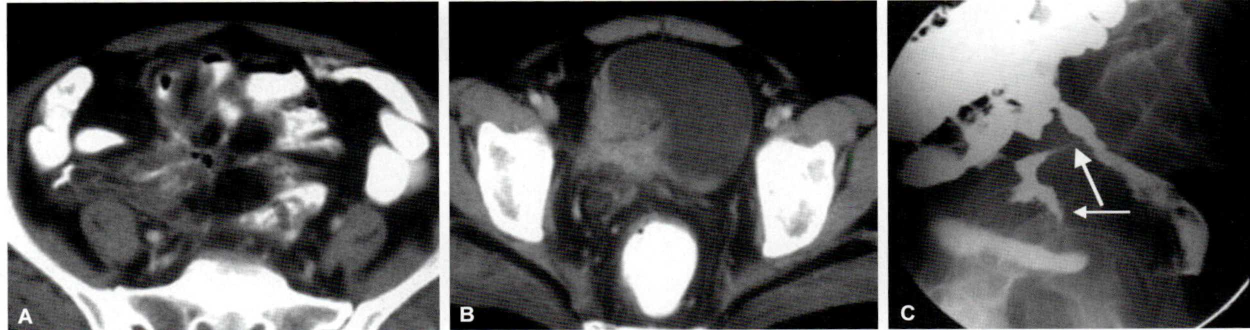

Figs 8.17A to C: CECT revealing multiple fistulous tracts from ileal loops (A) with inflammatory soft tissue at right lateral wall of urinary bladder (B). Barium examination confirms the presence of ileo vesical than (thin arrow) and ileo rectal (thick arrow) fistula (C)

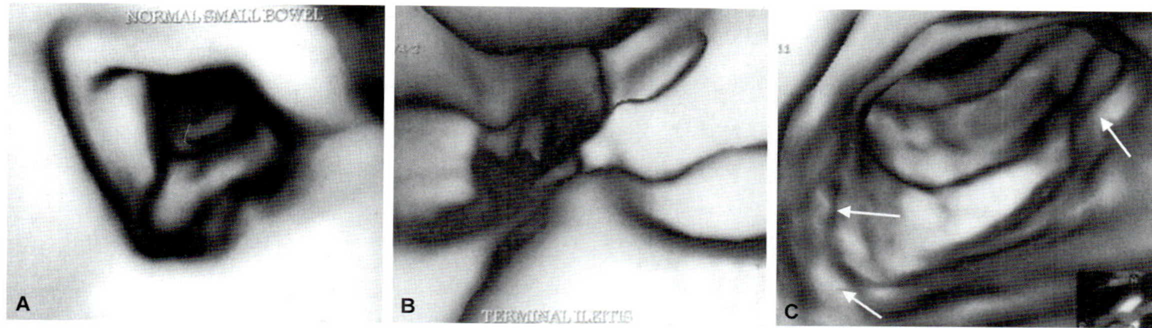

Figs 8.18A to C: Virtual ileoscopic images showing normal ileal mucosa (A), thickened folds (B), and nodular mucosa (C)

The degree of enhancement correlates with the disease activity and inflammation.[24] Mesenteritis appears as high signal on T2-weighted images which resolves with remission. Mesenteric vascular engorgement is evident as "Comb sign" (Fig. 8.19). In addition fibrofatty proliferation of mesentery and enlarged mesenteric lymph nodes which are of low signal intensity can also be present.[16]

In the fibrostenotic subtype MR readily differentiates fibrotic and edematous wall thickening which is useful for selecting patients for medical versus surgical treatment. Fibrotic wall thickening demonstrates low signal on both T1WI and T2WI sequences.[16] True FISP sequences are superior to HASTE for demonstration of sinuses and intramural tracts.

High resolution sonography may show bowel thickening with mural stratification and mesenteric lymphadenopathy. On Doppler examination hyper-vascularity of bowel wall can be seen which parallels the activity of inflammatory disease. Crohn's disease activity can also be determined by assessing the superior mesentery artery flow which is increased in the acute stage of disease. [25] Intensity of color Doppler signals and resistive index measurements of thickened bowel wall can be used as quantitative diagnostic tools in the assessment of disease activity. [26] Sinus and fistulous tracts are poorly visualized but power Doppler can demonstrate vascularity within the wall of tract. Recently a technique called "hydrogen peroxide enhanced US-fistulography" has been described in which a solution of 30% hydrogen peroxide and 70% providone/iodine is injected into the skin orifice of entero-cutaneous fistulae which enhances visualization of fistulous tract. [27]

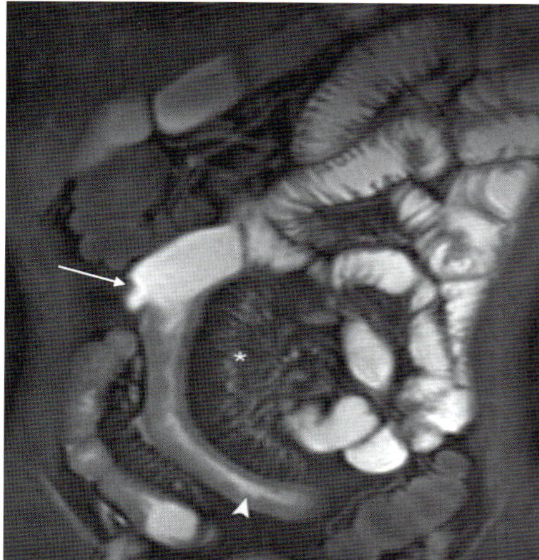

Fig. 8.19: MR enteroclysis showing increased mesenteric hypervascularity- comb sign (*), mural thickening (arrow head) and an ulcer (arrow). (With permission from Maglinte DD, et al: Classification of small bowel Crohn's subtypes based on multimodality imaging. RCNA 2003; 41: 285-303)

PET-CT is being evaluated in the evaluation of small bowel disease and PET-CT enteroclysis provides information of metabolic activity of inflammatory lesions of the intestine.[28]

In Crohn's colitis the earliest radiographic findings on DCBE are represented by aphthous ulcers that appear as punctate collection of barium surrounded by radiolucent halo of edema (Fig. 8.20). These lesions represent shallow erosion on the surface of hyperplastic lymphoid follicles in the lamina propria. Such ulcers, though characteristic of CD, can also be seen in other conditions (Table 8.2). As the disease progresses, aphthoid ulcers enlarge and coalesce to form linear areas of ulcerations with skip involvement resulting in segmental colitis (Fig. 8.21). Disease progression may lead to the development of cobblestone appearance caused by deep transverse and longitudinal ulcers separated by residual areas of edematous mucosa (Fig. 8.22). Other conditions resulting in cobblestone pattern are listed in (Table 8.3). Double tracking may be seen as longitudinal extra luminal tracked

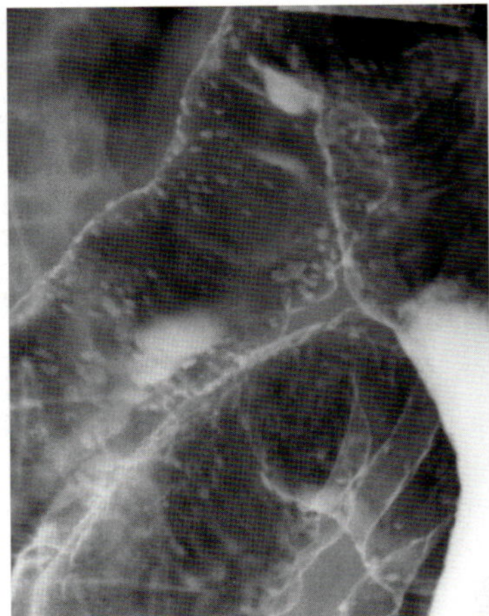

Fig. 8.20: DCBE showing aphthoid ulcers

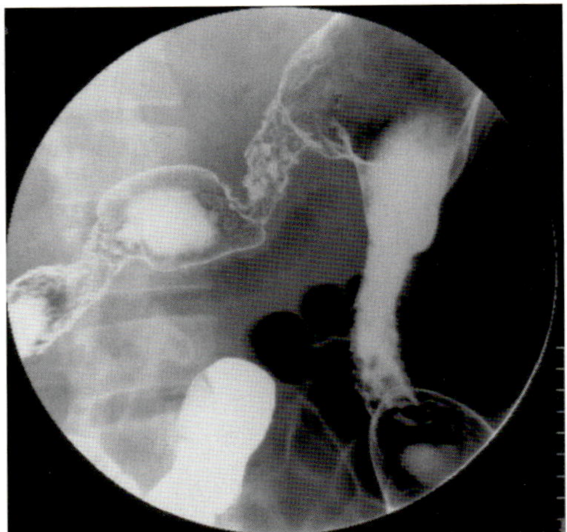

Fig. 8.21: Segmental colitis affecting descending and transverse colon

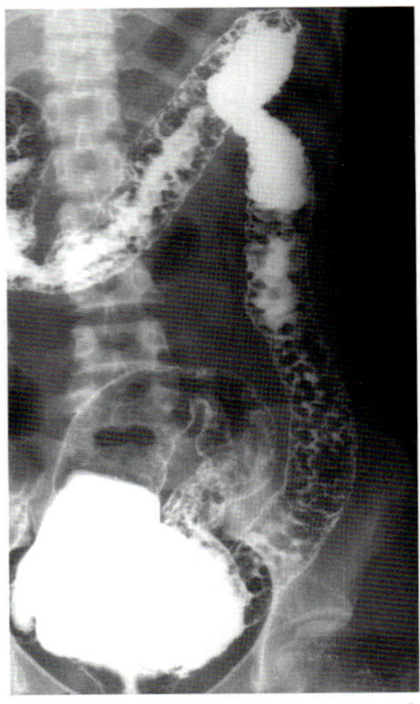

Fig. 8.22: Cobblestone appearance of colon

Table 8.2	Aphthoid ulcers
	• Crohn's disease • Tuberculosis • Yersinia • Amebiasis • Behcet's syndrome

Table 8.3	Cobblestone pattern
	• Crohn's disease • Ischemic bowel disease • Tuberculosis • Amebiasis • Salmonellosis

of barium parallel to the lumen of bowel loop (Fig. 8.23). In advanced CD, transmural ulcerations may lead to the development of fissures, sinus tracts, fistulae and abscess. In the chronic phase, CD is associated with transmural fibrosis with the development of strictures (Fig. 8.24).[2]

CT findings in Crohn's colitis include wall thickening which is eccentric, segmental and measures 10-20 mm (Fig. 8.25). It shows homogenous enhancement after IV contrast.[14] Ultrasound shows marked thickening of wall, presence of deep ulcers and serosal involvement with evidence of hypertrophic fat. In chronic stage there is loss of mural stratification due to fibrosis.[2-5] CT and MR colonoscopic findings are comparable to that of conventional colonoscopy.

Complications of IBD

Toxic megacolon, a potentially fatal complication is seen in less than 5% of patients and is characterized by both non-obstructive dilatation of the colon to more than 6 cm and evidence of systemic toxicity (Fig. 8.26).[29] This dilatation is most commonly observed in the transverse colon which has led to an erroneous impression that the process is specific of the transverse colon. In fact, the entire colon is involved, but the distribution of gas in the transverse colon is a result of anatomy and gravity since the plain X-ray abdomen is taken in supine position. Concomitant distension of the small bowel and less frequently, the stomach has also been reported. The pathogenesis of colonic and GI distension in severe colitis

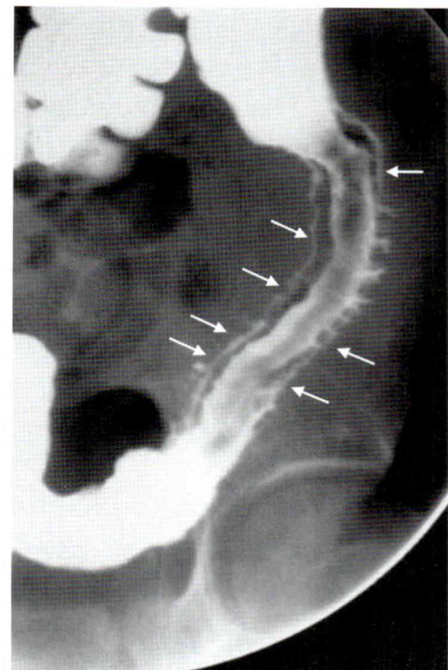

Fig. 8.23: Deep ulcers with double tracking of sigmoid colon (arrows)

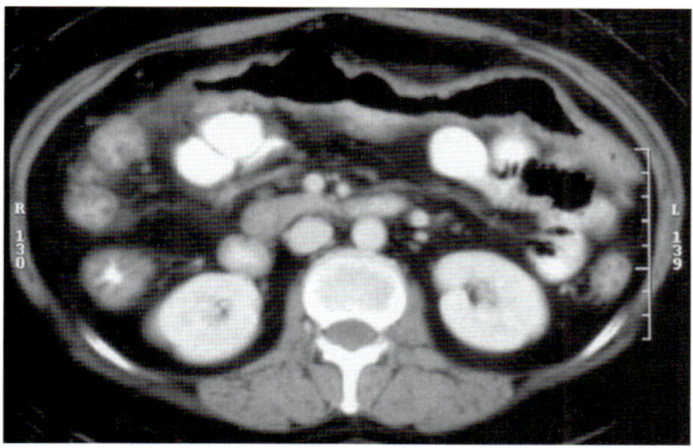

Fig. 8.24: CECT showing asymmetric mural thickening of transverse colon

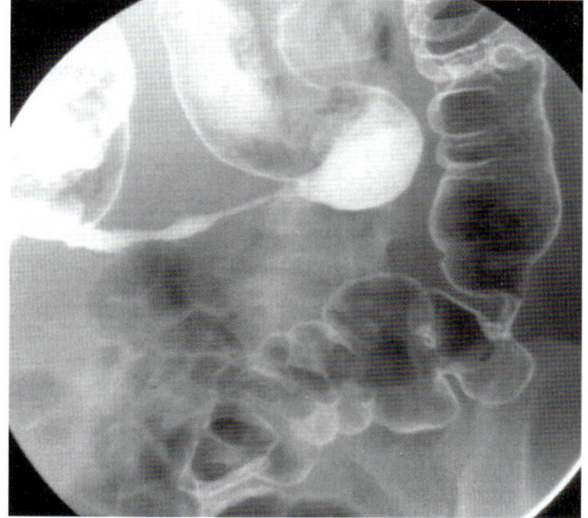

Fig. 8.25: DCBE showing strictures in descending and transverse colon

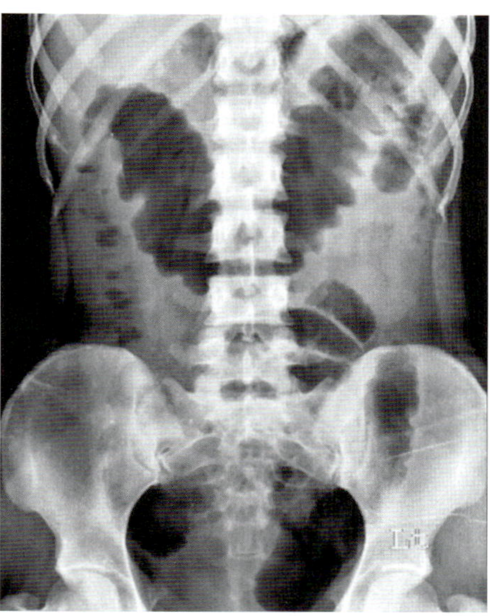

Fig. 8.26: Dilated transverse colon with thickened edematous bowel wall (toxic mega colon)

is still unclear. It seems to result from a combination of several factors such as increased release of soluble inflammatory mediators enhancing nitric oxide generation and activation of nerve endings of mucosal afferent fibres. Nitric oxide generation leads to muscle relaxation and colonic dilatation, whereas the activation of sensory fibres elicit inhibitory reflexes leading to distension of stomach and small bowel. While toxic megacolon is most frequently associated with ulcerative colitis, it can be seen in other conditions also (Table 8.4). Abscesses and fistula are detected almost exclusively in CD and not in UC. Imaging modalities can be used to diagnose these complications and for percutaneous drainage of these abscesses. Ulcerative colitis and Crohn's disease are associated with an increased colorectal cancer risk depending on the duration and extent of disease (more common in UC than CD).[29] Carcinoma complicating UC is seen as asymmetrical mural thickening, focal loss of mural stratification and mural thickening of more than 15 mm on CT. CT is also helpful in detecting and staging tumor.

Table 8.4	Toxic megacolon
	• Ulcerative colitis • Crohn's disease • Ischemic colitis • Amebic colitis • Typhoid fever • Pseudomembranous colitis

Extra Intestinal Complications

- Hepatobiliary — Fatty liver, sclerosing, cholangitis, cholangiocarcinoma, chronic active hepatitis
- Musculoskeletal — Arthritis, sacroilitis, osteoporosis, ankylosing spondylitis
- Ocular — Iritis, uveitis, conjunctivitis, etc.
- Dermatologic — Erythema nodosum, vitiligo, dermatitis
- Hematologic — Anemia, thromboembolic disease, etc.
- Renal disease — Urolithiasis, pyelonephritis
- Cardiovascular — Endocarditis, myocarditis, cardiomyopathy, vasculitis
- Pulmonary — Bronchitis, bronchiectasis, pulmonary embolism, etc.

Ulcerative Colitis vs Crohn's Disease

It is important to distinguish UC from CD as the complications, management and prognosis of these two diseases differ (Table 8.5). It is also important to differentiate Crohn's disease from tuberculosis because these two diseases closely resemble each other in their clinical presentations. Histopathological examinations are inconclusive in majority causing a great diagnostic dilemma. In such confusing situations radiological differentiation between tuberculosis and Crohn's disease is possible in majority of cases.

Table 8.5 Radiological features of ulcerative colitis and Crohn's disease

Radiological findings	*Ulcerative colitis*	*Crohns disease*
• Site of involvement	Colon (rectum)	Any part of GI tract
• Extent of involvement	Diffuse	Segmental (skip lesions)
• Small bowel involvement	Backwash ileitis	Common
Barium Examination		
• Mucosal pattern	Granular	Smooth
• Polyps	Frequent	Infrequent
• Cobblestoning	Infrequent	Frequent
• Thumb printing	Infrequent	Infrequent
• Perforation and fistulae	Rare	Extremely common
• Malignant change	High risk	Low risk
Ultrasound		
• Wall thickness	Moderate	Marked
• Wall echogenicity	Hypoechoic	Hypoechoic
• Anatomic five layers	Well preserved	Completely lost
Computed Tomography		
• Mural stratification	Present	Present (acute phase) Absent (chronic phase)
• Wall thickness	Moderate	Marked
• Wall attenuation	Inhomogeneous	Homogeneous (chronic phase)
• Mesenteric involvement	Not seen	Hypervascularity Fibrofatty proliferation

Crohn's Disease Vs Tuberculosis

Distribution of Disease

The most common location of intestinal tuberculosis is ileo-caecal region seen in 80-90% of cases followed by small bowel and colon.[30-31] Isolated involvement of ileo-caecal region is extremely uncommon in Crohn's disease though ileo-caecal area may be involved in direct contiguity with terminal ileum and colon.[32]

Barium Findings

Finding	*Intestinal Tuberculosis*	*Crohn's Disease*
Stricture	Short, concentric and smooth in outline with significant prestenotic dilatation **[Most Common]**	Strictures eccentric **[Asymmetric involvement]** with sacculations at anti-mesentric border without significant prestenotic dilatation
Ulcers	Longitudinally oriented—larger than Crohn's disease. Tend to be round to oval	**Aphthous** with thickened folds (Ulceronodular pattern **Segmental colitis.**
Complications	**Enteroliths-common** Perforation, Fistulae-rare Carcinoma- not seen	Enteroliths- rare **Perforation, Fistulae and Carcinoma - common**

CT Findings

Intestinal Tuberculosis	*Crohn's Disease*
Mural thickening without stratification	**Mural thickening with stratification in active inflammation**
Strictures concentric	Strictures eccentric
Fibrofatty proliferation of mesentery very rare	**Fibrofatty proliferation of mesentery**
Mesenteric inflammation but no vascular engorgement	Hypervascular mesentery (comb sign)
Hypodense lymph nodes with peripheral enhancement	Mild lymphadenopathy
High density ascites	**Abscesses**

OTHER INFLAMMATORY BOWEL DISEASES

Ischemic Bowel Disease

Mesenteric ischemia is a complicated disorder that occurs when blood flow to the intestine is compromised. Mesenteric ischemia can occur as a result of arterial occlusion, venous occlusion or low flow states. Mesenteric ischemia may be acute or chronic depending on the onset and clinical presentation. Acute mesenteric ischemia may be caused by either arterial or venous occlusion, although arterial occlusion is far more common. Thromboembolic arterial occlusion is the most common cause of acute mesenteric ischemia. Non-occlusive mesenteric ischemia is also acute ischemia and is usually segmental involving the splenic flexure or the sigmoid colon representing the "watershed" zones. Most cases of colonic ischemia occur as a result of sudden drop in blood flow because of low flow states. Chronic mesenteric ischemia results from atherosclerosis of the mesenteric arteries. The location of ischemic lesion varies with the site of occlusion. The radiological approach is tailored to the individual patient.[33, 34]

Duplex doppler sonography has been used as a preferred non-invasive modality for evaluation of stenosis of mesenteric arteries. Superior mesenteric artery (SMA) peak systolic velocity of 275 cm/sec or no flow signals are reliable indicators of 70% or greater stenosis.[33]

The important role of CT is to detect ischemic changes in the affected bowel loops and mesentery and to determine the cause of ischemia by allowing evaluation of the mesenteric vasculature.[33-36] Negative oral contrast agents with rapid intravenous administration of contrast make it possible to quantify small changes in bowel enhancement with 3D CT angiography. CT perfusion scanning is able to detect early changes in perfusion in ischemic segments before irreversible damage has occurred. The CT findings typically differ in patients with acute versus chronic ischemia.

MRI is comparable to CT for demonstrating bowel wall changes and the mesenteric vascular abnormalities. Both arterial and venous abnormalities can be seen. Intraluminal thrombus and collateral vessels can be readily identified. Additional abnormal findings consist of bowel wall thickening and increase in signal intensity from compromised bowel on T2W1. Vascular visualization is markedly improved by contrast enhanced MR angiography.[33]

Digital subtraction angiography remains the most accurate modality to evaluate the degree of stenosis. The diagnostic sensitivity of angiography is very high in assessing arterial occlusion.[34] It allows not only diagnosis but also interventional therapy. Percutaneous transluminal angioplasty with or without stent placement can be done.[37] Although angiography is considered the gold standard for diagnosing thromboembolism, it is an invasive and time consuming procedure.

In patients with acute ischemia, the most common CT finding is circumferential thickening of the bowel wall. The bowel wall may demonstrate low attenuation reflecting submucosal edema and inflammation; or high attenuation due to submucosal hemorrhage. It can appear homogeneous or may have a "halo" appearance. After the intravenous administration of contrast material affected loops may demonstrate decreased enhancement compared with normal loops due to compromised blood flow. In some patients, the affected loops may demonstrate increased enhancement due to hyperemia. In cases of infarction, pneumatosis may be present, signifying irreversible disease (Fig. 8.27). Pneumatosis with or without air in the mesenteric vessels or portal vein in an ominous finding in patients and suggests necrosis. CT is more sensitive than plain radiography in detection of pneumatosis and sometimes allows identification of the cause. Most cases of transient colonic ischemia due to hypovolemia are treated conservatively. The colon gradually returns to normal. However, some patients go on to develop scarring and stricture in the involved segment.

In addition to bowel wall thickening, ischemic small bowel may demonstrate luminal dilatation and mesenteric stranding. Inflammatory changes in the pericolic fat may also be present. In patients with acute mesenteric ischemia,

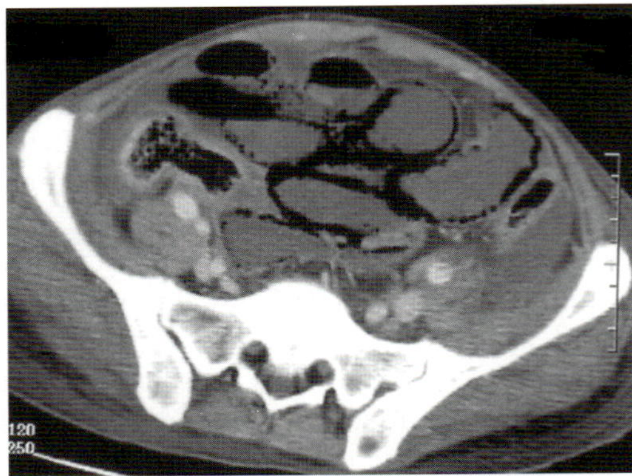

Fig. 8.27: CECT showing intra mural air in small bowel loops

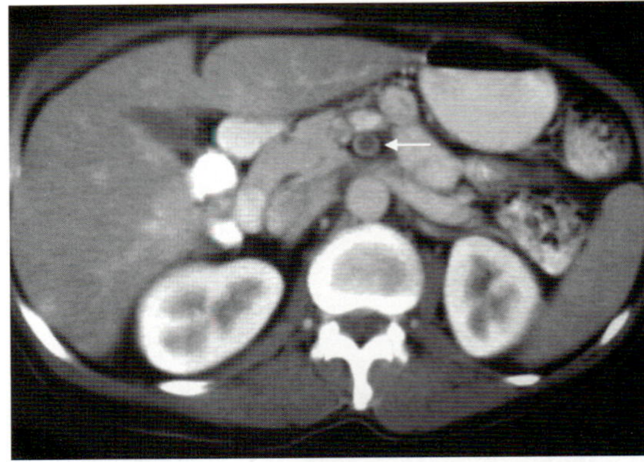

Fig. 8.28: CECT showing a thrombus in the superior mesenteric artery (arrow)

the portion of the intestine affected depends on the cause of the ischemia and the availability of collateral vessels. If a major artery or vein is compromised the entire mesenteric small bowel (i. e., the jejunum and ileum) may be involved as well as the right and transverse colon. In addition, multi-detector row CT with 3D reformatting can evaluate the mesenteric vessels in patients with acute mesenteric ischemia (Figs 8.28 and 8.29). In low-flow states causing mesenteric ischemia the mesenteric arteries may appear narrowed with limited opacification of branches due to hypovolemia and spasm. CT shows diffuse thickening of bowel wall with or without mucosal enhancement and increased intraluminal fluid (Fig. 8.30).

In contrast to acute ischemia, most cases of chronic mesenteric ischemia result from atherosclerosis of the mesenteric arteries. Patients with chronic mesenteric ischemia will typically develop collateral pathways in an effort to keep the intestine adequately perfused. CT can detect calcified plaque in the aorta and mesenteric arteries. Unlike in patients with acute mesenteric ischemia, the small intestine usually appears normal in patients with chronic mesenteric ischemia.

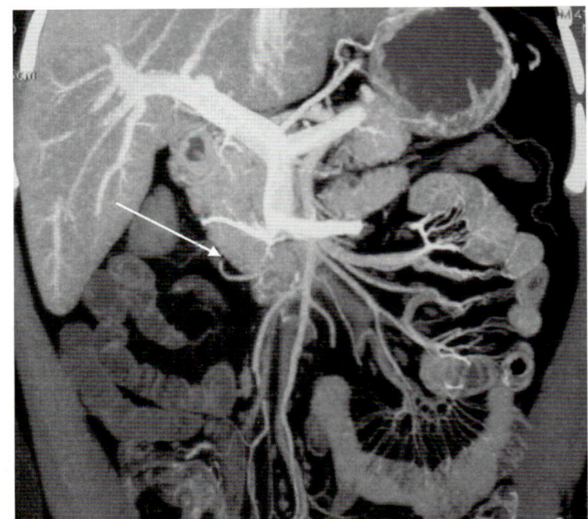

Fig. 8.29: CT angiography showing occlusion of superior mesenteric vein

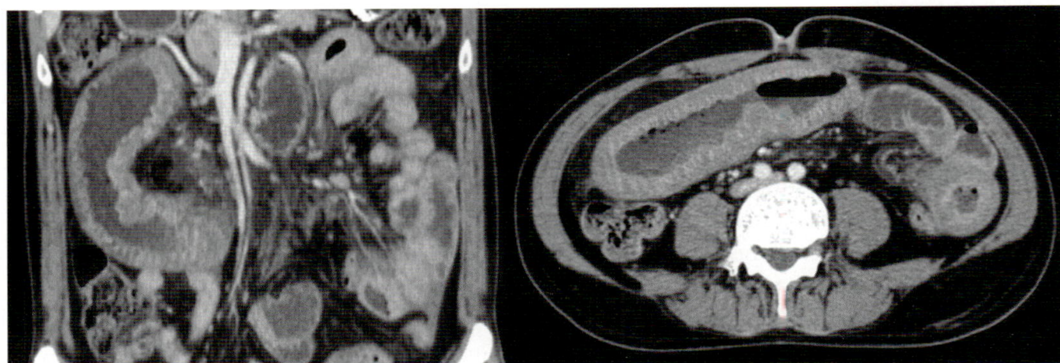

Fig. 8.30: Diffuse thickening of bowel wall with mural enhancement. CT angiographic image showing normal opacification of SMA and SMV

Barium studies should not be performed in cases of suspected acute mesenteric ischemia. In clinically unsuspected cases, barium findings include bowel dilatation, thumb printing, thickened folds, sub-mucosal edema and ulceration. There is uniform regular thickening of small bowel folds which produce a symmetric spike-like configuration simulating a 'stack of coins' or 'picket fence' (Fig. 8. 31).[38] In chronic cases, there may be formation of strictures which are usually smooth in outline (Fig. 8.32).

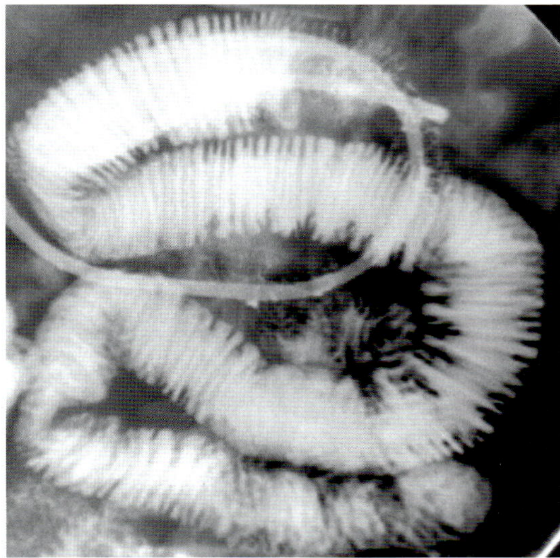

Fig. 8.31: Barium enteroclysis showing regular thickening of small bowel folds

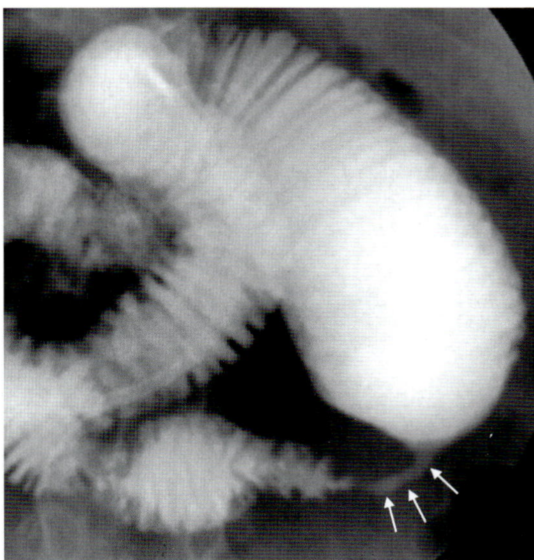

Fig. 8.32: A short smooth stricture with proximal dilatation seen in jejunum (arrows)

Appendicitis

Acute appendicitis occurs when the appendiceal lumen becomes occluded, resulting in an accumulation of fluid, appendiceal dilatation, inflammation, ischemia, and eventually perforation with possible abscess formation. Accuracy rates of spiral CT for diagnosis of appendicitis are as high as 98% .[14, 39] In acute appendicitis, appendix appears dilated (>6 mm in diameter) and unopacified with a thickened wall that homogeneously enhance after administration of intravenous contrast material. The appendix may be filled with fluid or debris. An appendicolith is detected in up to 25-40% of cases. The presence of an appendicolith along with pericecal inflammation or a mass is considered diagnostic for appendicitis. Changes in the adjacent cecum such as focal cecal apical thickening, the "arrowhead sign", or a cecal bar may be present and may help confirm the diagnosis. Focal cecal apical thickening occurs when appendiceal inflammation spreads contiguously to involve the cecal tip. The "arrowhead sign" is also caused by contiguous spread of inflammation from the appendix to the cecum, resulting in a triangular space between the thickened walls of the appendix. A cecal bar occurs when a curved soft-tissue bar is interposed between the cecal lumen and appendicolith. A hallmark of acute appendicitis is a varying degree of inflammatory thickening in the fat surrounding the diseased appendix with stranding of the pericecal fat. Perforation is a potential complication of appendicitis and appears as small pockets of extraluminal air. An appendiceal abscess appears as a pericecal fluid collection that may contain air or necrotic debris.

Compression-grade ultrasonography (US) a reliable technique for diagnosis of acute appendicitis, especially in children and thin adults.[39] On ultrasound inflamed appendix appears as a dilated (more than 6 mm), blind ending tubular structure which is seen in relation to the cecum and is noncompressible (Fig. 8.33). Periappendiceal fluid and increased vascularity of appendix are other supportive evidences in diagnosis of appendicitis. The presence of hyperemia in the appendiceal wall is a sensitive indicator of inflammation and can be well demonstrated on color Doppler (Fig. 8.34).

Epiploic Appendagitis

Epiploic appendagitis is a rare inflammatory and ischemic condition that results from torsion or spontaneous venous thrombosis of one of the appendices epiploicae. At CT, a

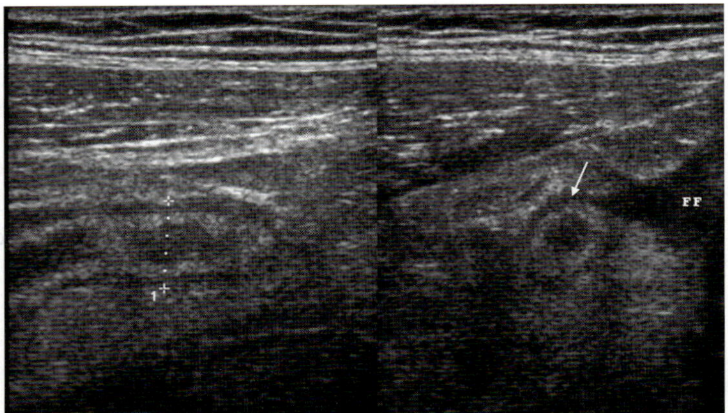

Fig. 8.33: High resolution sonography showing dilated tubular appendix (calipers and arrow) with peri appendiceal fluid collection (FF)

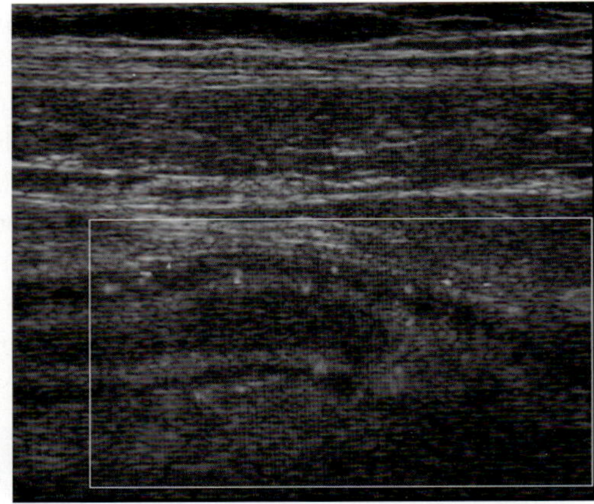

Fig. 8.34: Color Doppler showing increased vascularity in wall of appendix *(For color version see plate 1)*

1-4 cm, oval fatty pericolic lesion with surrounding mesenteric inflammation is considered to be diagnostic of epiploic appendagitis (Fig. 8.35). Rarely, a central high-attenuation "dot" can be identified within the inflamed appendage: this finding corresponds to the thrombosed vein. The CT appearance of epiploic appendagitis cannot be reliably distinguished from that of omental infarction.[14,39]

Diverticulitis

Acute diverticulitis occurs when the neck of a diverticulum is occluded by stool, inflammation or food particles, resulting in a microperforation of the diverticulum and surrounding pericolic inflammation. CT is well suited for evaluation of diverticular disease because it is able to demonstrate the wall of the colon as well as the surrounding pericolic fat.[14,39]

At CT, diverticulitis appears as segmental wall thickening and hyperemia with inflammatory changes in the pericolic fat. The key to distinguishing diverticulitis from other inflammatory conditions that affect the colon is the presence of diverticula in the involved segment. Also, diverticulitis typically occurs in the descending or sigmoid colon. CT allows detection of complications of diverticulitis such as diverticular abscess, colovesical fistula and perforation and is more sensitive than contrast enema examination. The CT staging system for diverticulitis has been proposed for the purpose of management (Fig. 8.36).[40] When an abscess is detected, CT can provide guidance for percutaneous drainage, which can eliminate the need for emergent surgery. One potential pitfall of diagnosis of diverticulitis with CT is overlapping imaging findings in diverticulitis and colon cancer. The presence of fluid in the

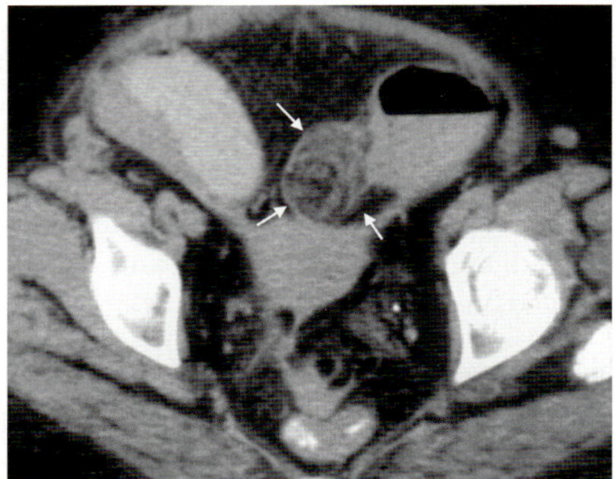

Fig. 8.35: A well defined mass lesion with specks of fat seen in peri-colonic area (arrows)

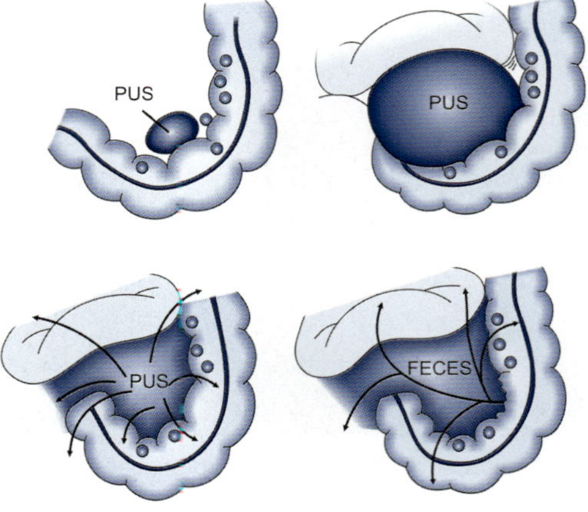

Fig. 8.36: CT staging system of diverticulitis

root of the sigmoid mesentery and engorgement of adjacent sigmoid mesenteric vasculature favours the diagnosis of diverticulitis. Conversely, the presence of pericolic lymph nodes suggests the diagnosis of colon cancer rather than diverticulitis. However, in some cases it may not be possible to distinguish diverticulitis from colon cancer with CT alone and histologic samples will be required.

Radiation Colitis

Patients receiving more than 3, 000cGy of radiation therapy to the pelvis experience acute proctitis. Acute radiation injury to the small intestine and colon occurs during or within a few weeks of radiation exposure. Imaging is typically not necessary for diagnosis. If CT is performed during the acute phase of radiation injury, nonspecific wall thickening and inflammatory stranding will be demonstrated in the affected region.

Chronic radiation injury leads to a variety of complications with most patients presenting 6-24 months after completion of radiation therapy. Such injury is the result of radiation-induced endarteritis. The sigmoid colon and rectum are the most commonly affected because radiation therapy is often given for pelvic disease. Barium exam is an excellent method to evaluate the site and extent of involvement, even though the findings are non-specific. These are in the form of thickened mucosal folds, ulcers, strictures, sinuses and fistulae (Fig 8.37). CT findings include nonspecific wall thickening, increased pelvic fat and thickening of the perirectal fibrous tissue.[14] The clinical history is the key to suggesting the diagnosis because the CT findings can be nonspecific.

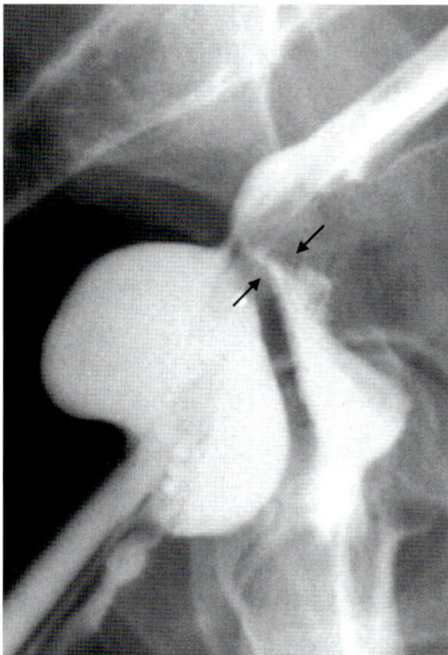

Fig. 8.37: Barium enema showing a stricture in proximal rectum with recto vesical fistula (arrows)

Pseudomembranous Colitis

Pseudomembranous colitis results from toxins produced by an overgrowth of the organism *Clostridium difficile*. Barium enema examination is contraindicated in severely ill patients. In mild cases, a low pressure barium enema may be performed which shows pseudomembranes as elevated plaques. Radiologists should be familiar with the CT findings because the diagnosis may not be suspected clinically. [14] The most common CT finding is thickening of the colonic wall, which may be circumferential or eccentric. The colonic wall thickness ranges from 3-32 mm (mean, 14. 7mm). Amount of bowel wall thickening in pseudomembranous colitis is greater than in any other inflammatory or infectious disease of the colon except Crohns disease; this is a helpful differential point. The wall thickening in pseudomembranous colitis is often more irregular and shaggy than in Crohns disease, bowel wall may have low attenuation due to edema or may enhance significantly after intravenous administration of contrast material secondary to hyperemia. In addition to wall thickening the colon is often dilated, probably due to the transmural inflammation. Mild pericolic stranding may also be present. The pericolic stranding in pseudomembranous colitis is often disproportionately mild relative to the marked colonic wall thickening, since the condition predominantly affects the mucosa and submucosa. The target sign originally described in ulcerative colitis and Crohns disease, has also been reported in pseudomembranous colitis. When haustral folds are significantly thickened, they can appear as broad transverse bands that may trap oral contrast material. This appearance is known as the "accordion sign". The accordion sign is very suggestive of pseudomembranous colitis but typically occurs only in severe cases and is therefore not a sensitive indicator.[39] In its classic form, pseudomembranous colitis is a pancolitis. Ascites has been reported in upto 35% of patients with pseudomembranous colitis. Thus ascites may be another helpful differentiating point between pseudomembranous colitis and Crohns disease.

Amebic Colitis

Entameba histolytica is a simple protozoan which invades the mucosa and causes cell destruction. The cecum is involved in 70-90% of cases. The radiological findings in amebiasis are as varied as its clinical presentation. Barium examination may show collar button ulcers, cobblestoning pattern or thumb printing (Fig.8.38). Concentric narrowing resulting in coned cecum with shaggy contour may be seen with disease progression. The direct extension through bowel wall due to extrinsic bowel necrosis results in a large mass called ameboma. Fulminant amebic colitis may rarely lead to toxic megacolon and perforation. CT exam may show edematous bowel wall thickening, polypoidal ameboma masses and liver abscesses (Fig. 8.39).[39]

Typhilitis

Typhilitis formerly known as neutropenic enterocolitis or as the ileocecal syndrome is now referred to as neutropenic typhilitis. It is characterized by edema and inflammation of cecum, ascending colon and rarely the terminal ileum. CT findings in typhilitis include bowel wall thickening with adjacent fat stranding and areas of low attenuation due to edema and necrosis, pneumatosis and pericolonic fluid (Fig. 8.40).[14]

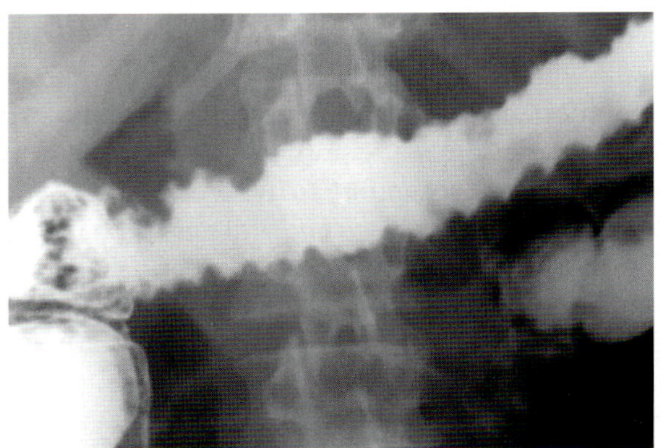

Fig. 8.38: Barium enema showing mucosal edema and loss of haustrations

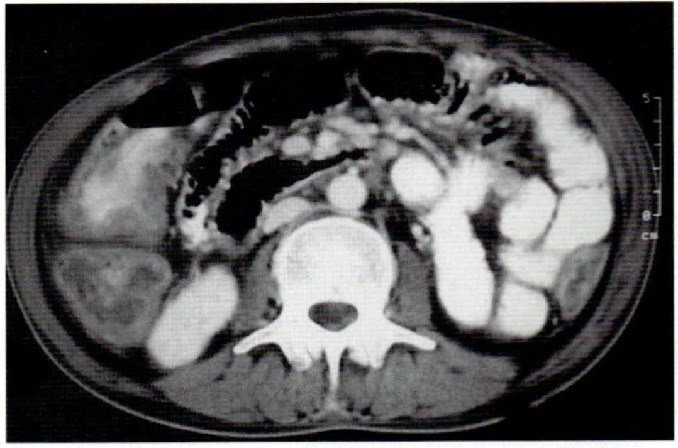

Fig. 8.40: Mural thickening of cecum and ascending colon with mild peri-colonic soft tissue stranding

Celiac disease

Celiac disease is a gluten-sensitive malabsorption syndrome. Barium and MR enteroclysis in the majority of patients may provide positive evidence for the diagnosis or exclusion of celiac disease.[41] With lumen distension, mucosal folds are well delineated. Five folds or more per inch in jejunum and two to four folds per inch in ileum are described as normal. A decrease in number of jejunal folds and an increase in number of ileal folds (Jejuno-ileal fold pattern reversal) is a striking and common feature seen in celiac disease (Fig. 8 41). Increased number of ileal folds represents a compensatory response to prolonged villous

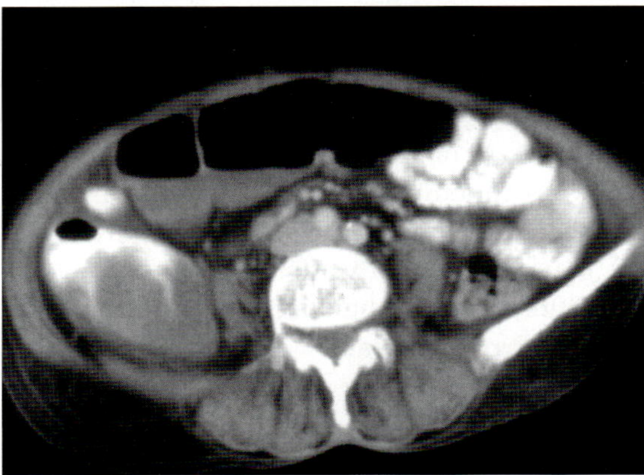

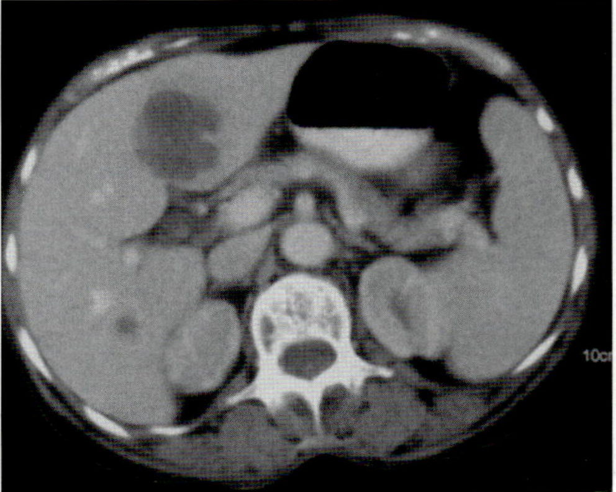

Fig. 8.39: CECT showing a polypoidal mass in cecum with liver abscesses

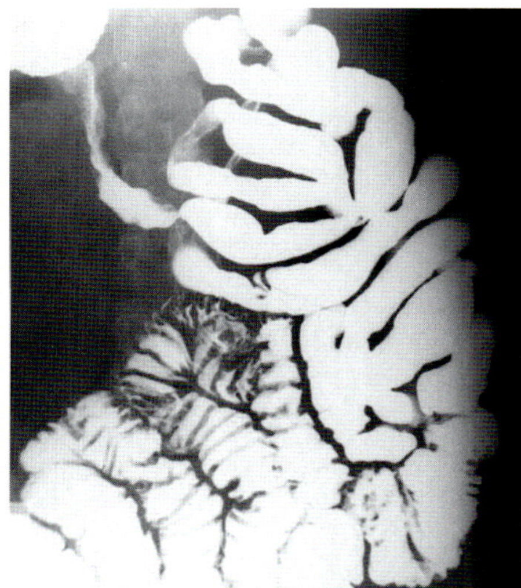

Fig. 8.41: Barium examination showing reversal of fold pattern

atrophy in proximal jejunum. If there is any alteration in the clinical condition, while still on gluten-free diet, enteroclysis may reveal mucosal irregularity with nodular fold thickening or a narrowed segment suggestive of lymphoma complicating celiac disease. The value of enteroclysis has been further extended to the management outcome of these patients by observing the return of normal number of jejunal folds after successful therapy and persistence of fold separation in refractory celiac disease.

Doppler measurement of resistive index differences of SMA in fasting and postprandial state can be an effective way to express severity of celiac disease and to document its regression after diet therapy.[42] CT examination may show dilatation of bowel loops with increased intraluminal fluid and mild adenopathy in mesentery and retroperitoneum.[43]

Eosinophilic Enteritis

Eosinophilic enteritis is characterized by eosinophilic infiltration of wall of small bowel with marked peripheral eosinophilia. Barium examination shows thickened and distorted folds in the proximal small bowel (Fig. 8.42). CT scan also shows thickening and nodularity of folds.[43]

Amyloidosis

Small bowel is involved in more than 70% of cases of generalized amyloidosis. Amyloid is deposited in submucosa around blood vessels or in muscular layer of bowel wall. Barium examination shows diffuse fold thickening with nodularity throughout the entire small bowel. Thickening of folds in ileum has been described as "jejunization" of ileum (Fig. 8.43). Enteroclysis shows 3-4 mm mucosal nodules with fold irregularity. CT findings are non-specific and show diffuse wall thickening. Mild adenopathy may be present.[43]

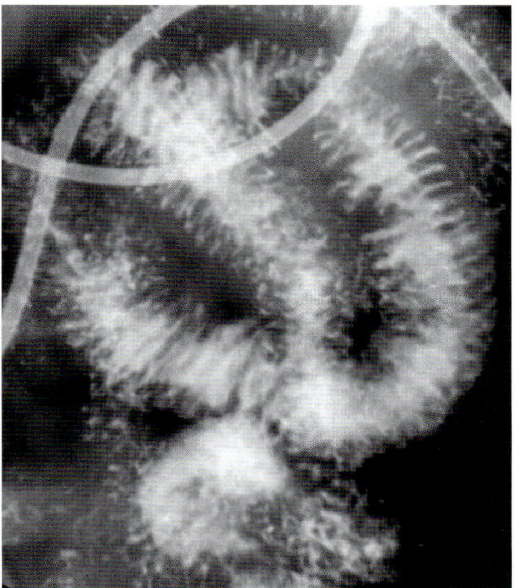

Fig. 8.42: Barium enteroclysis showing thickened distorted folds of jejunum

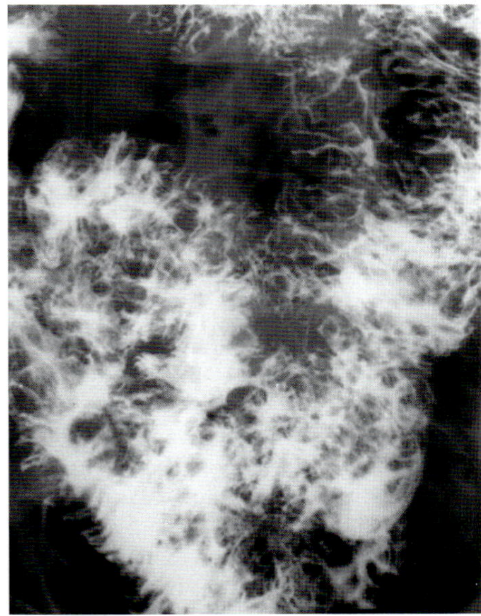

Fig. 8.43: Gross thickening of ileal folds (jejunization) with nodular filling defects

REFERENCES

1. Herlinger H, Caroline DF. Crohn's disease of the small bowel. In: Gore RM, Levine MS, Textbook of gastrointestinal radiology. Philadelphia: Saunders, 2000; 2:726-45.
2. Carucci LR, Levine MS. Radiographic imaging of inflammatory bowel disease. Gastroenterol Clin N Am 2002;31:93-117.
3. Horsthuis K, Stokkers CF, Stoker J. Detection of inflammatory bowel disease: diagnostic performance of cross-sectional imaging modalities. Abdom imaging 2008;33:407-16.
4. Meisner RS, Spier BJ, Einarsson S et al. Pilot study using PET/CT as a novel, noninvasive assessment of disease activity in inflammatory bowel disease. Inflamm Bowel Dis. 2007;13:993-1000.
5. Mackalski BA, Bernstein CN. New diagnostic imaging tools for inflammatory bowel disease, Gut 2006;55: 733-41.
6. Ambrosini R, Barchiesi A, Mizio VD et al. Inflammatory chronic disease of the colon: how to image. European Journal of Radiology, 2007;61:442-48.
7. Gore RM. CT of inflammatory bowel disease. Radiol Clin North Am 1989;27:717-23.
8. Carrascosa P, Castiglioni R, Capunay C et al. CT Colonoscopy in inflammatory bowel disease. Abdom Imaging: 2007;32:596-601.
9. Wong SH, Wong, VWS, Sung JJY. Virtual colonoscopy-induced perforation in a patient with Crohn's disease. World J Gastroenterol 2007; 13: 978-79.
10. Schreyer AG, Scheibi K, Heiss P et al. MR colonography in inflammatory bowel disease. Abdom Imaging 2006;31:302-07.
11. Valelette PJ, Rioux M, Pillentl F et al. Ultrasonography of chronic inflammatory disease. Eur Radiol 2001;11: 1859-66.
12. Limberg B and Osswald B. Diagnosis and differential diagnosis of ulcerative colitis and Crohn's disease by hydrocolonic sonography. Am J Gastroenterol 1994;89:1051-57.
13. Long Sun, Hua Wu, Yong-Song Guan. Colonography by CT, MRI and PET/CT combined with conventional colonoscopy in colorectal cancer screening and staging, World J Gastroenterol 2008;14:853-63.
14. Horton KM, Corl FM, Fishman KE. CT evaluation of the colon: inflammatory disease. Radiographics 2000;20: 399-418.
15. Gore MR, Balthazar JF, Ghahremani GF et al. AJR 1996;167:3-15.
16. Maglinte DD, Gourtsoyiannis N, Rex D et al. Classification of small bowel Crohn's subtypes based on multimodality imaging. Radiol Clin North Am. 2003;41:285-303.
17. Kale DB, Joet GF, Craing A et al. Crohns Disease. Mural attenuation and thickness at contrast enhanced CT enterography - correlation with endoscopic and histologic findings of Inflammation. Radiology 2006;238:505-16.
18. Maglinte DT, Kumaresan S, John C L. CT Enteroclysis: Techniques and Applications. Radiol Clin North Am 2007;45:289-301.
19. Saibeni S. , Rondonotti E, Iozzelli A et al. Imaging of the small bowel in Crohn's disease: A review of old and new techniques. World J Gastroenterol 2007;13:3279-87.
20. Furukawa A, Saotome T, Yamasaki M et al. Cross sectional imaging in Crohn's disease. Radiographics 2003;24: 689-702.
21. Meyers MA, McGuire PV. Spiral CT demonstration of hypervascularity in Crohn's disease. Vascular jejunization in Crohn's disease or the comb sign. Abdom Imaging. 1995;20:327-32.
22. Hara AK, Alam S, Heigh RI et al. Using CT enterography to monitor Crohn's disease activity: a preliminary study, AJR 2008;190: 1512-16.
23. Wiarda BM, Kuipers EJ, Heitbrink MA et al. MR enteroclysis of inflammatory small bowel disease. AJR 2006;187:522-31.
24. Florie J, Wasser NNJM, Cieslik KA et al. Dynamic contrast enhanced MRI of the bowel wall for assessment of disease activity in Crohn's disease. AJR 2006;186:1384-92
25. Franceasco G, Daniele D, Piatro Vernia. Doppler Sonography of the Superior Mesenteric Artery in Crohn's Disease. AJR 1998;170:123-26.
26. Sjekavica I, Babic VB, Krznaric Z et al. Assessment of Crohn's disease activity by Doppler ultrasound of mesenteric artery and mural arteries in thickened bowel cross sectional study. Croat Med J 2007;48:822-30.
27. Maconi G, Parente F, Bianchi PG. Hydrogen peroxide enhanced ultrasound- fistulography in the assessment of enterocutaneous fistulas complicating Crohns disease. Gut 1999;45:1-6.
28. Das CJ, Makharia G, Kumar R et al. PET-CT enteroclysis: a new technique for evaluation of inflammatory diseases of the intestine. Eur J Nucl Med Mol Imaging 2007;34: 2106-14.
29. Roggeveen MJ, Tismennetsky M and Shapiro R. Ulcerative colitis. Radiographics 2006;26:947-51.
30. Gilinsky NH, Marks IN, Kotler RE, Price SK. Abdominal tuberculosis: a 10 year review. S Afr Med J 1983;64:849-57.
31. Ludstedt C, Nyman R, Brismar J, et al. Imaging of tuberculosis II. Abdominal manifestations in 112 patients. Acta Radiol 1996;37:489-595.
32. Werbeloff L, Novis BH, Bank S, etal. The radiology of tuberculosis of gastrointestinal tract. Br J Radiol 1973;46:329-36.
33. Kim YA and Ha KH. Evaluation of suspected mesenteric ischemia: efficacy of radiologic studies. Radiol Clin N Am 2003;41:327-42
34. Wolf EL, Sprayregen S, Bakal CW. Radiology in Intestinal Ischemia, surgical clinics of North America, 1992;72: 107-24.
35. Horton KM, Fishman EK. Multi-detector row CT of mesenteric ischemia: can it be done? Radiographics 2001;21:1463-73.
36. Horton KM, Fishman EK. Multidetector CT angiography in the diagnosis of mesenteric ischemia. Radiol Clin North Am. 2007;45:275-88.

37. Schaefer PJ, Schaefer FKW, Huelsbeck SM et al. Chronic mesenteric ischemia: stenting of mesenteric arteries. Abdom Imaging 2007;32:304-09.
38. Nolan DJ, Herlinger H. Vascular disorders. In: Gore RM, Levine MS, Textbook of gastrointestinal radiology. 1st Ed Philadelphia: Saunders, 1994;967-73.
39. Thoeni RF and Cello PI. CT imaging of colitis. Radiology 2006;240:623-38
40. Neff CC, vanSonnenberg E. CT of diverticulitis. Radiol Clin North Am 1989;27:743-52.
41. Barlow JM, Johnson CD, Stephens DH. Celiac disease: How common is jejunoileal fold pattern reversal found at small bowel follow through? AJR 1996;166:575-77.
42. Giovagnorio F, Picarelli A, Di Giovambattista F et al. Evaluation with Doppler sonography of mesenteric blood flow in celiac disease. AJR 1998;171:629-32.
43. Horton KM, Fishman EK. Uncommon inflammatory disease of the small bowel: CT findings. AJR 1998; 170: 385-88.

Chapter Nine

Colorectal Malignancies

Naveen Kalra, Mandeep Kang

Epidemiology

Colorectal cancer is the third most common cancer overall in both men and women and the second leading cause of cancer deaths following lung cancer.[1] In women it is the third most common cancer after lung and breast cancer while in men it is the third most common cancer after lung and prostate cancer. [2] The distribution of colon cancer varies widely throughout the globe. While the incidence is high in North America, Europe and New Zealand, it is low in South America, Africa and Asia.[3] The reported incidence of colon cancer from eight population registries in India is 0.7-3.7/100,000 in men and 0.4-3/100,000 in women with a higher incidence of rectal cancer(1.6-5.5/ 100,000 in men, 0-2.8/100,000 in women).[4] In general colon cancer is more common in economically affluent populations exhibiting Western lifestyle practices like high intake of dietary fat, low intake of dietary fiber and sedentary life style.[5] Only 5.4% of colorectal cancers occur in patients younger than 40 years.[5] The incidence of colorectal cancer rises after the age of 40 years with 90% of these cancers occurring in persons older than 50 years.[6] The reported median age at the time of diagnosis of colon and rectal cancer is 71 and 69 years respectively. Approximately one half of the colon cancers occur in the rectum and sigmoid colon and can be detected by the flexible sigmoidoscope.[7] It has been observed that there has been an increase in right-sided lesions as opposed to the left-sided lesions. More distal lesions are found in men than in women.

Risk Factors

There are numerous risk factors which predispose to the development of colorectal cancer. These include dietary factors, hereditary factors, inflammatory bowel disease and other miscellaneous causes.

High calorie, low fiber diet rich in animal fats, primarily beef is an important risk factor for the colon carcinogenesis. Excess intake of fat increases the level of fatty acids and free bile acids in the feces which irritates the colonic mucosa and causes epithelial reparative proliferation.[8] High fiber decreases exposure to the carcinogens by decreasing the fecal transit time. It also decreases the bacterial mediated conversion of primary to secondary bile acids by lowering the pH of the stool.[9]

There is an inverse relationship between the dietary intake of calcium and ingestion of antioxidants like vitamins A, C, E, selenium and colon cancer.[10] On the other hand there is a direct relationship between heavy alcohol consumption, smoking, hypergastrinemia in pernicious anemia patients, increased growth hormone level in patients with acromegaly and increased parathyroid hormone in patients with parathyroid adenomas, and the incidence of colorectal malignancy.

Prior cholecystectomy may increase the risk of developing right-sided colon cancer in women by 1.5 times.[11] This is due to the deposition of potential carcinogens like bile salts and neutral sterols while the distal colon is spared on account of their absorption in the proximal colon into the enterohepatic circulation.

Prior ureterosigmoidostomy following cystectomy is also a potential risk factor for the development of adenocarcinoma at the anastomatic site.

Occupational and environmental risk factors include exposure to asbestos, oils, printing materials, halogens, metal fumes, organic solvents, paint and dyes.

Radiation induced colorectal cancers arise in rectum and sigmoid colon of patients with carcinoma of cervix, bladder and prostate. The latent period for such cancers is longer than 10 years with 3000 rad threshold value.[12] 1.5-9% of patients with colorectal cancer have a second synchronous cancer[13] and 5-8% subsequently develop a metachronous cancer.[14,15] The time interval between initial and metachronous cancer varies but the majority arises within 5 to 7 years of the index cancer.

Hereditary factors have been a subject of interest for colorectal cancer. Heredity plays a role in 5-6% of all colorectal cancers.[3] Familial adenomatous polyposis (FAP) is an autosomal dominant syndrome caused by the germline mutation of the adenomatous polyposis coli gene. Colorectal cancer always occurs if a prophylactic colectomy is not performed in a patient with FAP. Turcot's syndrome is a variant of FAP in which the extracolonic lesion is a brain tumor such as medulloblastoma.

There is a high incidence of colorectal neoplasia (dysplasia and adenocarcinoma) found in upto 20% patients at a relatively younger age (37 years) in juvenile polyposis coli which is an autosomal dominant trait.[10] Screening should be performed periodically in patients with Cronkhite-Canada syndrome, which is characterized by multiple juvenile polyps throughout the gastrointestinal tract except the esopahgus. These can undergo adenomatous and carcinomatous degeneration.

Hereditary non-polyposis colorectal cancer (Lynch syndrome), accounts for 4-6% of all colorectal cancers. In Lynch syndrome I, colorectal cancer is inherited as autosomal dominant susceptibility with more metachronous and synchronous lesions. In Lynch syndrome II, there is an increased incidence of adenocarcinoma of endometrium, ovary and other organs in addition to colorectal cancer. The precursor lesion in Lynch related colon cancer is a discrete proximal colonic adenoma. Right-sided colon cancer occurring at young age is the hallmark of Lynch syndrome. Lynch colon cancers have a better prognosis than other colorectal cancer varieties.[10]

Carcinoma in ulcerative colitis is uncommon, occurs in patients with pancolitis and is responsible for only 1% of colorectal cancers. Patients with left-sided disease are at less risk. The risk begins to increase after 7-10 years of colitis. Actual risk of developing colorectal cancer is 0.5-2% after the first 10 years of disease, 6.6% after 26 years, 11.4 after 32 years. Disease activity does not increase the risk of long term colorectal cancer and lack of activity does not have a protective effect. The mean age of presentation is 40-45 years.[10]

The risk of developing adenocarcinoma of large and small bowel has been estimated to be 4 to 20 times greater than that of general population in Crohn's disease. Most cancers develop in inflamed segments, segments having strictures and fistulae. Excluded colon and rectum as well as bypassed small bowel segments are at particular risk. Multifocal carcinomas may be seen and are discovered late as they cannot be distinguished from benign strictures.[10]

Pathogenesis

Most colorectal cancers arise in adenomatous polyps.[16] The risk of malignant transformation is higher in adenomas more than 1 cm in size. The transition from benign adenoma to cancer may take 7 to 10 years. This adenoma-carcinoma sequence suggests that colon cancer is preventable if polypoid lesions larger than 1 cm are detected and removed. The importance of screening programs for colon cancer also needs to be stressed here.

In patients with inflammatory bowel disease, carcinoma evolves through a sequence of inflammation, dysplasia and carcinoma.

The malignant potential of an adenomatous polyp has four major determinants. These include size, presence of a stalk, villous architecture and degree of cellular atypia and dysplasia. Polyps less than 5 mm have virtually no risk of malignant transformation, those between 1-2 cm carry a 5% risk and those more than 2cm carry a 50% risk of harboring malignancy.[10] Sessile polyps are at higher risk for malignancy (> 50%) than pedunculated polyps. In case a pedunculated polyp turns malignant the invasion of the colonic wall by the cancer is rare if the length of the stalk is more than 2 cm. Adenomatous polyps are of three types, tubular, villous and tubulovillous. Villous adenomas are more likely to have malignant transformation than tubular adenomas.[17] This is because villous adenomas are usually sessile and penetration of the muscularis mucosa is more likely in a sessile polyp. Polyps with a greater degree of cellular atypia and dysplasia are more likely to become malignant.

Clinical Features

As colorectal cancer is a slow growing tumor, symptoms may be absent or minimal at the time of diagnosis. Symptomatic colorectal cancers usually present with evidence of bleeding. This may be in the form of occult blood in the stool, passage of bright red blood per rectum or development of iron deficiency anemia. The patient's symptoms are related to size and location of the tumor. Right-sided colon cancers usually grow to a large size before symptoms develop. This is because the right colon is more capacious and the contents are relatively fluid in consistency. Anemia and disorded bowel function are earlier findings in right-sided colon cancer. On the other hand sigmoid cancers present early as sigmoid colon is the narrowest portion of the large bowel and the tumor obstructs the passage of solid fecal matter early. These patients present with colicky, crampy abdominal pain that is relieved by a bowel movement. Left-sided colon cancers usually present with per rectal bleeding or intestinal obstruction.

A feeling of incomplete bowel evacuation, persistent constipation or diarrhea and change in stool calibre should arouse suspicion of colorectal carcinoma in patients older than 40 years. Weight loss and anemia are seen in 50% of patients with colorectal carcinoma.

Physical examination is usually normal in patients with colorectal carcinoma. Patients may present with a palpable mass or signs of intestinal obstruction. Palpable supraclavicular nodes may be seen with left-sided colon cancer and hepatomegaly may be present due to metastases. Among the laboratory investigations measurement of carcinoembryonic antigen (CEA) levels is a useful test. CEA is an antigen shed from the surface of tumor cells. Although not specific, CEA is a very sensitive marker for colorectal cancer. The elevation of serum CEA correlates with cancer stage and tumor size. Elevated preoperative CEA level predicts shorter disease free survival.

Pathology

The gross morphology of the colorectal adenocarcinoma is related to its location. Large, polypoidal bulky masses overgrowing their vascular supply are found in the cecum and ascending colon. They may also undergo necrosis. Tumors in the transverse and descending colon are ulcerative and infiltrative and have a large intramural component. Thus they are more invasive in nature. Tumors in the more distal colon and rectum are also infiltrative and produce an annular constricting or 'napkin ring' appearance. These tumors are the most biologically aggressive. In the setting of inflammatory bowel disease colon cancers are scirrhous, plaque like or finely nodular.[18]

Malignancies of the large bowel are predominantly adenocarcinoma. Mucinous/colloid carcinomas are seen in patients with inflammatory bowel disease and hereditary non-polyposis related carcinoma in early age. They constitute 10 to 15% of the cancers with large lakes of mucin containing scattered collection of tumor cells with signet ring cells. As the mucin is secreted within the interstitium of the gut wall it dissects the wall, helps in the extension of the malignancy and worsens the prognosis. Calcification may occur in these tumors. Tumors that arise at the anorectal junction include squamous cell carcinoma, cloacogenic carcinoma, transitional cell carcinoma and melanocarcinoma.[10] They comprise less than 5% of malignant tumors of large bowel. Primary lymphomas, carcinoid tumors and leiomyosarcomas comprise less than 0.1% of all large bowel neoplasms.[19] In addition lymphoma, leiomyosarcoma and cancers of the breast, ovaries, prostate, lung and stomach can metastasize to the colon.

Route of Spread

There are five methods of tumor spread after the tumor has become invasive.

1. *Direct extension*: Direct invasion may occur along the tissue layers that provide least resistance. As peritoneum represents a relative barrier, direct spread to neighboring intraperitoneal organs is rare. After invading the visceral peritoneum the tumor can spread to stomach, greater omentum, spleen, small bowel, another portion of the colon, uterus, bladder, fallopian tubes and ovaries. Retroperitoneal tumor may involve kidneys, pancreas, ureters and posterior truncal musculature. Rectal carcinoma after breaching fascia of Waldeyer may invade sacral plexus, sacrum and coccyx.[20] It may also invade internal iliac vessels and obturator musculature posterolaterally, and prostate, seminal vesicles, bladder, vagina and cervix anteriorly after compromising the fascia of Denonvillier's.

2. *Lymphatic spread*: Lymphatic spread occurs after the invasion of muscularis through submucosal lymphatics. Intramural spread of colorectal malignancy occurs to submucosal, muscular and subserosal lymphatics. The epiploic and paracolic lymph nodes are usually the first sites of involvement. The intermediate lymph nodes (along vascular branches) and principal lymph nodes (at origins of colonic blood vessels) generally show involvement later in the course of disease. The prognosis worsens with increasing number of involved lymph nodes.
3. *Hematogenous metastases*: There exists the potential for hematogenous metastases if colorectal malignancy invades the rich capillary network of lamina propria. The most common route is through branches of portal vein. Thus liver is the organ which is most commonly involved by metastases. Distal rectum drains through tributaries of internal iliac vein, which drain into the inferior vena cava. Batson's vertebral venous plexus is another path of hematogenous spread. Liver is the sole site of metastases in 20-40% colorectal carcinoma patients. Metastases to the lung are seen in 20% of patients. The lungs are the sole site of metastases in 4% of patients. Other sites are less common and include adrenal glands, bone, kidney, pancreas, spleen and central nervous system.
4. *Peritoneal seeding*: Intraperitoneal seeding may occur during operation because of breach in serosa. Seeded metastases may occur especially on the anterior wall of rectosigmoid junction. Eventually, both the parietal and visceral peritoneal surfaces will be involved leading to malignant ascites.
5. *Intraluminal implantation*: Intraluminal tumor spillage at surgery is a likely source of implantation metastases and anastomotic recurrence. [21] Anastomotic recurrences may also be due to incomplete tumor excision or a metachronous tumor.

Staging

Colorectal cancer staging has evolved over many years. In 1932, Dr Cuthbert E Dukes, a London based pathologist, detailed a study of 215 patients with rectal cancers in which he found direct relationship between survival and depth of tumor penetration into the intestinal wall and lymph node metastasis. [22] The Astler and Coller modification of the Dukes classification is commonly employed to stage colonic neoplasm.

This classification uses the following designations:

A Tumor limited to the mucosa

B1 Tumor extending into, but not through, the muscularis propria

B2 Tumor penetrating the bowel wall, but without any lymph node involvement

C Tumor with regional lymph node involvement. This is divided into CI in which the primary tumor is limited to the bowel wall and C2, in which the primary tumor has penetrated the bowel wall

In 1967 Turnball introduced an additional staging category as stage D, further divided into stage D1, which included fixed cancers that had invaded adjacent organs and stage D2, in which, distant metastases had occurred. Currently the American Joint Committee on Cancer (AJCC) and International Union against Cancer (UICC) have designated staging by TNM classification. [23] Local tumor staging (T staging) is based on the depth of tumor penetration into the bowel wall. The extent of mural invasion is important, as it has shown to influence prognosis independent of lymph node involvement.

Primary Tumor (T)

Tx Primary tumor cannot be assessed

T0 No evidence of primary tumor

Tis Carcinoma *in situ*

T1 Tumor invades submucosa

T2 Tumor invades muscularis propria

T3 Tumor extending through the muscularis propria into subserosa or non-peritonealized pericolic or perirectal tissue

T4 Tumor directly invades other organs or structures (T4a) or perforates the visceral peritoneum (T4b)

Regional Lymph Node (N)

Nx Regional lymph nodes cannot be assessed

N0 No regional lymph node metastasis

N1 Metastasis in 1-3 pericolic or perirectal lymph nodes

N2 Metastasis in 4 or more pericolic or perirectal lymph nodes

Distant Metastasis (M)

Mx Presence of distant metastasis cannot be assessed

M0 No distant metastasis

M1 Distant metastasis

Stage Grouping[24]

Stage 0	Tis	N0	M0
Stage I	T1	N0	M0
	T2	N0	M0
Stage II	T3	N0	M0
	T4	N0	M0
Stage III A	Any T	N1	M0
B	Any T	N2	M0
Stage IV	Any T	Any N	M1

Role of Radiology

Radiology plays an important role in screening for colorectal carcinoma. The goal of imaging studies in patients with colorectal carcinoma is to provide the surgeon and the oncologist complete and accurate assessment of the primary tumor, local and distant spread of the disease, synchronous lesions and to detect clinically occult complications. Radiology has a critical role after treatment of colorectal carcinoma in the detection of recurrent or residual disease, local and distant metastases and metachronous cancers.

Screening for Colorectal Cancer

The American Cancer Society has recommended that beginning at the age of 50 years, one of the following five testing schedules should be adopted:[25]

1. Yearly fecal occult blood test (FOBT) or fecal immunochemical test (FIT)
2. Flexible sigmoidoscopy every 5 years
3 Yearly FOBT or FIT, plus flexible sigmoidoscopy every 5 years
4. Double contrast barium enema every 5 years
5. Colonoscopy every 10 years

FOBT is the most widely available and least expensive screening test for colorectal cancer. Colorectal cancers bleed intermittently and the blood that is lost into the stool is broken down into hematin. Hematin reacts with guaiac and the commonly used Hemoccult test is based on the guaiac reaction. False positive reactions are caused by ingestion of meat, certain vegetables and aspirin. False negative results occur as cancers only bleed intermittently. Moreover it is thought that a polyp must be over 2 cm in size before it bleeds regularly. The sensitivity for detection of colon cancer is lower than 50% and nearly 90% of polyps are undetected by FOBT.[26]

Flexible sigmoidoscopy visually inspects the rectum and distal sigmoid colon. Therefore approximately only half of the colorectal cancers can be detected by flexible fibreoptic sigmoidoscopy alone. Though it is a safe and well tolerated procedure and does not require sedation, it is relatively expensive and has the potential for transmission of disease by contaminated instruments.

Double contrast barium enema (DCBE) is an inexpensive and simple test. However, in a study comparing DCBE to colonoscopy it was found that the sensitivity of DCBE was only 32% for polyps less than 0.5 cm, 53% for polyps 0.6 to 1 cm and 48% for polyps greater than 1 cm.[27]

Colonoscopy can directly visualize most colon cancers. The National Polyp Study and the Italian Mutlicenter Study showed reduction in colorectal cancer incidence among patients who had adenomas detected and removed on colonoscopy.[28,29] Colonoscopy is regarded as the gold standard for determining sensitivities of other examinations of the colon. However in a review of tandem or back-to-back colonoscopies an average of 21% of adenomas were missed.[30] Of these adenomas, 26% were 1 to 5 mm and 2% were 10 mm or more in size. There are blind spots in the colon behind folds and around flexures. Colonoscopy also has the risk of perforation or hemorrhage in 1:500 examinations and a fatality rate of 1:5000 examinations. The completion rate of colonoscopy ranges from 55 to 95%.

Virtual colonoscopy is a new noninvasive method wherein a three-dimensional endoluminal image is generated after processing data acquired by multidetector helical CT using specialized computer software. In the American College of Radiology Imaging Network (ACRIN) study conducted at 15 study centers on 2600 asymptomatic participants it was found that CT colonography has a 90% sensitivity and 86% specificity for detection of polyps measuring 10 mm or more in diameter.[31] Thus virtual colonoscopy performs well in detecting lesions larger than 1cm which are actually clinically significant lesions. The entire colon is also evaluated by virtual colonoscopy. However, patients found to have significant lesions must undergo optical colonoscopy. The reported rate of complications with this technique is relatively small (0.08%).

Double contrast barium enema and virtual colonoscopy will be discussed in detail in subsequent sections.

Diagnostic Methods

Imaging modalities available are plain abdominal radiographs, barium enema, ultrasound including endoluminal and Doppler ultrasound, computed tomography/CT colonography, MRI/MR colonography and angiography.

Plain Radiographs

These are usually not very informative except for depicting complications of advanced colorectal malignancy like obstruction and perforation. Dilatation of colon and small bowel in cases of obstruction, thumb printing suggestive of ischemic colitis proximal to an obstructing lesion and free intraperitoneal air in cases of perforation and pericolonic abscess formation may be detected on plain films. There may be a fistula with gall bladder or urinary bladder. Calcification of carcinomatous lesion or hepatic metastases may be evident. When advanced, invasion of bone is easily diagnosed by identifying destruction of bone and presence of soft tissue mass. Lung metastases may be seen on chest skiagram.

Barium Enema

The major advantage of barium enema is its ability to examine the entire colon. It is reasonably accurate, minimally invasive and requires no sedation. Complications related to the investigation are rare. DCBE has a 20% better sensitivity than single contrast barium enema for detecting adenomatous polyps less than 1cm in size.[32] However, there is no difference in the sensitivity of the two types of barium enema for the detection of colorectal carcinoma. Recent studies have reported the sensitivity of barium enema in the range of 90 to 95% for the detection of significant (1 cm) size polyps and cancer.[33] Thorough bowel preparation is the most important prerequisite for an accurate radiological examination with selection of an appropriate technique, careful quality control during the study and meticulous interpretation of the radiographs. Combination of dietary manipulation, oral catheters and cleansing enema is the most effective regimen. 10 to 40% of colonic carcinomas can be missed on initial barium enemas due to poor colon preparation.[34,35] Presence of fecal matter can mimic or mask polyps and cancers and is the most common reason for false positive findings on barium enema. The single contrast barium enema is simpler in concept than the double contrast study, but requires meticulous technique. Indication for the examination, sensitivity for detecting specific diseases and the age and physical condition of the patient helps to select the type of barium enema to be performed.

DCBE give better information of mucosa with better detection of smaller lesions. Therefore it is the procedure of choice in patients who are older than 40 years, who have a personal or family history of colonic polyps, cancer or inflammatory bowel disease, and a positive FOBT. Other indications are patients with previous ovarian, breast or cervical carcinoma and with prior pelvic irradiation.

Single contrast barium enema is simpler and does not require rigorous maneuvers. Therefore it is indicated in patients older than 70 years of age, debilitated or uncooperative patients and in those patients where barium study is indicated for exclusion of obstruction or diverticulitis. Young patients with low likelihood of colon disease may also be candidates for single contrast study. Manual or mechanical compression of the colon during fluoroscopy and spot radiographs of the various segments are critical in detecting small polypoid lesions. Technique protocols should be followed, the adequacy of colon cleansing assessed, careful fluoroscopy performed, poor quality films repeated and additional films of questionable lesions should be obtained when needed.

Meticulous interpretation of the barium enema films is needed to avoid diagnostic errors due to presence of stool, air bubbles and diverticulae, or confusion of normal anatomic structures for an abnormality. False negative errors are caused by perceptive lapses, technical problems, interpretive mistakes, or a combination of these factors. Perceptive errors can be reduced by close scrutiny, second review or retrospective review of the films especially for diagnosing colonic polyps and sigmoid colon malignancies. Accuracy of DCBE for evaluation of colorectal polyps depends on the location of lesion and size of the colonic polyps. The sensitivity of DCBE is poor for polyps under 5mm, improving for polyps 5 to 9 mm and is best for diagnosing polyps over 1 cm.

Complications of barium enema are uncommon. The rates of perforation for barium enema are documented at 1:2500 to 1:12,500 and for mortality at 1:50,000.[36,37] Subsequent to a biopsy performed through a rigid scope, enema should be deferred for 2 weeks due to risk of perforation. Enema need not be postponed if biopsy is performed through a flexible sigmoidscope or colonoscope as the depth of biopsy does not extend beyond the muscularis mucosa. Recent endoscopic polypectomy precludes enema for 2-3 weeks. Barium and latex sensitivity, barium impaction, transient bacteremia, dehydration and inadvertent placement of the enema tip into vaginal vault are other complications which may also be encounted. Despite the risk of transient bacteremia there is presently no recommendation to give prophylactic antibiotics.

Colorectal malignancies show a broad spectrum of radiographic appearances reflecting various morphologic types. The mucosal surface can be seen en face, either in the barium pool or in air contrast. The normal mucosal surface is smooth. An abnormal mucosal surface may have a granular, finely nodular or ulcerated surface. Early carcinoma usually presents as a sessile polypoid mass. The radiologic detection of early carcinoma is mainly an exercise in the detection of small polyps. There are two common types of colonic polyps, hyperplastic and adenomatous. Hyperplastic polyps have no malignant potential. Small polypoidal carcinomas may have a smooth outline and be radiographically indistinguishable from benign tumors (Figs 9.1 and 9.2). Barium enema cannot determine accurately, whether polypoid lesions in the size range of 0.5 to 3 cm are benign or malignant. Whenever, possible polyps more than 1 cm in size are found they must be removed by colonoscopic polypectomy followed by histological examination.

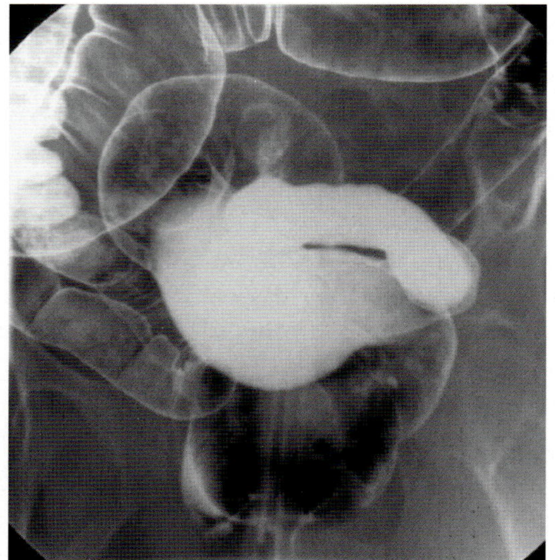

Fig. 9.1: DCBE shows a solitary, small, smooth polypoid lesion in the sigmoid colon which was malignant on histopathology

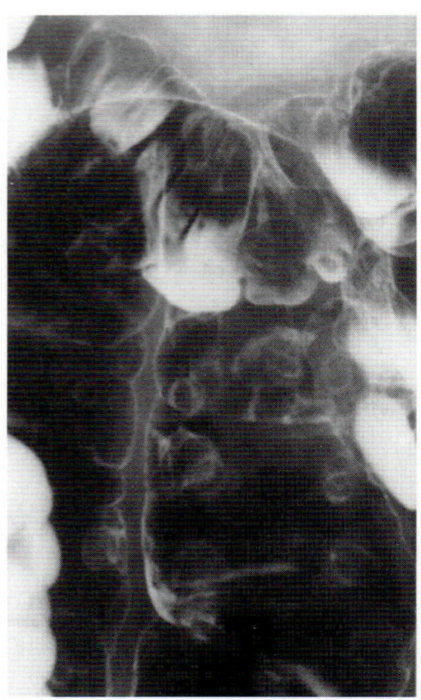

Fig. 9.2: DCBE in a patient with familial adenomatous polyposis showing multiple polyps in the colon

Pedunculated polyps are best demonstrated on erect or lateral decubitus views of the colon. Those arising from the non-dependent wall of the colon give the appearance of 'Mexican hat' sign[38] where the central ring represents the stalk and the outer ring represents the head of polyps. In these cases a change in position of patients shows the stalk in profile and confirms the diagnosis.

Sessile polyps may vary in appearance from a small, smooth polypoidal lesion to a bulky, lobulated mass forming acute angles with the adjacent colonic wall. When viewed en face, they appear as filling defects in the thin barium pool if they arise from dependent wall and etched in white if present on the non-dependent surface. However, they may be missed if too much of high density barium is present in the lumen, obscuring the lesion. When viewed in oblique projections sessile polyps manifest as 'Bowler hat' sign,[39] with the dome representing the head of polyps and brim representing base of the polyp. Although the 'Bowler hat' sign can be produced by a diverticulum, the direction of the dome distinguishes a polyp from a diverticulum. When the dome points away from the axis of the bowel the lesion is a diverticulum and when it points towards the lumen of the bowel it is a polyp.

Certain criteria have been described to assess the risk of malignancy of polyps based on their imaging features which include sessile versus pedunculated appearance, size of the polyp, number of polyps, basal indentation and surface contour. 1 cm is the threshold size for increased cancer risk of a polyp. In case of pedunculated polyps a stalk length >2 cm is not associated with malignant invasion into the adjacent wall. Smooth basal indentation is related to geometric factors and can be seen in both benign and malignant lesions. Presence of basal irregularity is most predictive of malignant lesion when it is broad and irregular in larger polyps. The smooth surface contour is unreliable is distinguishing benign from malignant polyps. Lesions that have an irregular, 'soap bubbly' surface generally have villous elements and are likely to have malignant degeneration in at least 50% of lesions.[40,41] Most colonic adenomas are tubular adenomas. They have varying degrees of villous change which increases as the polyp increases in size. At the other end of the spectrum are villous adenomas which have a frond like surface. There may be a transition from tubular adenoma to tubulovillous adenoma to villous adenoma. The risk of malignancy is related to the proportion of villous change in an adenoma. As the barium gets caught in the frond like protusions which go hand in hand with the villous change, the surface of the polyp assumes a 'soap bubbly' or a 'lacy' pattern. The term 'carpet lesion' has also been used to describe a flat lobulated lesion that manifests due to an alteration in surface texture of the bowel. These are again tubular adenomas with varying degrees of villous change.

Once a polyp is detected there is a 3.5% risk of synchronous cancer and a 20% chance of an additional polyp.[42] Therefore the remainder of the colon should be examined meticulously.

Advanced colorectal cancers have various morphological types. These include polypoidal, annular, scirrhous and flat lesions. The polypoidal lesions protrude into the lumen and have an irregular outline (Figs 9.3A to D). They may cause bowel obstruction or intussusception. Annular cancers are short in length with abrupt transition between normal and tumor mucosa (Figs 9.4 and 9.5). The mucosa is destroyed and there may be heaped up edges or ulceration. A focal area of spasm may cause confusion on DCBE but the mucosal folds remain intact within the area of the spasm. The differential diagnosis of annular colonic narrowing

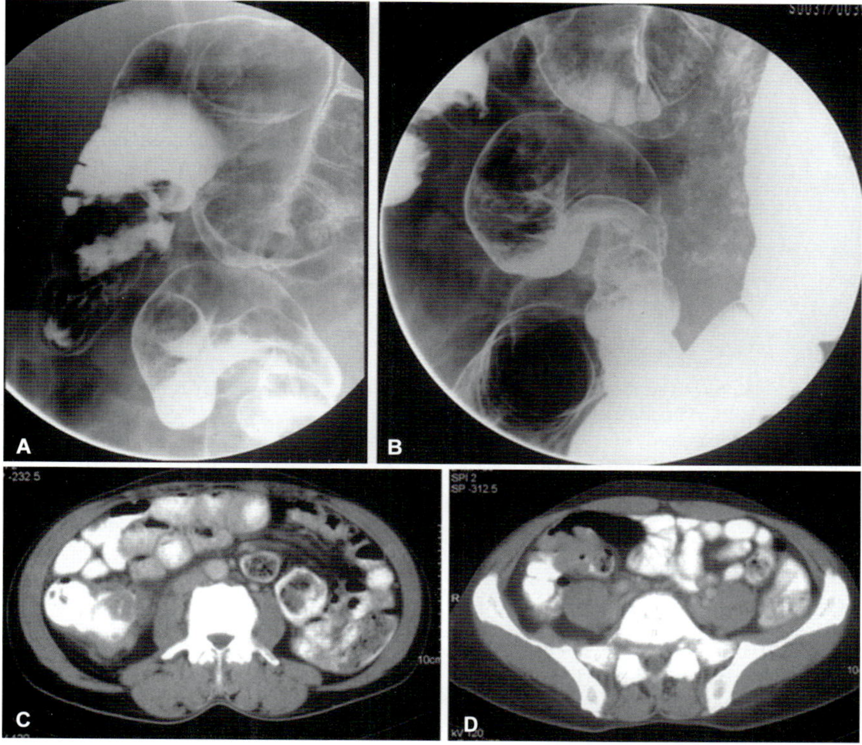

Figs 9.3A to D: DCBE showing synchronous cancers in the ascending colon (A) and sigmoid colon (B). There is a short segment stricture in the ascending colon with a polypoidal component protruding into the colon. The sigmoid colon also shows a segment of narrowing. Axial CECT sections in the same patient showing circumferential mural thickening with a polypoidal component in the ascending colon (C). A similar lesion is also seen in the sigmoid colon with presence of ulcerations (D)

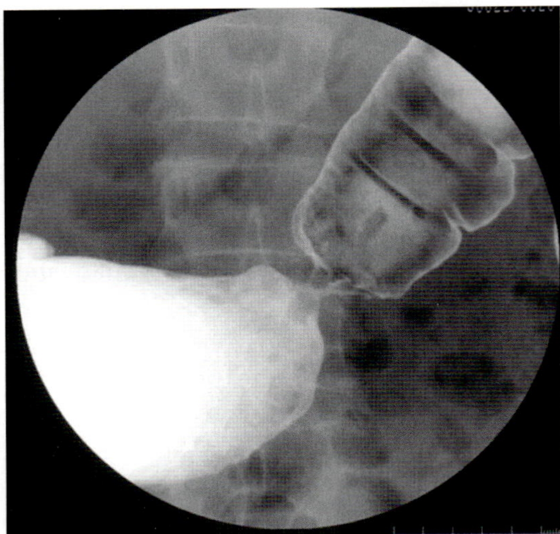

Fig. 9.4: DCBE showing a short annular stricture in the transverse colon with mucosal irregularity in a patient with colon cancer

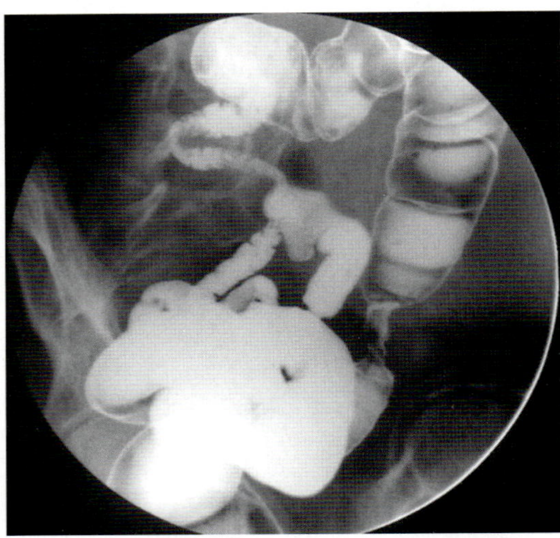

Fig. 9.5: Barium enema showing a stricture with mucosal irregularity in the descending colon in a patient with metachronous cancer. The patient had previous history of right hemicolectomy and ileo-transverse anastomosis for carcinoma of ascending colon (Courtesy: Dr. B. Nagi, Department of Gastroenterology, PGIMER)

includes adhesions, inflammation, diverticulitis, endometriosis, radiation changes, metastatic disease and primary adenocarcinoma. Semiannular or 'saddle' tumor involves only a portion of the wall and result in asymmetry of bowel lumen. En face, these tumors produce overlapping lines with an abnormal orientation on double contrast studies. Scirrhous tumor causes marked mural thickening and smooth strictures with submucosal and muscular invasion. Flat lesions are uncommon and usually occur in patients with long-standing ulcerative colitis. They can just result in abnormal lines on DCBE.

Problem Areas in Barium Studies

1. Distal rectum: The catheter tip in the rectum can itself obscure plaque like or polypoidal lesions. Large internal hemorrhoids may mimic carcinoma, which appear on DCBE as thickened lobulated folds extending 3 cm or less from the anal verge or as cluster of small submucosal nodules in the rectum. However, low lying rectal cancers that spread through the submucosa mimic hemorrhoids, but asymmetry of lesion and extent of rectal involvement suggests the diagnosis.
2. Ileocaecal valve: Tumors arising in this area have subtle findings which include widening, splaying, straightening or asymmetric lobulation of the valve. These may be missed on initial observation.
3. The presence of diverticulosis may obscure lesions. In patients who have equivocal lesions in the sigmoid colon, a 'sigmoid flush' may be performed at the end by introducing a small amount of low-density barium into the rectum to demonstrate polypoidal lesions as filling defects in the thin barium pool.[43] Common errors in barium interpretation can be due to:
   a. Failure to detect small filling defects in a pool of barium.
   b. Insufficient distension or overdistension.
   c. Incomplete cleansing prior to the study.
   d. Poor adherence of barium resulting in poor mucosal coating.
   e. Failure to detect a synchronous lesion in presence of one lesion. Satisfaction or distraction by finding one lesion may result in overlooking a synchronous lesion.
   f. Lesions may be obscured by haustral folds or overlying bowel loops.
   g. Perceptive errors, because of extraneous material such as feces, anatomic variation such as redundant bowel loops or presence of diverticulae.

As most colorectal carcinomas are slow growing it is assumed that if a carcinoma is found within 3 years of a previous normal barium enema study, the tumor was missed. [33,44,45]

Ultrasound

The appearance of bowel on ultrasound depends not only upon the structures of the individual segment but more importantly upon its content and degree of distension. The bowel may be collapsed, containing only a small amount of mucus (the mucus pattern), or may contain fluid or gas. The mucus pattern is the classical target appearance. Large bowel tends to produce a more complex pattern, because it contains small amount of fluid and gas even in the fasting state. Sometimes the colonic contents are reflective with distal shadows due to suspended fecal material. In case of colorectal malignancy, bowel wall thickening may be visualized by ultrasound resulting in a target or 'pseudokidney' configuration (Figs 9.6A to C). Normal bowel wall thickness in the non-distended state is 5 mm, reducing to about 3 mm when bowel is distended. When the bowel wall is thickened, the mucus pattern changes to a thickened, sometimes irregular 'halo' of bowel wall, with highly reflective irregular centre giving a 'pseudokidney' sign.[45] This sign is nonspecific but strongly suggests bowel pathology. The site of the involved bowel must be inferred from the position of the lesion in the abdomen. In inflammatory processes of bowel wall the multiple layers are retained with a large segment of involvement. However, in neoplastic process a short segment involvement with obliteration of bowel wall layers is seen. The exception is lymphoma in which the wall layers are preserved. The diagnostic accuracy of transabdominal ultrasound is improved by retrograde instillation of fluid into the colon. This procedure known as sono-colonography, enables an accurate evaluation not only of the colonic lumen but also of colonic wall and surrounding connective tissue. According to a study done by Bernd[46] the sensitivity of the technique in the detection of colonic carcinomas was 94% and the specificity was 100% . Ultrasound (US) screening of abdomen helps to find out liver metastasis and retroperitoneal lymphadenopathy. Fine needle aspiration and core biopsy technique is possible using US guidance. It is particularly valuable in patients where confirmatory studies are either technically difficult or the findings are nonspecific.

Endorectal ultrasound (ERU): Evaluation of rectum with an endosonic probe was first done by Wilde and Reed in 1956.[45] The procedure is performed with an endorectally placed, rotating, high frequency transducer. If possible, the transducer should be passed proximal to the visualized tumor for complete assessment of mural involvement. The five layers of the rectal wall can be demonstrated as layers of alternating echogenicity with high frequency transducers allowing an assessment of the depth of invasion of rectal tumors. The innermost ring is hyperechoic and represents the interface of the probe and the mucosa. The second ring is hypoechoic and is due to the muscularis mucosa. The third ring is hyperechoic and represents the submucosa. The fourth ring is again hypoechoic and is formed by the muscularis propria. The fifth ring is hyperechoic and is due to the perirectal fat or in areas of peritoneal reflection by the serosa and fat. Rectal carcinoma appears as a hypoechoic mass with irregular borders interrupting the normal five-

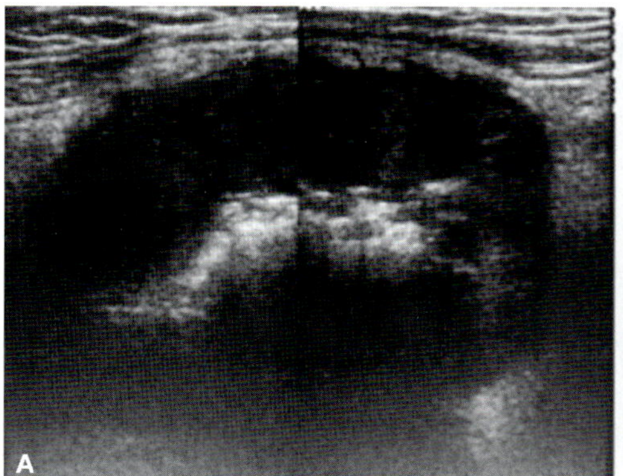

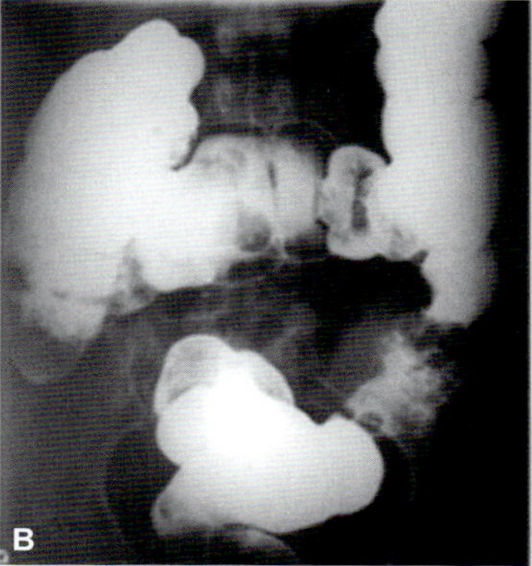

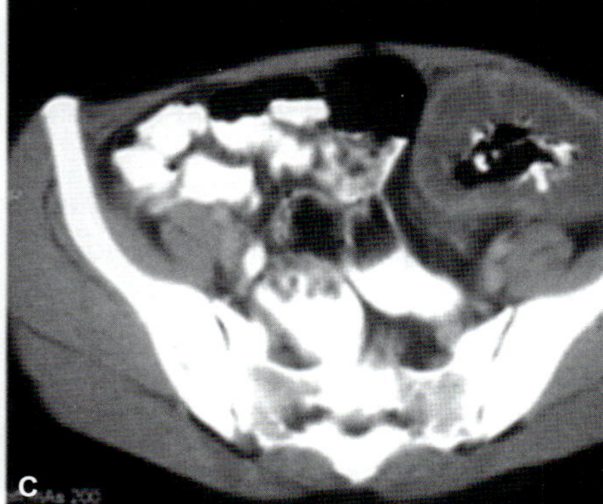

Figs 9.6A to C: (A) Ultrasound of the lump in the left iliac fossa shows thickened bowel wall with highly reflective centre consistent with 'pseudokidney' sign, (B) Barium enema in the same patient shows a mass like lesion with deep ulcerations in the region of descending colon, (C) Axial CECT section shows concentric mural thickening with ulcerations in the same segment

layer wall pattern. The accuracy of ERU in staging of colorectal carcinoma varies from 64 to 93%. Most of the errors are due to overestimates of the depth of invasion possibly as a result of co-existing inflammation. Tumor confined to the muscularis mucosa can be differentiated from tumor extending into the perirectal fat with invasion of adjacent structures and metastatic involvement of the perirectal lymph nodes.

ERU has been used with some success in differentiating benign villous adenomas from those with focal areas of invasive carcinoma. Glaser et al[47] reported that benign villous adenoma appears hyperechoic and areas of invasive carcinoma appear hypoechoic. Hulsmans et al[48] used involvement of the muscularis propria by the mass to determine the presence of invasive carcinoma within a villous adenoma. Perirectal lymph nodes as small as 5 mm can be reliably shown by ERU but size cannot be used to predict nodal involvement by malignancy. Studies evaluating nodal metastasis based on size have rather low accuracy rates. Nodal echotexture and morphology are the most often used criteria. Nodes with sharply demarcated borders and an inhomogenous hypoechoic pattern strongly suggest malignancy unlike nodes with indistinct borders and a hyperechoic pattern. Limitation of ERU is in evaluating distant metastasis, stenosing rectal carcinomas and tumors near the anal verge, which are difficult to visualize and may be missed. Other limitations of ERU include the inability to assess depth of penetration beyond the colonic wall as well as possible overestimation of tumor size in patients with extensive peritumoral inflammation or with preoperative radiation. Failure of the technique occurs in upto 15% of all rectal carcinomas.[45]

Transrectal US can distinguish three stages of disease based on TNM classification:

1. T1 tumor confined to mucosa and submucosa which does not interrupt the middle echogenic ring.
2. T_2 tumor confined to rectal wall in which the outermost echogenic interface is intact.
3. T_3 tumor which penetrates the perirectal fat and leads to disruption of outermost echogenic ring.

Doppler US may complement the US imaging by showing increased color flow, increased diastolic flow within tumor with low resistance waveform, as tumor vessels lack smooth muscle layer, thus offering little resistance. A cut-off peak systolic velocity (PSV) of more than 25 cm/s is used to differentiate T3 and T4 tumors from T1 and T2 tumors and a PSV of more than 20 cm/s in lymph nodes is classified as malignant.

Computed Tomography

The primary role of computerized tomography in imaging colorectal carcinoma is for preoperative staging, in assessing postoperative complications and in detection of tumor recurrence. It is estimated that upto 25% of patients with colorectal carcinoma have metastatic disease at the time of diagnosis.[49] Therefore staging technique should include both the primary colorectal neoplasm and sites of potential metastases.

Barium studies and colonoscopy/sigmoidoscopy provide excellent visualization of the mucosa. However, they cannot determine the depth of mural invasion by the tumor or the extent of metastatic involvement. Preoperative staging aims to accurately assess tumor extent to individualize therapy, assess risk of disease recurrence, and determine prognosis. By virtue of their cross-sectional imaging format and ability to demonstrate the extent of wall invasion, extraluminal tumor spread, lymph node and distant metastasis, CT and MRI have become the primary means for radiologic staging of colorectal carcinoma. Complications of primary colonic malignancies such as obstruction, perforation and fistula formation can also be readily visualized with CT.

The accuracy of CT for colonic evaluation can be improved with several additional techniques including adequate cleansing of colon, administration of IV smooth muscle relaxants, distension of the colon with either air (CT colonography) or water and by having thin sections through the areas of tumor (Fig. 9.7). A rectal enema may be given to delineate the descending colon and rectosigmoid region.

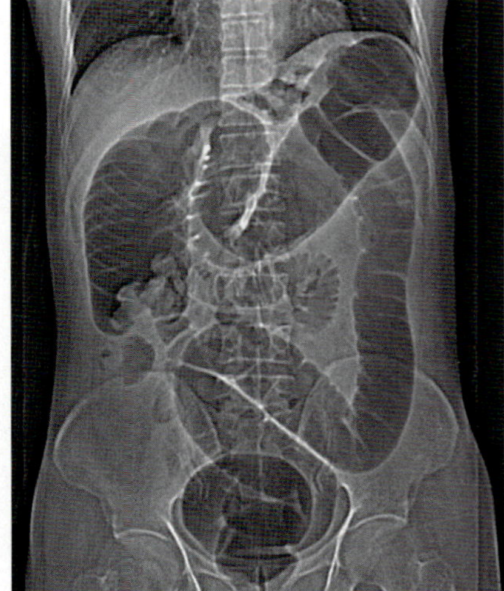

Fig. 9.7: Topogram obtained before acquiring data for CT colonography shows the polypodial mass lesion in the cecum. The rest of the colon is well distended with air

The normal wall thickening in a well-distended colonic segment is 3 mm, 3-6 mm is considered indeterminate, measurement greater than 6 mm is considered abnormal. Both the mucosal margin and outer colonic margin should be smooth and delineated by air/ water soluble contrast or pericolonic fat respectively. The rectum, rectosigmoid region, ascending and descending segments of the colon are relatively fixed structures and were therefore easily evaluated by conventional CT. Tumors in the flexures and transverse colon were less readily examined by conventional CT because colonic peristalsis and diaphragmatic excursion made these parts more difficult to evaluate. This has been overcome by the advent of fast helical CT scanners.

The primary bowel tumor is identified on CT as focal or circumferential wall thickening (> 6 mm) with contour distortion or more frequently as a discrete mass. Occasionally an intraluminal polypoid mass without wall thickening is seen (Figs 9.8A to C). CT cannot depict the various layers of the bowel wall and cannot distinguish T1 from T2 stage. Sometimes contrast enhanced CT scan with rectal contrast can demonstrate a typical 'napkin ring' lesion of annular contricting malignancy and plaque like lesion. Large masses may undergo central necrosis and appear as a soft tissue mass with central low attenuation. Mucinous primary adenocarcinoma may rarely contain calcification, however, this occurs more often in hepatic metastasis than in the primary tumor. Rectal and sigmoid cancers may appear as asymmetric nodular wall thickening that narrows the lumen. This appearance may mimic diverticulitis, especially if the tumor involvement of the wall has resulted in infiltration of the pericolic fat. However, presence of fluid in the root of the sigmoid mesentery and engorgement of adjacent sigmoid mesenteric vasculature, favors the diagnosis of diverticulitis and presence of pericolic lymph nodes raises the suspicion of colon cancer. Pericolic lymph node adjacent to a segment of thickened colonic wall are seen much more frequently in cases of colon cancer than with diverticulitis. Thickening can occasionally appear symmetric and involve the entire circumference of the bowel wall. In such cases, malignancy can be difficult to differentiate from benign causes of wall thickening, including inflammation and mural edema.

The pericolonic and perirectal fat appear uniformly low in density without soft tissue stranding on CT. Thickening of the perirectal fascia produces the 'halo sign' which can be seen with extension of tumor into perirectal fat. Invasion beyond the bowel wall should be suspected if a focal mass deforms the contour of the outer colonic wall with an advancing nodular margin with or without pericolonic soft tissue stranding (Figs 9.9A to C). Extracolonic tumor spread is also suggested by loss of fat planes between the large bowel and the surrounding muscles like levator ani, obturator internus, piriform, coccygeous and gluteus. Unfortunately as the loss of fat plane is a nonspecific sign in cross-sectional imaging and can also be seen with cachexia and lymphatic or vascular congestion, this interpretation must be made with caution. However, invasion is definite when a tumor mass is seen to extend directly into the adjacent muscle with obliteration of fat planes with enlargement of the individual muscle. Occasionally an enhancing intramuscular mass is seen.

Spread to contiguous organs in the pelvis should also be cautiously diagnosed and considered definite only if a major portion of the viscera is enveloped or if an obvious

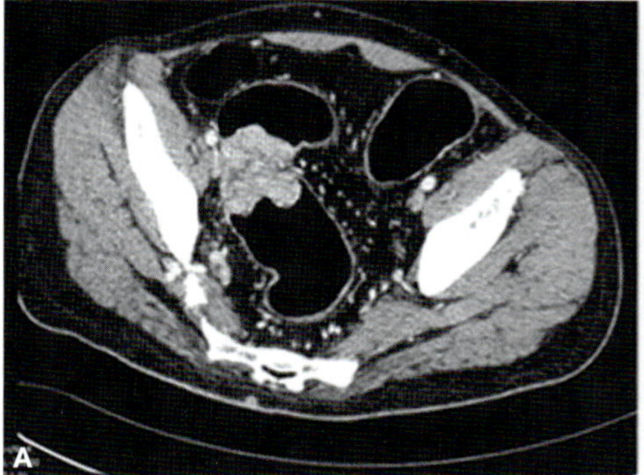

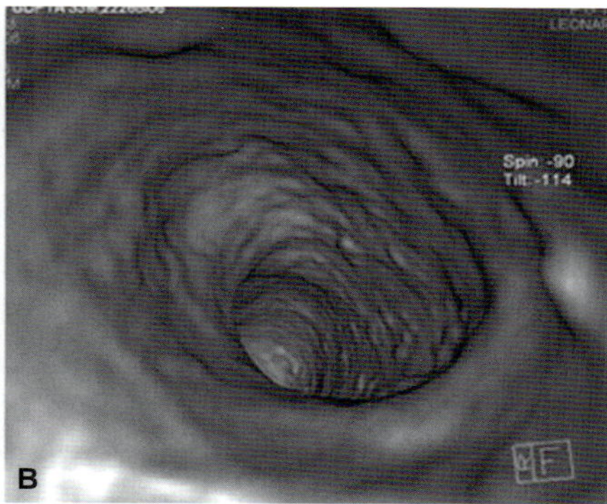

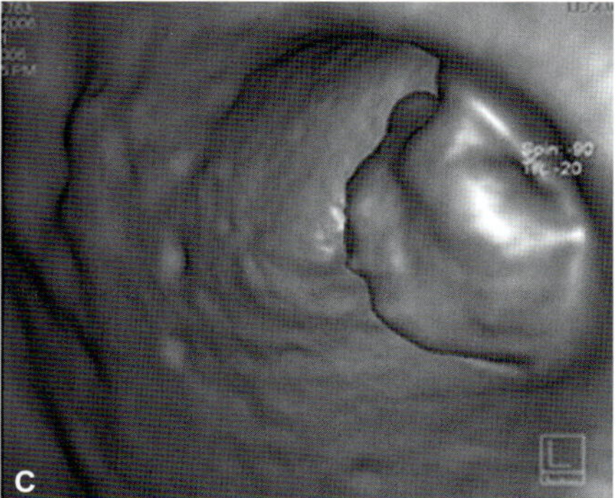

Figs 9.8A to C: (A) Axial CECT section shows a large polypoidal obstructive growth in the colon with increased vascularity in the adjacent mesentery. No pericolonic lymphnodes or stranding is seen. Actual colonoscopy was not possible in this patient, (B) CT colonography shows multiple pseudopolyps suggestive of ulcerative colitis and (C) the polypoidal growth in the sigmoid colon *(For color version see plate 1)*

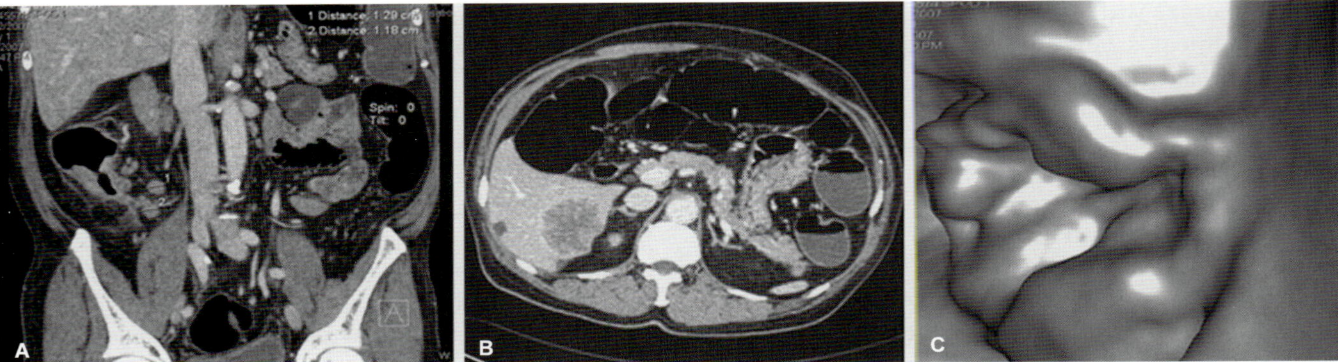

Figs 9.9A to C: (A) Coronal MPR image shows concentric mural thickening with a polypoidal component in the cecum. Pericolonic stranding and multiple enlarged pericolonic lymph nodes are also seen, (B) Axial CECT section of the upper abdomen shows hypodense lesions in segment VI of liver suggestive of metastases, (C) CT colonography endoluminal image shows the intraluminal irregular polypoidal growth *(For color version see plate 2)*

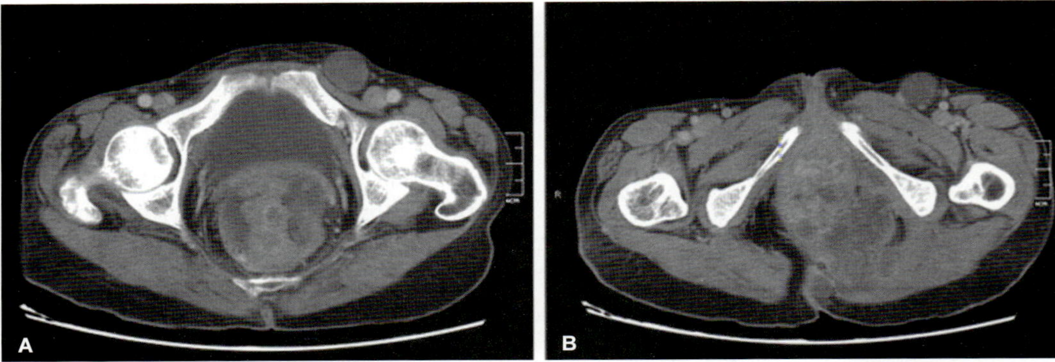

Figs 9.10A and B: Axial CECT sections show a large heterogeneous mass in the rectum obliterating the lumen. The planes of the mass with the vagina, lateral pelvic wall and gluteal muscles on the left side are lost consistent with invasion. A large left inguinal lymph node is also seen

mass involves an adjacent organ (Figs 9.10A and B). Primary or recurrent colonic cancers can invade the small and large bowel, the seminal vesicles, sciatic nerve, prostate, bladder, uterus and ovaries and can produce hydronephrosis by obstructing the ureters. Fistula between tumor and adjoining viscera such as bladder can be demonstrated by either direct visualization of fistulous tract on CECT or demonstration of air within bladder. Fistulation into uterovaginal areas, ischiorectal fossa and small bowel can occur. Colonic cancers can destroy the adjacent bone. Minor invasion of bone can present as cortical destruction. In advanced cases soft tissue mass with destruction of bones of sacrum, coccyx and ilium can be seen.

Regional lymph nodes are the most common metastatic site of colorectal carcinoma. CT cannot distinguish benign from malignant lymphadenopathy. Many metastatic foci are found in normal sized lymph nodes (< 1 cm). Likewise reactive inflammatory lymph nodes are frequently larger than 1 cm resulting in false positive assessment of nodal disease. Only lymphangiography or guided biopsy can give a definite diagnosis. Any non-enhancing mass in the perirectal fat should be considered to be malignant lymphadenopathy irrespective of the size as hyperplastic lymph nodes do not occur in this region.

Sites of distant metastasis generally include the liver, lung, adrenals, peritoneum, kidneys and bone marrow. The liver is the most common site of extranodal metastasis. On non-contrast CT scans, hepatic metastasis are typically discrete, hypodense lesions of variable size, although foci of calcification can be seen within metastatic mucinous adenocarcinoma. Following a bolus IV injection of iodinated contrast, deposits often show early peripheral enhancement or become uniformly hyperdense, go through an isodense phase and finally again become hypodense lesions. Scanning early in the dynamic phase to maximize liver-lesion contrast is critical to increase lesion conspicuity.

Peritoneal carcinomatosis caused by spread of tumor over peritoneal surface, is usually well demonstrated by CT and appears as linear or nodular peritoneal thickening which enhances with contrast and is associated with ascites. In patients with disseminated disease, careful analysis of chest CT may reveal metastatic nodules. In women with an advanced stage of colon carcinoma masses in the ovaries may be detected (Krukenberg's tumor).

CT scan is quite accurate in staging patients with advanced disease. Pitfalls occur in interpretation of scans in patients with less advanced tumors. Perforation/ ulceration of colonic cancer can result in an inflammatory mass or abscess which obscures the underlying cancer. CT scan obtained after surgery or radiation therapy can demonstrate edema or hemorrhage of the pelvic structures simulating residual/recurrent disease.

CT staging is based on an analysis of thickness of the colon wall and the presence or absence of tumor spread to adjacent and distant organs. Earlier studies have shown low accuracy (41-64%) for staging with conventional CT owing to low sensitivity of local tumor extent (53-77%) and of lymph node metastases (22-73%).[50] Recent studies have shown MDCT to be very useful in preoperative staging for colon cancer with accuracy of 4-slice CT being 83% for T-staging and 85% for N-staging.[51,52] In a study conducted at our Institute which was presented at the World Cancer Congress of UICC in 2008, the diagnostic accuracy for T-staging was 92.3% and for N-staging was 42.3%. [53] The lower specificity for lymph node metastases accounted for the lower accuracy of N-staging in this study.

CT Colonography

CT colonography is an innovative technique that entails CT examination of the entire colon and computerized processing of the raw data acquired after colon cleansing and colonic distension. It was in 1994 that Vining and Gelfand from Bowman Gray University introduced CT colonography and exhibited the first CT colonography fly-through video at the annual meeting of the Society of Gastrointestinal Radiologists.[54]

The accepted indications for CT colonography are as follows:

A. Incomplete colonoscopy due to an occlusive mass or stricture preventing examination of the proximal colon.
B. Incomplete colonoscopy due to colonic tortuosity, adhesions, severe diverticular disease or patient intolerance of colonoscopy.
C. Inability to perform colonoscopy due to requirement for anticoagulant therapy or risks of sedation.
D. Patients who adamantly refuse to undergo colonoscopy but have a strong indication for diagnostic colonoscopy.

CT colonography is under analysis as a screening tool for colorectal cancer because of its relative safety and greater patient acceptance as compared with other available screening methods.

The contraindication for CT colonography are allergy to contrast, suspected colonic perforation, acute colonic infection (acute diverticulitis, severe infective colitis), acute lower GI bleeding, complete colonic obstruction, very recent colonic surgery (< 1 week), medically unstable patients and refusal to undergo colonic preparation.

The technique involves colonic cleansing, colonic distension, image acquisition and post-processing of acquired data. For 'wet preparation' polyethylene glycol is used while for 'dry preparation' phospho-soda is used. Adequate colonic distension is critical for increasing polyp conspicuity. This can be achieved by using room air or carbon dioxide. Colonic perforation is extremely rare (0.59-0.08%).[55] The risk factors for perforation are advanced age and underlying colonic pathology. Image acquisition is done after colonic insufflation in supine and prone positions on a helical CT scanner using low dose technique. The radiation dose is about half of the dose of a barium enema.[55] Intravenous contrast improves detection of medium sized polyps (6-9 mm) especially in a suboptimally prepared colon. After acquiring supine and prone scans, various software packages are used to display images in both 2D and 3D (endoluminal) views.

There are various mimickers of polyps which are potential pitfalls of CT colonography. These include adherent fecal matter, lipomas, inverted appendiceal stump, prominent ileocecal valve, inverted diverticulum and bulbous colonic folds. While some of these are due to technical errors on account of inadequate colon preparation or distension, others are due to perceptive errors.

In the first published study from India the sensitivity and specificity of CT colonography has been reported to be 65% and 77% respectively for lesions 1-5 mm, 97% and 83% respectively for lesions 6-9 mm and 100% and 100% respectively for lesions 10 mm or larger.[56] CT colonography scores over optical colonoscopy as it provides information about extracolonic findings. The incidence of significant extracolonic findings ranges from 6.8 to 21%.[55] A reporting system for CT colonography has been devised by the Working Group on Virtual Colonoscopy and has been termed 'C-RADS' or CT Colonography reporting and Data System.[57] The aim of this reporting system is to achieve standardization of reporting. The advances in CT colonography include fluid and fecal tagging to achieve 'prepless' studies by digital bowel cleansing using subtraction techniques. Computer-aided detection (CAD) software and novel 3D views that slice open and flatten the colonic wall are being developed.

MR Imaging

MRI can be used to detect and stage rectosigmoid tumors more accurately than tumors in the rest of the colon. This increased accuracy is due to the fixed position of the rectosigmoid colon in relation to the pelvis. Many refinements have been described including MRI using an endorectal coil, addition of IV gadolinium chelate and the use of oral and rectal contrast agents to achieve bowel distension. High performance gradient, faster pulse sequences, and high resolution MRI are now routinely available, producing additional improvement in MRI quality.

Presently MRI using thin sections and phased-array coils can distinguish tumors localized to mucosa and submucosa (T1) and those that infiltrate the entire colonic wall (T_2) with a reasonable accuracy (65-85%).[58] Detection of tumor improves if proper colon cleansing and adequate distension can be obtained with administration of air, water or supraparamagnetic contrast medium. Imaging in prone position helps to decrease motion artifacts with better depiction of rectal tumors.

The different layers comprising the bowel wall on gadolinium enhanced T1-weighed fat-suppressed spin echo images are the high signal intensity mucosa, low signal intensity muscularis mucosa and lamina propria, high signal intensity submucosa and low signal intensity muscularis propria.

In T1W SE images, rectosigmoid tumors appear as wall thickening with signal intensity similar to or higher than skeletal muscles (long T1). Perirectal fat has short T1 and hence appears bright on T1WI and rectal air has no signal, thus these tumors are very well delineated on T1W images and their extension beyond the colonic wall is well visualized. If polyps or tumor contain a large amount of mucin, signal intensity can be higher on T1WI.

Gadolinium enhancement makes lesions more conspicuous (Figs 9.11A to C). On gadolinium enhanced SGE MR images with oral and rectal contrast the lesion is depicted as an enhancing soft tissue mass or as mural thickening.

On T2W images, the lesion is hyperintense to the muscle, but as fat is also hyperintense, contrast between the tumor and perirectal fat is not adequate and hence T2W images are not as useful as T1W images for diagnosing extracolonic extension. T2W images provide good contrast between tumor tissue and surrounding pelvic wall muscles as tumor is hyperintense and muscle hypointense on T2WI.

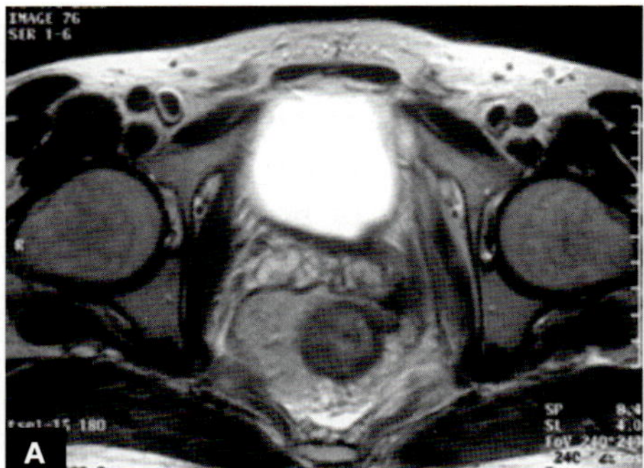

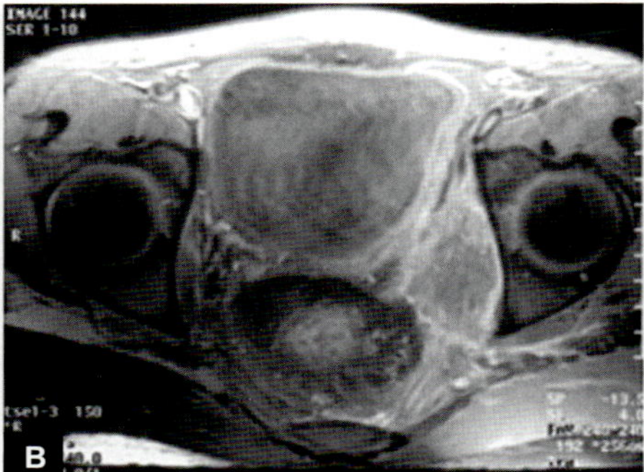

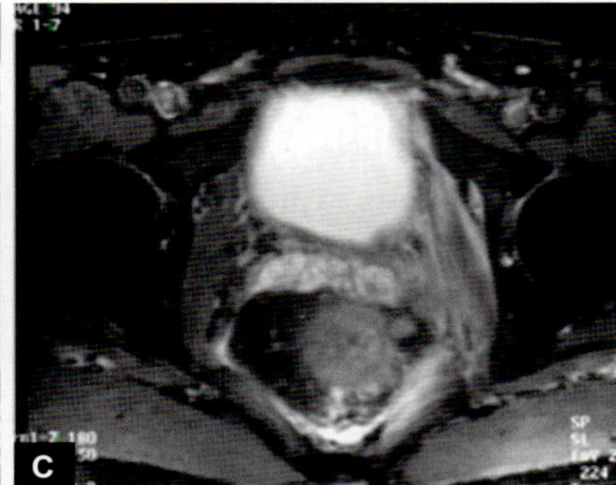

Figs 9.11A to C: T_2W and T_2W fat suppressed images show concentric mural thickening of the rectum. There is presence of perirectal lymph node, thickening of left mesorectal fascia and infiltration of the lateral pelvic wall with enhancement seen on CEMR (C)

Recent studies have shown that T2WI is superior to T1WI for evaluating the extent of tumor in relation to the rectal wall layers and the mesorectal fascia. [59,60] T2WI can demonstrate the mesorectal fascia better than T1WI. This has assumed importance since the introduction of total mesorectal excision (TME) for rectal cancer. In this the entire mesorectal compartment is removed which includes rectum, surrounding mesorectal fat with the perirectal lymph nodes and a thin fascia that envelopes the two former structures and is known as mesorectal fascia. The recurrence rate of cancer after TME is reported to be less than 10%.[61]

For evaluation of cancers involving the anal sphincter, images in the coronal plane are particularly useful. Routine MR imaging cannot recognize tumor foci in normal sized lymph nodes. A T1W SE sequence with fat suppression, readily demonstrates lymph nodes. Depicting tumor in normal sized lymph nodes may require the use of additional contrast agent directed at imaging nodal metastasis. Invasion of adjacent organs is demonstrated best by transverse or coronal MR images. Neither CT nor MRI can detect microinvasion.

Liver and adrenal metastases are as well demonstrated on MR as on helical CT. All extrahepatic anatomic sites must be evaluated carefully to assess for possible metastatic tumor. Peritoneal carcinomatosis is difficult to detect on MR images. Fat suppressed, gadolinium enhanced SGE MR images are most useful for extrahepatic imaging. Peritoneal deposits enhance slowly with gadolinium and are most conspicuous on delayed images obtained after 5 minutes delay. Surface implants on the liver may be detected by T2 WI without IV contrast material. The ability of MRI to depict subtle osseous metastases is an advantage compared with helical CT. MR imaging is superior to CT at distinguishing between fibrosis and recurrent cancer and could eliminate the need for biopsies.

More advanced MR technique includes the use of an endorectal surface coil which has the potential to allow differentiation of the bowel wall layers and thus permit more accurate 'T' stage determination. Comparison of endorectal MR (ERMRI), ERUS and 3D-ERUS have shown an overall similar accuracy for depicting the transmural extent of the rectal cancer, 91%, 84% and 88% respectively.[62] In a comparison of ERUS, ERMRI and CT in rectal cancer, Kim et al[63] have shown comparable accuracies of 81% for both ERUS and ERMRI for depth of tumor penetration which was superior to CT (65%).

Endorectal MRI does have some limitations. This technique cannot be performed in patients with severely stenotic infiltrating lesions. It is a rigid device with a small radial area of acceptable signal to noise imaging. It cannot adequately assess the mesorectal fascia and the circumferential resection margin (CRM).

MR Colonography

MR colonography is based on the acquisition of MR datasets of the abdomen which optimizes visualization of the large bowel. Data is acquired during single breath-hold scans. The bowel is distended per rectally with water, barium, room air or CO_2. Spasmolytics are given intravenously before rectal filling. Patient preparation involves use of cathartics and enemas. 2D and/or 3D fast imaging with steady-state precession (FISP) is a useful sequence for MR colonography. 3D TIW images are also acquired before and after administration of gadolinium intravenously. A T1W 2D FLASH (fast low-angle shot) sequence is also acquired in the axial plane for evaluation of adjacent abdominal organs. Axial, MPR and 'fly through' images are analyzed in both antegrade and retrograde directions. MR colonography has been reported to have 100% sensitivity for lesions larger than 10 mm and 89% for lesions 5 to 10 mm in size.[64] However, it has very limited accuracy for detecting lesions smaller than 5 mm.

The advantage of MR colonography over CT colonography is lack of ionizing radiation and superior soft tissue contrast. The disadvantages are lower spatial resolution, high susceptibility to motion artifacts, longer examination time and limited availability.

Arteriography

Arteriography has a limited value in colonic cancers. Its application is restricted to the investigation of patients with acute bleeding of apparent colonic origin with therapeutic embolization. The bleeding site may be demonstrated in patients with chronic low-grade blood loss. Arteriography with chemoembolization or radio-frequency ablation is also used for treating metastatic liver deposits in patients with colonic malignancies who are not surgical candidates.

Immunoscintigraphy

Labeled anticarcinoembryonic antigen (CEA) monoclonal antibodies (MoAbs) have been used as in vivo tumor localizing agents. Primary adenocarcinoma of colon and metastatic foci are seen as areas of increased radioactivity (hot spots). Depending on the size of tumor necrosis, liver metastases may appear as areas of intense, absent or intermediate uptake. The reported sensitivity of monocolonal antibody staging of colorectal cancer is 65 to 86% with specificity for detection of primary tumor, local recurrence and distant metastasis varying between 77 to 92%. [65]

PET

Fluorine 18- labeled deoxyglucose (18FDG) is used, and there is a remarkably close correlation between tumor grade and glucose utlization. This method can be used for detection of distant, residual or recurrent disease. Malignant tissue demonstrates more rapid uptake with accumulation compared with normal tissue. Time activity curves of glucose utilization are generated for region of interest and pathologic areas are compared with surrounding normal tissue by generating a differential absorption ratio.

Recent Advances

These include PET/CT colonography and CT perfusion imaging for colorectal tumors. PET/CT colonography involves the combination of 18F-FDG PET with CT colonography. It provides both anatomic and functional information. It has been used both for staging of colon cancer as well as for screening purposes.[66,67] The standard uptake value of malignant tumors has been reported to be between 4 and 20 with a mean of 9.[67]

Tumor perfusion of rectal cancer has been measured with first pass perfusion CT. Rectal cancers show higher blood flow (BF) and shorter mean transit time (MTT) compared with those of normal rectum. After chemotherapy and radiotherapy, responders show significant reduction in BF and increase in MTT. [68,69] Significant difference in baseline BF and MTT is seen between responders and nonresponders.

Other Malignant Tumors of Colon

Squamous cell carcinomas are rare except in the rectum. Radiographic appearance is similar to adenocarcinima and differentiation from other tumors is possible only by biopsy.

Cloacogenic carcinomas arise from transitional cloacogenic remnants of the anorectal junction. Radiographically the lesions are plaque like and have a smooth or finely irregular surface. In profile the borders form a tapered obtuse angle with the bowel wall. Ulceration is usually present. Since the lesions lie in the distal rectal areas, the catheter tip may completely obscure the lesion.

Gastrointestinal stromal tumors (GISTs) arise from the interstitial cells of Cajal and express CD34. Only 1% of all GI tumors are of stromal origin and these are least commonly located in the colon. Small tumors are seen as sessile or pedunculated polyps. Large tumors may be seen as cavitating masses with a large extraluminal component or as submucosal masses with or without central ulceration (Fig. 9.12). These lesions may mimic colonic lymphoma or carcinoma.

Carcinoid tumors present as submucosal lesions. The most common sites of colonic carcinoids are the rectum and cecum. They are seen as round, well circumscribed masses (Figs 9.13A and B). Invasion of the bowel wall by tumor mass produces intense desmoplastic reaction and proliferation of fibrous tissue, resulting in contraction and kinking of the large bowel. Carcinoid tumors located in cecum and ascending colon are indistinguishable from adenocarcinoma on imaging.

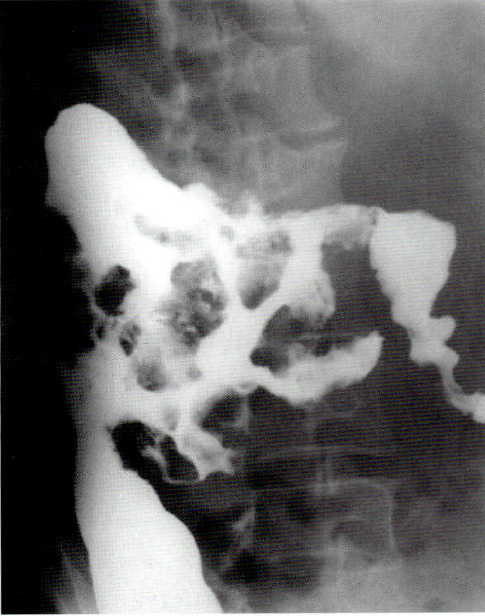

Fig. 9.12: Barium enema shows a large cavitatory mass lesion in the hepatic flexure with presence of deep ulcerations in a patient with leiomyosarcoma (Courtesy: Dr B Nagi, Department of Gastroenterology, PGIMER)

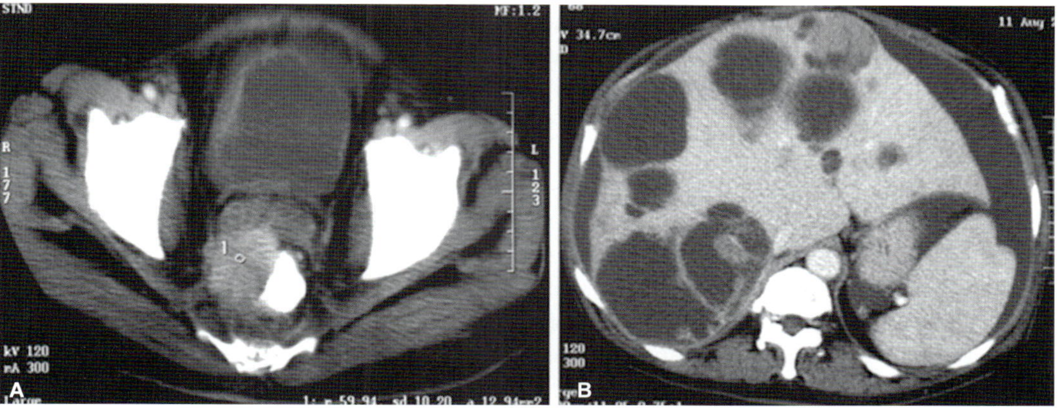

Figs 9.13A and B: Axial CECT sections show a well-defined mass lesion along the right lateral wall of the rectum (A) with multiple cystic focal lesions in the liver (B) some of which are showing solid component in a patient with biopsy proven carcinoid

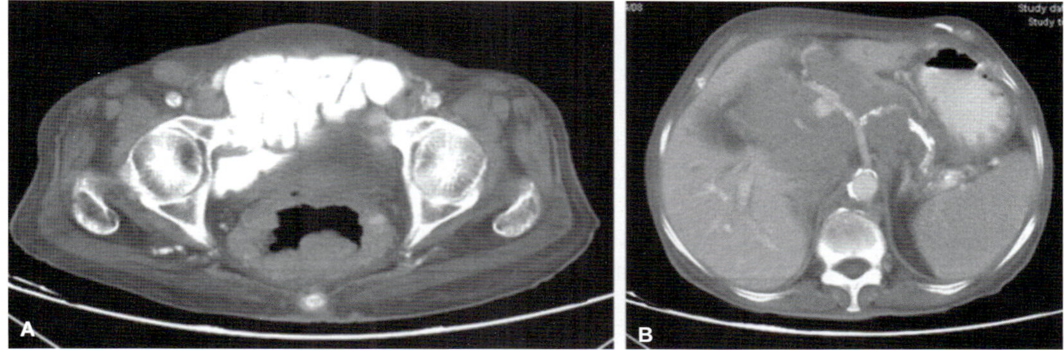

Figs 9.14 A and B: Axial CECT sections show concentric nodular mural thickening of the rectum (A) with conglomerate lymph nodal mass encasing the celiac trunk (B) in a patient with disseminated lymphoma

Mesodermal sarcomas of the large bowel are uncommon. They have a predilection for the rectal region. The lesions are usually rounded and lobulated but may be pedunculated. The tumors may grow extramurally and when the overlying mucosa ulcerates, necrosis and cystic cavitations can develop. Kaposi's sarcoma can involve any part of the gastrointestinal tract and presents as typical extramucosal mass or masses. On imaging Kaposi's sarcoma is seen as a flat or plaque like lesion, a small polypoid nodule or a polypoid submucosal lesion with or without umbilication.

Lymphoma of the colon is rare. The colon is the third most common primary site of lymphoma involving the gastrointestinal tract after stomach and the small bowel. As a primary lesion, lymphoma accounts for only 0.5% of all malignant tumors. Secondary involvement is usually widely distributed and often multicentric (Figs 9.14A and B). The radiographic pattern may be localized or diffuse. In the localized form the lesion is either a polypoid mass that protrudes into the colonic lumen or a constricting lesion that simulates an annular carcinoma. In the diffuse form multiple small nodular lesions are seen. The defects are submucosal in origin with intact overlying mucosa. When lymphoma involves the mesentery, large masses may compress the colon.

Tumors that commonly metastasize to colon include stomach, breast, pancreas and gynecologic pelvic malignancies. Infiltration of the colon by secondary tumors produces thickening of the colonic wall and mucosal folds. The classic radiographic appearances include indentations, spiculation, angulation, narrowing, displacement and fixation. Lymphogenous spread of tumors to the colon is characterized by the involvement of long segments, variable narrowing and loss of haustral markings. When metastases occur by the hematogenous route, as in melanoma, lesions present as smoothly marginated submucosal masses.

CONCLUSION

Colorectal cancer is a unique malignancy as it represents a preventable disease. The adenoma-carcinoma sequence reiterates the need for screening for polyps which are precursors of colorectal cancer. Screening is of immense importance in countries which have high prevalence of colorectal cancer. Though this malignancy has a low prevalence in the Indian subcontinent, it is expected to increase as more people are adopting Western lifestyle and dietary habits.

Imaging plays a key role in the screening programe as well as for detection and staging of colorectal cancer. For screening purpose the radiological options include, DCBE and CT colonography. CT colonography is presently under evaluation as a possible technique which could replace actual colonoscopy for the purpose of screening. The high sensitivity of CT colonography for detecting clinically significant polyps >1 cm has been possible due to the spectacular advances in CT technology.

Endoscopic sonography, CT and MRI are the primary cross-sectional techniques used for staging of colorectal cancer. Of these modalities MDCT is preferred due to its ability to evaluate the entire colon, better spatial resolution, wider availability and limited cost.

Among the recent advances, PET/CT colonography and perfusion CT are promising techniques as they provide anatomical as well as functional information and are very useful for evaluating residual or recurrent tumor.

REFERENCES

1. Jemal A, Siegel R, Ward E, et al. Cancer statistics, 2007. CA Cancer J Clin 2007;57:43-66.
2. Seidman H, Mushinski MH, Gelb SK, et al. Probability of eventually developing and dying of cancers: United States, 1995. CA Cancer J Clin 1985;35:36-56.
3. Theoni RF, Laufer I. Polyps and carcinoma of the colon. In Gore RM, Levine MS (Eds): WB Saunders, Philadelphia. Textbook of Gastrointestinal Radiology 2008;1121-1166.
4. Mohandas KM, Desai DC. Epidemiology of digestive tract cancers in India. Ind J Gastroenterol 1999;18:118-21.
5. Potter JD, Slattery ML, Bostick RM, et al. Colon cancer: A review of the epidemiology. Epidemiol Rev 1993;15: 499-545.
6. Fleshner B, Slater G, Aufses AH. Age and sex distribution of patients with colorectal cancer. Dis Colon Rectum 1989;32:107-11.
7. Bond JH. Colonic tumors. Endoscopy 1998;30:150-157.
8. Kritchevsky D. Colorectal cancer- the role of dietary fat and caloric restriction. Mutat Res 1993;290:63-70.
9. Heilbrum LK, Nomura A, Hankin JH, et al. Diet and colorectal cancer with special reference to fiber intake. Int J Cancer 1989;44:1-6.
10. Gore RM. Colorectal cancer: Clinical and pathologic features. Radiologic Clinics of North America 1997;35: 403-29.
11. McFaralane MJ, Welch KE. Gallstones, cholecystectomy and colorectal cancer. Am J Gastroenterol 1992;87: 1120-24.
12. Wilson RE, Donohue JH. Neoplasia of the colorectum. In Phillips SF, Pemberton JH, Shorter RG (eds). Raven Press, New York. The large intestine: Physiology, pathophysiology and disease. 1991;521-47.
13. Fenlon HM, McAneny DB, Nunes DP, et al. Occlusive colon carcinoma: Virtual colonoscopy in the preoperative evaluation of the proximal colon. Radiology 1999;210: 423-28.
14. Bulow S, Svendsen LB, Mellemgaard A. Metachronous colorectal carcinoma. Br J Surg 1990;77:502-5.
15. Cali RL, Pitsch RM, Thorson AG, et al. Cumulative incidence of metachronous colorectal cancer. Dis Colon Rectum 1993;36:388-93.
16. Lane N, Fenglio CM. The adenoma-carcinoma sequence in the stomach and colon: I. Observation on the adenoma as precursor to ordinary large bowel carcinoma. Gastrointest Radiol 1976;1:111-19.
17. Cooper HS, Deppisch LM, Gourley WK, et al. Endoscopically removed malignant colorectal polyps: Clinicopathologic correlations. Gastroenterology 1995;108:1657-65.
18. Lev R, Lee M. Colorectal carcinoma: Pathology. In Rustgi AK (Ed). Gastrointestinal cancers: Biology, diagnosis, and therapy. Lippincott- Raven: Philadelphia 1995;379-98.
19. Dodd GD. Malignancies In: Alimentary tract radiology. Margulis AR, Burhenne HJ (Eds) 4th ed: The CV Mosby Company 1989;1051-92.
20. Gore RM, Meyers MA. Pathways of abdominal and pelvic disease spread. In Gore RM, Levine MS, Laufer I (Eds): Textbook of Gastrointestinal Radiology. WB Saunders: Philadelphia 1994;2352-66.
21. Turnbull RB. The no-touch isolation technique of resection. JAMA 1975;231:1181-85.
22. Johnson RD, Geisinger KR. Colorectal adenocarcinoma: Staging and histopathology. Seminars in Roentgenology 1996;31:94-102.
23. Berlin JW, Gore RM, Yaghmai V, et al. Staging of colorectal cancer. Seminars in Roentgenology 2000;35:370-84.
24. Silva AC, Hara AK, Leighton JA, et al. CT colonography with intravenous contrast material: varied appearance of colorectal carcinoma. Radiographics 2005;25:1321-34.
25. Mandel JS. Screening for colorectal cancer. Gastroenterol Clin N Am 2008;37:97-115.

26. Pamela M, McMahon G, Scott G. The case for colorectal screening. Seminars in Roentgenology 2000;35:325-32.
27. Winawer SJ, Stewart ET, Zauber AG, et al. A comparison of colonoscopy and double-contrast barium enema for surveillance after polypectomy. National Polyp Work Group. N Engl J Med 2000;342;1766-72.
28. Winawer SJ, Zauber AG, Ho MN, et al. Prevention of colorectal cancer by colonoscopic polypectomy. N Eng J Med 1993;329:1977-81.
29. Citarda F, Tomaselli G, Capocaccia R, et al. Efficacy in standard clinical practice of colonoscopic polypectomy in reducing colorectal cancer incidence. Gut 2001;48: 812-15.
30. van Rijn JC, Reitsma JB, Stoker J, et al. Polyp miss rate determined by tandem colonoscopy: a systemic review. Am J Gastroenterol 2006;101:343-50.
31. Johnson CD, Chen MH, Toledano AY, et al. Accuracy of CT colonoscopy for detection of large adenomas and cancers. N Engl J Med 2008;359;1207-17.
32. Gelfand DW. Colorectal cancer: Screening strategies. Radiology Clinics of North America 1997;35:431-38.
33. Brady AP, Stevenson GW, Stevenson I. Colorectal cancer overlooked at barium enema examination and colonoscopy: A continuing perceptual problem. Radiology 1994;192;373-78.
34. Ott DJ, Gelfand DW. How to improve the efficacy of the barium enema examination. AJR Am J Roentgenol 1993;160;491-95.
35. Ott DJ, Gelfand DW, Ramquist NA, et al. Causes of error in gastrointestinal radiology: II Barium enema examination. Gastrointest Radiol 1980;5;99-105.
36. Gelfand DW, Ott DJ. Cost-effective screening for colorectal cancer. The radiologist's view. Primary Care and Cancer 1992;12:11-3.
37. Stevenson GW. Normal anatomy and technique of examination of the colon: Barium, CT and MRI. In Freeny PC, Stevenson GW (Eds) : Margulis and Burhenne's Alimentary Tract Radiology. Mosby and company, St Louis 1994;692.
38. Laufer I, Kressel HY. Principles of double contrast diagnosis. In Laufer I, Levine MS (Eds). Double contrast gastrointestinal radiology. WB Saunders, Philadelphia 1992;9-54.
39. Youker JE, Welin S. Differentiation of true polypoid tumors of the colon from extraneous material: A new roentgen sign. Radiology 1985;84;610-15.
40. Buetow PC, Buck JL, Carr NJ, et al. Colorectal adenocarcinima: Radiologic-pathologic correlation. Radiographics 1995;15:127-46.
41. Delamarre J, Descombes P, Marti R, et al. Villous tumors of the colon and rectum: Double-contrast study of 47 cases. Gastrointest Radiol 1980;5:69-73.
42. Bond JH. Polyp guideline: Diagnosis, treatment, and surveillance for patients with nonfamilal colorectal polyps. Ann Intern Med 1993;119:836-43.
43. Lappas JC, Maglinte DDT, Kopecky KK, et al. Diverticular disease: Imaging with post-double contrast sigmoid flush. Radiology 1988;168;35-7.
44. Kelvin FM, Gardiner R, Vas W, et al. Colorectal carcinoma missed on double contrast barium enema study: A problem in perception. AJR Am J Roentgenol 1981; 137;307-13.
45. Dubbins PA. The small bowel and colon. In Abdominal and general ultrasound. Cosgrove D, Meire H, Dewbury K (Eds). Churchill Livingstone 1993;2:765-76.
46. Bernd L. Diagnosis of large bowel tumors by colonic sonography. The Lancet 1990;20:144-46.
47. Glaser F, Schalg P, Harfarth C. Endorectal ultrasonography for the assessment of invasion of rectal tumors and lymph node involvement. Br J Surg 1990;77:883-87.
48. Hulsmans FH, Tio TL, Mathus-Vliegen EMH, et al. Colorectal villous adenoma: Transrectal US in screening for invasive malignancy. Radiology 1992;185;193-96.
49. Scharling ES, Wolfman NT, Bechtold RE. Computed tomography evaluation of colorectal carcinoma. Seminars in Roentgenology 1996;31:142-53.
50. Regina GH, Beets T, Beets GL. Rectal cancer: Review with emphasis on MR imaging. Radiology 2004;232:335-46.
51. Filippone A, Ambrosini R, Fuschi M, et al. Preoperative T and N staging of colorectal cancer. Accuracy of contrast enhanced multidetector row CT colonography-Initial experience. Radiology 2004;231;83-90.
52. Chung DJ, Huh KC, Choi WJ, et al. CT colonography using 16-MDCT in the evaluation of colorectal cancer. AJR Am J Roentgenol 2005;184:98-103.
53. Kalra N, Narayanan S, Wig JD, et al. Staging of colon cancer by contrast enhanced multidetector computed tomographic colonography (CEMDCTC) Presented in the World Cancer Congress (UICC), Geneva (Switzerland) 2008.
54. Vining DJ, Gelfand DW. Non-invasive colonoscopy using helical CT scanning, 3D reconstruction and virtual reality. Presented in the syllabus of the 23rd annual meeting. Society of Gastrointestinal Radiologists. Maui (Hawaii) 1994.
55. Summerton S, Little E, Cappell MS. CT colonography: Current status and future promise. Gastroenterol Clin N Am 2008;37:161-89.
56. Kalra N, Suri S, Bhasin DK, et al. Comparison of multidetector computed tomographic colonography and conventional colonoscopy for detection of colorectal polyps and cancer. Ind J Gastroenterol 2006;25;229-32.
57. Zallis ME, Barish MA, Choi JR, et al. CT colonography reporting and data system: A consensus proposal. Radiology 2005;236;3-9.
58. Brown G, Radcliffe AG, Newcombe RG, et al. Preoperative assessment of prognostic factors in rectal cancer using high-resolution magnetic resonance imaging. Br J Surg 2003;90:355-64.
59. Beets-Tan RG, Beets GL, Vliegen RF, et al. Accuracy of magnetic resonance imaging in prediction of tumor-free resection margin in rectal cancer surgery. Lancet 2001;357:497-504.
60. Brown G, Kirkham A, Williams GT, et al. High-resolution MRI of the anatomy important in total mesorectal excision of the rectum. AJR Am J Roentgenol 2004;182:431-39.

61. Heald RJ, Ryall RD. Recurrence and survival after total mesorectal excision for rectal cancer. Lancet 1986;1: 1479-82.
62. Hunerbein M, Pegios W, Rau B, et al. Prospective comparison of endorectal ultrasound, three dimensional endorectal ultrasound and endorectal MRI in the preoperative evaluation of rectal tumors. Preliminary results. Surg Endosc 2000;14:1005-09.
63. Kim NK, Kim MJ, Yan SH, et al. Comparative study of transrectal ultrasonography, pelvic computerized tomography and magnetic resonance imaging in preoperative staging of rectal cancer. Dis Colon Rectum 1999;42:770-75.
64. Ajay W, Pelster G, Treichel U, et al. Dark lumen magnetic resonance colonography: Comparsion with conventional colonoscopy for the detection of colorectal pathology. Gut 2003;52:1738-43.
65. Britton KE, Granowska M. The diagnostic role of radiolabelled antibodies. In Murrary IPS, EII PJ (Eds): Nuclear medicine in clinical diagnosis and treatment. Churchill Livingstone: Edinburgh 1998;871-92.
66. Kinner S, Antoch G, Bockisch A, et al. Whole-body PET/CT colonography: a possible new concept for colorectal cancer staging. Abdom Imaging 2007;32:606-12.
67. Gollub MJ, Akhurst T, Markowitz AJ, et al. Combined CT colonography and 18F- FDG PET of colon polyps: potential technique for selective detection of cancer and precancerous lesions. AJR Am J Roentgenol 2007;188: 130-8.
68. Sahani DV, Kalva SP, Hamberg LM, et al. Assessing tumor perfusion and treatment response in rectal cancer with multisection CT: initial observations Radiology 2005;234;785-92.
69. Bellomi M, Petralia G, Sonzogni A, et al. CT perfusion for the monitoring of neoadjuvant chemotherapy and radiation therapy in rectal carcinoma: initial experience. Radiology 2007;244;486-93.

Chapter Ten

Lymphoma of the Gastrointestinal Tract

Anupam Lal, Mahesh Prakash

INTRODUCTION

Extranodal lymphomas may arise anywhere outside the lymph node regions. Gastrointestinal lymphoma is an uncommon disease but is the most frequently occurring extranodal lymphoma constituting 2-4% of all malignant tumors of the gastrointestinal tract.[1] The gastrointestinal tract (GIT) may be involved by lymphoma as a primary tumor or as a part of generalized disease process. Secondary involvement is common because of the frequent occurrence of lymphomas in the mesenteric or retroperitoneal nodes and the abundance of lymphoid tissue in the gastrointestinal tract and may be seen in up to 50% of cases of disseminated lymphomas.[2] Generally, the lymphoma is considered "primary" in the gastrointestinal tract, when the initial symptoms of the disease are in the abdomen and present as gastrointestinal disturbances.

Dawson *et al*[3] have cited five criteria for diagnosis of primary gastrointestinal lymphoma as follows:

1. No palpable superficial lymph nodes
2. Normal chest radiograph (no adenopathy)
3. Normal white cell count (both total and differential)
4. At laparotomy, the alimentary lesion must predominate and lymph node involvement, if any, must be confined to the drainage area of the involved segment of gut
5. No involvement of liver and spleen.

Primary GI lymphoma in advanced stage may eventually disseminate widely and be clinically, radiologically, and pathologically indistinguishable from secondary GI lymphoma.[4]

Risk factors predisposing to lymphoma include HIV infection, Helicobacter pylori infection, celiac disease, inflammatory bowel disease, congenital immunodeficiency states and immunosuppression after solid organ transplantation.

Lymphoma generally occurs in 5th and 6th decade in both sexes, but a double peak has also been reported–below 10 years. Thus though rare, they are reported to be most common GI tumors in children.[5]

In both primary and secondary forms, stomach is most commonly affected (51%), followed by small bowel (33%), large bowel (16%) and esophagus (< 1%).

Pathology

Lymphoma is a general term for a group of cancers that originate in the lymphatic system. The lymphomas are divided into two major categories: Hodgkin lymphoma (HL) and non-Hodgkin lymphoma (NHL). In 2001, the World Health Organization published a comprehensive classification system for lymphoid neoplasm incorporating entities like morphology, immunology, genetic features, and clinical features. The three large groups are (1) the B-cell tumors, (2) the T-cell and natural killer cell tumors, and (3) HL.

Majority of lymphomas involving GIT are non-Hodgkin's lymphomas and of B-cell origin. In 1982, working formulation of clinical usage was formulated classifying NHL into three prognostic groupings (i) low grade, (ii) intermediate, and (iii) high grade.[6] Low grade lymphomas are follicular or small lymphocytic type, diffuse infiltrative lymphomas constitute the intermediate grade whereas the high grade lymphomas include lymphoblastic and immunoblastic lymphomas (derived from immunoblasts which are formed by maturation and transformation of B-lymphocytes).

The B-cell lymphoma can be subdivided into (MALT) lymphoma, immunoproliferative small-intestinal disease (IPSID), and Burkitt lymphoma.

It is now well accepted that most low grade B-cell primary gastrointestinal lymphomas arise from mucosa associated lymphoid tissue (MALT). These tumors form a distinct pathological entity as they remain localized for a long time and have a much better prognosis. This type of GI lymphoma usually affects adults, has no gender predilection, and may arise anywhere in the gut. Stomach is the most common site of involvement which is normally devoid of any lymphoid tissue, but as a result of chronic infection by *Helicobacter pylori* (*H. pylori*) there is proliferation of lymphoid tissue in the gastric mucosa with accumulation of lymphoid follicles in the lamina propria which later transform into low grade B-cell MALT lymphoma.[7] These may subsequently undergo transformation into intermediate or high grade lymphoma if left untreated. More than 80% of patients having gastric MALT lymphoma have been shown to have chronic H.pylori infection. Following eradication of infection with antibiotics, low grade MALT lymphoma is known to undergo complete remission.[8]

IPSID also referred to as Mediterranean lymphoma commonly affects the children and young adults without any sex predilection. A high proportion of patients have malabsorption and weight loss preceding the development of the lymphoma.

Less common lymphomas of GIT are the T-cell type (often associated with enteropathy); Burkitt lymphoma; and the slow-growing types, mantle cell and follicular lymphoma.

Enteropathy-type intestinal T-cell lymphoma represents one end of a spectrum of disorders including refractory sprue and ulcerative jejunitis characterized by a proliferation of phenotypically abnormal mucosal T-cell clones.

Some investigators have also attempted to classify T-cell lymphoma of the intestine, including enteropathy-associated T-cell lymphoma, enteropathy-associated T-cell–like lymphoma without enteropathy, and non–enteropathy-associated T-cell lymphoma, according to the histopathologic findings.[9] The incidence of malabsorption and intestinal recurrence is high in enteropathy-associated T-cell lymphoma. A history of autoimmune or lymphoproliferative disorders or celiac disease has been reported in a minority of cases.[10]

Staging

The Ann Arbor staging system, introduced in 1970 and routinely used in nodal non-Hodgkin's lymphoma has also been used for gastrointestinal lymphoma with several modifications and alternatives.

Ann Arbor Staging of Extranodal Lymphoma (Modified by Musshoff)[11]

- IE Lymphoma restricted to GI tract on one side of diaphragm
- IE1 Infiltration limited to mucosa and submucosa
- IE2 Infiltration extending beyond submucosa
- IIE Lymphoma infiltrating lymph nodes on same side of diaphragm
- IIE1 Infiltration of regional lymph nodes
- IIE2 Infiltration of lymph nodes beyond regional nodes
- IIIE Lymphoma infiltrating GIT and/ or lymph nodes on both sides of diaphragm
- IV Diffuse or disseminated involvement of liver, spleen, lung, brain

However, neither differentiation of stage IE1 (confinement of lymphoma to the mucosa and submucosa) from stage IE_2 nor discrimination of stage IIE1 (involvement of regional lymph nodes) from stage IIE2 (node involvement beyond the regional area, as assessed in the Musshoff modification[11] is sufficiently serving the demand for documenting all features of lymphoma. To meet these shortcomings, the Lugano classification was constructed by Rohatiner and colleagues[12] introducing stage IIE for "serosa penetration" without lymph node involvement into the Ann Arbor system. This represents a change in meaning of stage IIE that originally indicated lymph node involvement.

TNM staging for tumors of epithelial origin has also been proposed as an alternative in gastrointestinal lymphoma to describe localized disease. The 'T' part of this system pertains to the anatomical structure of the organs and sufficiently fulfills the requirements for staging of local extent of the disease.

Recently a modified TNM staging system has been proposed by European Gastrointestinal Lymphoma Study Group (EGILS), named after the first venue of the group in Paris.[13] The staging system adequately records: (1) depth of tumor infiltration; (2) extent of nodal involvement; as well as (3) specific lymphoma spreading.

It is adjusted to the gastrointestinal origin of the lymphoma, considering histopathological characteristics of extranodal B and T-cell lymphomas.

Paris staging system for primary gastrointestinal lymphomas*†

TX	Lymphoma extent not specified
TO	No evidence of lymphoma
T1	Lymphoma confined to the mucosa/submucosa
T1m	Lymphoma confined to mucosa
T1sm	Lymphoma confined to submucosa
T2	Lymphoma infiltrates muscularis propria or subserosa
T3	Lymphoma penetrates serosa (visceral peritoneum) without invasion of adjacent structures
T4	Lymphoma invades adjacent structures or organs
NX	Involvement of lymph nodes not assessed
NO	No evidence of lymph node involvement
N1‡	Involvement of regional lymph nodes
N2	Involvement of intra-abdominal lymph nodes beyond the regional area
N3	Spread to extra-abdominal lymph nodes
MX	Dissemination of lymphoma not assessed
MO	No evidence of extranodal dissemination
M1	Non-continuous involvement of separate site in gastrointestinal tract (e.g., stomach and rectum)
M2	Non-continuous involvement of other tissues (e.g., peritoneum, pleura) or organs (e.g., tonsils, parotid gland, ocular adnexa, lung, liver, spleen, kidney, breast, etc.)
BX	Involvement of bone marrow not assessed
B0	No evidence of bone marrow involvement
B1	Lymphomatous infiltration of bone marrow
TNM	Clinical staging: status of tumor, node, metastasis, bone marrow
pTNMB	Histopathological staging: status of tumor, node, metastasis, bone marrow
pN	The histological examination will ordinarily include 6 or more lymph nodes

Radiological staging of primary gastrointestinal lymphoma is best made with the classification system adopted at the consensus conference in Luguano in 1993.[12]

Stage I—Tumor confined to GI tract, single primary site or multiple noncontiguous lesions.

Stage II—Tumor extends into the abdominal cavity from the primary GI site.

II1—Local nodal involvement

II2—Distant nodal involvement.

Stage III—Penetration through serosa to involve adjacent organs or tissues.

Stage IV—Disseminated extranodal involvement or a GI tract lesion with supradiaphragmatic nodal involvement.

Clinical Presentation

Clinical presentation depends on the gross morphological type. Abdominal pain is the most common presenting symptom.[14] Patients may also have features of malabsortion, anorexia and weight loss with a palpable abdominal mass with or without GI hemorrhage depending upon the presence or absence of ulceration.

Imaging Modalities

Diagnostic imaging studies play an important role in documenting lymphoma, staging and re-staging the disease, evaluating treatment response and performing follow-up evaluations.

*Valid for lymphomas originating from the gastroesophageal junction to the anus (as defined by identical histomorphological structure).

†In case of more than one visible lesion synchronously originating in the gastrointestinal tract, give the characteristics of the more advanced lesion.

‡Anatomical designation of lymph nodes as "regional" according to site:

a. stomach: perigastric nodes and those located along the ramifications of the coeliac artery (that is, left gastric artery, common hepatic artery, splenic artery) in accordance with compartments I and II of the Japanese Research Society for Gastric Cancer (1995);
b. duodenum: pancreaticoduodenal, pyloric, hepatic, and superior mesenteric nodes;
c. jejunum/ileum: mesenteric nodes and, for the terminal ileum only, the ileocolic as well as the posterior caecal nodes;
d. colorectum: pericolic and perirectal nodes and those located along the ileocolic, right, middle, and left colic, inferior mesenteric, superior rectal, and internal iliac arteries.

Barium Studies and Computed Tomography (CT)

The barium examination and CT are commonly used imaging modalities for evaluation of GI lymphomas. Both are complementary however, CT is more useful for overall staging of disease. Gastrointestinal lymphoma has a variable imaging appearances and definite diagnosis relies on histopathological analysis however certain imaging findings like bulky mass or diffuse infiltration with preservation of fat planes, no obstruction, multiple site involvement and associated bulky lymphadenopathy can suggest the diagnosis. Imaging also has important role in detection of complications associated with disease process such as obstruction, perforation and fistulization.

CT Enteroclysis

Computed tomography (CT) enteroclysis is a new technique consisting of helical CT of the abdomen after administration of water through a nasojejunal tube and intravenous contrast, resulting in adequate distension and visualization of the small bowel wall thus the technique is useful to characterize the lesions as endoluminal, exophytic, or mixed. Tumor characterization and staging can be performed using a single examination. CT enteroclysis is less invasive than enteroscopy and definitely more sensitive than SBFT and conventional CT examination for detection of small bowel tumors.[15, 16]

MRI

The accuracy of MR imaging in detecting lymph node and organ involvement in GIT lymphoma is similar to that of CT.[17] MR imaging reveals the lymphoma masses to be low to iso-signal intensity onT1-weighted images and moderately high signal on T2-weighted. Active untreated tumor tissue contains an excess of free water, which increases the signal intensity on T2-weighted imaging. With successful treatment, cellular elements and the water content of the tumor are reduced. Tumor masses are hyper intense onT2-weighted images, and chronic fibrosis or scar is often hypo intense.

The mucosa of gastrointestinal tract can strongly enhance after intravenous gadolinium contrast administration. The wall is composed of three zones: high-intensity mucosa, intermediate-intensity submucosal tumor infiltration, and a low-intensity proper muscular layer. This three-zone appearance may be useful in differentiating a submucosal tumor from the ones arising from the mucosa.[18] In addition to the detection of gastrointestinal tract abnormalities, MRI offers further information about extraluminal tumor extent, mesenteric or retroperitoneal Lymphadenopathy, and other organ involvement similar to CT scan.

Radionuclide Imaging

Anatomical imaging modalities including computed tomography (CT) and magnetic resonance (MR) imaging have some limitations, especially when defining the viability of the residual mass, treatment response or both.

Gallium-67 scintigraphy has been proposed as a functional imaging modality to assess remission and to evaluate the nature of residual masses in patients with lymphoma. However, gallium-67 scintigraphy is of little use in the abdomen because of the high hepatic uptake and excretion into the bowel and should be performed before treatment to determine whether the patient has a gallium-fixing tumor and whether the absence of fixation after treatment corresponds to a residual mass.

PET using 2-(18)F-fluoro-2-deoxy-D-glucose (FDG), a radioactive derivative of glucose, is an advanced imaging tool, based on the increased glucose consumption of cancer cells. Recently, it has been shown that PET imaging may provide valuable information with respect to diagnosis, extent and evaluation of therapy in patients of lymphoma. Nodes considered to be benign on CT scan based on size criteria are often positive on PET suggesting lymphomatous involvement.[19] PET is superior to both US and CT in differentiation of metastatic lymph nodes from reactive lymphadenopathy as well as for detection of tumor in normal sized lymph nodes.[20]

Fluorodeoxyglucose positron emission tomography (FDG-PET) is now considered the most accurate tool for the assessment of treatment response and prognosis in patients with Hodgkin lymphoma and aggressive non-Hodgkin lymphoma. However, there are some limitations, such as low FDG uptake in some cancers, substantial FDG uptake in inflammatory cells, and the lack of anatomical information and poor imaging quality of PET. A recently developed integrated PET/computed tomography (CT) system, which combines a PET camera and CT scanner in a single session, has overcome these drawbacks by providing both anatomical and functional imaging at the same position. PET-CT fusion images improve the accuracy of primary staging and development of recurrent disease and can directly guide biopsies and interventional procedures.[21]

Radiological Findings

Esophagus

Esophageal involvement in lymphoma is rare and more often seen as secondary involvement by enlarged mediastinal lymph nodes compared to intrinsic involvement. Barium swallow shows a smooth extrinsic impression on the esophagus with or without displacement.

In intrinsic involvement, distal esophagus is affected most frequently. Barium swallow may show a smooth tapered stricture simulating achalasia or a large filling defect involving the fundus and gastroesophageal junction indistinguishable from carcinoma. These tumors can manifest with polypoidal mass, ulceration and nodularity. Rarely the lesions may appear as thickened folds simulating varices seen best in double contrast studies. Barium swallow better demonstrates mucosal and submucosal abnormalities; however, CT better defines the extent of local disease, staging and complication if any.

Stomach

Stomach is the most frequent site of extranodal disease accounting for 50-70% of all primary GI lymphomas and constitutes 1-5% of all gastric malignancies.[22] Five gross pathological types have been described.

1. Infiltrative form–may be localized or diffuse.
2. Polypoidal form – usually associated with ulceration.
3. Ulcerative form–presenting as shallow ulceration with overhanging edges.
4. Nodular form–comprising of single or multiple nodular masses. Mucosa is usually intact.
5. A combination of the above.

Findings on barium meal reflect the above mentioned gross pathological appearances and are best seen on primary double contrast studies.

Infiltrative form presents as diffuse enlargement of gastric folds. Normal gastric folds measure 0.5 to 1cm. Presence of large serpiginous folds that have a nodular appearance and are rigid and not effaced after hyoscine butyl bromide injection should suggest the possibility of lymphoma (Fig. 10.1). The capacity of the stomach is usually not reduced and the organ retains its distensibility. Endoscopic biopsy may yield false negative results in as many as 30% of these cases due to disease being primarily submucosal. Other causes of generalized hypertrophy of rugae such as Menetrier's disease and hypertrophic gastritis need to be considered in differential diagnosis. Hodgkin's disease and rarely non-Hodgkin's lymphoma involving the stomach may produce a linitis plastica appearance by inciting a desmoplastic response and fibrosis.

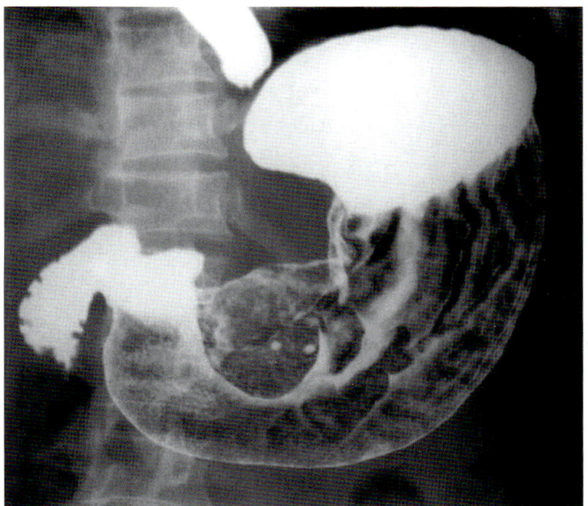

Fig. 10.1: Barium meal study showing hypertrophied gastric folds due to infiltrating form of gastric lymphoma

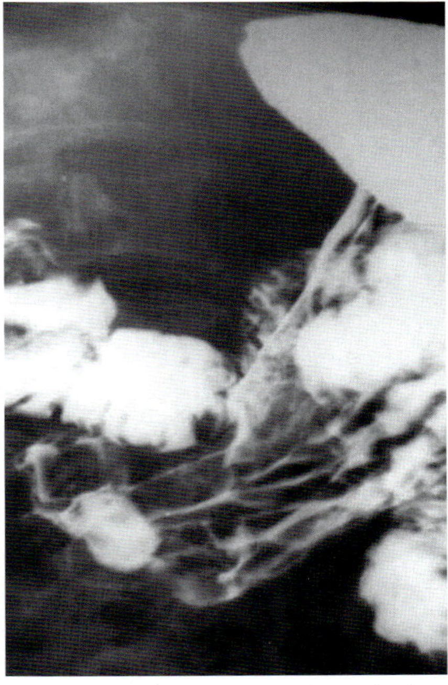

Fig. 10.2: Submucosal polypoidal filling defect with central ulceration in the antrum of stomach in polypoidal form of lymphoma

Polypoidal form presents as smooth submucosal filling defect or lobulated intraluminal mass with or without ulceration. The adjacent folds may also reveal thickening (Fig. 10.2).

Ulcerative form is generally seen in combination with polypoidal form. Rarely it may be seen as a simple ulcer without any surrounding mass. Absence of areae gastricae in the region of ulcer should suggest malignant nature (Fig. 10.3).

Nodular form is seen as multiple submucosal nodules or masses. They often ulcerate producing typical 'bull's eye' or target lesions.

Transpyloric and transcardiac spread of lymphoma to involve the duodenum or the esophagus is seen in 30-40% and 10% of patients respectively (Fig. 10.4).

Low grade MALT lymphoma are superficial spreading lesions with or without ulceration. They are seen on double contrast studies as variable sized, rounded nodules, shallow ulcer or mild fold thickening. CT scan shows mild wall thickening (0.8 cm) with lymphadenopathy seen in approximately 14% of cases only.[23]

High grade MALT lymphoma/advanced gastric lymphoma generally presents as polypoidal mass like lesions or severe fold thickening. Although the entire stomach may be infiltrated by tumor, most cases involve the antrum and body.

Differentiation of gastric lymphoma from carcinoma is often not possible. Features that should suggest lymphoma include presence of enlarged folds, large submucosal component with massive ulceration, minimal change in the capacity of the stomach, and CT showing generalized wall thickening of the stomach with preserved fat planes.

On routine grey scale ultrasound markedly thick gastric wall is usually seen. Spectrum of findings includes smooth or nodular thickening of the hypoechoic submucosal layer or presence of transmural bulky tumor (Figs 10.5A to C).

Endoscopic ultrasound (EUS) by virtue of its ability to demonstrate the different layers of the gastric wall as well as the adjacent lymph nodes is an ideal technique to assess the depth of tumor infiltration and differentiate stage I and II disease. Lymphoma of stomach is seen as a hypoechoic mass that disrupts the normal five layered wall pattern or may be seen as diffuse thickening of all

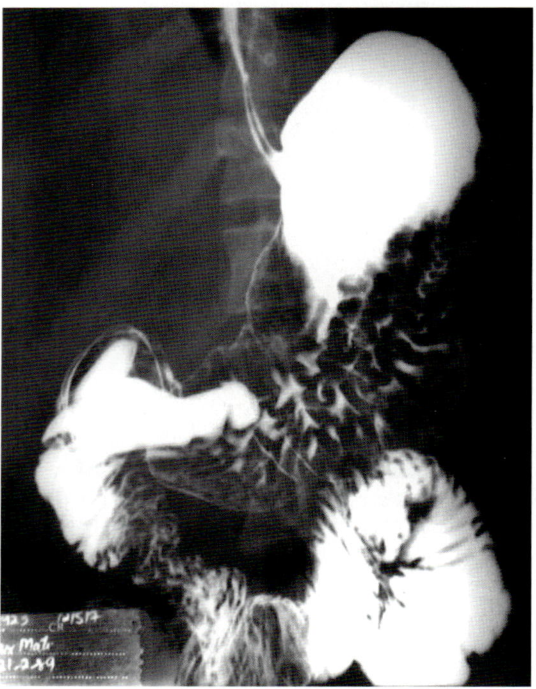

Fig. 10.3: Barium meal showing a simple ulcer along lesser curvature with absence of areae gastricae in the adjacent body of stomach-ulcerative form of lymphoma

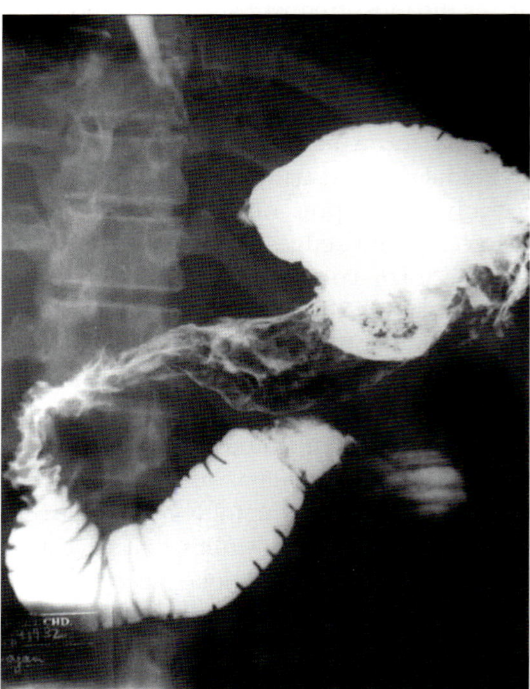

Fig. 10.4: Infiltrating type of lymphoma of stomach showing traspyloric spread

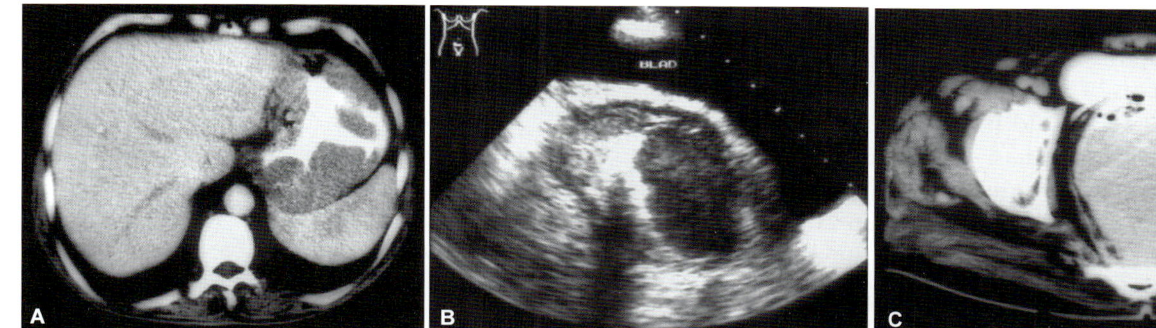

Figs 10.5A to C: Gastrointestinal lymphoma with multicentric involvement. (A) Showing gross mural thickening of stomach with preserved adjacent fat planes (B and C) Ultrasound showing extensive hypoechoic mural thickening with central echogenic focus suggestive of bowel mass involving rectum. CT of the same patient shows similar findings

five layers. Gastric MALT lymphoma has been classified on endoscopic ultrasound as:

- T1a : When the tumor is limited to superficial mucosa (the 1st hyperechoic layer).
- T1b : When the tumor involves the deeper mucosa upto muscularis mucosa (2nd hypoechoic layer).
- T2 : When the tumor extends to submucosa (3rd hyperechoic layer).
- T3 : When the tumor extends beyond submucosa (muscularis propria–4th hypoechoic layer and serosa 5th hyperechoic layer).

Endoscopic ultrasound remains the best method to detect 1perigastric lymphadenopathy, but it cannot differentiate metastatic lymphadenopathy from reactive hyperplasia and false positive diagnosis is high. In a multicentre study, comparing EUS with histopathological stage sensitivity for defining stage T1, T2 and T3 was 67%, 83% and 71% respectively.[24]

CT has only limited value in the assessment of local tumor staging and perigastric lymphadenopathy. CT may reveal focal or diffuse wall thickening or multiple submucosal masses. CT features of gastric lymphoma and adenocarcinoma may be similar in advanced cases. Both may exhibit wall thickening, mural mass, ulceration, extension into perigastric fat, regional lymphadenopathy and spread to peritoneum. However, thickening of the gastric wall >3 cm involving most or all of the stomach circumference strongly suggests lymphoma (Gossios, 2000 #59). Outer wall of the gastric lesion is often smooth in contor with preservation of fat planes between tumor and adjacent organs (Figs 10.5A to C). In addition, the stomach remain pliable even with extensive lymphomatous infiltration and gastric outlet obstruction is rarely seen.

Small Intestine

Lymphomas of the small intestine constitute one half of all malignant tumours of the small bowel.[5] Ileum is the most common site due to increased concentration of Payer's patches in the submucosa of the distal ileum followed by jejunum and duodenum. About 50% of the lesions are confined to the intestine as primary neoplasm (arising from mucosa associated lymphoid tissue – MALT). Twenty to thirty percent have nodal involvement and remainder show widespread dissemination. Great majority are NHL of B-cell origin. T-cell lymphomas are less common with increased incidence in celiac disease. The preferential site of peripheral T-cell lymphoma of GIT is the upper part of jejunum with a high incidence of multifocal bowel involvement. It shows only mild bowel thickening with non-bulky lymphadenopathy. The incidence of bowel perforation is high (40-50%).[25]

Clinically, patients may present with mass (30%), perforation (15%) and intussusception. Malabsorption may occur due to obstruction of mesenteric lymphatics or may be related to villous atrophy which could be a precursor to development of lymphoma.

Lesions of lymphoma may be single or multiple. Marshak et al[26] classified radiographic manifestations into five patterns: (i) multiple nodules, (ii) an infiltrating tumor, (iii) a polypoidal mass, (iv) an endoexoenteric form with excavation, and (v) mesenteric form with extraluminal mass.

Infiltrating form: This is considered the most common type and reveals focal or diffuse thickening of the bowel wall with alternating areas of dilatation or constriction of the bowel lumen (Figs 10.6A and B). Folds in the affected segment are thickened, nodular, effaced and may show ulceration. Occasionally, the involved segment may appear featureless or devoid of mucosal folds. The lumen may be narrowed, normal or widened (aneurysmal dilatation due to destruction of the nerve plexuses in the wall) (Fig. 10.7).

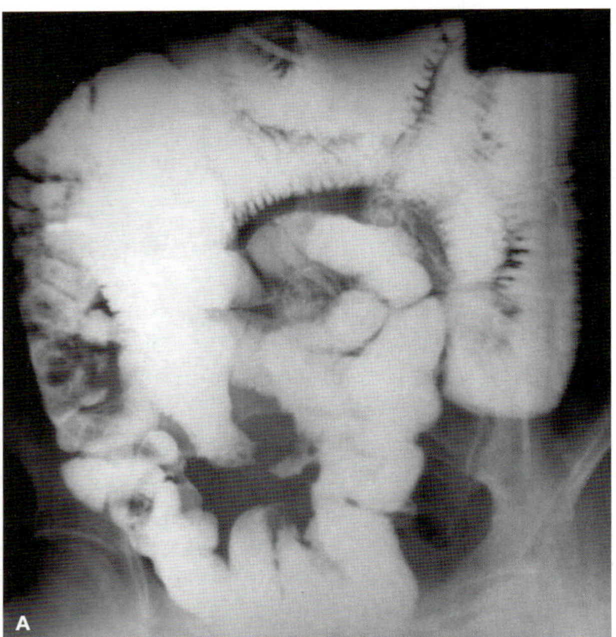

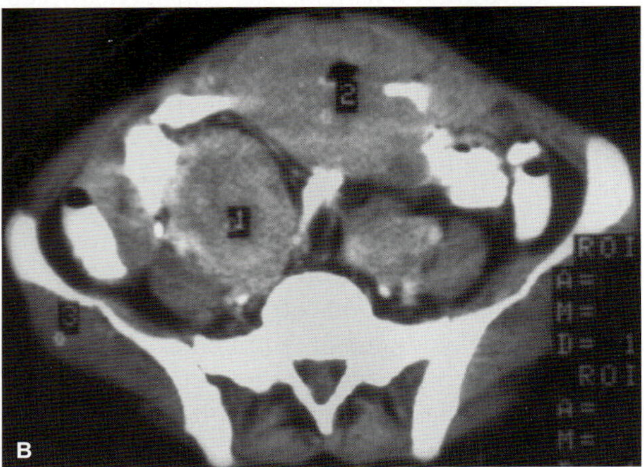

Figs 10.6A and B: (A) Focal infiltrative form of lymphoma showing tight stricture involving the ileum (B) CT showing extensive mural thickening2 suggestive of lymphoma. Huge lymphadenopathy is also seen1. Histology confirmed the diagnosis of non-Hodgkin's lymphoma

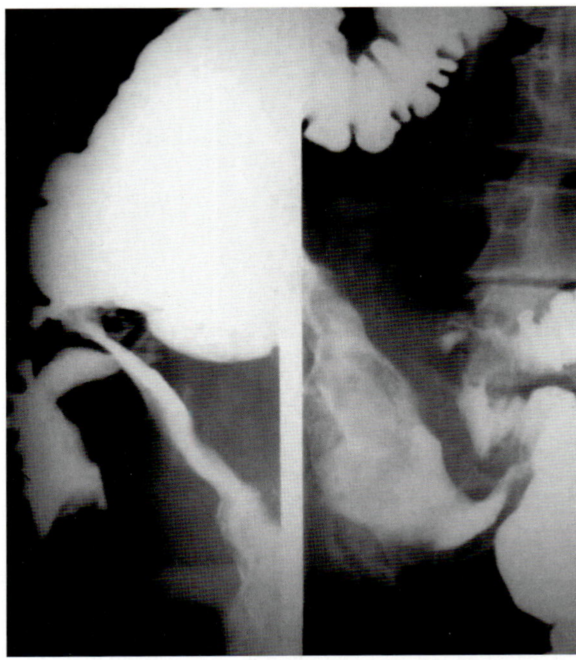

Fig. 10.7: BMFT in a 50 years old female presenting with mass abdomen. A long segment of distal ileum showing loss of normal folds and gross dilatation suggesting aneurismal form of lymphoma. Terminal ileum is narrowed because of mural thickening

Endoexoenteric form: Second common pattern has been described as endoexoenteric form. In this, the affected segment shows irregular collection of barium due to central ulceration, associated with displacement of adjacent bowel loops. There may be associated mesenteric abscess or fistula between the tumor and adjacent bowel loops (Figs 10.8A to C).

Multiple nodular pattern: It is usually seen in T-cell lymphoma complicating celiac disease and is considered most infrequent (Fig. 10.9).

Polypoid form: It causes submucosal filling defect and is often associated with intussusception (Figs 10.10A to 10.11C).

Mesenteric form: In the mesenteric form, the large nodal mass indents the mesenteric border of the small bowel and causes wide separation of the bowel loops.

Differentiation of lymphoma from adenocarcinoma and other malignant lesions of intestine is not always possible. However, detection of irregular nodules with thickened folds, presence of polypoidal filling defect with dilatation of the lumen, bizarre irregular areas of ulceration with marked separation of bowel loops are features which should suggest lymphoma. Adeno-

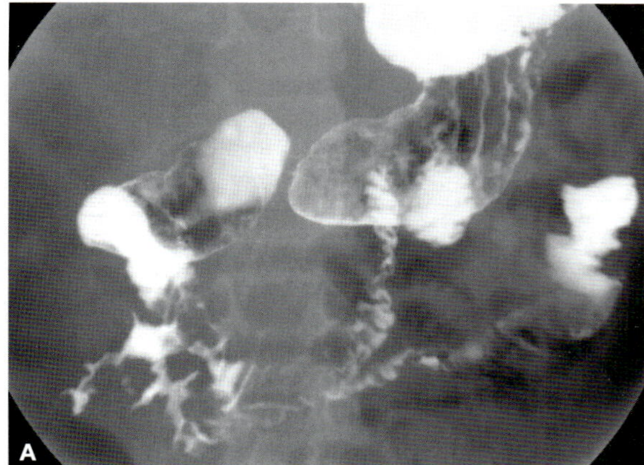

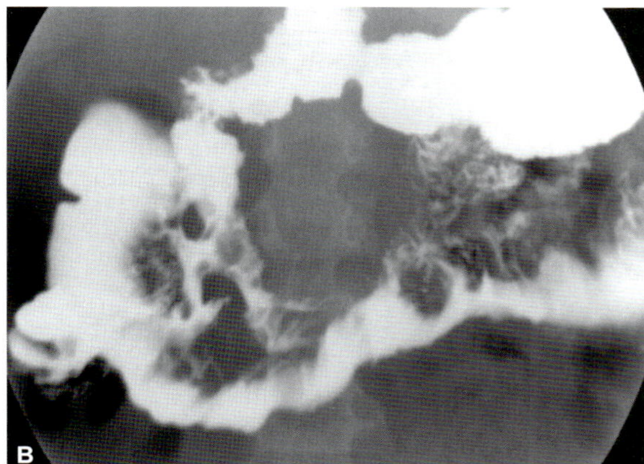

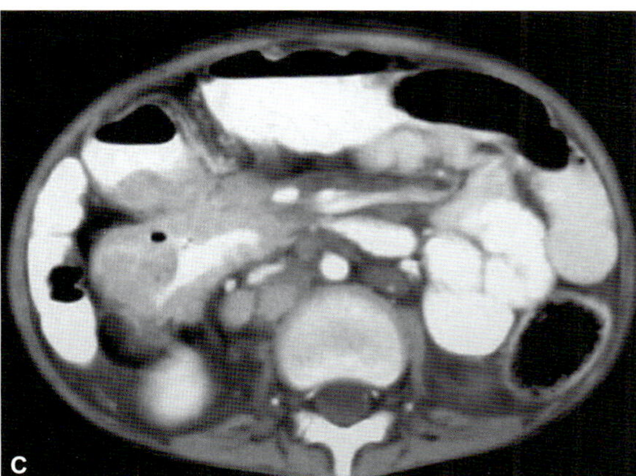

Figs 10.8A to C: Endoexoenteric form of lymphoma with duodenocolic fistula in a 8 year male. (A and B) Barium study shows mucosal distortion and nodularity in the second part of duodenum with extravasation of barium from the lateral aspect. This fistulous tract was seen to communicate with the transverse colon. (C) CECT shows extensive mural thickening of the duodenum with presence of air in the lateral wall suggestive of ulceration

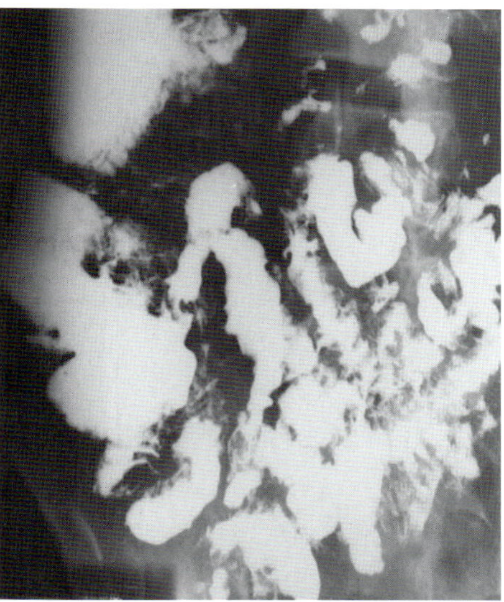

Fig. 10.9: Primary small bowel lymphoma showing diffuse nodular thickening of folds in distal ileum

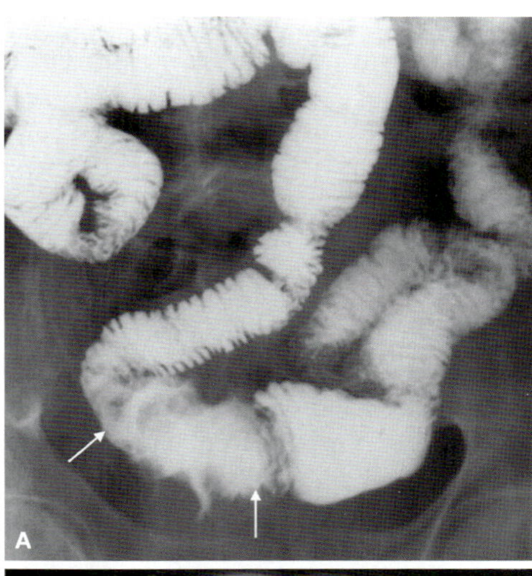

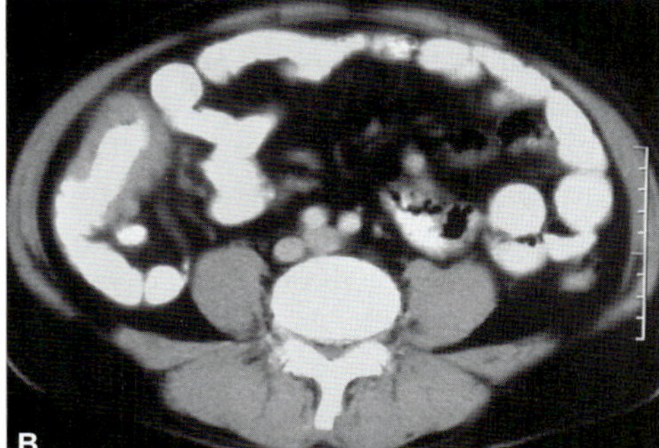

Figs 10.10 A and B: Primary jejunal lymphoma in two different patients. Note dilated featureless involved segment of jejunum in baium study and homogenous mural thickening with preserved adjacent fat planes in CT image

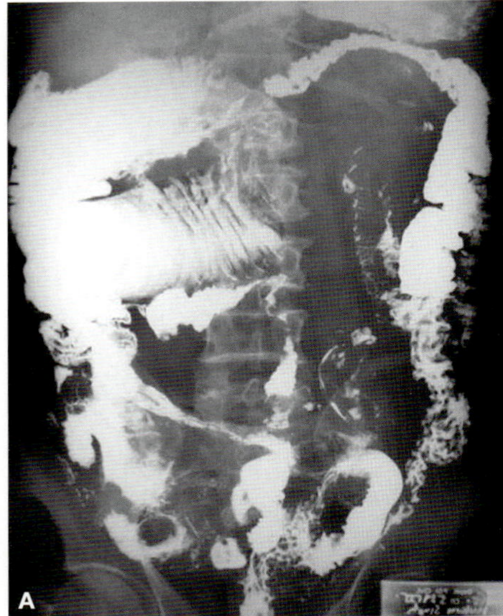
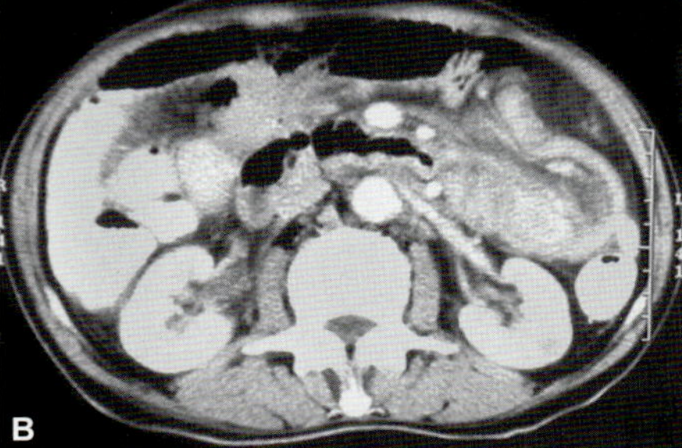
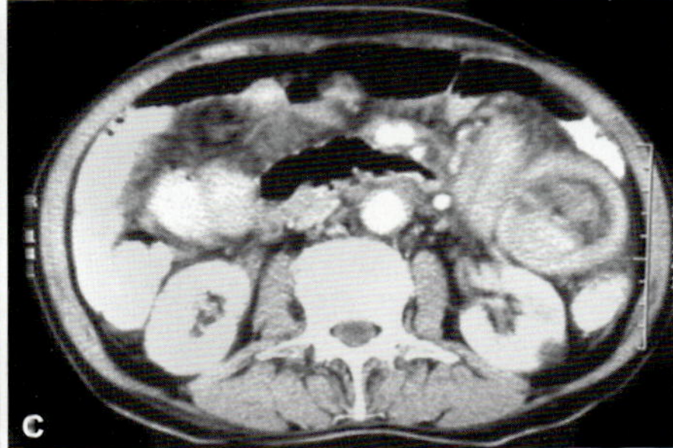

Figs 10.11 A to C: Multifocal lymphoma with diffuse involvement of small and large bowel: (A) Barium study shows grossly dilated loop of proximal jejunum with intussusception. A mid ileal loop shows narrowing with mucosal distortion and cecum shows polypoidal filling defects. In addition descending colon and rectum reveal diffuse mucosal nodularity due to lymphomatous nodules, (B) CECT shows the presence of an intussusception in the proximal jejunum due to lymphoma

carcinoma usually involves short segments of bowel with stricturous lesion. Strictures in lymphoma are rare except in Hodgkin's disease. Perforation is seen in 15% cases of lymphoma while it never occurs in carcinoma of bowel.

Peritoneal lymphomatosis from primary gastrointestinal lymphoma is rare compared to peritoneal carcinomatosis. The patterns of involvement of mesentry, omentum and peritoneum are difficult to differentiate from those seen in peritoneal carcinomatosis or tuberculous peritonitis.

Appendix

Involvement of appendix is seen in 1 to 3% of cases of GI lymphoma. Patient presents with signs and symptoms of appendicitis. CT shows markedly diffuse mural soft tissue thickening (2.5-4.0 cm). Vermiform shape is usually maintained and aneurysmal dilatation is sometimes seen. Stranding of periappendicial fat may be seen. Co-existent lymphadenopathy may or may not be seen.[27]

Colon and Rectum

Primary colonic lymphoma constitutes 0.05% of colonic tumors and 0.1% of all rectal tumors. Cecum and rectum are affected more frequently than other parts of the colon.[28] In secondary involvement, colon is affected in 10% of patients with GI lymphoma and the lesions are often multicenteric. Clinical picture and radiological findings are similar to changes seen in lymphomatous involvement of other parts of the GI tract. A large submucosal mass in the cecum may be present with signs of intussusception (Fig. 10.12). Adjacent terminal ileum may also be involved. Rectum may be involved by perirectal disease with displacement and narrowing by enlarged lymph nodes.

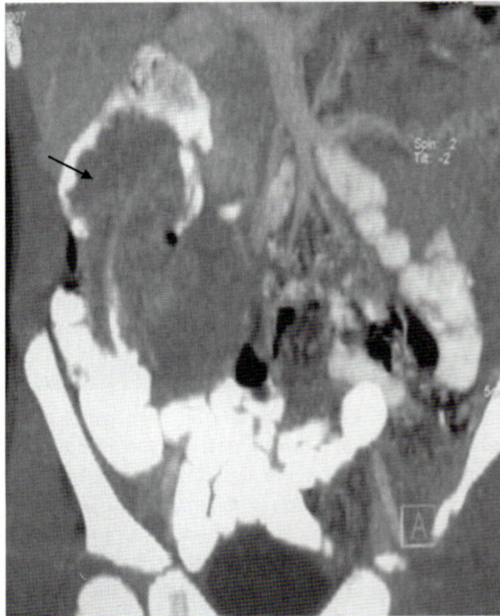

Fig. 10.12: CT reconstructed image showing large polypoidal mass (Histologically proven NHL) causing intussusception of ascending colon

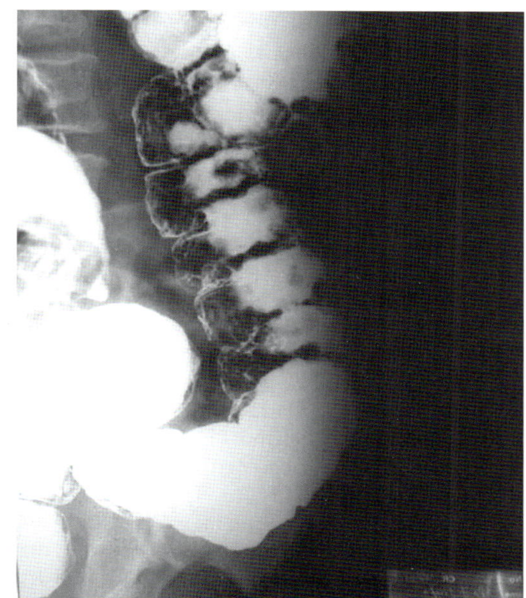

Fig. 10.13: Barium enema showing multiple polypoidal filling defects in colon

In the diffuse form, smooth sessile small nodules 0.2 to 2 cm in size are scattered throughout the colon. Some of the lesions may show umbilication (Fig. 10.13).

Rarely colonic lymphoma presents as markedly thickened folds with loss of contraction of colon on the post-evacuation film. Focal strictures, aneurysmal dilatation or large ulcerating masses with fistula formation have also been described.

Features that help differentiate lymphoma from adenocarcinoma include extension into terminal ileum, preservation of fat planes, absence of invasion of adjacent structures and perforation with no desmoplastic response. Obstruction is also less likely features of lymphoma.

Lymphoma Variants

Burkitt's Lymphoma

Burkitt's lymphoma is a tumor of B lymphocytes that is seen in younger patients of less than 30 years of age. Ileocecal region is most frequently involved. Large rapidly growing masses with mesenteric lymphadenopathy may be encountered.[29]

Mediterranean Lymphoma

Mediterranean lymphoma affects younger persons. There is marked thickening of the mucosal folds with nodules due to massive infiltration by plasma cells (Fig. 10.14). The unaffected intestinal loops show features of malabsorption in the form of flocculation, segmentation and dilatation.[30]

Multiple Lymphomatous Polyposis

Multiple lymphomatous polyposis is a rare form of lymphoma in which multiple polypoid lesions of malignant lymphoma are distributed throughout the GI tract[31] (Figs 10.15A and B).

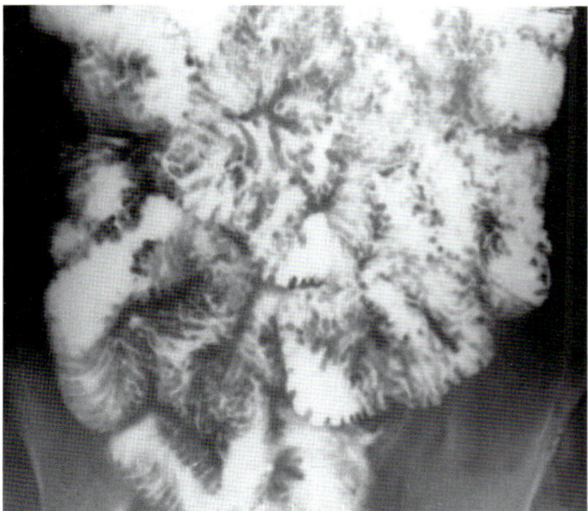

Fig. 10.14: Small bowel enema showing nodular fold thickening of jejunal loops in a case of Mediterranean lymphoma

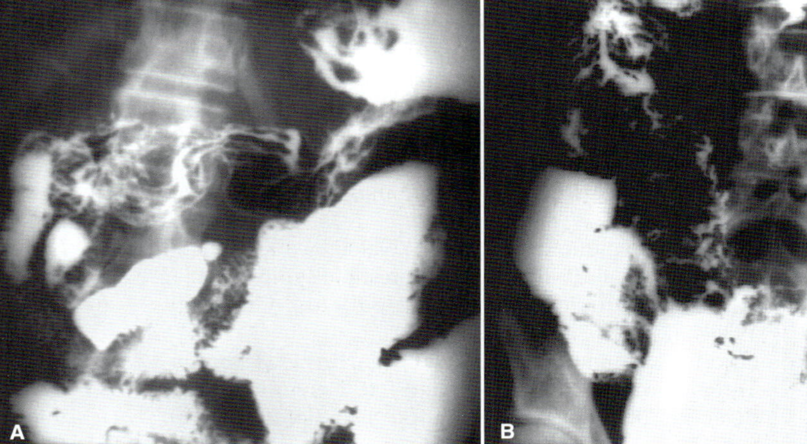

Figs 10.15A and B: (A) Barium study showing thickened folds in body of stomach extending into duodenum and a polypoid lesion in the fundus, (B) Terminal ileum is enlarged with multiple nodular filling defects distorting the mucosa. Histology confirmed the diagnosis of multiple lymphoid polyposis

REFERENCES

1. Loehr WJ, Mujahed Z, Zahn FD, Gray GF, Thorbjarnarson B. Primary lymphoma of the gastrointestinal tract: a review of 100 cases. Ann Surg 1969;170(2):232-8.
2. Ehrlich AN, Stalder G, Geller W, Sherlock P. Gastrointestinal manifestations of malignant lymphoma. Gastroenterology 1968;54(6):1115-21.
3. Dawson IM, Cornes JS, Morson BC. Primary malignant lymphoid tumours of the intestinal tract. Report of 37 cases with a study of factors influencing prognosis. Br J Surg 1961;49:80-9.
4. Yoo CC, Levine MS, McLarney JK, Rubesin SE, Herlinger H. Value of barium studies for predicting primary versus secondary non-Hodgkin's gastrointestinal lymphoma. Abdom Imaging 2000;25(4):368-72.
5. Dodd GD. Lymphoma of the hollow abdominal viscera. Radiol Clin North Am 1990;28(4):771-83.
6. National Cancer Institute sponsored study of classifications of non-Hodgkin's lymphomas: summary and description of a working formulation for clinical usage. The Non-Hodgkin's Lymphoma Pathologic Classification Project. Cancer 1982;49(10):2112-35.
7. Eidt S, Stolte M, Fischer R. Helicobacter pylori gastritis and primary gastric non-Hodgkin's lymphomas. J Clin Pathol 1994;47(5):436-9.
8. Bayerdorffer E, Neubauer A, Rudolph B, Thiede C, Lehn N, Eidt S, et al. Regression of primary gastric lymphoma of mucosa-associated lymphoid tissue type after cure of Helicobacter pylori infection. MALT Lymphoma Study Group. Lancet 1995;345(8965):1591-4.
9. Chott A, Dragosics B, Radaszkiewicz T. Peripheral T-cell lymphomas of the intestine. Am J Pathol 1992;141(6):1361-71.
11. Musshoff K. [Clinical staging classification of non-Hodgkin's lymphomas (author's transl)]. Strahlentherapie 1977;153(4):218-21.
12. Rohatiner A, d'Amore F, Coiffier B, Crowther D, Gospodarowicz M, Isaacson P, et al. Report on a workshop convened to discuss the pathological and staging classifications of gastrointestinal tract lymphoma. Ann Oncol 1994;5(5):397-400.
13. Ruskone-Fourmestraux A, Dragosics B, Morgner A, Wotherspoon A, De Jong D. Paris staging system for primary gastrointestinal lymphomas. Gut 2003;52(6):912-3.
14. Aozasa K, Tsujimoto M, Inoue A, Nakagawa K, Hanai J, Kurata A, et al. Primary gastrointestinal lymphoma. A clinicopathologic study of 102 patients. Oncology 1985;42(2):97-103.
15. Orjollet-Lecoanet C, Menard Y, Martins A, Crombe-Ternamian A, Cotton F, Valette PJ. (CT enteroclysis for detection of small bowel tumors). J Radiol 2000;81(6):618-27.
16. O'Brien A, Cruz JP, Berrios C, Melipillan Y, Butte JM, Alvarez M. (Advances in radiography of the small intestine: computed tomography enteroclysis). Gastroenterol Hepatol 2006;29(9):528-33.
17. Anis M, Irshad A. Imaging of abdominal lymphoma. Radiol Clin North Am 2008;46(2):265-85.
18. Chou CK, Chen LT, Sheu RS, Yang CW, Wang ML, Jaw TS, et al. MRI manifestations of gastrointestinal lymphoma. Abdom Imaging 1994;19(6):495-500.
19. Jerusalem G, Beguin Y, Najjar F, Hustinx R, Fassotte MF, Rigo P, et al. Positron emission tomography (PET) with 18F-fluorodeoxyglucose (18F-FDG) for the staging of low-grade non-Hodgkin's lymphoma (NHL). Ann Oncol 2001;12(6):825-30.
20. Endo K, Oriuchi N, Higuchi T, Iida Y, Hanaoka H, Miyakubo M, et al. PET and PET/CT using 18F-FDG in the diagnosis and management of cancer patients. Int J Clin Oncol 2006;11(4):286-96.
21. Schoder H, Larson SM, Yeung HW. PET/CT in oncology: integration into clinical management of lymphoma, melanoma, and gastrointestinal malignancies. J Nucl Med 2004;45 Suppl 1:72S-81S.
22. Gossios K, Katsimbri P, Tsianos E. CT features of gastric lymphoma. Eur Radiol 2000;10(3):425-30.
23. Park MS, Kim KW, Yu JS, Park C, Kim JK, Yoon SW, et al. Radiographic findings of primary B-cell lymphoma of the stomach: low-grade versus high-grade malignancy in relation to the mucosa-associated lymphoid tissue concept. AJR Am J Roentgenol 2002;179(5):1297-304.
24. Ahmad A, Govil Y, Frank BB. Gastric mucosa-associated lymphoid tissue lymphoma. Am J Gastroenterol 2003; 98(5):975-86.
25. Byun JH, Ha HK, Kim AY, Kim TK, Ko EY, Lee JK, et al. CT findings in peripheral T-cell lymphoma involving the gastrointestinal tract. Radiology 2003;227(1):59-67.
26. Marshak RH, Lindner AE, Maklansky D. Lymphoreticular disorders of the gastrointestinal tract: roentgenographic features. Gastrointest Radiol 1979;4(2):103-20.
27. Pickhardt PJ, Levy AD, Rohrmann CA, Jr., Abbondanzo SL, Kende AI. Non-Hodgkin's lymphoma of the appendix: clinical and CT findings with pathologic correlation. AJR Am J Roentgenol 2002;178(5):1123-7.
28. Richards MA. Lymphoma of the colon and rectum. Postgrad Med J 1986;62(729):615-20.
29. Jeen YT, Chung RS, Chun HJ, Kim CD, Ryu HS, Hyun JH. Small intestine Burkitt's lymphoma. Gastrointest Endosc 2002;56(5):731.
30. Cooper DL, Doria R, Salloum E. Primary gastrointestinal lymphomas. Gastroenterologist 1996;4(1):54-64.
31. Hotta K, Oyama T, Kitamura Y, Tomori A, Miyata Y, Mitsuishi T. Mantle cell lymphoma presenting as multiple lymphomatous polyposis spreading widely to the small intestine and diagnosed by double-balloon endoscopy. Endoscopy 2007;39 Suppl 1:E347-8.

Chapter Eleven

Imaging of Appendix

Anju Garg

The vermiform appendix is present only in man, certain anthropoid apes and the wombat. Morphologically, it is the undeveloped distal end of the large caecum found in many lower animals. It usually arises from the posteromedial wall of the caecum about 2.5-4 cm below the ileocecal valve[1] (Fig. 11.1). Although the relationship of the base of the appendix to the caecum is essentially constant, the remainder of the appendix is free, which accounts for its variable location in the abdominal cavity. If the caecum occupies a relatively normal position, the retrocecal position of the appendix is the most frequent. More than 50% of the appendices are retrocecal or retrocolic in position as judged from both operative and postmortem reports. The next most frequent position is pelvic and rarer situations are preileal, post ileal, splenic and pericolic (Fig. 11.2). A recent imaging based study showed that only in 4% cases is the appendix located at the classic McBurney point[2] (junction of the lateral and middle third of the line between the anterior superior iliac spine and the umbilicus).

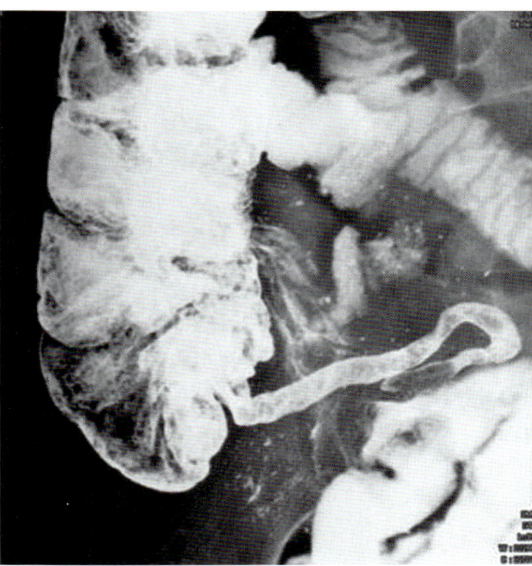

Fig. 11.1: Barium meal follow through study shows the origin of the appendix from the cecum below the ileocecal valve. A well defined intraluminal filling defect is seen at its distal end due to a fecalith

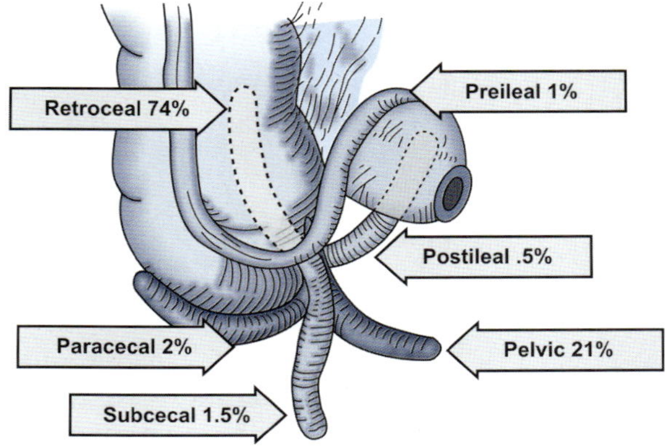

Fig. 11.2: The variable positions of the appendix

The appendix is invested with a mesentery called the "mesoappendix". The wall of the appendix is composed of the mucosa, submucosa, muscularis and serosa, similar to the rest of the intestine. There is a 'valve' at its orifice in the caecum which probably does not function in life. At postmortem examination total occlusion of the lumen of the appendix is seen in 3-4% cases, whereas almost total/partial obliteration is found in an additional 25%. In persons greater than 60 years of age, the lumen is obliterated in more than 50% cases and may represent a retrogressive normal change with age.[3]

NORMAL IMAGING APPEARANCE

On *plain films* a normal appendix cannot be visualized. A calcified appendicolith may sometimes be detected, incidentally, as a laminated density of variable size (0.5-6 cm) in the right lower quadrant (Fig. 11.3). It may occur in unusual locations when the appendix is in an abnormal position.

The normal appendix fills with barium in 80-90% of *barium studies* and is seen as a thin, tubular structure with a convex, rounded tip. There may be filling defects seen within the barium filled appendix which can be due to non-calcified fecaliths, air bubbles, or mucus (Fig. 11.1). The presence of air bubbles within the lumen may be a normal finding specially in the subhepatic, vertically directed appendix.

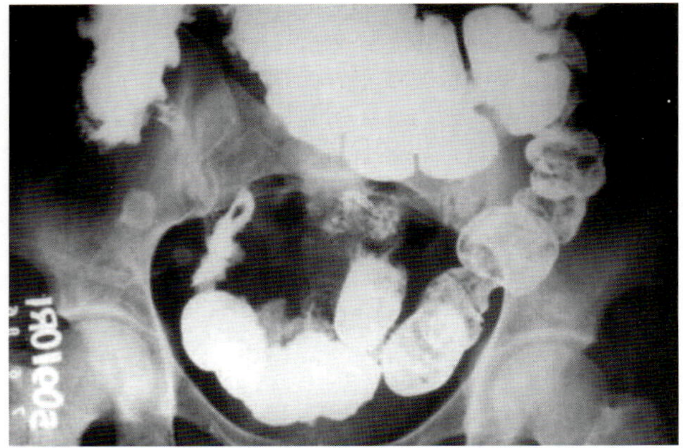

Fig. 11.3: Two appendicoliths can be seen in a non-contrast filled appendix on a barium study

Occasionally the appendix may not fill immediately at the time of a barium examination but may be seen to contain barium in delayed films. In approximately 10% of cases the normal appendix may not fill at all. In some cases barium may be persistently retained in the appendix for a period of weeks or months after the barium examination (Figs 11.4A and B). Retention of barium can rarely predispose to the development of acute appendicitis.[4,5]

Sonography: In 1986, Puylaert[6] described a specific technique of graded compression applied with a high frequency transducer (> 5 MHz) for examination of the appendix. Using this technique the fat and bowel are displaced or compressed. This eliminates artefacts from bowel contents and reduces the distance from the transducer to the appendix, allowing the use of a high frequency probe with better image quality.

The normal appendix, when identified, is seen as a compressible, tubular, blind ended structure, of double layer wall thickness ≤ 6 mm, with or without echogenic intraluminal material (gas or feces) with no evidence of peristalsis.[7] The typical lamellated appearance may be seen even in the normal appendix representing (from outer to inner) the echogenic outer serosa, the hypoechoic muscular layer, the echogenic submucosa, followed by the hypoechoic muscularis mucosae and the innermost echogenic mucosal lining[8] (Fig. 11.5).

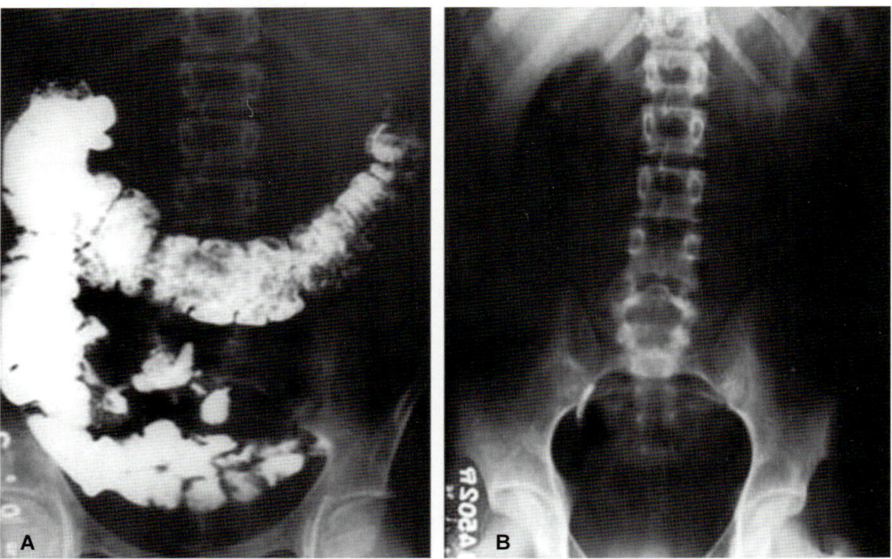

Figs 11.4A and B: (A) Barium study showing a normally filling appendix, (B) Plain radiography done one month later shows retention of barium within the appendix

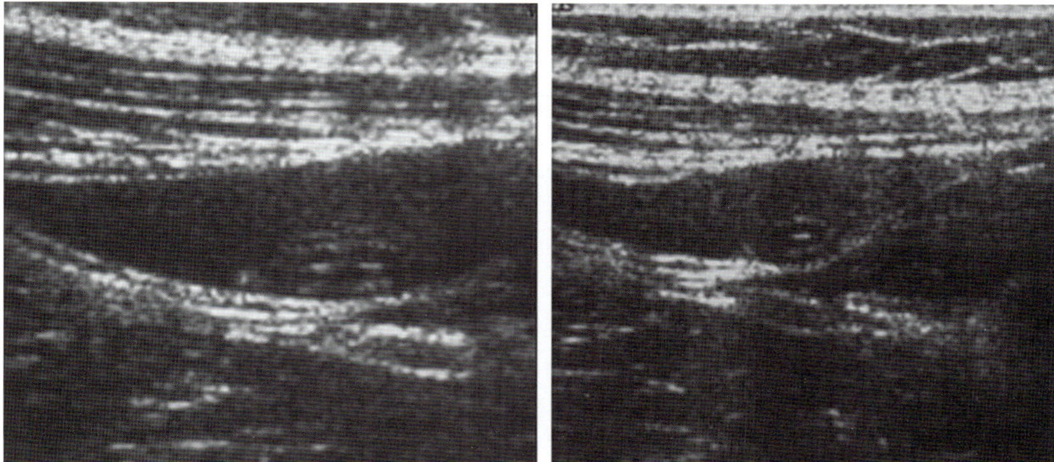

Fig. 11.5: Sonographic visualization of the normal appendix in a case of ascites – longitudinal and transverse scans. The appendiceal wall shows the typical laminated appearance – the central hyperechoic interface of collapsed lumen, surrounded by the inner hypoechoic mucosa, echogenic muscularis propria bounded by the thin echogenic serosa. The total AP thickness of the appendix measured 3.8 mm

During *computed tomography (CT)* of the abdomen visualization of a normal appendix depends in great measure on the amount of intraperitoneal fat, the adequate opacification of terminal ileal loops and caecum, the type and quality of CT examination, and the diligence of the examiner. The normal appendix can be identified in 67-100% of adults who undergo dedicated thin-section (5 mm) helical CT scan.[9-11] Although the normal appendix may be seen in most cases even on unenhanced scans, intravenous and oral contrast do increase the detection rate.

Depending on its orientation, the appendix appears as a small tubular or ring-like density in the right lower abdomen which is either collapsed or can be fluid or air filled and has a thin wall with a sharp outer contour (Fig. 11.6). It is enveloped by the homogenous fat density of normal mesenteric structures and may be located in the pelvis or posterior to the right colon in the retrocaecal position. The diameter of the appendix has been seen to range from 3-10 mm which overlap the values used to diagnose appendicitis.[12] Appendicoliths may be seen in asymptomatic individuals presenting as ring like or homogenous calcific densities associated with a normal-looking appendix. The presence of air, fecal matter, or calcifications in the appendix has no immediate clinical implications without the expected inflammatory changes indicative of appendicitis.

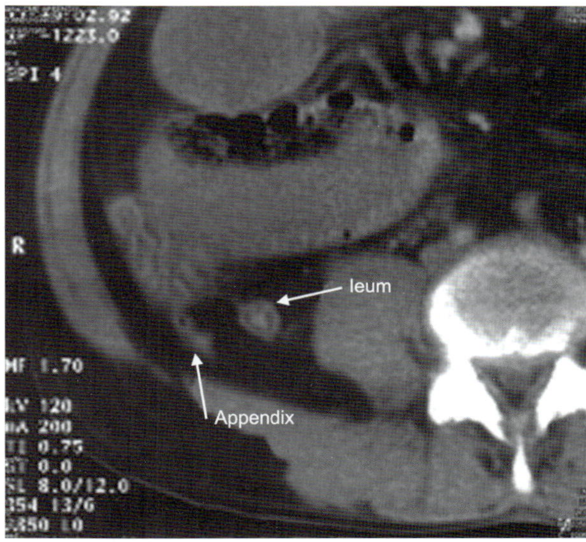

Fig. 11.6: CECT shows the appendix as a thin tubular structure in right iliac fossa. A small air lucency can be identified within the lumen. The collapsed terminal ileum is seen in cross-section medial to the appendix

ACUTE APPENDICITIS

Acute appendicitis is the most common cause of acute abdominal pain requiring surgery. Early diagnosis is crucial to the success of therapy, which consists of surgical removal of the inflamed appendix before it perforates.

Pathophysiology

The pathogenesis of acute appendicitis is thought to relate to obstruction of its orifice.[13,14] Mechanical obstruction by fecalith or solid faecal material in the caecum is demonstrated in one third of the cases. Occasionally tumours, parasites, foreign bodies etc. may be incriminated. However, no obstruction is demonstrated in upto half of the patients with appendicitis.

Fecaliths, which result from the inspissation of fecal material and inorganic salts within the appendiceal lumen, are the most common cause of obstruction and are present in 11-52% of patients with acute appendicitis.[15,16] True appendiceal calculi (hard, non-crushable, calcified stones) are less common than appendiceal fecaliths (hard but crushable concretions) but have been shown to be associated more commonly with perforating appendicitis and periappendiceal abscess.[15]

As the secretions distend the obstructed appendix, the intraluminal pressure rises, eventually leading to ischemia, mucosal ulceration and invasion of the wall by intestinal bacteria. The inflammation commences as a catarrhal appendicitis with congestion of the mucous membrane and variable reaction in the submucosal, muscular and peritoneal layers. It progresses rapidly, specially in the presence of a fecalith and the infected, necrotic wall becomes gangrenous which may perforate within 24-48 hours.[17]

Rupture of the appendix with spillage of pus into the peritoneal cavity results in localized or generalized peritonitis. In most cases, the spill of pus is limited, being walled off by omentum, mesentery, bowel loops and adhesions. If this protective measure is successful an "appendicular mass" is formed which may be a phlegmon or, in cases of circumscribed pus collection, an appendiceal abscess. The abscess may be intra-peritoneal or retroperitoneal. It is most often located in the proximity of the appendix, so that the inflammatory mass usually lies adjacent to the caecum and terminal ileum. Depending on the position of the appendix, this may be in the right iliac fossa or in the pelvis. When the appendix is abnormally located or is unusually long, the abscess can be anywhere in the abdomen. Abscesses have been described in the left lower quadrant, the right flank, the anterior abdominal wall, the lesser sac, and in the subhepatic and subdiaphragmatic spaces.

Clinical Picture

Acute appendicitis typically presents with diffuse abdominal pain, anorexia, nausea and vomiting with subsequent migration of pain to the right iliac quadrant. However this typical presentation is seen in only 50-60% of patients. The cardinal signs of appendicitis are localized abdominal tenderness, muscle guarding, pain on percussion and rebound tenderness. Laboratory abmnormalities include leucocytosis and an elevated C-reactive protein. The differential diagnosis of appendicitis includes a long list of common gastrointestinal and genitorurinary disorders (Table 11.1).

IMAGING

Conventional Radiography

Though *plain films* of the abdomen are abnormal in approximately 50% of patients with acute appendicitis, they are not specific. The presence of calcified fecaliths (appendicoliths) is the single most important sign of appendicitis. Not only is their detection on the plain abdominal radiograph strong evidence of acute appendicitis, but their presence suggests perforation early in the course of the disease. Localised ileus, air-fluid level in caecum, cecal wall thickening and small bowel obstruction are other findings that can be seen on plain

Table 11.1	Differential diagnosis of appendicitis
Acute mesenteric adenitis	
Acute gastroenteritis	
Pelvic inflammatory disease	
Urinary tract infection	
Ureteral stone	
Ruptured Graafian follicle	
Epiploic appendagitis	
Endometriosis	
Ovarian torsion	
Ruptured ectopic pregnancy	
Meckel's diverticulitis	
Intussusception	
Crohn's disease	
Yersinosis	
Perforated peptic ulcer	
Henoch-Schonlein purpura	

films.[18,19] Generalised paralytic ileus may occur in cases of perforated appendicitis but pneumoperitoneum is rare.

When an abscess is present, plain abdominal radiographs show a poorly defined mass, with displacement of the adjacent loops of bowel. Irregular radiolucencies in the mass due to bubbles of gas produced by the bacteria in the abscess often produce a mottled pattern radiographically. In some cases, the abscess may form a unilocular mass containing gas and pus and a single fluid level may be seen which should be differentiated from air-fluid levels in the bowel.

On *barium studies* an adequate visualization of a normal caecum with filling of the appendix to its smooth, rounded tip excludes the diagnosis of appendicitis. Non-filling of the appendix occurs in patients with appendicitis, but this finding alone is not conclusive, since the appendix may not fill on barium enema in as high as 10-20% of normal patients. Sehey found that the normal appendix fills in 92% of children, so failure of the appendix to fill in symptomatic children is a significant finding.[20] Much more conclusive evidence of appendicitis is provided by non-filling of the appendix associated with an external or intramural mass impressing the medial aspect of the caecum (Fig. 11.7). The mass is the abscess/ inflammatory reaction surrounding the inflamed appendix and may be associated with spasm or irritability of the adjacent caecum which can be visualized fluoroscopically. The terminal ileum may be displaced or narrowed by the adjacent inflammatory mass and there may be thickening of the mucosal folds of the terminal ileum. Occasionally barium extravasates into a peri-appendiceal abscess, indicating that the appendiceal lumen is not obliterated in every case. US and CT have replaced barium examinations as the primary means of examining patients suspected to have appendicitis. Barium enema examination is not obsolete however, and may be useful in evaluating complex colonic abnormalities detected with cross-sectional imaging.

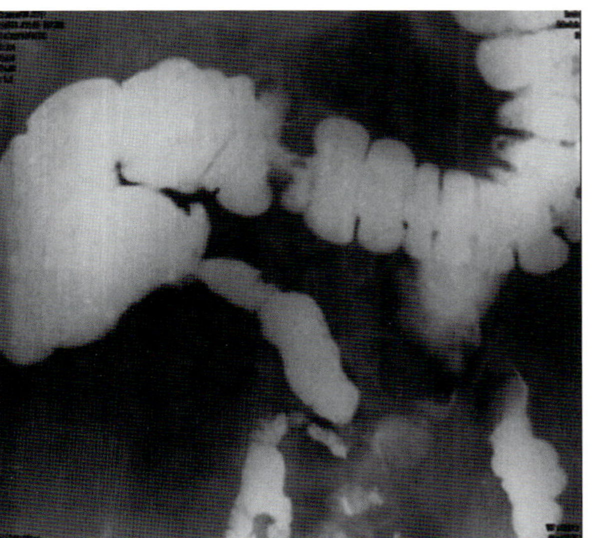

Fig. 11.7: Smooth impression on the inferomedial aspect of the caecum with medial displacement of the terminal ileum suggests an appendicular mass

Ultrasonography

Ultrasonography is a widely available and inexpensive modality with the potential for highly accurate imaging in the patient suspected to have acute appendicitis.[21] In experienced hands US has reported sensitivities of 75 to 90%, specificities of 86-100%, accuracies of 87-96%, positive predictive values of 91-94% and negative predictive values of 89-97% for the diagnosis of acute appendicitis.[7, 22-24]

US Technique

Puylaert's technique of using graded compression US[6] is the most popular method of examination. It has a number of advantages. Firstly, it allows normal and gas filled loops of gut to be displaced from the field of view or compressed between the layers of musculature of the anterior and posterior abdominal wall. In contrast, abnormal loops of gut, or the obstructed appendix will be non-compressible and well seen on the graded compression image. This technique also allows for a successful examination of the patient who may have peritoneal irritation and sensitivity, as the compression is slow and gentle. Thirdly, the patient is able to provide input as to the point of maximal tenderness, which is often useful in focussing the examination in the correct area.[25] When a patient can self localize the site of maximal tenderness, there is a significant sonographic finding at this site in 94% of cases.[26]

Several additional manouvres have been shown to facilitate visualization of the appendix, e.g. applying pressure posteriorly to improve the degree of compression[27] or applying forceful upward sweeps with the transducer to displace the caecum and appendix upwards specially when the appendix is low lying or pelvic.[28] Turning the patient into the left lateral decubitus position maybe helpful in visualizing the retrocecal appendix.

Although high frequency linear probes are in wide use in patients suspected to have acute appendicitis, it has been reported that curvilinear probes work equally well and provide a slightly larger field of view and greater penetration. Transducers with a variable short focal zone and a frequency of 5-9 MHz have been recommended.[29] The use of harmonic imaging has also been shown to falicitate visualization of the appendix and the relevant surrounding structures.[30]

Sonographic Findings

The inflamed appendix is seen as a blind ending, lamellated, aperistaltic tubular structure which is fixed, non compressible and appears round on transverse sections. Traditionally appendicitis was diagnosed when its transverse diameter exceeded 6 mm. The threshold of 6 mm has a reported sensitivity of 98%,[31] however, sonographic studies of normal individuals show that upto 23% of normal patients have appendicular sizes > 6 mm.[32] Thus, the diameter of the appendix should be correlated with the associated findings, alongwith the clinical picture before a diagnosis of appendicitis is considered.

In early acute appendicitis-catarrhal stage-five layers can be identified (Figs 11.8A and B):

- A central, thin hyperechoic line representing the collapsed lumen and mucosal lining
- Hypoechoic layer (2-3 mm) representing the edematous lamina propria and muscularis mucosa
- Hyperechoic submucosa (2-3 mm)
- Hypoechoic muscular layer (2-3 mm)
- Outer most thin hyperechoic line representing the serosa.

In the later suppurative stages, the lumen of the appendix gets distended with pus/fluid (Fig. 11.9) and there may be an increase in the thickness of the submucosa and muscular layer in the range of 3-6 mm.

Appendicoliths are seen as bright, echogenic foci with clean distal acoustic shadowing (Fig. 11.10). Their identification within the appendix or in the adjacent perienteric soft tissue after perforation is highly associated with a positive diagnosis. Failure to see an appendicolith is non-contributory. Inflammatory change in the adjacent fat appears bright and noncompressible and is a sonographic clue to the presence of appendicitis in doubtful cases. Enlarged mesenteric lymph nodes may be identified.

An asymmetric thickening of the appendiceal wall with a focal/circumferential lack of visualization of the echogenic submucosa indicates perforation of the inflamed appendix. The lumen may or may not be distended.

An appendiceal mass is seen as a complex paracecal mass of mixed echogenicity and thickened paracecal fat. Phlegmonous change manifests as hypoechoic zones with poor margination within the inflamed fat. Liquefaction and abscess formation will manifest as an actual fluid component (Fig. 11.11). Gas bubbles within a

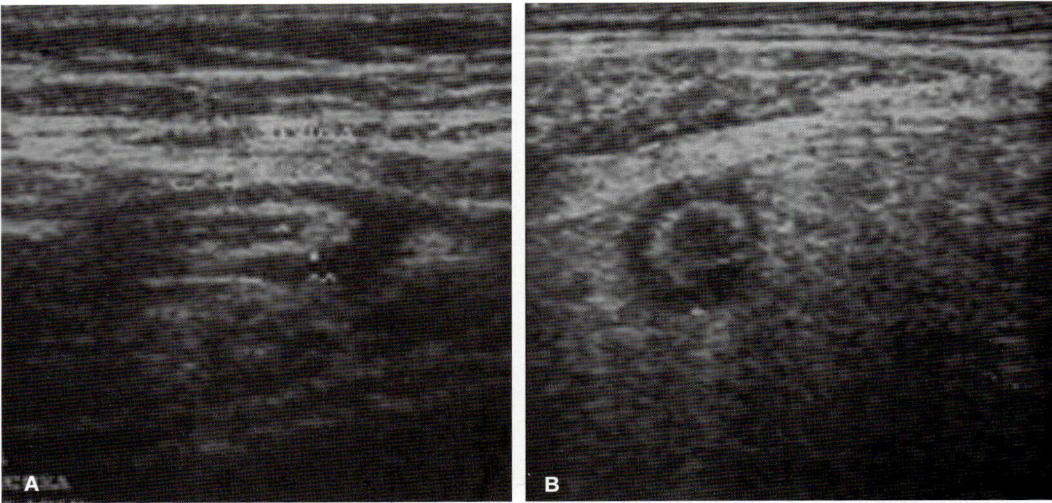

Figs 11.8A and B: Sonographic appearance of early acute appendicitis. (A) Longitudinal scan shows an enlarged (maximal diameter 11 mm), non compressible appendix with maintained wall layering, (B) On transverse section it appears round. Inflammatory changes can be seen as diffuse hyperechogenicity in the surrounding fat

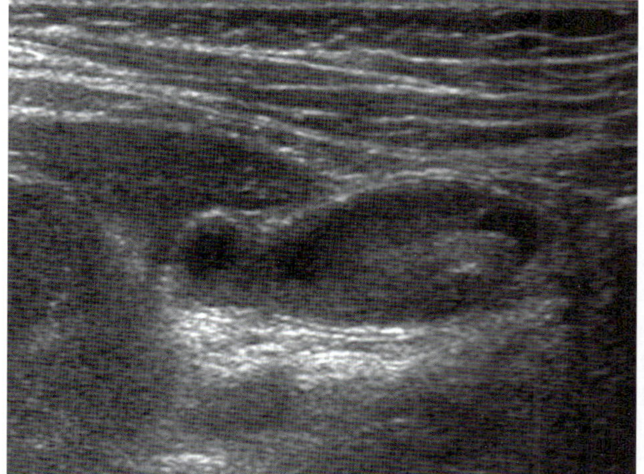

Fig. 11.9: Suppurative appendicitis. Longitudinal image showing a markedly distended appendiceal lumen with a fluid-debris level

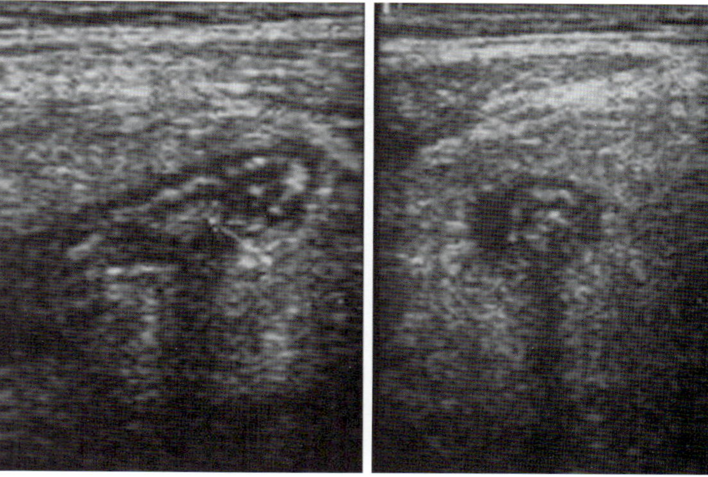

Fig. 11.10: Acute appendicitis with appendicolith. Longitudinal and transverse sonographic images show an inflamed appendix with an appendicolith seen as an echogenic focus with distal shadowing within the lumen

collection suggest either perforation or gas forming organisms. Sympathetic thickening of the adjacent terminal ileum and ascending colon can often be seen.[29]

Doppler Imaging

In cases of appendicitis, the presence of hyperaemia in the appendiceal wall and adjacent meso–appendix (Fig. 11.12) is a sensitive indicator of inflammation and can be well demonstrated on colour Doppler.[33] The contribution of Doppler US is most evident in cases of equivocal grey scale US examination in which it is uncertain as to whether the imaged appendix is inflamed or normal.[34] When gangrenous changes supervene, colour Doppler sonography may show decreased or no perfusion.

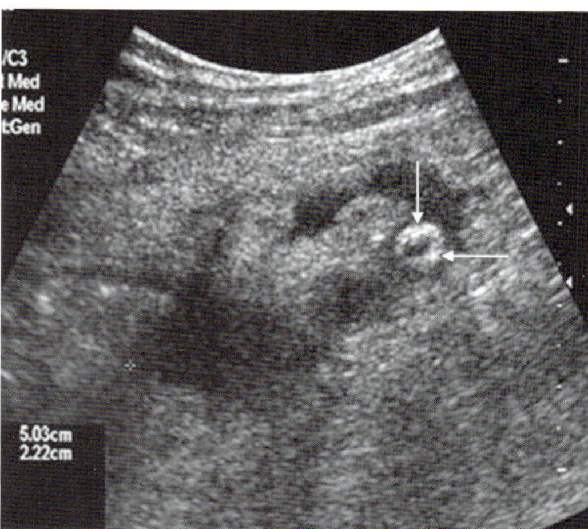

Fig. 11.11: Appendiceal mass. Sonography shows an ill-defined fluid collection and hyperechoic inflamed fat in the right iliac fossa with a small ring shaped structure within it – the appendiceal remnant (arrows)

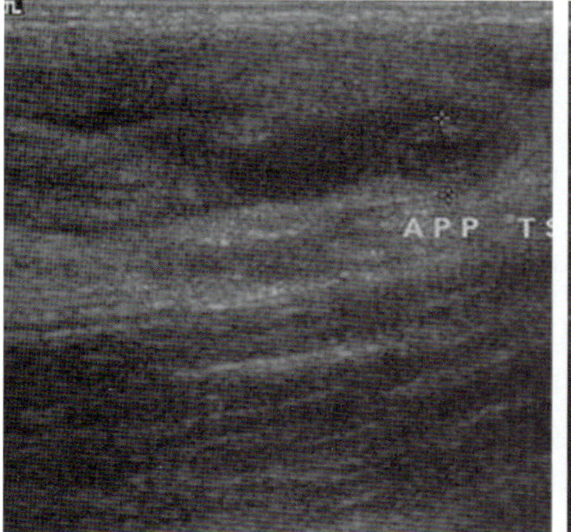

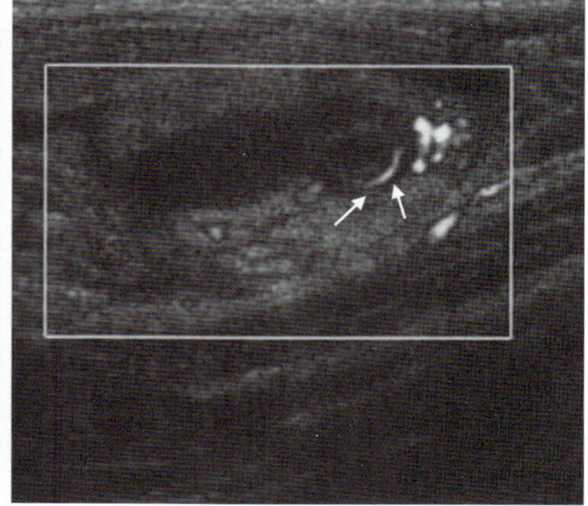

Fig. 11.12: Color Doppler in acute appendicitis. Doppler demonstrates focally increased flow in the appendiceal wall and in the adjacent inflamed fat

Pitfalls in Sonographic Diagnosis

Although ultrasound is highly specific for diagnosis of acute appendicitis, it requires considerable expertise. The most important cause for a false negative result is overlooking of the appendix. Other causes are obesity and a retrocecal position of the appendix. Peritonism may prevent graded compression in patients with perforation, or the dilated, air filled loops of adynamic ileus can hide the appendix from view. The appendix may be relatively thickened in cases of perforated peptic ulcer or sigmoid diverticulitis and a false positive diagnosis is possible. In some cases the terminal ileum may be misinterpreted as the inflamed appendix.

Computed Tomography

Computed tomography is a highly accurate and effective cross-sectional imaging technique for diagnosing and staging acute appendicitis. CT is readily available, operator independent and relatively easy to perform. It has reported sensitivities of 90-100%, specificities of 91-99%, accuracies of 94-98%, positive predictive values of 92-98% and negative predictive values of 95-100% for diagnosis of acute appendicitis.[29]

CT Technique

Appendiceal CT protocols differ considerably with regard to the anatomic area to be included in the scan and to the use of intravenously, orally and rectally administered contrast material. The most popular and conservative approach is to perform helical CT scanning of the entire abdomen and pelvis with intravenous and oral contrast material. The main advantage of this technique is its ability to establish alternative or concurrent diagnoses. Scanning the entire abdomen also allows easy visualization of appendices in the non-standard positions, including the right upper quadrant. The disadvantage of this technique is the time taken for the oral contrast to reach the caecum, which is essential for best results.

To overcome this drawback, simultaneous administration of rectal contrast has been recommended.[35] Not only does it shorten the delay of diagnosis, but the excellent visualization of the large bowel is helpful in identifying the appendix in difficult cases, in distinguishing bowel pathology from appendicitis and in distuingishing pelvic organs from bowel loops.

Rao et al advocated a focussed appendiceal CT technique in which a limited helical CT study of the right lower quadrant is performed after the rapid administration of colonic contrast material.[10] This technique has proved to be as accurate as those techniques in which intravenous and oral contrast material are administered, while allowing scanning to be completed within 15 minutes in the majority of patients examined. A limitation of this scanning method is that a minority of patients will require additional scanning of the proximal abdomen or of the distal pelvis to identify disease not included in the scanning field of view.

The fastest CT protocol has been promoted by Lane et al[36, 37] who have advocated use of non-enhanced helical CT of entire abdomen and pelvis. This examination may be performed in less than 10 minutes, does not expose the patient to the potential risks associated with iodinated contrast agents, requires no bowel preparation and represents the most cost effective imaging alternative to ultrasound. This procedure is most effective in patients with large body habitus, as diagnostic accuracy may be compromised in patients with little abdominal and intrapelvic fat.

CT Findings in Acute Appendicitis

A definitive CT diagnosis of acute appendicitis can be made if an abnormal appendix is identified or if a calcified appendicolith is seen in association with pericecal inflammation.[38, 39] The inflamed appendix is seen as an enlarged, fluid filled, tubular structure associated with inflammatory stranding in the surrounding fat. Circumferential and symmetric wall thickening is nearly always present and is best demonstrated on images obtained with intravenous contrast enhancement (Figs 11.13A to C). The thickened wall usually enhances homogenously, although mural stratification in the form of a target sign may be noted. Traditionally, the threshold diameter of 6 mm was used for diagnosis of appendicitis. However, it has been suggested that this may be too low, as studies in healthy adults have shown that the normal range of appendiceal size varies between 3-10 mm.[40] When the appendix diameter measures between 6-10 mm associated secondary changes such as fat stranding or cecal thickening should be present for a definitive diagnosis of appendicitis on CT. In the absence of secondary changes, a luminal diameter of 9 mm has been advocated as the threshold size for appendicitis.[41]

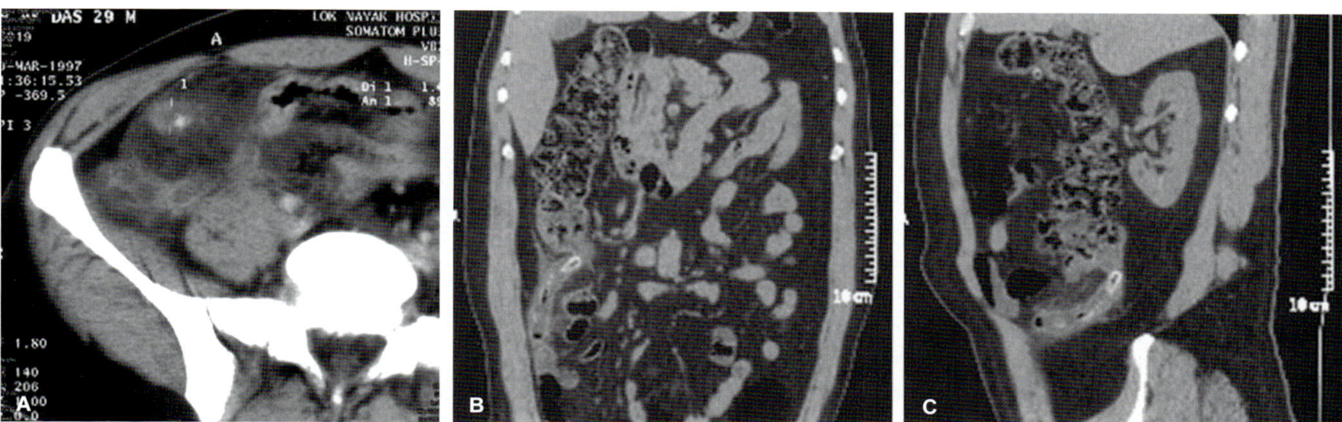

Figs 11.13A to C: CT in a case of acute appendicitis.Axial section (A) The appendix is seen as a thick walled fluid filled structure (measuring 1.4 cm) with a small hyperdense focus within it – an appendicolith. Hazy, ill-defined, linear and streaky densities are seen in the adjacent mesentery due to severe peri-appendiceal inflammation.(B and C) Coronal and sagittal sections in another patient show the entire length of an enlarged, enhancing appendix arising from the cecum with an appendicolith and few air lucencies within the lumen

Linear fat stranding, local fascial thickening, and subtle clouding of the mesentery (Figs 11.13A to C) are characteristic findings of periappendiceal inflammation in non-perforated appendicitis; they may also be seen with microperforation. Other important findings include cecal apical thickening and the arrow head sign (Fig. 11.14). The latter finding occurs when cecal contrast material funnels symmetrically at the cecal apex to the point of appendiceal occlusion due to focal inflammatory thickening.[42] Another rare sign is the cecal bar sign, which is seen when the inflamed cecal wall is interposed between cecal contents and a proximal obstructing appendicolith. Both, the arrowhead sign and the cecal bar sign can be seen only if positive contrast is present in the cecum.

Perforated appendicitis is usually accompanied by pericecal phlegmon or abscess formation (Fig. 11.15). Associated findings include extraluminal air, marked ileocecal thickening, localised lymphadenopathy, peritonitis, and small-bowel obstruction. Contrast-enhanced CT may be useful in cases of perforation by

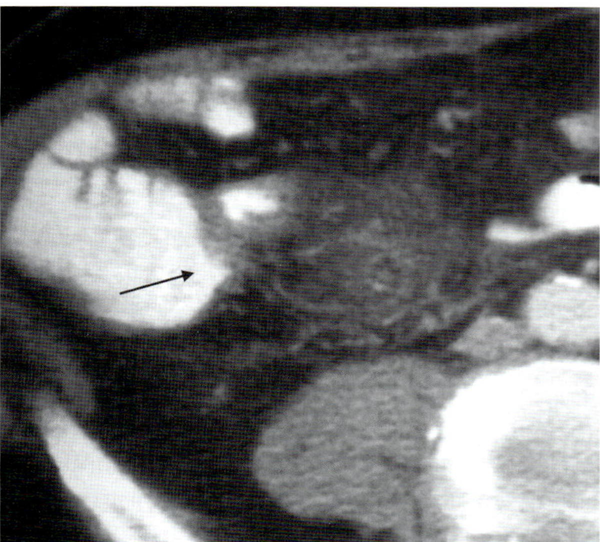

Fig. 11.14: Cecal arrowhead sign on CT. The focally thickened wall of the cecum seems to "funnel" the contrast material (arrow) towards the origin of the inflamed appendix

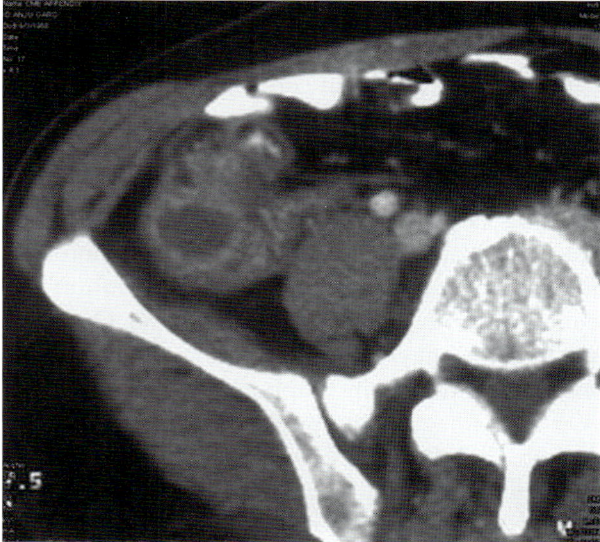

Fig. 11.15: CT of appendiceal abscess seen as a soft-tissue density mass with a central area of decreased attenuation in the right iliac fossa

demonstrating the remains of a fragmented appendix. If the abnormal appendix is not seen, a specific diagnosis of appendicitis can be made by identifying an appendicolith with a periappendiceal abscess or phlegmon. Appendicolith detection rates for helical CT are approximately twice those for conventional CT.[9, 10, 36]

Although a pericecal phlegmon or abscess is strongly suggestive of appendicitis, these are nonspecific findings that may be seen with other disease entities. If substantial inflammation is present within the right lower quadrant, it may be difficult to differentiate primary appendicitis with secondary inflammation of the cacum and terminal ileum from ileocolitis with secondary inflammation of the appendix.

The CT findings of recurrent and chronic appendicitis are identical to those of acute appendicitis.[43] Distal appendicitis is diagnosed when CT reveals appendicitis that involves the distal, "upstream" aspect of the appendix, with a normal appearance of the proximal appendix and cecal apex. An obstructing appendicolith often is identified at the transition point between the normal and abnormal appendiceal segments. The proximal appendix in these cases may be collapsed or partially filled with contrast material or with air.

Magnetic Resonance Imaging (MRI)

MRI is not routinely advocated in cases of suspected appendicitis, it can be useful in cases where sonography is equivocal and CT is not possible or contraindicated such as pregnant women.

On MRI acute appendicitis is best seen in T2W sequences in the axial and coronal planes. T2W images are superior to T1W images because of better visualization of the bright signal intensity of inflammatory change associated with acute appendicitis.[44] The fat suppressed sequence in the axial plane shows the location of inflammation and free fluid collections better than other sequences although spatial resolution is less as compared with T1W and T2W sequences. On fat saturated, gadolinium enhanced T1W images enhancement of the wall of the inflamed appendix is well seen.[45]

On T2W imaging,the thickened appendiceal wall is seen as a slightly hyperintense ring with a markedly hyperintense centre representing intraluminal fluid (Figs 11.16 and 11.17). The cutoff threshold of the appendix is the same as for CT. Periappendiceal inflammation gives a marked hyperintense signal. Appendicoliths are difficult to demonstrate on MRI as they are seen as intraluminal structures without signal intensity on all sequences.

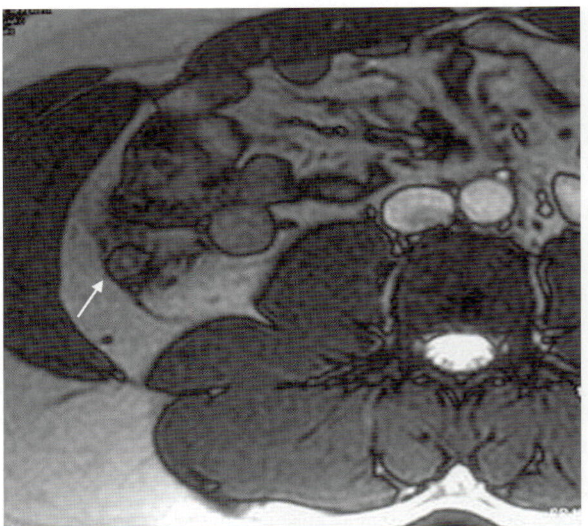

Fig. 11.16: MR-T2 weighted axial image showing a thickened, inflamed appendix in cross-section (arrow)

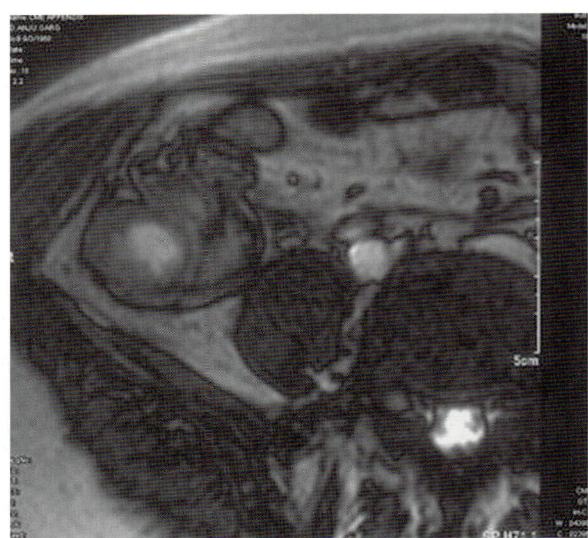

Fig. 11.17: MR-T2 weighted axial image in a case of appendiceal abscess shows a hyperintense fluid collection with a thick wall of lesser intensity

Although MR has the advantage of good visualization of the abnormal appendix and adjacent inflammatory process, the ability to identify appendicitis in atypical locations and operator independence. However, its drawbacks are long scan time, high cost, limited availability and the inability to visualize a normal appendix and appendicolith.

WHICH MODALITY AND WHEN

In almost 80% of the cases, acute appendicitis presents with typical findings and no imaging is required. In the rest of the patients, who are usually young, old or pregnant the clinical picture may be obscure and diagnosis is sometimes impossible until laparotomy. It is in this group of patients that imaging plays an important role and cross sectional imaging has a distinct advantage over clinical assessment.

In an effort to assess the comparative accuracy of US and CT, Doria et al performed a meta analysis of the studies published between 1986 and 2004.[46] CT had a pooled sensitivity and specificity of 94% and 95% respectively in children and 94% and 94% respectively in adults. Ultrasound had a pooled sensitivity and specificity of 88% and 94% respectively in children and 83% and 93% respectively in adults. Also, studies which compared US and CT directly confirmed that CT was more sensitive than ultrasound.

Although CT seems to have an advantage over ultrasound in detection of acute appendicitis, US is substantially less expensive than CT and does not use ionising radiation. It is also more universally available in our country. However, it is operator dependent and a small but finite number of false negative results occur regardless of expertise. Nevertheless, it is still recommended as the initial imaging modality specially in children, followed by CT only if sonographic diagnosis is uncertain. This approach seems to have excellent accuracy with reported sensitivity of 94% to 99% and specificity of 94% to 95%.[47-49]

Computed tomography, being the best modality for showing the extent of inflammatory process, should be used in patients with a high likelihood of perforation. This includes elderly, immunosuppressed patients and those with prolonged clinical symptoms (> 72 hours duration) or a high fever and marked leucocytosis. CT is also the preferred modality for obese patients, patients with right lower quadrant masses and in those with persistent pain but a negative ultrasound.

Ultrasound is also the initial imaging modality in pregnant women with suspected appendicitis. However several factors may limit its usefulness; the appendix may be displaced and adequate graded compression maybe difficult in the presence of the gravid uterus. In these cases MRI has emerged as a useful second line modality and has a reported high accuracy and low failure rate.[45]

MUCOCELE OF APPENDIX

Mucocele of the appendix is a descriptive term for an abnormal sterile, mucus accumulation distending the appendiceal lumen, regardless of the underlying cause. A precursor to the formation of a mucocele is obstruction of the appendiceal lumen which can occur due to fecalith, foreign body, carcinoid tumour, adhesions, endometriosis and mucinous cystadenoma or cystadenocarcinoma.[50] Mucoceles associated with primary mucinous cystadenoma or mucinous cystadenocarcinoma, are also termed malignant mucoceles.

There is formation of a globular or reniform smooth walled, broad based mass invaginating the caecum, with frequent calcification in the wall or substance of the mass. It may be asymptomatic or patients may present with vague abdominal pain—acute or chronic, and rarely intermittent colicky pain caused by intussusception of the mucocele into the caecum.

Plain films may show a soft tissue mass, with or without rim calcification. Barium studies will show non-filling of the appendix with a globular, smooth, broad based filling defect that invaginates into the caecum.[51] The caecum may be displaced laterally and/or cephalad depending on the size of the mucocele. Ultrasound demonstrates a cystic mass extrinsic to the solid viscera in the right lower quadrant, which may show internal echoes, layering or polypoid excrescences (Figs 11.18A and B). Peripheral rim calcification may be seen in some cases.[52, 53] On computed tomography a round, sharply defined mass with or without calcification or septation is seen. Attenuation values range from near water density to soft tissue density (0-40 H) similar to the attenuation values seen in mucinous ascites and other proteinaceous fluids[54] (Figs 11.18C and D).

Myxoglobulosis is a rare variant of mucocele in which the appendix is filled with clusters of pearly white mucus balls intermixed with mucus.[55] These mucus balls may calcify to form spherules 1-10 mm in diameter which can be seen on plain films. Unlike appendiceal calculi, the calcified spherules in myxoglobulosis are usually annular and non laminated, shift within the mucocoele and can layer in the upright position.

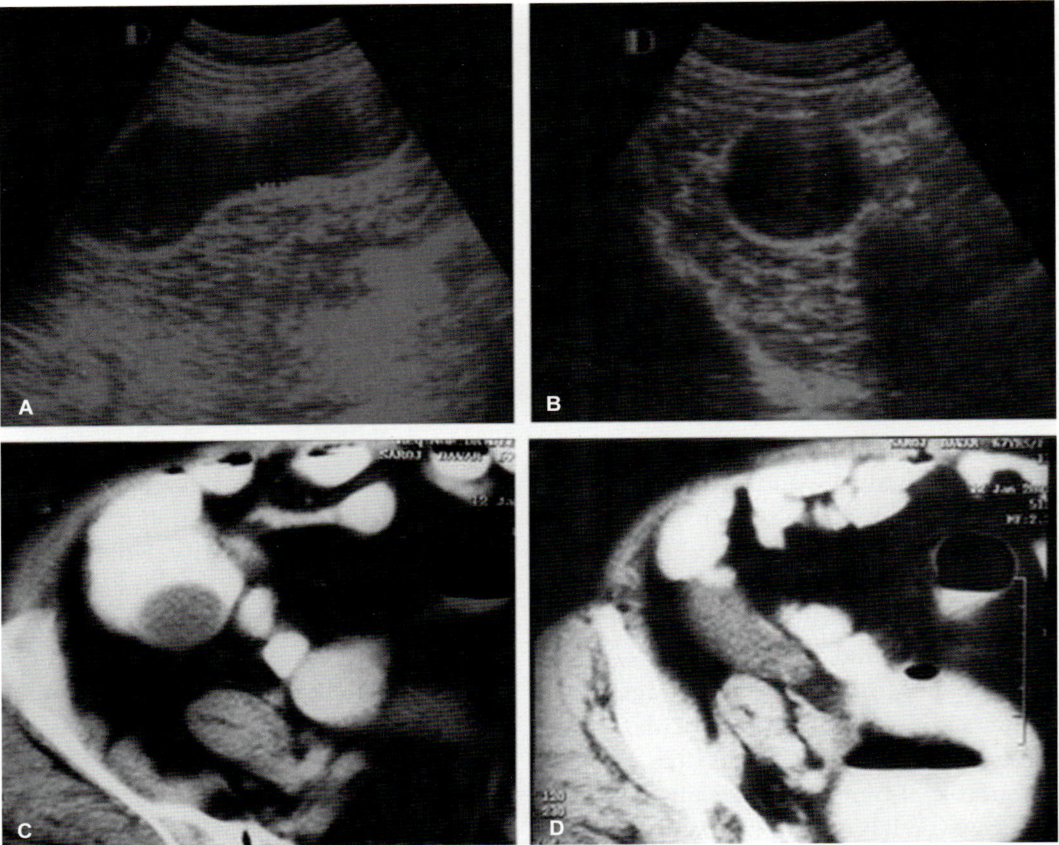

Figs 11.18A to D: Mucocele of the appendix. (A and B) Axial and longitudinal views on sonography show a well defined, thin walled, tubular, fluid filled mass in the right iliac fossa, (C and D) Axial CECT scans show the mucocele invaginating into base of caecum

PRIMARY APPENDICEAL INTUSSUSCEPTION (PAI)

This may present as an acute surgical emergency without time for preoperative diagnostic studies, or as a subacute recurring condition. PAI can also be asymptomatic and may be noted only during a barium enema examination (Figs 11.19A to F). It produces an oval, round, or finger like filling defect projecting from the medial wall of the caecum alongwith non visualization of the appendix.[56]

The radiographic pattern of PAI must be differentiated from mural and intramural cecal defects due to other causes like benign and malignant tumors of the caecum, inverted appendiceal stumps, appendiceal tumors or abscesses. Such a differentiation may be greatly aided if a specific attempt is made to fill and visualize the appendix by appropriate pressure over the caecum during the barium enema examination. Should the defect remain constant and homolateral to the ileocecal valve

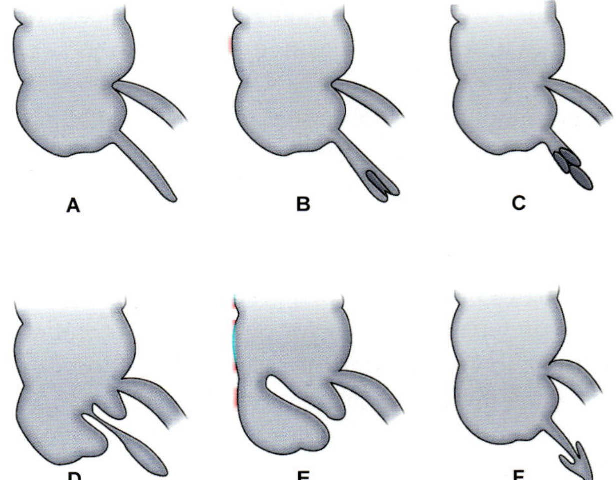

Figs. 11.19A to F: Types of simple primary appendiceal intussusseption (A) The normal appearance (B,C and F) Variations of the appendico-appendiceal intussusceptions. (D) Incomplete appendiceal intussusception into the caecum (E) Complete appendiceal intussusception into the caecum. Only types D and E are visualized radiographically

on two examinations, definite differentiation cannot be made between irreducible intussusception, appendiceal and cecal masses.

POSTOPERATIVE APPENDICEAL DEFECTS

Postoperative defects in the caecum following appendicectomy may be secondary to inversion of the appendiceal stump, ligation of the stump without inversion or complete resection of the appendix.[56]

The inverted appendiceal stump produces a filling defect in the tip of the caecum at the base of the appendix on barium enema examination which varies widely in size from several millimetres to 3 cm. The inverted stump is particularly prominent for several weeks after surgery owing to persistent oedema and inflammation. The surface may be smooth, lobulated or irregular, so that differentiation from a mucosal lesion of the caecum is often difficult, if not impossible.

The importance of recognising the defect lies in differentiating an inverted appendiceal stump from a significant lesion. The inverted stump rarely causes symptoms, although cases of ulceration and intussusception have been reported.

TUMORS OF THE APPENDIX

Primary appendiceal neoplasms are uncommon, being found in approximately .5-1% of appendicectomy specimens at pathological evaluation.[57] Approximately 30-50% of all appendiceal neoplasms will manifest clinically with signs and symptoms of acute appendicitis. Other clinical manifestations include an asymptomatic palpable mass, incidental imaging findings, intussusception, GI bleeding, ureteral obstruction or hematuria or increasing abdominal girth from pseudomyxoma peritoneii.

Although rare, a variety of primary neoplasms can arise from the appendix (Table 11.2). Collins reported an incidence of carcinoid 0.5%, adenocarcinoma 0.08% and benign tumors 4.3%.[3] Benign tumors are rarely picked up preoperatively because of their small size. The diagnosis is usually an incidental finding at surgery.

Carcinoids are the most common and represent upto 80% of all appendiceal neoplasms. They are commonly seen in young adults. Over 70% of these tumors are found in the distal third of the appendix and are < 1 cm in size.[59, 60] Most carcinoids are discovered in appendices removed incidentally at surgery for another procedure or because of acute appendicitis. Although carcinoid tumors are considered potentially malignant, metastatic deposits and carcinoid syndrome with an appendiceal primary site are exceedingly rare.

Table 11.2	Primary neoplasms of the appendix[58]
Adenoma or adenocarcinoma (epithelial)	
Mucinous	
Nonmucinous (colonic type)	
Carcinoid tumor	
Classic	
Tubular	
Goblet cell	
Lymphoma	
Other tumors (rare)	
Ganglioneuroma	
Pheochromocytoma	
Mesenchymal tumors	
Kaposi sarcoma	

Mucinous cystadenomas and cystadenocarcinomas commonly present as mucoceles in case they cause luminal obstruction, or pseudomyxoma peritoneii in case of rupture of mucocele or direct tumor extension into the peritoneal cavity.

On imaging it is rarely possible to see the tumor as it is generally very small. Features of mucocoele (described above) or pseudomyxoma peritoneii may be seen. Pseudomyxoma peritoneii is a diffuse intraperitoneal accumulation of gelatinous ascites. Some investigators posit that nearly all true cases of pseudomyxoma peritoneii are appendiceal in origin and that associated ovarian lesions usually represent metastatic disease, although this is controversial.[61, 62] Ultrasound shows multiple solid appearing intraperitoneal masses displacing the bowel posteriorly, or a multiseptaed ascites. Scalloping of the surface of the liver and spleen is a pathognomonic feature (Figs 11.20A and B). Computed tomography shows characteristic low attenuation (< 20 HU) masses throughout the peritoneal space displacing the bowel loops centrally and scalloping the surfaces of the liver and spleen. MRI additionally enables differentiation between mucinous and fluid ascites on T2W images. Synchronous metastatic ovarian tumours maybe seen in almost 40% of cases.

The *colonic (non-mucinous) adenocarcinomas* are much rarer than the mucinous adenocarcinomas. These tend not to form mucococles, rather they manifest clinically

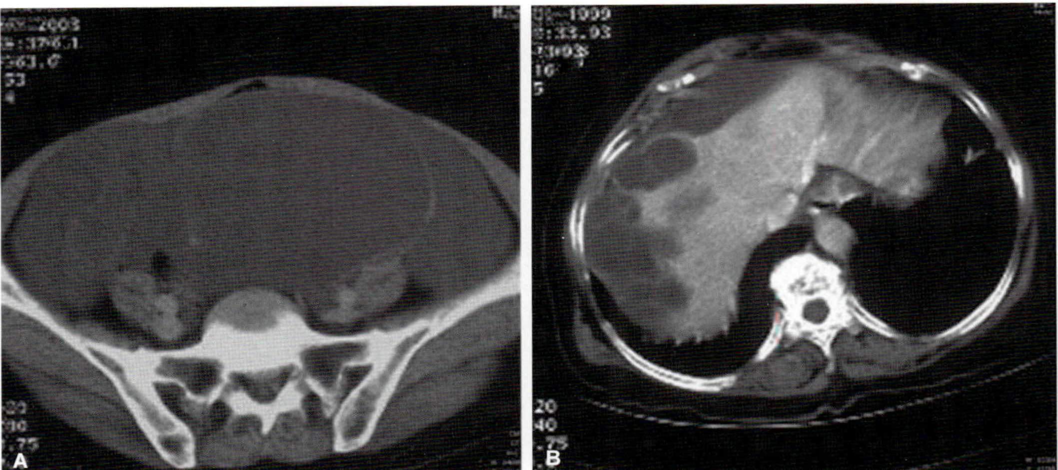

Figs 11.20A and B: Pseudomyxoma peritoneii from mucinous adenocarcinoma of appendix manifesting as increasing abdominal girth. (A) Axial CECT scan shows large locules of high density intraperitoneal fluid, (B) A higher section shows scalloping of the liver margins by the mucin locules

with appendicitis, related to malignant luminal obstruction.[58] At CT, a focal soft tissue mass that involves the appendix but does not show a mucocele formation is most characteristic.

Lymphoma of the appendix is mostly of the non Hodgkin's variety. The appendix becomes massively enlarged but typically maintains its vermiform appearance. On US, diffuse hypoechoic mural thickening with a soft tissue attenuation on CT can be seen. Aneurysmal dilatation of the appendiceal lumen has also been described.[63]

REFERENCES

1. Buschard K, Kjaeldfaard A. Investigation and analysis of the position, fixation, length and embryology of the vermiform appendix. Acta Chir Scand 1973;139:293-8.
2. Oto A, Ernst RD, Mileski WJ, et al. Localisation of appendix with MDCT and inference of findings on choice of appendecectomy incision. AJR 2006;186:987-90.
3. Collins DC. 71,000 human appendix specimens. A final report summarising 40 years' study. Am J Proctocol 1963;14:265.
4. Totty WG, Koehler RE, Cheung LY. Significance of retained barium in the appendix. AJR 1980;135:753.
5. Vukmer GJ, Trummer MJ. Barium appendicitis. Arch Surg 1965;91:630.
6. Puylaert JB. Acute Appendicitis: US evaluation using graded compression. Radiology 1986;158:355-60.
7. Abu-Yousef MM, Bleichaer JJ, Maher JW, et al. High resolution sonography of acute appendicitis. AJR 1987;149:53-8.
8. Rioux M. Sonographic detection of Normal and Abnormal Appendix. AJR 1992;158:733-78.
9. Rao PM, Rhea JT, Novelline RA, et al. Helical CT technique for the diagnosis of appendicitis: prospective evaluation of a focussed appendix CT examination. Radiology 1997;202:139-44.
10. Rao PM, Rhea JT, Novelline RA, et al. Helical CT combined with contrast material administered only through the colon for imaging of suspected appendicitis. AJR 1997;169:1275-80.
11. Stillman CA, Katz DS, Lane MJ. The normal appendix: Evaluation with unenhanced helical CT (abstr) AJR 1999;172(Suppl):58.
12. Karabulut N, Boyaci N, Yagci B, et al. Computed tomography evaluation of the normal appendix : Comparison of low-dose and standard dose unenhanced helical computed tomography. JCAT 2007;31:732-40.
13. Wangensteen OH, Denins C. Experimental proof of the obstructive origin of appendicitis in man. Ann Surg 1939;110:629-47.
14. Pieper R, Kager L, Tidefelt U. Obstruction of the appendix vermiformis causing acute appendicitis: An experimental study in the rabbit. Acta Chir Scand 1982;148:63-72.
15. Nitecki S, Karmeli R, Sarr MG. Appendiceal calculi and faecoliths as indicators for appendicectomy. Surg Gyn Obstet 1990;171:185-8.
16. Shaw RE. Appendix calculi and acute appendicitis. Br J Surg 1965;52:451-59.
17. Trimaur—Dahl J. Roentgen Examinations in Acute Abdominal Diseases. Springfield, IL, Charles C Thomas, 1960.
18. Soter CS. The contribution of the radiologist to the diagnosis of acute appendicitis. Semin Roentgen 1973;8:375.
19. Graham AD, Johnson HF. The incidence of radio-graphic findings in acute appendicitis compared to 200 normal abdomens. Milit Med 1966;131:272.

20. Sehey WL. Use of barium in the diagnosis of appendicitis in children. AJR 1973;118:95.
21. Jeffrey RB Jr, Laing FC, Townsend RR. Acute appendicitis: Sonographic criteria based on 250 cases. Radiology 1988;167:327-29.
22. Jeffrey RB Jr, Laing FC, Lewis FR. Acute Appendicitis: High-resolution real time US findings. Radiology 1987;168:11-4.
23. Puylaert JBCM, Rutgers PH, Laosang RI, et al. A prospective study of ultrasonography in the diagnosis of appendicitis. N Engl J Med 1987;317:666-9.
24. Sivit CJ, Newman KD, Boenning DA, et al. Appendicitis: Usefulness of US in diagnosis in a paediatric population. Radiology 1992;185:549-52.
25. Chesbrough RM, Burhard TK, Balsara EN, et al. Self-localisation in US of appendicitis: An addition to graded compression. Radiology 1993;187:349-51.
26. Chesbrough RM, Burkhard TK, Balsara ZN, et al. Self-localization in US of appendicitis : an addition to graded compression. Radiology 1993;187:349-51.
27. Lee JH, Jeong YK, Hwang JC et al. Graded compression sonography with adjuvant use of a posterior manual compression technique in the sonographic diagnosis of acute appendicitis. AJR Am J Roentgenol 2002;78:863-8.
28. Lee JH, Jeong YK, Park KB, et al. Operator-dependent techniques for graded compression sonography to detect the appendix and diagnose acute appendicitis. AJR Am J Roentgenol 2005;184:91-7.
29. Birnbaum BA, Wilson SR. Appendicitis at the Millenium. Radiology 2000;215:337-48.
30. Rompel O, Huelsse B, Bodenschatz K, et al. Harmonic US imaging of appendicitis in children. Pediatr Radiol 2006;36(12):1257-64.
31. Kessler N, Cyteval C, Gallix B et al. Appendicitis: evaluation of sensitivity, specificity, and predictive values of US, Doppler US, and laboratory findings. Radiology 2004;230:472-8.
32. Rettenbacher T, Hollerweger A, Macheiner P, et al. Outer diameter of the vermiform appendix as a sign of acute appendicitis: evaluation at US. Radiology 2001;218: 757-62.
33. Quillin SP, Siegel MJ. Appendicitis: Efficacy of colour Doppler sonography. Radiology 1994;191:557-60.
34. Lim HK, Lee WJ, Kim TH, et al. Appendicitis: Usefulness of colour Doppler US. Radiology 1996;201:221-25.
35. O'Malley ME, Halpert E, Mueller PR, et al. Helical CT protocols for the abdomen and pelvis: a survey. AJR Am J Roentgenol 2000;175:109-13.
36. Lane MJ, Katz DS, Ross BA, et al. Unenhanced helical CT for suspected acute appendicitis. AJR 1997;168: 405-09.
37. Lane MJ, Liu DM, Huynh MD. Unenhanced helical CT for suspected acute appendicitis: Experience in 300 consecutive patients (abstr) AJR 1999;172 (suppl):114.
38. Birnbaum BA, Balthazar EJ. CT of appendicitis and diverticulitis. Radiol Clin North Am 1994;32:885-98.
39. Balthazar EJ, Megibow AJ, Siegel SE, et al. Appendicitis: Prospective evaluation with high resolution CT. Radiology 1991;180:21-4.
40. Tamburrini S, Brunetti A, Brown M, et al. CT appearance of normal appendix in adults. Eur Radiol 2005;15: 2096-103.
41. Daly CP, Cohan RH, Francis IR, et al. Incidence of acute appendicitis in patients with equivocal CT findings. AJR Am J Roentgenol 2005;184:1813-20.
42. Rao PM, Wittenberg J, McDowell RK, et al. Appendicitis: Use of arrow head sign for diagnosis at CT. Radiology 1977;202:363-6.
43. Rao PM, Rhea JT, Novelline RA, et al. The computed tomography appearance of recurrent and chronic appendicitis. Am J Emerg Med 1998;16:26-33.
44. Hoerman M, Paya K, Eibenberger K, et al. MR imaging in children with non-penetrated acute appendicitis: Value of unenhanced MR imaging in sonography selected cases. AJR 1998;171:467-70.
45. Inceseu L, Coskun A, Seleuk MB, et al. Acute appendicitis: MR imaging and sonographic correlation. AJR 1997; 168:669-74.
46. Doria AS, Moineddin R, Kellenberger CJ, et al. US or CT for diagnosis of appendicitis in children and adults? A meta-analysis. Radiology 2006;241:83-94.
47. Garcia Pena BM, Mandl KD, Kraus SJ, et al. Ultrasonography and limited computed tomography in the diagnosis and management of appendicitis in children. JAMA 1999;282(11):1041-6.
48. Smink DS, Finkelstein JS, Garcia-Pena BM, et al. Diagnosis of acute appendicitis in children using a clinical practice guideline. J Pediatr Surg 2004;35:392-5.
49. Hernandez JA, Swischuk LE, Angel CA, et al. Imaging of acute appendicitis. US as the primary imaging modality. Pediatr Radiol 2005;35:392-5.
50. Higa E, Rosai J, Pizzimbono CA, et al. Mucosal Hyperplasia, Mucinous cystadenoma and Mucinous Cystadenocarcinoma of the Appendix. Cancer 1973;6:1525-41.
51. Marohak RH, Gerson A. Mucocele of the appendix. Am J Digest Dis 1960;5:49.
52. Dachman AH, Lichtenstein JE, Friedman AC. Mucocele of the appendix and pseudomyxoma peritoneii. AJR 1985;144:923-9.
53. Kim SH, Lim HK, Lee WJ, et al. Mucocele of the appendix: Ultrasonographic and CT findings. Abdominal Imaging 1998;23:292-6.
54. Madwed D, Mindelzun R, Jeffrey RB Jr. Mucocele of the Appendix: Imaging findings. AJR 1992;159:69-72.
55. Lubin J, Berle S. Myxoglobulosis of the appendix. Arch Pathol 1972;94:533.

56. Berk RN. Radiology of the appendix. In Taveras JM, Ferucci JT (Eds) Radiology–Diagnosis—Intervention. Philadelphia: JB Lippincott Co. 1986;4(41).
57. Connor SJ, Hanna GB, Frizelle FA. Appendiceal tumors: retrospective clinicopathologic analysis of appendiceal tumors from 7,970 appendicectomies. Dis Colon Rectum 1998;41:75-80.
58. Pickhardt PJ, Levy AD, Rohrmann CA. et al. Primary neoplasms of the appendix: Radiologic spectrum of disease with pathologic correlation. Radiographics 2003;23:645-62.
59. Deans GT, Spence RA. Neoplastic lesions of the appendix. Br J Surg 1995;82:299-306.
60. Moertel CG, Weiland LH, Nagomey DM et al. Carcinoid tumor of the appendix: treatment and prognosis. N Eng J Med 1987;317:1699-1701.
61. Carr NJ, Sobin LH. Unusual tumors of the appendix and pseudomyxoma peritoeii. Semin Diagn Pathol 1996; 13:314-25.
62. Hinson FL, Ambrose Ns. Pseudomyxoma peritoneii. Br J Surg 1998;85:1332-9.
63. Pickhardt PJ, Levy AD, Rohrmann CA et al. Non Hodgkin Lymphoma of the appendix: Clinical and CT findings with pathological correlation. AJR 2002;187:1123-7.

Part Two

Hepatobiliary and Pancreatic Imaging

Chapter Twelve

Liver Anatomy and Techniques of Imaging

Smriti Hari

INTRODUCTION

The segmental anatomy of the human liver has become a matter of increasing interest to the radiologist especially in view of the need for an accurate preoperative localization of focal hepatic lesions. Presently, the type of surgical resection chosen depends largely on the segmental localization of the hepatic lesion.[1] Depiction of arterial, portal venous and hepatic venous anatomy and identification of important vascular variants is critical for surgical guidance. This chapter outlines the gross and segmental liver anatomy along with the imaging and surgical implications. It introduces the various imaging techniques that are used to evaluate this organ which today occupies the center stage of gastrointestinal radiology.

NORMAL ANATOMY

The liver is the largest gland in the body weighing about 1.4 kg in an adult. It occupies the right hypochondrium and part of the epigastrium.Its left lobe may extend a variable distance into the left hypochondrium. The anatomy of the liver can be detailed based on its external appearance or based on its vascular and biliary architecture. The liver is covered by peritoneum, except along a portion of its posterosuperior surface known as the bare area and the fossae for gall bladder and the inferior vena cava (IVC). It has two major surfaces, a superior or diaphragmatic surface and an inferior or visceral surface.

On the superior surface, the falciform ligament separates the liver into a larger right lobe and a smaller left lobe. At the porta hepatis the main portal vein, the proper hepatic artery, and the common bile duct are contained within investing peritoneal folds known as the hepatoduodenal ligament. The main portal vein divides into a short right and a longer left branch. The right portal vein has an anterior branch that lies centrally within the anterior segment of the right lobe and a posterior branch that lies centrally within the posterior segment of the right lobe. The left portal vein initially courses anterior to the caudate lobe. The ascending branch of the left portal vein then travels anteriorly in the left intersegmental fissure to divide the medial and lateral segments of the left lobe.

BISMUTH AND COUINAUD'S SEGMENTAL NOMENCLATURE

The Bismuth and Couinaud classification of liver anatomy divides the liver into four sectors and eight functionally indepedent segments based on the hepatic veins and branches of the portal vein (Fig. 12.1).[2, 3] Each segment has its own vascular inflow, outflow, and biliary drainage. In the center of each segment there is a branch of the portal vein, hepatic artery and bile duct. In the periphery of each segment there is vascular outflow through the hepatic veins. Right hepatic vein divides the right lobe into anterior and posterior segments. Middle hepatic vein divides the liver into right and left lobes (or right and left hemiliver). This plane runs from the inferior

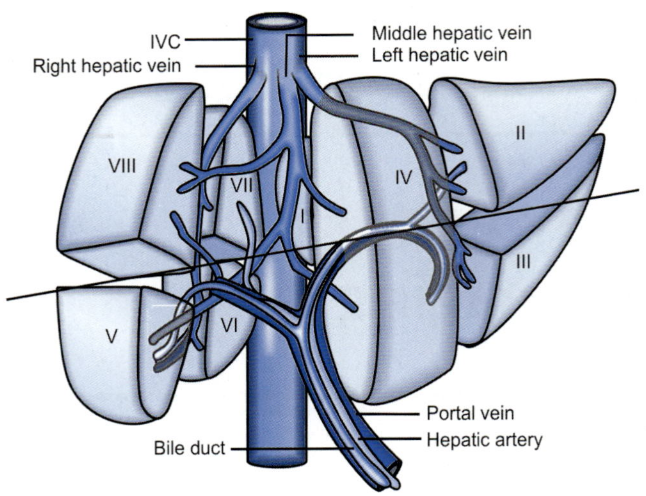

Fig. 12.1: Segmental liver anatomy according to Bismuth-Couinaud's classification. The liver is divided into eight functionally independent segments based on the hepatic veins and branches of the portal vein. The dashed line represents the transverse plane intersecting the liver at the level of the portal vein bifurcation separating the superior from the inferior hepatic segments

vena cava to the gallbladder fossa. Left hepatic vein divides the left lobe into medial and lateral segments.

The Bismuth-Couinaud classification also defines a so called portal vein plane as the transverse plane intersecting the liver at the level of the portal vein bifurcation into the right and left branches. This plane divides the hepatic segments into superior (II, IVa, VII, VIII) and inferior (III, IVb, V, VI) segments. In the functional left lobe of liver, segment II lies above the portal vein plane to the left of and lateral to the left hepatic vein. Segment III lies below the portal vein plane also to the left of and lateral to the left hepatic vein. Segement IV lies between the middle and left hepatic veins and is further subdivided into segements IVa (above the portal vein plane) and IVb (beneath this plane).

The functional right lobe of liver is composed of segments V through VIII, which lie to the right and lateral to the middle hepatic vein. Segment V lies between the middle and right hepatic veins below the portal vein plane. Segment VI also lies below the portal vein plane but posterolateral to the right hepatic vein. Segment VII lies directly cranial to segment VI that is above the portal vein plane. Lastly Segment VIII lies between the middle and right hepatic veins above the portal vein plane.[3, 4] Middle hepatic vein divides the liver into right and left lobes (or right and left hemiliver). This plane runs from the inferior vena cava to the gallbladder fossa.

Segment I (caudate lobe) is bordered posteriorly by the IVC, laterally by the ligamentum venosum, and anteriorly by the left portal vein. Unlike the other segments of the liver, it receives branches from the main trunk as well as both the right and left branches of the portal vein. The caudate lobe has one or more veins that drain directly into the IVC, separately from the three main hepatic veins. This special vascularization is a distinctive characteristic of segment I and is the reason for its hypertrophy in patients with cirrhosis and hepatic venous outflow tract obstruction.

Segments II and III correspond to the superior and inferior subsegments of the lateral segment of left lobe and segment IV correponds to the medial segment of the left lobe. Segments V and VIII correspond to inferior and superior subsegments of anterior segment of right lobe, whereas segment VII and VI correspond to the superior and inferior subsegments of the posterior segment of right lobe respectively.[3]

Couinaud's nomenclature provides critical information regarding the potential resection planes. Recent advances in hepatic surgery have made anatomic resections along these planes possible while minimizing morbidity and blood loss. This nomenclature is an invaluable tool for both the radiologist and surgeons, allowing them to define the location of tumors and their relationship with major vascular structures. Major resections of up to 75% of the liver can be performed provided the future liver remnant is not functionally compromised. The liver regenerates following extended hepatectomies provided two or three adjacent segments remain.

The segmental hepatic anatomy can be readily identified on cross-sectional imaging techniques including CT and MRI, and to a lesser extent sonography.[2, 4]

ULTRASONOGRAPHY (US)

Sonography is a versatile, noninvasive and inexpensive modality for evaluating the liver. It is usually the initial imaging modality used for suspected liver pathology.[5] It plays a vital role in the evaluation of focal liver lesions, screening for liver metastases in a patient with known malignancy, screening for hepatocellular carcinoma in the setting of hepatitis/cirrhosis, portal hypertension, surgical obstructive jaundice, hepatic veno-occlusive disease and preoperative work up and postoperative follow up of liver transplant patients. Sonography is ideally suited to study the internal architecture of a focal mass, and distinguish a solid from a cystic lesion.

Some lesions are known to have characteristic sonographic morphology and the technique helps to narrow the differential diagnosis and triage patients for further imaging workup. The major drawback of this technique is that it is highly operator dependent. The details of sonographic features of different pathologies will be discussed in subsequent chapters. The addition of color Doppler flow imaging further helps in characterizing mass lesions and assessing patency of vessels.[2] Doppler is particularly helpful in liver transplants, Budd-Chiari syndrome and cirrhosis.

Technique

The liver is usually scanned in the supine or left decubitus position with a 3.5-5 MHz convex transducer in the transverse, sagittal and oblique planes, from a subcostal approach. The sub-costal approach may not suffice in all patients and intercostal scanning may have to be done with a small footprint transducer.[2] This is especially true in shrunken cirrhotic livers. An attempt is made to delineate the venous landmarks so that all the liver segments are sequentially scanned.

The porta is an area that needs special attention. The portal vein, common duct and hepatic artery need to be evaluated and if available, color Doppler should be used for this purpose. Color Doppler and particularly power Doppler are very useful to assess the vascularity of focal liver lesions aiding in the characterization of these lesions.

The recent advances in ultrasound technology include multifrequency electronic transducers which have multiple and variable focal zones, tissue harmonic imaging and ultrasound contrast agents. These advances have all contributed to better resolution and have enhanced the capability of US even in difficult patients.[5]

Ultrasound Contrast Agents

Intravenous contrast agents in the form of microbubbles have found major clinical application in the liver for detecting and characterizing focal lesions. These agents flood the blood pool after IV injection and remain confined to the vascular compartment. Both the gas they contain (usually air or a perfluoro compound) and their stabilizing shell (denatured albumin, surfactants or lipids) are critical to render them sufficiently stable so that they survive for several minutes after injection. Microbubbles are easily destroyed by acoustic pressure. Low mechanical index and intermittent imaging are employed to obtain sufficient contrast enhancement. Harmonic color and power Doppler imaging and pulse inversion techniques are powerful sonographic contrast-specific techniques.[5] The characteristics of dynamic enhancement pattern of tumors, such as hepatocellular carcinoma, hemangioma, focal nodular hyperplasia and adenoma are very similar to those with contrast enhanced CT and MR imaging.[6]

Sonographic Anatomy

Liver parenchyma is imaged as fine homogeneous mid-level echoes interrupted only by fissures and vessels. The liver echogenicity is usually greater but may be equal to renal echogenicity. Hepatic veins are well-defined tubular structures without significant marginal echoes (Fig. 12.2A), whereas portal veins invariably have echogenic walls due to fibrous and fatty tissue (Figs 12.2B and C). Bile ducts run parallel to portal vein branches, but their location in relation to veins is variable, and the axiom that ducts are always anterior to portal vein branches is not correct. The state of art electronically focused ultrasound equipment demonstrates normal intrahepatic biliary radicles quite well and a bile duct must be atleast 40% of the size of its neighboring portal vein branch for it to be considered dilated. Therefore the mere visualization of parallel channels in the liver parenchyma does not indicate biliary dilatation.[2]

The gallbladder is located in the interlobar fissure and is ideally suited for sonographic evalution. The wall of the gallbladder should not be greater than 3 mm in the fasting state. The common duct lies anterior to the portal vein at the porta hepatis and is measured at the place where the hepatic artery crosses perpendicularly between them (Fig. 12.2C). This level has been used because of the consistent acoustic window provided by the surrounding liver which ensures reproducibility of the measurement. The common duct should not be greater than 6 mm at this point.

On Doppler examination the normal hepatic vein trace reflects the transmitted right heart pressure changes leading to flow reversal during the right atrial contraction (Fig. 12.2D). The portal vein trace is normally continuously antegrade with a mean peak velocity of 15-22 cm/s. The portal venous flow shows slight undulation related to the cardiac cycle and respiration (Fig. 12.2E).[2]

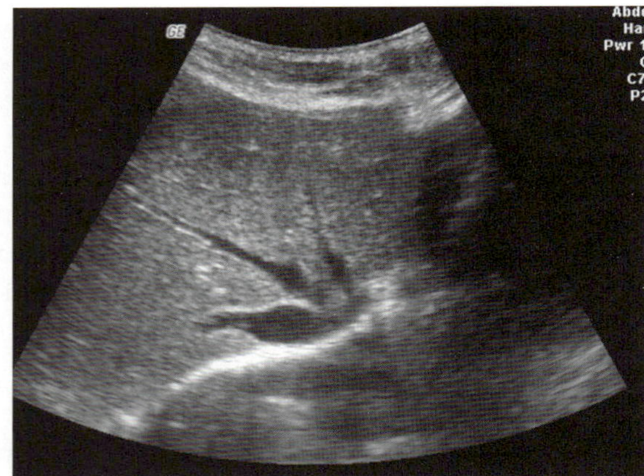

Fig. 12.2A: Transverse US scan showing the three hepatic veins joining the IVC

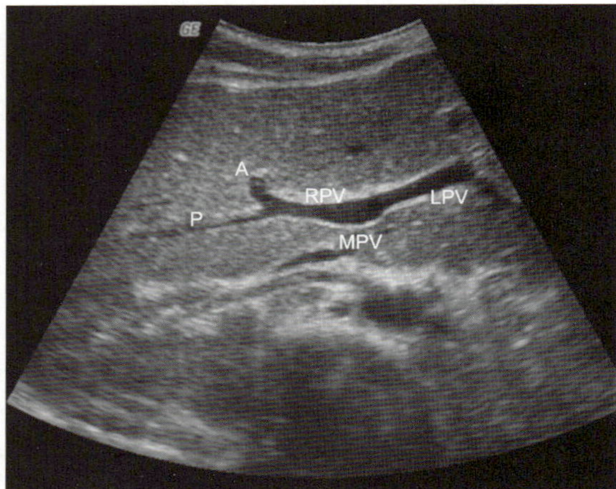

Fig. 12.2B: US scan showing the bifurcation of main portal vein (MPV) into the right (RPV) and left portal veins (LPV). Right portal vein is further dividing into the anterior (A) and posterior (P) segmental branches

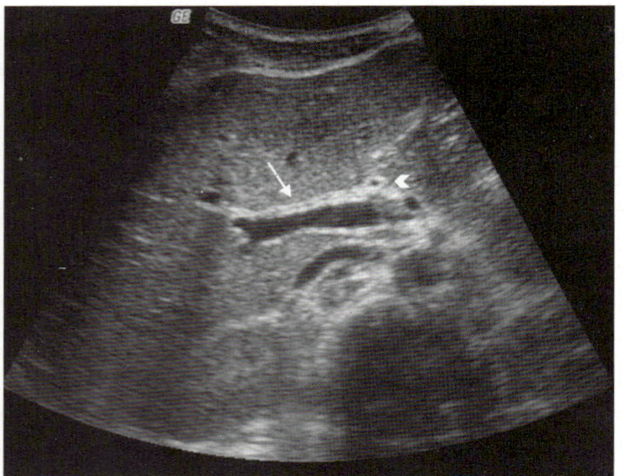

Fig. 12.2C: US scan at the level of porta hepatis showing the portal vein and the collapsed common duct (arrow) anterior to it. The circular structure anterior to the portal vein is the hepatic artery seen in cross-section (arrowhead)

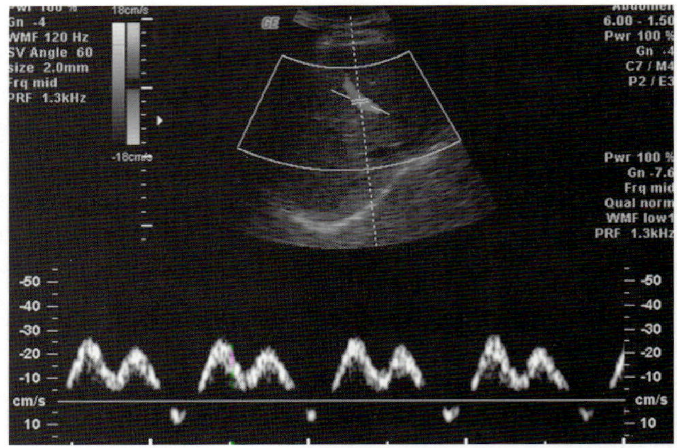

Fig. 12.2D: Color Doppler flow imaging of hepatic vein showing normal triphasic flow pattern with a short phase of reversed flow *(For color version see plate 2)*

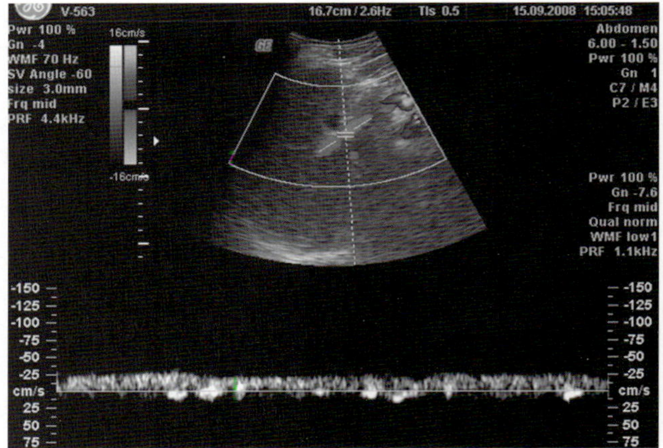

Fig. 12.2E: Color Doppler flow imaging of portal vein showing continuous antegrade flow with minimal phasicity *(For color version see plate 2)*

Intraoperative Ultrasonography (IOUS)

Intraoperative and laparoscopic US are very useful techniques that have had major impact on patient management. IOUS has superior lesion detection rate as compared to CT and MRI. Its major impact has been in patients with colorectal malignancy with liver metastases undergoing surgery. IOUS is used to accurately identify liver metastases and guide surgical resection. It can demonstrate tumor nodules as small as 3-5 mm. It is also useful to localize deep seated lesions that have been localized on preoperative imaging but cannot be palpated by the surgeon.[2]

A 5-7 MHz T-shaped linear array probe is used for intraoperative scanning. The probe can be sterilized using ethylene oxide gas sterilization. The probe is applied directly to the liver surface and no gel or acoustic coupling agent is necessary. The liver is scanned from the dome to the caudal edge and from left to right in a sequential manner. Color Doppler can be coupled with the gray scale scan and is very useful to identify vascular landmarks and assess their patency.

IOUS provides the operating surgeon with useful real-time diagnostic and staging information that may result in an alteration in the planned surgical approach. Current applications for this technique include tumor staging, metastatic survey, guidance for metastasectomy and various tumor ablation procedures, documentation of vessel patency, evaluation of intrahepatic biliary disease, and guidance for liver transplantation.[7]

Computed Tomography

CT has for long been the modality of choice for evaluation of focal liver lesions. The helical CT scan allows the entire liver to be scanned in a breath-hold leading to the routine use of, "dual-phase" scanning, in which first an arterial dominant phase is acquired 20 seconds after the beginning of an intravenous injection of the contrast material bolus, and subsequently, beginning 60 seconds after the start of the contrast material injection, a portal venous phase is acquired. Multidetector computed tomography (MDCT), based on different row configuration of detectors, together with the development of sub-second gantry rotation time, has further reduced scanning time and improved the z-axis resolution.

With MDCT systems, the initial admixed arterial dominant phase used with a single-detector CT system can be subdivided into a pure early arterial phase and a late arterial phase (Figs 12.3A to C).[8] The early arterial phase exquisitely displays the hepatic arterial system. The late arterial phase corresponds to initial opacification of the portal venous system. The enhancement of hypervascular neoplasms is maximized during this phase. In both primary and metastatic hypervascular neoplasms (e.g. hepatocellular carcinoma, islet cell tumor, carcinoid, sarcoma), approximately 30% more lesions are detectable during this phase than during the later portal venous phase. The phase of maximum hepatic parenchymal enhancement and hepatic venous opacification occurs about 45 seconds after the beginning of the pure early arterial phase. This circulatory phase has been entitled the portal venous phase. During this phase, enhancement of background hepatic parenchyma is maximized.

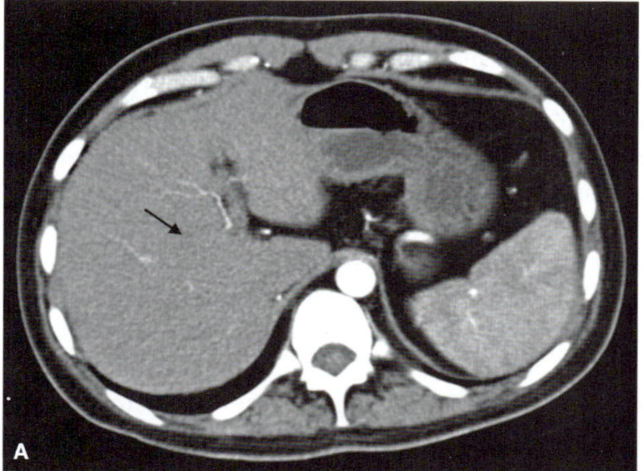

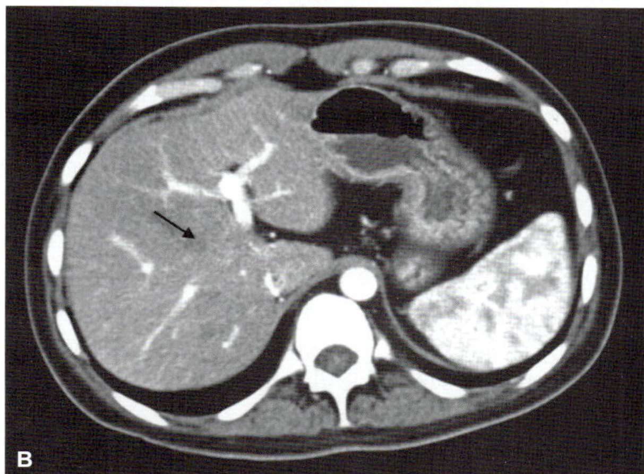

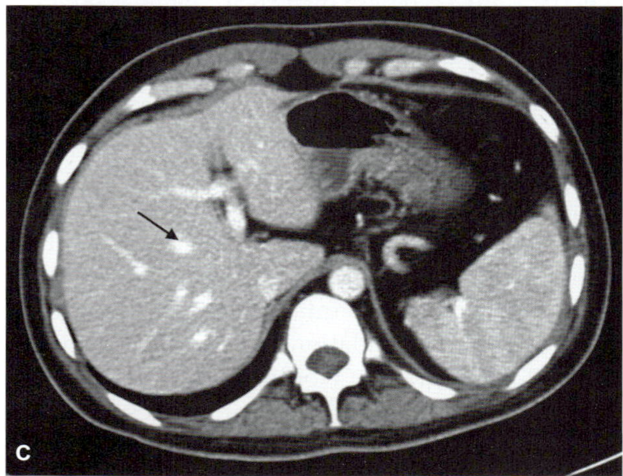

Figs 12.3A to C: Triphasic CT examination. Axial sections at the same level following a bolus of IV contrast demonstrating clearly the hepatic vessels and phases of enhancement. Early arterial phase (A), late arterial phase (B), portal venous phase (C). Note the hepatic vein appears as a focal lesion on the early and late arterial phases but normally fills in during the portal venous phase (arrows)

For triphasic hepatic imaging, about 150 ml of iodinated contrast is injected at 3-4 ml/sec via a pressure injector. Acquisition parameters, specifically, table speed per rotation and scan rotation speed are set to allow full coverage of the liver in less than 8 seconds. Three image acquisitions are performed, one each during the early arterial phase (20 seconds after injection of contrast medium), late arterial phase (30 seconds after the initiation of injection), and portal venous phase (60 seconds after the start of injection). A fourth delayed phase is added when required at 3-5 minutes and is especially useful in the evaluation of hemangiomas. Accurate acquisition timing for multiphasic imaging depends on the assessment of circulation time in individual patients. This assessment is made by using either a preliminary injection of a small bolus of contrast material ("mini-bolus injection") or online bolus tracking software. The early arterial-phase scan for CT angiography is started at the time of peak aortic enhancement or at aortic enhancement of arbitrary numbers between 100 and 150 Hounsefield units (HU). If only two phases are planned through the liver (late arterial and portal venous), then the late arterial-phase scan can be triggered following a delay of 10 seconds after peak aortic enhancement time. For a single portal-venous phase scan, a region of interest can be placed over the liver parenchyma and the scan can be triggered at 30 to 55 HU hepatic enhancement over the baseline. Using fixed delay times (i.e. 30 seconds for late arterial phase and 60–70 seconds for portal venous phase) does not take into account patient related factors, such as weight and cardiac output. In patients without circulatory disturbances, however, they can still be used. Water is used as the enteric contrast agent in the upper gastrointestinal tract to allow a three-dimensional volume data set to be used for multiplanar CT angiography.[8, 9]

Early arterial phase imaging of the hepatic and mesenteric arterial circulation is reserved for patients in whom CT angiography would be of benefit, such as potential transplant recipients, candidates for hepatic resection or cryoablation, or candidates for chemoembolization.[8] CT angiography images can be created through three-dimensional reconstructions of the thin-slice, isotropic images obtained in the early arterial phase. Maximum intensity projection, surface-shaded display, and volume-rendered techniques have been applied to the production of CT angiography to depict vascular anatomy (Fig. 12.4). A combined CT angiogram/CT

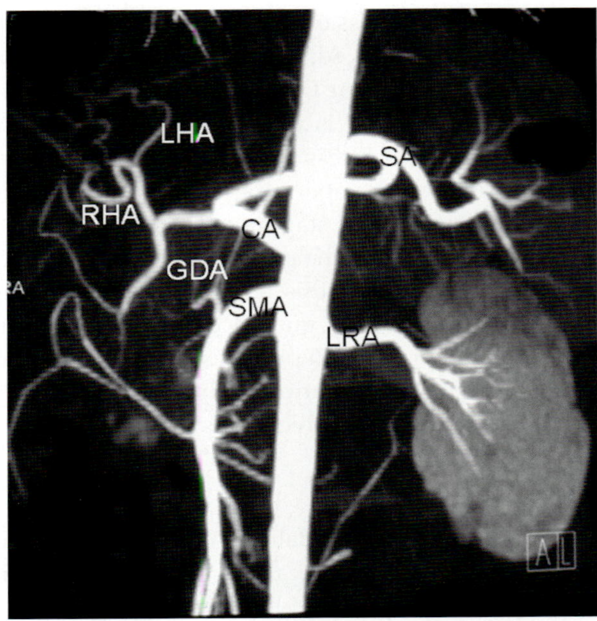

Fig. 12.4: Coronal maximum intensity projection (MIP) reconstructed from the axial MDCT images obtained during early arterial phase of contrast enhancement demonstrates abdominal aorta and its branches, celiac axis (CA), superior mesenteric artery (SMA) left gastric artery (LGA), gastroduodenal artery (GDA), right hepatic artery(RHA), left hepatic artery (LHA), left renal artery (LRA)

portogram can be obtained from the late arterial imaging phase. This study is valuable for mapping the extrahepatic portal venous system in patients with suspected pancreatic or bile duct malignancy and in patients who are potential transplant recipients.[8] Venous compression, venous stenosis or thrombosis, and portal systemic venous collateral vessels can be displayed.

MDCT scanners permit acquisition of thin slices with isotropic voxel size. The advantages of thinner, isotropic slices are less partial volume averaging and, more importantly, superior quality, true isotropic, three-dimensional, multiplanar reconstructions (MPR) (Fig. 12.5).[9, 10] Superior quality MPRs obtained in various planes improve the detection of small subcapsular lesions, can show the feeding arteries and venous drainage of detected lesions, or help in the characterization of lesions by better demonstrating their enhancement patterns.

Virtual hepatectomy with volume-rendered images and liver volume estimation before surgery is useful in planning the extent and nature of hepatic resection (Fig. 12.6).[8] Estimation of liver volume using three-

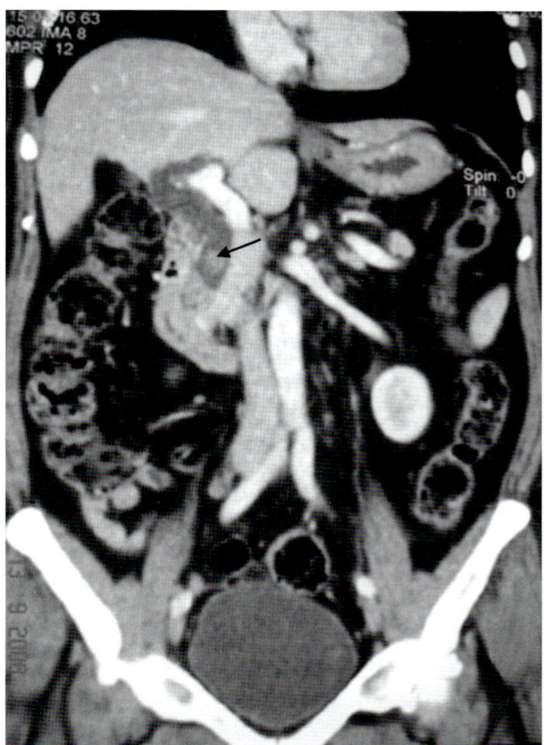

Fig. 12.5: Coronal maximum intensity projection (MIP) reconstructed from the axial MDCT images obtained during the portal venous phase of contrast enhancement shows a dilated common duct with a calculus at the distal end (arrow)

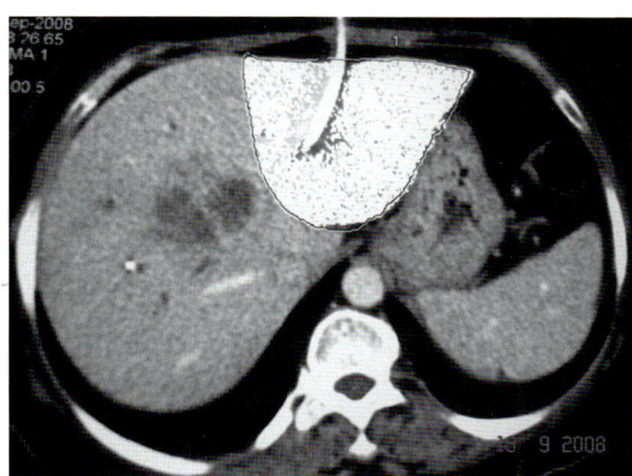

Fig. 12.6: CT volumetry in a patient with cholangiocarcinoma planned for partial liver resection. Segments II and III are manually mapped out on contiguous axial slices and the volume is calculated using volumetric software

dimensional techniques, when combined with clinical and laboratory evaluation of liver function, can facilitate the prediction of postoperative liver failure in patients undergoing resection, assists in embolization procedures, and aids planning of staged hepatic resection for bilobar disease.[11]

CT Anatomy

The CT attenuation value of liver on non-contrast enhanced studies ranges between 40 and 80 HU. The normal liver appears homogenous and has a density greater than spleen, pancreas and kidneys due to the high concentration of glycogen in liver. Increased density of liver may be seen in hemochromatosis and glycogen storage diseases, whereas decreased density is most often related to fatty infiltration of the liver.[2]

The hepatic veins are well visualized on axial sections through the superior part of the liver. They can be seen coursing towards the inferior vena cava and help to delineate the segmental anatomy (Fig. 12.7A). Just inferior to this level, axial scans show the left portal vein (Fig. 12.7B). The fissure of the ligamentum venosum separates the left lobe and the caudate lobe. Further inferior sections show the bifurcation of portal vein into its right and left branches (Fig. 12.7C). Horizontal portion of the right portal vein dividing into its anterior and posterior branches is seen more caudally (Fig. 12.7D). Most caudal scans show the gallbladder (Fig. 12.7E).

Magnetic Resonance Imaging

MR imaging offers major advantages due to its high contrast resolution, multiplanar capability, sensitivity to blood flow and lack of ionizing radiation. Technical advances in MR hardware and software have allowed the introduction of faster pulse sequences void of motion artifacts that previously posed limitations to abdominal MR imaging. It has evolved into a robust problem solving technique for liver lesions.

Technique

Liver imaging is ideally done on a high field system (> 1.0 T) with fast gradients. Phased array multicoils are used which provide high signal to noise ratio.

Fast gradient echo sequences (such as FLASH on a Siemens scanner and spoiled GRASS on a GE scanner) are generally used to obtain T1 weighted sequences (Figs 12.8A and B)) and echo-train sequences (such as Turbo spin echo on Siemens scanner and Fast spin echo on a GE scanner) are used for T2 weighted sequences (Fig. 12.8C).[12] Echo-train spin echo sequences acquired as contiguous thin 2D sections or as a thick 3D volume slab, also form the basis for MR cholangiography (Fig. 12.8D). Fat suppression is frequently used with these echo train sequences because fat has very high signal intensity on

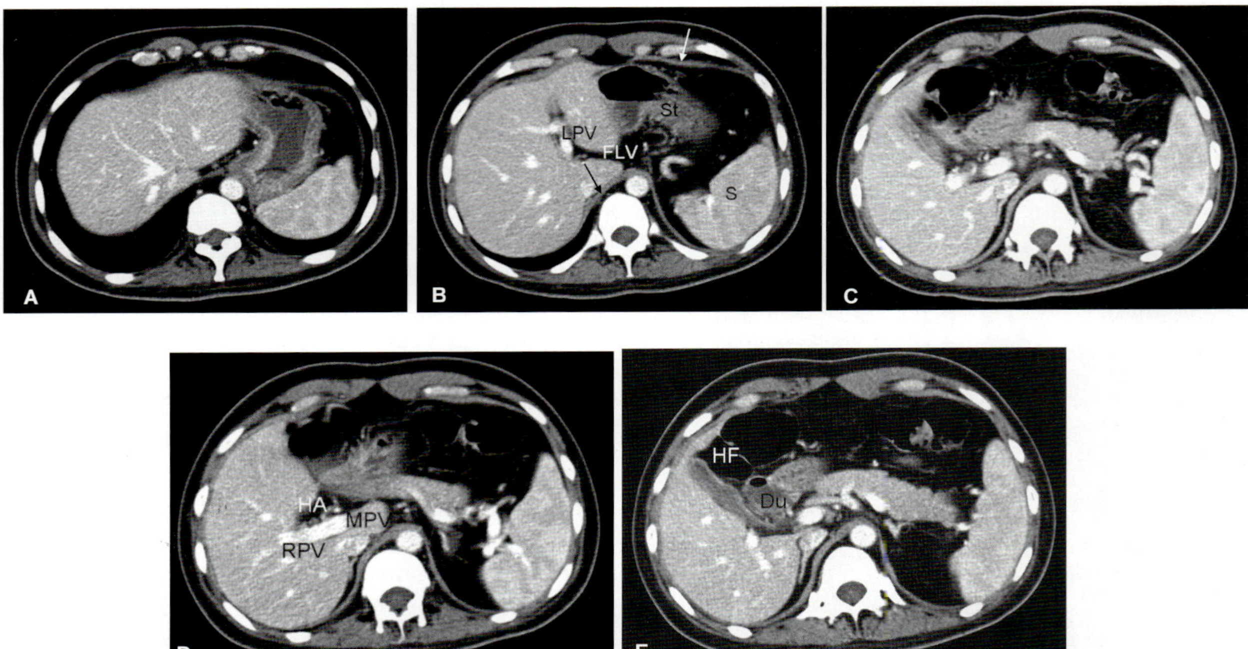

Figs 12.7A to E: Liver anatomy on contrast enhanced (portal venous phase) scans at different levels. A: The hepatic venous branches are clearly identified coursing towards the IVC. B: Level 30 mm caudal to A shows the left portal vein (LPV). The adjacent organs at this level can be easily identified with the stomach (St) to the left and the diaphragm seen posteriorly (black arrow) as well as anteriorly (white arrow), S, spleen. The fissure of the ligamentum venosum (FLV) separates the left lobe and the caudate lobe. C: Level 20 mm caudal to B shows the portal bifurcation. According to the Bismuth classification, this is the craniocaudal demarcation level, separating the superior segments (2,4a,7,8) and the inferior segments(3,4b,5,6).D: Level 20 mm caudal to C shows the main portal vein (MPV) giving rise to the right portal vein (RPV) which bifurcates into anterior and posterior branches. The hepatic artery (HA) can be seen anterior and medial to the main portal vein. E: Level 20 mm caudal to D shows the gallbladder. Hepatic flexure (HF) of the colon and second part of duodenum (Du) are seen medially

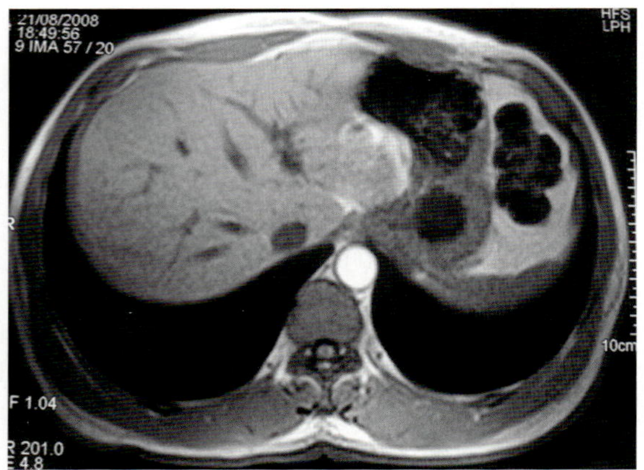

Fig. 12.8A: Gradient echo breath-hold axial T1W MR image showing hepatic veins as tubular flow voids

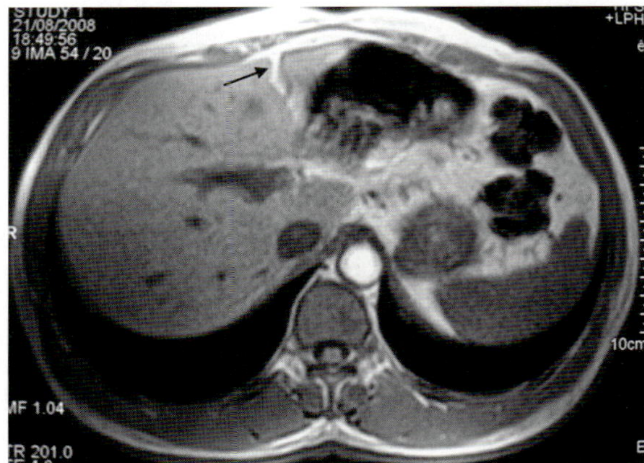

Fig. 12.8B: Gradient echo breath-hold axial T1W MR image at a more caudal level showing right branch of the portal vein. The fissure for ligamentum teres is clearly seen as a fatty cleft arrow

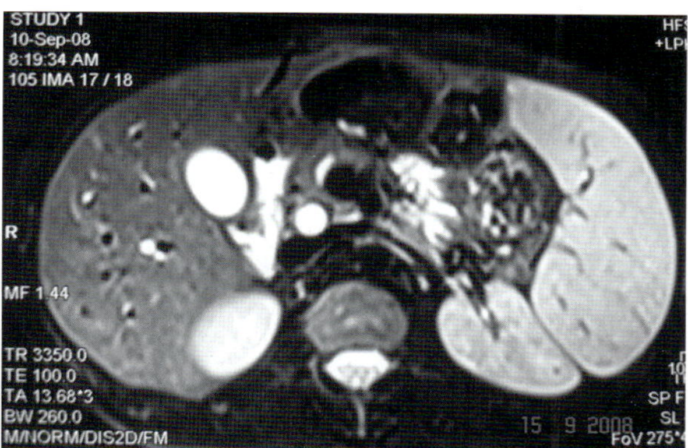

Fig. 12.8C: Turbo spin echo T2W MR image showing the liver to be dark as compared to the spleen

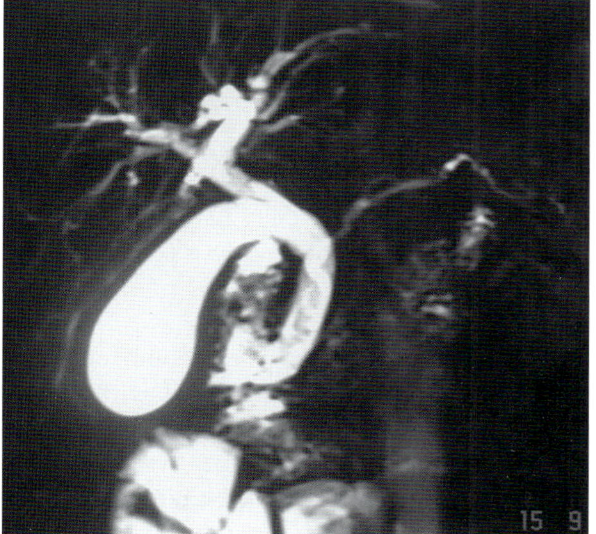

Fig. 12.8D: MRCP image showing dilated intrahepatic biliary radicles, common bile duct and pancreatic duct in a case of periampullary carcinoma

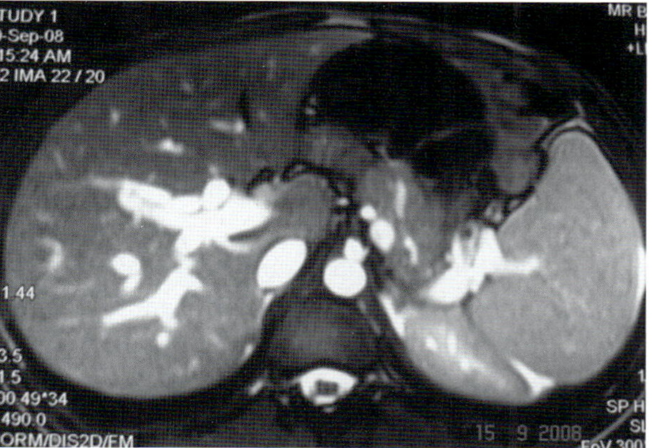

Fig. 12.8E: Axial Fast imaging employing steady state acquisition (True FISP). Anatomical details can be visualized in a single breath hold. Tissues like blood, fat and bile appear bright due to their high T2/T1 ratio

these images. To evaluate intracellular lipid content in focal lesions, fatty sparing or fatty infiltration, TE may be set in phase (4.4 ms at 1.5T) or out of phase (2.2 ms at 1.5T). Signal intensity drop out is present in out of phase images if fat and water are present in the same voxel.[12] True fast imaging with steady state free precession (true FISP), a GRE sequence keeps TR and TE as short as possible to minimize motion and susceptibility artifacts. In true FISP the contrast is related to the T2/T1 ratio; thus the tissues with a high T2/T1 ratio like blood, fat and bile appear bright (Fig. 12.8E).

T1-weighted 2D gradient echo sequences are used to perform dynamic post contrast imaging of the liver. Volumetric interpolated breath-hold examination(VIBE) permits the acquisition of isotropic pixels of 2 mm in all dimensions with an acquisition time of less than 25 seconds.[13] The volumetric dataset can be reconstructed in any plane, producing MR angiography and venography images. Single shot echo-planar imaging (EPI), which allows the acquisition of T2-weighted images in a very short time, is useful for new applications such as diffusion and perfusion imaging. These techniques provide additional functional and qualitative information regarding the liver lesions. Some recent studies have shown that benign lesions such as hepatic cysts and hemangiomas have higher ADCs than malignant lesions (hepatocellular carcinoma and metastases).[14]

MR Imaging Contrast Agents

MR contrast agents are currently used to accentuate the difference in signal intensity between the liver lesion and adjacent normal tissue and to highlight different enhancement patterns. According to the biodistribution, the contrast agents available for liver imaging can be divided into three categories: extracellular contrast agents; hepatobiliary contrast agents and reticuloendothelial system (RES) targeted contrast agents.

Extracellular contrast agents are hydrophilic, small molecular weight gadolinium chelates. Gd-DTPA, Gd-DOTA and the more recent nonionic agents gadodiamide, gadobutrol and gadoteridol, provide information on vascularization and perfusion similar to that of iodinated contrast media at CT examination.[15] Using breath-hold T1-weighted GRE sequences, a dynamic contrast enhanced study of the liver is performed during the arterial (20-30 s after injection), portal venous (70-80s after injection), and the delayed (2-3 min after injection) phase of enhancement. Fat saturation is recommended to decrease motion artifacts and to homogenize the images. For accurate timing of image acquisition, either a timing bolus of 1-2 ml of a Gd-chelate or automatic triggering based on the detection of vessel enhancement (Smartprep, Carebolus) may be used.

Hepatobiliary agents are either only hepatocyte selective, such as mangafodipir trisodium (Mn-DPDP), or are Gd chelates (gadobenate dimeglumine [Gd-BOPTA] and Gd-ethoxybenzyl [Gd-EOB]) that are both distributed in the extracellular space and are hepatocyte selective.[16] The hepatocyte specific Gd-chelates and Mn-DPDP are T1 agents, which shorten T1 time and result in increased signal on T1-weighted images.They demonstrate enhancement of the normal liver parenchyma on T1-weighted imaging. Mn-DPDP is injected at a dose of 0.5 mmol/kg as a slow intravenous infusion and maximum liver enhancement is observed within 15-20 minutes after the infusion. On postcontrast images, most tumors of nonhepatocellular origin including metastases, benign liver cysts, and hemangiomas typically are hypointense relative to enhanced liver parenchyma on T1-weighted images and are more conspicuous than on unenhanced images. Tumors of hepatocellular origin, such as FNH, adenoma, and well differentiated HCC, have been shown to accumulate Mn-DPDP.[17]

Gd-BOPTA is the only contrast agent currently available in India for clinical use. It combines the properties of a conventional nonspecific Gd agent with that of a hepatocyte selective agent. Gd-BOPTA is mainly eliminated by the kidneys and the biliary excretion rate is only 3 to 5%. Gd-BOPTA is administered intravenously in a lower dose of 0.05 mmol/kg compared to the extracellular contrast agents. Serial contrast-enhanced liver imaging can be performed with the use of Gd-BOPTA after bolus injection, in the same fashion as with other nonspecific extracellular contrast agents (Fig. 12.9). Since an increased fraction of Gd-BOPTA is taken up by the hepatocytes, the detection and delineation of hypovascular lesions on delayed (40-120 min post-injection) or static hepatobiliary liver imaging is improved.[18] Differentiation between hepatocellular adenomas and FNH is possible with the use of Gd-BOPTA during the hepatobiliary phase. FNH contains biliary ducts, whereas hepatocellular adenoma does not have biliary ducts. In the hepatobiliary phase FNH reveals increased enhancement as compared with hepatocellular adenomas. In contrast to Gd-BOPTA, Gd-EOB-DTPA has a high biliary excretion rate of 50%. Hepatobiliary contrast enhancement with Gd-EOB-DTPA reaches the maximum level at about 10 to 20 minutes postinjection and is followed by a plateau phase that has duration of 2 hours. The highest liver-to-lesion contrast is observed during the imaging window of 20 to 45 minutes after injection of Gd-EOB-DTPA.

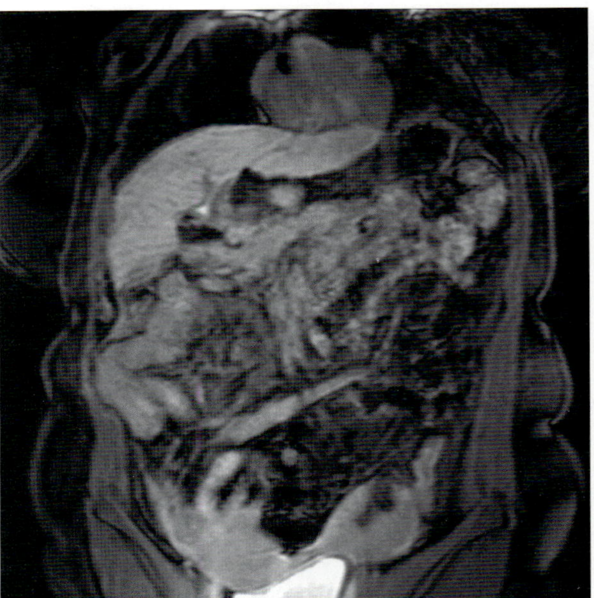

Fig. 12.9: Gd-BOPTA (MultiHance) enhanced imaging of biliary-enteric anastomosis. T1W scan obtained 1 hour after contrast injection shows diffuse persistent contrast uptake and enhancement of the liver. Additionally, contrast agent is opacifying the anastomosis. Approximately 3% of Gd-BOPTA clearance is from liver uptake and excretion into bile

RES targeted contrast agents are superparamagnetic particles of iron oxide (SPIO), which produce signal loss on T2-weighted images. Kupffer cells take up more than 80% of these particles allowing liver-specific phase imaging 10 min after injection. Malignant focal lesions usually do not contain Kupffer cells and therefore appear as bright nodules against the markedly hypointense liver parechyma.[19]

MRI and MR angiography examinations are commonly requested for patients with endstage liver and renal disease to evaluate for transplant eligibility, visualization of vascular anatomy, and post transplant complications. Gadolinium-enhanced MRI traditionally has been preferred over contrast-enhanced CT because many of these patients have impaired renal function. Gadolinium-based contrast media (at doses of 0.1-0.2 mmol/kg) are considered less nephrotoxic than iodinated contrast agents. Recently, however, there have been many reports of incidence of nephrogenic systemic fibrosis (NSF) triggered by IV injection of double-dose gadodiamide for MRI and MR angiography examinations in patients with acute or chronic renal insufficiency who are usually, but not always, on dialysis.[20] NSF is a fibrosing skin condition with systemic manifestations including fibrosis of the skeletal muscle, bone, lungs, pleura, pericardium, myocardium, kidney, muscle, bone, testes, and dura. This condition can be quite disabling because the skin tightening and musculotendinous involvement result in joint contractures, muscle weakness, and arthralgia. To date, the only gadolinium-based contrast agent reported to be associated with NSF is gadodiamide. However, the reporting of this association is still quite immature and other gadolinium agents may be found to have a similar association. Therefore, it is advisable to follow the recommendations of the European Society of Urogenital Radiology: "In patients with CKD [chronic kidney disease stage] 4 and 5 (GFR < 30 mL/min), always use the smallest possible amount of the contrast agent to archieve an adequate diagnostic examination, and never use more than 0.3 mmol/kg of gadolinium-based contrast medium."[21] It would be prudent to screen patients scheduled for contrast-enhanced MRI examinations by obtaining a recent serum creatinine level and calculated creatinine clearance if they have a history of kidney disease or diabetes mellitus.

MR Anatomy

The liver parenchyma appears homogeneous on both T1 and T2 weighted scans. The liver shows moderate signal intensity on T1W images, similar to the pancreas but brighter than spleen and kidneys (Figs 12.8A and B). On T2W scans the liver appears dark and has signal intensity less than that of pleen (Fig. 12.8C).

The anatomy is similar to that seen on CT except that it can be displayed in the coronal and sagittal planes also. The intrahepatic venous structures are well delineated on both spin echo and gradient echo sequences.

The left and right hepatic ducts and the common bile duct can be demonstrated on MRCP images (Fig. 12.8D).

ANGIOGRAPHY

The high quality of images provided by cross-sectional imaging techniques has led to a dramatic change in the indications for hepatic angiography. This technique is now seldom used for diagnostic purpose, but is widely used for vascular interventions used in the management of liver lesions.

Technique

Prior to the procedure, coagulation profile and serum creatinine are obtained. The femoral artery is the preferred approach and Seldinger technique is used for the puncture. Angiography of the liver is performed by selective injections of the coeliac axis and superior mesenteric artery (SMA) or one or more of their branches. A 5 French right angle or reverse curve catheter such as Cobra is commonly used. The volume of contrast used is about 20-30 cc injected at a rate of 5-6 cc per second.[2] Visualization of the portal venous system is done by injecting the splenic artery or SMA coupled with prolonged filming.

Anatomy

The common hepatic artery is a branch of the coeliac axis (Fig. 12.10). It gives rise to the gastroduodenal artery after which it becomes the proper hepatic artery. The proper hepatic artery divides into the right and left hepatic arteries, both of which divide into two major branches supplying the corresponding segments. Congenital variants are commonand are seen in 25-50% of patients. The common variants include a replaced or accessory right hepatic artery arising from the SMA (11-17%) (Fig. 12.11) and a replaced or accessory left hepatic artery

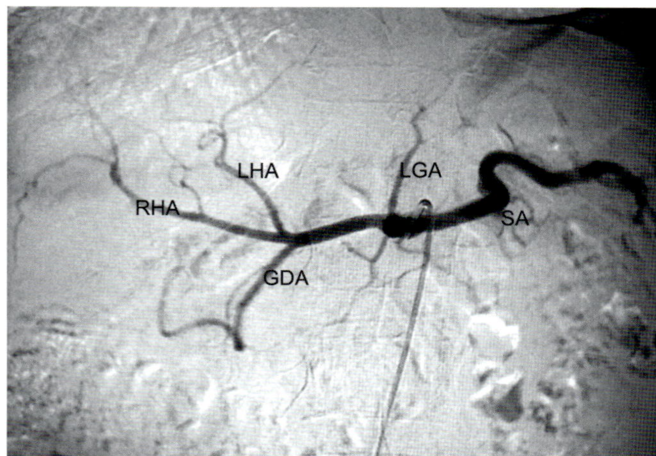

Fig. 12.10: Intra-arterial DSA showing selective celiac axis injection, splenic artery (SA), left gastric artery (LGA), gastroduodenal artery (GDA), right hepatic artery (RHA), left hepatic artery (LHA)

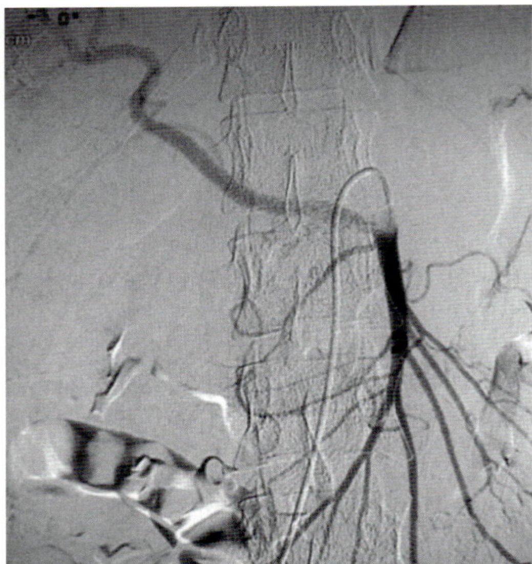

Fig. 12.11: Selective superior mesenteric artery injection during Intra-arterial DSA showing anomalous origin of right hepatic artery from superior mesenteric artery

arising from the left gastric artery.[2] The vascular anatomy and hemodynamics of liver is needed in order to select the appropriate angiointerventional treatment and in hepatic surgeries. In accessory or a replaced right hepatic artery, whether it is originated from the superior mesenteric artery or the celiac trunk, it is still running in the hepatoduodenal ligament and ascends behind the portal vein and posterolateral to the common hepatic duct and reaches the porta hepatis. In accessory or a replaced left hepatic artery, originating from the left gastric artery, in runs in the gastro-hepatic ligament and enters the umbilical fissure via the fissure of the ligamentum venosum to reach the left lobe of liver. Many other less common anomalies are also described.

PET

PET is an imaging modality that uses positron emitters, such as fluorine-18, to visualize tissues, such as cancers with increased glucose metabolism. The most commonly used radiotracer for PET is 2-[18F] fluoro-2-deoxy-d-glucose (FDG). FDG-PET has been proved to be highly sensitive in detecting hepatic metastases from various primaries, such as colon, pancreas, esophagus, sarcoma, and parotid (Fig. 12.12). Additionally, in the case of suspected recurrent colorectal cancer, FDG-PET may be more sensitive than CT for discovering hepatic metastases, with the potential of detecting disease earlier than CT, so that metastatic disease is more amenable to curative resection. FDG-PET should be considered in the setting of increasing serum carcinoembryonic antigen level to assess for hepatic metastases, because it has been shown to be more sensitive than CT for this purpose.[22]

The sensitivity of FDG-PET for HCC is about 50%. Although FDG-PET can fail to detect many HCCs and their extrahepatic metastases, it does detect many of the poorly differentiated HCC. For benign primary liver lesions, like hemangioma, hepatocellular adenomas, and focal nodular hyperplasia, FDG-PET is also not suitable. The ability of FDG-PET quantitatively to estimate metabolic rates makes it a potentially valuable tool for monitoring response to therapy, which will likely assume an expanding role for this modality. PET has limited spatial resolution compared with CT and MR imaging, and the intrinsic heterogeneous activity in normal background liver further limits the ability of FDG-PET to show small malignant lesions.[23]

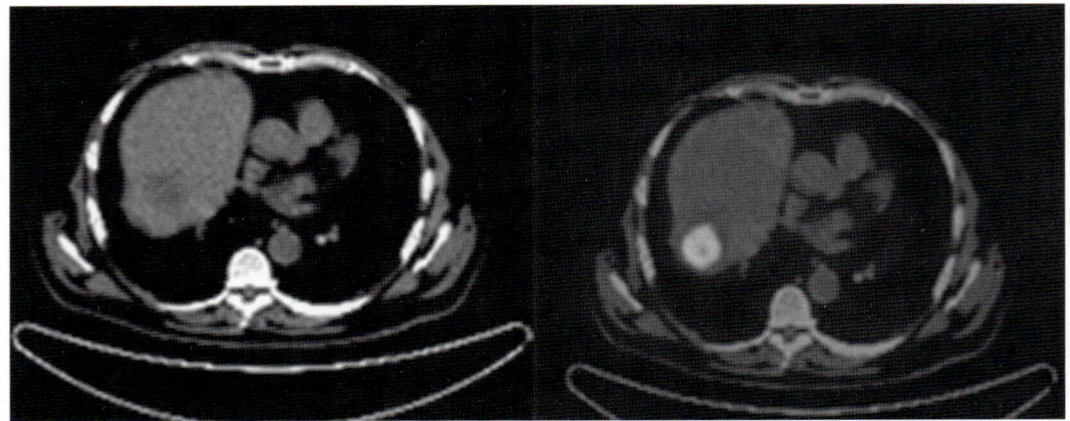

Fig. 12.12: FDG-PET image showing a metastatic lesion in the segment 8 of liver in a newly diagnosed case of carcinoma colon *(For color version see plate 3)*

REFERENCES

1. Taylor HM, Ros PR. Hepatic Imaging: An overview. The Radiologic Clinics of North America 1998;6:2:237-45.
2. Gazelle GS, Saini S, Mueller PR, eds. Hepatobiliary and Pancreatic Radiology: Imaging and Intervention. New York, NY, USA: Thieme Medical Publishers, 1998.
3. Gazelle GS, Haage JR. Hepatic neoplasms: Surgically relevant segmental anatomy and imaging techniques. Am J Roentgen 1992;158:1015-18.
4. Lafortune M, Madore F, Patriquin H, et al. Segmental anatomy of the liver: A sonographic approach to the Couinaud's nomenclature. Radiology 1991;181:443-48.
5. Kono Y, Mattrey RF. Ultrasound of the liver. The Radiologic Clinics of North America 2005;43(5):815-26.
6. Wilson SR, Jang HJ, Kim TK et al. Diagnosis of Focal Liver Masses on Ultrasonography: Comparison of Unenhanced and Contrast-Enhanced Scans. J Ultrasound Med 2007;26(6):775-87.
7. Kruskal JB, Kane RA. Intraoperative US of the liver: techniques and clinical applications. Radiographics 2006;26(4):1067-84.
8. Oto A, Tam EP, Szklaruk J. Multidetector Row CT of the Liver. The Radiologic Clinics of North America 2005; 43(5):827-48.
9. Ji H, McTavish JD, Mortele KJ et al. Hepatic Imaging with Multidetector CT. Radiographics 2001;21:S71-S80.
10. Foley WD. Special focus session: Multidetector CT: abdominal visceral imaging. Radiographics 2002;22: 701-19.
11. Wigmore SJ, Redhead DN, Yan XJ, et al. Virtual hepatic resection using three-dimensional reconstruction of helical computed tomography angioportograms. Ann Surg 2001;233:221-6.
12. Martin DR, Danrad R, Hussain SM. MR Imaging of the Liver. The Radiologic Clinics of North America 2005; 43(5):861-86.
13. Rofsky NM, Lee VS, Laub G, et al. Abdominal MR imaging with a volumetric interpolated breath-hold examination. Radiology 1999;212:876-84.
14. Parikh T, Drew SJ, Lee VS, et al. Focal liver lesion detection and characterization with diffusion-weighted MR imaging: comparison with standard breath-hold T2-weighted imaging. Radiology 2008;246(3):812-22.
15. Semelka RC, Martin DR, Balci NC, et al. Focal liver lesions: comparison of dual-phase CT and multisequence multiplanar MR imaging including dynamic gadolinium enhancement. J Magn Reson Imaging 2001;13:397-401.
16. Reimer P, Schneider G, Schima W. Hepatobiliary contrast agents for contrast-enhanced MRI of the liver: properties, clinical development and applications. Eur Radiol 2004;14:559-78.
17. Braga HJV, Choti MA, Lee VS, et al. Liver lesion: manganese-enhanced MR and dual-phase helical CT for preoperative detection and characterization. Comparison with receiver operating characteristic analysis. Radiology 2002;223:525-31.
18. Ferrucci JT. Advances in abdominal MR imaging. Radiographics 1998;18:1569-86.
19. Reimer P, Jahnke N, Fiebich M, et al. Hepatic lesion detection and characterization: value of nonenhanced MR imaging. Superparamagnetic iron oxide-enhanced MR imaging, and spiral CT: ROC analysis. Radiology 2000;217:152-8.
20. Broome DR. Nephrogenic systemic fibrosis associated with gadolinium based contrast agents: a summary of the medical literature reporting. Eur J Radiol 2008;66(2): 230-4.
21. ESUR guideline: gadolinium based contrast media and nephrogenic systemic fibrosis. European Society of Urogenital Radiology (ESUR) Web site.http://www.esur.org/Nephrogenic_Fibrosis.39.0.html.
22. Flanagan FL, Dehdashti F, Ogunbiyi OA, et al. Utility of FDG-PET for investigating unexplained plasma CEA elevation in patients with colorectal cancer. Ann Surg 1998;227:319-23.
23. Bohm B, Voth M, Geoghegan J, et al. Impact of PET on strategy in liver resection for primary and secondary liver tumors. J Cancer Res Clin Oncol 2004;130:266-72.

Chapter Thirteen

Benign Focal Lesions of Liver

Sapna Singh, Veena Chowdhury

A focal liver lesion is, by definition, a discrete abnormality arising within the liver. Benign focal lesions of the liver in the adult can be classified as developmental, neoplastic, inflammatory and miscellaneous. Although in some cases, it is difficult to distinguish these entities with imaging criteria alone, certain focal liver lesions have classic ultrasonic, computed tomographic (CT) and magnetic resonance (MR) imaging features, which are important for the radiologist to understand and recognize. An understanding of the classic imaging appearances of focal liver lesions allows more definitive diagnosis and shortens the diagnostic work up. Lesions with such features include simple (bile duct) cyst, autosomal dominant polycystic liver disease, biliary hamartoma, biliary cystadenoma, pyogenic and amoebic abscesses, hemangiomas, intrahepatic hydatid cyst, extrapancreatic pseudocyst, and intrahepatic hematoma and biloma. Specific CT and MR imaging findings that are important to recognize are the size of the lesion; the presence and thickness of a wall; the presence of septa, calcifications, or internal nodules; the enhancement pattern; the MR signal intensity spectrum and the cholangiographic appearance. The development of multidetector row CT MDCT technology has helped CT to continue to excel in its already established indication i.e. hepatic lesion detection and characterization and to add new clinical indication i.e., CT angiography for pre-procedure mapping and liver perfusion. With MDCT there is faster scanning. In liver imaging faster scanning decreases respiration artifacts and improves multiphase imaging.[1]

MDCT allows improved spatial resolution allowing high quality multiplanar reconstructions and 3D reconstructions. Acquisition of very thin collimation scan provides improved detection rate of small liver lesions.[2]

Pathologic Classification of Benign Liver Tumors (Based on Cell of Origin)[3]

Hepatocyte

- Hepatocellular adenoma
- Hepatocellular hyperplasia
- Focal nodular hyperplasia
- Macroregenerative nodules
- Nodular regenerative hyperplasia

Bile Duct Epithelium (Cholangiocellular)

- Hepatic cysts
- Simple hepatic cysts
- Polycystic liver disease/congenital hepatic fibrosis
- Biliary cystadenoma
- Bile duct adenoma

Mesenchymal Cells

- Mesenchymal hamartoma
- Hemangioma
- Infantile hemangioendothelioma
- Lymphangioma
- Lipoma/angiomyolipoma/myelipoma
- Leiomyoma
- Fibroma

Heterotopic Cells

Hepatic Cysts

Hepatic cysts are developmental benign lesions in the liver that do not communicate with the biliary tree. The current theory regarding the origin of true hepatic cysts is that they originate from hamartomatous tissue.[4]

A simple hepatic cyst, or bile duct cyst, is defined as a solitary unilocular cyst with a lining composed of a single primary layer of cuboidal bile duct epithelium. They are seen in about 5-14% of the general population with a female male ratio of 5:2. Its wall is less than 1 mm thickness layer of fibrous tissue, surrounded by normal hepatic parenchyma. Usually asymptomatic, if symptomatic surgical excision or guided percutaneous aspiration or sclerotherapy may be done.

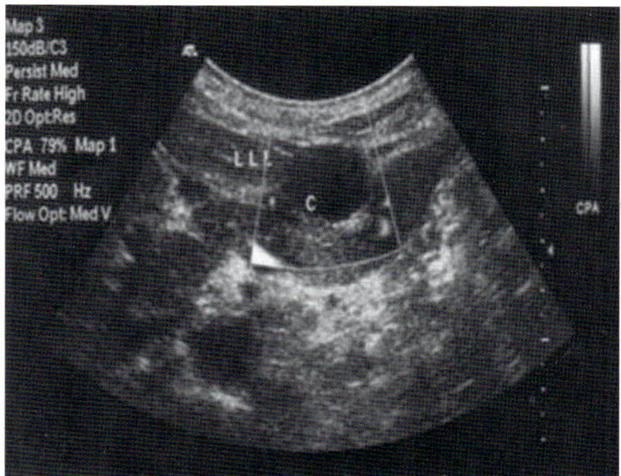

Fig. 13.2: Simple liver cyst seen as an anechoic lesion on Color Doppler imaging *(For color version see plate 3)*

IMAGING FEATURES

US

US is highly accurate in the demonstration of cystic lesions in any organ and its diagnostic accuracy in the diagnosis of simple liver cysts approaches 100%. Simple liver cysts appear as defined echo-free lesions with almost imperceptible walls and enhanced through transmission[5] (Figs 13.1 and 13.2). Thin septations can be present. The presence of internal echoes, debris, thick septations, mural calcification or nodules suggests an alternative diagnosis or a complicated cyst.

CT

A simple hepatic cyst appears on CT scan as a well-defined intrahepatic lesion having water attenuation (0-15 HU). It is round or oval in shape, has smooth thin walls and homogeneous appearance. There are no internal structures and no enhancement after contrast administration (Fig. 13.3). These are usually solitary and peripheral but may be multiple which occur more centrally. When more than 10 cysts are present, a polycystic disease should be considered. Cysts that become complicated by hemorrhage or infection may have septations and internal debris as well as wall enhancement.

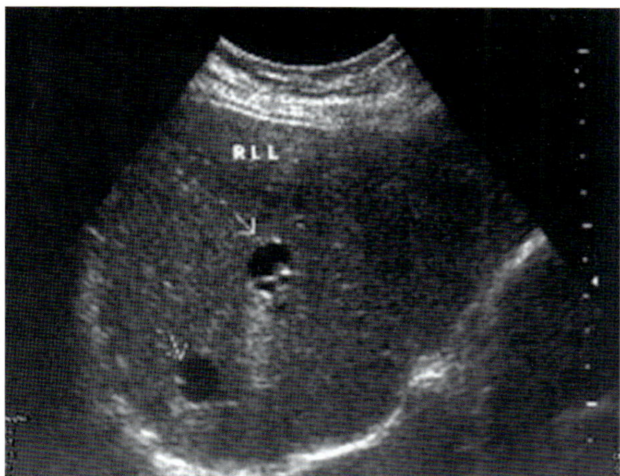

Fig. 13.1: Conventional US showing hypoechoic lesions in the right lobe of liver with posterior acoustic enhancement and enhanced through transmission—simple liver cysts

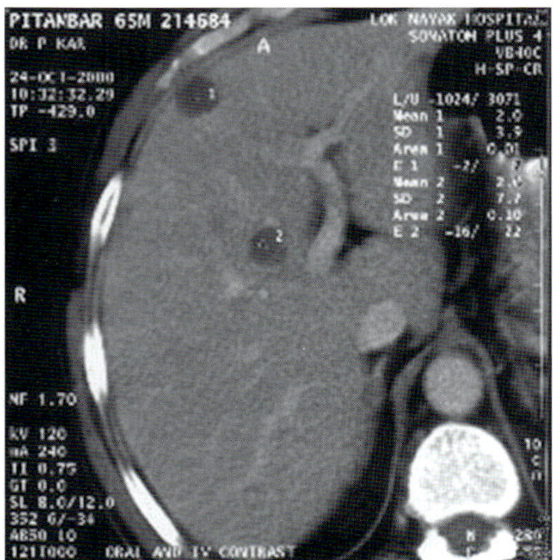

Fig. 13.3: Computed Tomography (CT) image revealing small markedly hypodense lesions in the liver—simple liver cysts

Small cysts often demonstrate attenuation values greater than water density as a result of volume averaging with adjacent liver parenchyma. Using spiral CT accurate densitometry can be obtained more easily by selecting reconstruction intervals to centre the lesion in a single slice. Multiphase spiral CT including pre- and post-contrast phases or portal phase and delayed phase is 100% specific for hepatic cyst.[6]

Nuclear Scintigrams

Cysts appear as cold lesions on nuclear scintigrams because there is no uptake of any radiotracer.

Angiogram

On angiograms simple hepatic cysts are noted to be avascular.

MRI

Hepatic cysts appear as homogeneous, sharply marginated masses hypointense on T1 and markedly hyperintense on T2-images (Figs 13.4A and B). Owing to the fluid content, an increase in signal intensity is seen on heavily T2-weighted images. This allows differentiation of these lesions from metastatic disease. No enhancement is seen after administration of gadolinium chelates. In cases of intracystic hemorrhage, a rare complication in simple hepatic cysts, the signal intensity is high, with a fluid level, on both T1 and T2-weighted images as mixed blood products are present.[7]

On the basis of these features in most cases either CT or MR imaging alone is sufficient to establish an accurate diagnosis of a simple hepatic cyst. However, guided percutaneous aspiration with cytological analysis may still be required in doubtful cases.

Congenital Hepatic Fibrosis and Polycystic Liver Disease

Congenital hepatic fibrosis and polycystic liver disease are part of the spectrum of fibropolycystic disease of the liver. Congenital hepatic fibrosis is characterized by periductal fibrosis and aberrant bile duct proliferation. In the polycystic disease variant, numerous large and small cysts which are pathologically identical to simple hepatic cysts are present with fibrosis. In polycystic liver and/or kidney disease, the liver, which surrounds the cysts, is not normal and frequently contains von Mayenburg's complexes and increased fibrous tissue. Hepatic involvement occurs in approximately 30 to 40% of patients with autosomal dominant adult polycystic kidney disease.[8] Though, hepatic cysts can occur without radiologically evident renal cysts; approximately 70% of patients with polycystic liver disease also have autosomal dominant polycystic kidney disease.

Imaging Features

MDCT scanners permit acquisition of thin slices with isotropic voxel size. A 64 detector scanner allows coverage of the liver with isotropic slices of 0.4 mm resolution in less than 5 seconds. MDCT allows for thin section images to be obtained during peak hepatic enhancement in the portal venous phase minimizing partial volume averaging artificat, while imaging simple hepatic cysts and

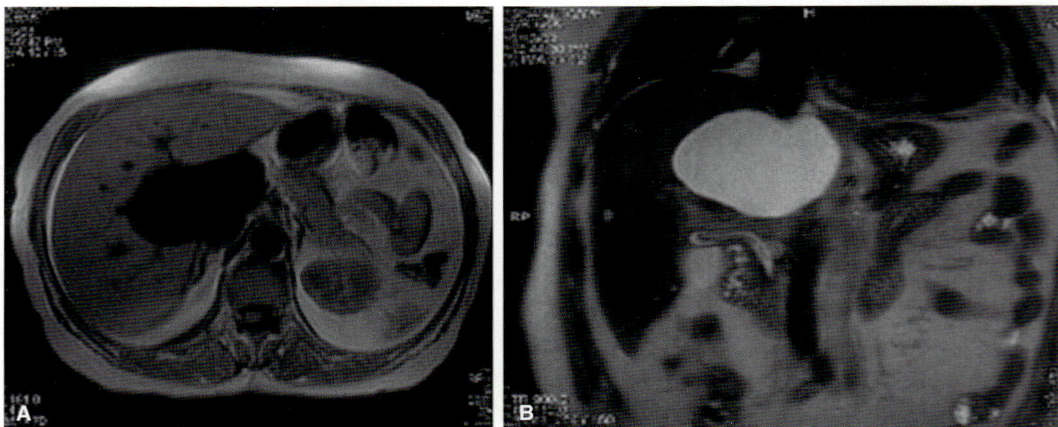

Figs 13.4A and B: (A) T_1W MR image showing a hepatic cyst as a homogeneous sharply marginated hypointense lesion (B) T_2W image reveals the cysts to be markedly hyperintense. Few smaller cysts are also seen in the periphery of the right lobe

maximizing the detection of subtle enhancement in the case of cystic metastases or abscess.[9]

US and CT demonstrate multiple cysts in liver. Calcification may be seen in the cyst wall. Hemorrhage may occur into the cyst resulting in increased attenuation of the cyst contents. Contrast enhancement of the cysts does not occur unless they become complicated by infection. MR imaging is more sensitive for the detection of complicated cysts.

Biliary Cystadenoma

Biliary cystadenomas are rare usually slow growing, multilocular cystic tumors that represent less than 5% of intrahepatic cystic masses of biliary origin. Eighty-five percent are generally intrahepatic although extrahepatic lesions have been reported.[10] Among intrahepatic cystadenomas, 55% occur in the right lobe, 29% in the left lobe and 16% occur in both lobes. They occur predominantly in middle-aged women (mean age 38 years) and are considered premalignant lesions.[11] The lesions are usually large ranging in diameter from 1.5-35 cm well-defined, solitary masses that are multiloculated and hypodense relative to liver. Rarely they may be multifocal. At microscopy, a single layer of mucin secreting cells lines the cyst wall.

IMAGING FEATURES

US and CT: Biliary cystadenoma appears as a solitary cystic mass with well-defined, thick fibrous capsule, mural nodules, internal septa and rarely capsular calcification.[10,11] Polypoid, pedunculated excrescences are seen more commonly in biliary cystadenocarcinomas than in cystadenomas. The septa in cystadenomas are thin and enhance on CT scans.The fluid within the tumor is usually mucin, but the cystic spaces vary in density, as the content can be proteinaceous, gelatinous, purulent or hemorrhagic due to trauma. They may communicate with the intrahepatic bile ducts and secrete mucinous material into the duct. Calcifications may be present in the septations. When coarse and associated with nodular projections, they are more suggestive of cystadenocarcinomas

MR Imaging: The appearance is typical for a fluid containing multilocular mass with homogeneous low signal on T1 and high signal on T2-weighted images. Variable signal intensities on both T1 and T2-weighted images depend on the presence of solid components, hemorrhage and protein content (Figs 13.5A and B).

The differential diagnosis of these lesions would include a complex benign cyst, abscess, hematoma, echinoccocal cyst, mesenchymal hamartoma, undifferentiated embryonal sarcoma, and cystic metastases. Diagnosis can be performed with percutaneous biopsy. Resection of these lesions is usually complete and leads to cure.

Bile Duct Hamartoma

Bile duct hamartomas, also called von Meyenburg complexes, originate from embryonic bile ducts that fail to

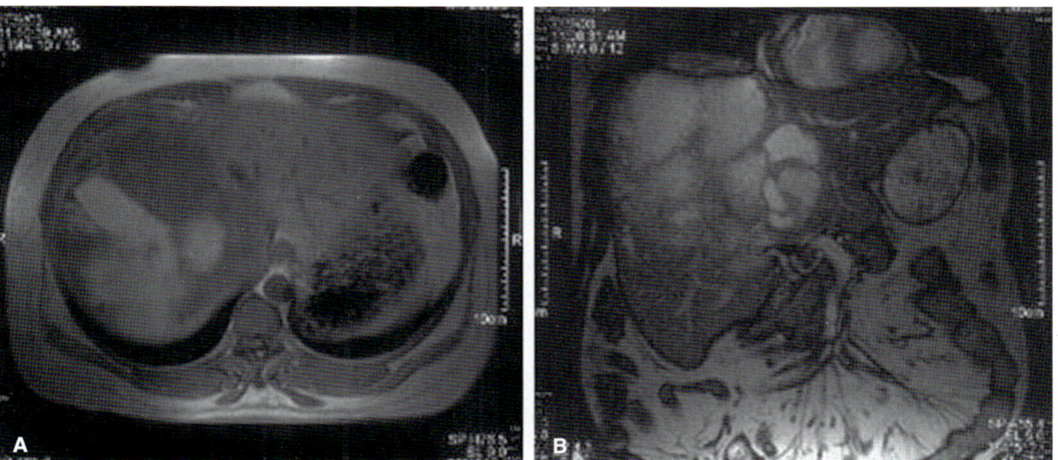

Figs 13.5A and B: (A) T1W MR image depicting a multilocular cystic mass with variable signal due to the presence of fluid and hemorrhage/protein content, (B) T2W image showing the lesion to be high signal—biliary cystadenoma

involute. They are generally without clinical manifestations and usually an incidental finding at imaging, laparotomy, or autopsy. At pathologic analysis, they appear as grayish-white nodular lesions 0.1-1.5 cm in diameter that do not communicate with the biliary tree and are scattered throughout the liver parenchyma.[12]

Non-enhanced CT shows multiple hypoattenuating, cyst like hepatic nodules occurring throughout both lobes of the liver and typically measuring less than 1.5 cm in diameter. The latter feature is the most essential one in the differential diagnosis from multiple simple cysts. Furthermore, typical simple cysts are regularly outlined, whereas bile duct hamartomas have a more irregular outline. Bile duct hamartomas do not exhibit a characteristic pattern of enhancement after intravenous administration of iodinated contrast material. Although homogeneous enhancement of the lesions has been noted in some cases mostly no enhancement is seen on contrast-enhanced CT images.

MR imaging is superior to CT in demonstrating the cystic nature of the lesions. On MR imaging, lesions are hypointense relative to liver parenchyma on T1-weighted images and strongly hyperintense on T2-weighted images. On heavily T2-weighted images, the signal intensity increases further, almost reaching the signal intensity of fluid. At MR cholangiography, bile duct hamartomas appear as multiple tiny cystic lesions that do not communicate with the biliary tree. After intravenous administration of gadolinium contrast material, thin rim enhancement may be seen. This rim enhancement is considered to correlate with the compressed liver parenchyma that surrounds the lesions at histopathologic analysis.[13]

At both CT and MR imaging, multiple small (< 1.5 cm diameter) cystic lesions in the liver without renal involvement should favor the diagnosis of biliary hamartomas.

Hemangioma

Hemangiomas are small, asymptomatic lesions seen in all age groups that are most often discovered incidentally on routine cross-sectional imaging studies. Symptoms, when present, are most commonly due to tumor enlargement. It is the most common benign neoplasm of the liver and the second most common hepatic tumor, exceeded only by metastases. Its incidence in the adult population has been reported to range between 0.4 and 20%. Hemangiomas are reported to be more common in women than in men, and are usually found within the right lobe of the liver. Although they may arise anywhere within the hepatic parenchyma, they frequently do so in either a subcapsular location or adjacent to intrahepatic vessels. They may range from a few millimetres to greater than 20 cm in diameter and may occasionally be pedunculated. Giant cavernous hemangiomas are by convention defined as lesions larger than 10 cm in size.

Pathology

Hemangiomas are mesodermal in origin. Histologically, they are composed of blood-filled cavernous vascular spaces of variable size and shape that are lined by a single layer of flat endothelium. These vascular channels are separated by thin fibrous septa that are often incomplete and project into the cavernous loculi. Slow blood flow within these spaces predisposes to the development of thrombosis, and organized thrombi may undergo fibrosis, calcification or ossification. Hemangiomas typically appear as soft reddish purple or bluish purple lesions at gross inspection.When the size exceeds 3 cm they are more likely to undergo involution, resulting in the formation of central fibrocollagenous scars as the thrombi and hemorrhage organize centrally and then spread peripherally until vascular occlusion is complete. Partial necrosis may develop as this occurs. Rarely, there is total sclerosis of a cavernous hemangioma, leading to the formation of a densely fibrotic nodule.

Spontaneous rupture with subsequent life- threatening hemorrhage is rare, as is acquired thrombocytopenia due to platelet sequestration and hypofibrinogenemia due to the intravascular deposition of fibrin clots within the hemangioma. A hormonal influence has also been noted, as some hemangiomas enlarge during pregnancy while treatment with corticosteroids has been observed to promote involution.

IMAGING FEATURES OF CAVERNOUS HEMANGIOMAS

Plain Film Findings

Most hepatic hemangiomas are too small to be identified on plain film of the abdomen. Very large lesions may exhibit nonspecific finding, with abdominal radiographs revealing either hepatomegaly or a large upper abdominal mass. Characteristic plain film findings have been described but are rarely seen. These include the presence of multiple calcified phleboliths and numerous calcified "trabeculations and spicules" that arise from a central point and radiate out toward the periphery of the lesion.[14] This latter finding signifies the presence of a hemangioma that has undergone extensive involution, resulting in the ultimate formation of a calcified central scar.

US and CT

The majority of hemangioma, less than 2 cm in diameter have a very distinctive pattern. They appear as sharply defined, highly reflective round tumor with a homogeneous echo pattern (Fig. 13.6). The high reflectivity is most likely due to the multiple interfaces between the vascular spaces. Lesions may occur anywhere within the liver but are most common in the posterior segment of the right lobe of the liver (Fig. 13.7). There is a tendency towards a peripheral location while those occurring centrally usually lie close to the main hepatic veins.

Larger tumors may develop a lobular margin. Haemangiomas larger than 2.5 cm in diameter are reported to show posterior acoustic enhancement which probably relates to the vascularity. As the haemangioma undergoes degeneration and fibrous replacement the reflectivity becomes more heterogeneous.

Microbubble Enhanced US

Hemangiomas demonstrate a reproducible and apparently specific pattern of enhancement at contrast enhanced US. Lesions rarely show linear vessels, instead they show peripheral puddles and pools of enhancement that expand in a centripetal pattern during the portal venous phase and beyond after progressing to a complete fill in of the lesion. Sustained enhancement in which the lesion has an echogenicity equal to or greater than that of the liver through the portal venous phase and beyond is a requisite to confident diagnosis.[15]

Hemangiomas are best evaluated with dynamic bolus CT by performing repeated scanning for 2-15 minutes at a single level. Following contrast administration large feeding vessels cause peripheral enhancement of the lesion with centripetal fill in of the lesion within 15 minutes. Most hemangiomas demonstrate a characteristic initial pattern of peripheral nodular enhancement that progresses to central enhancement (Figs 13.8A to C). Eventually, most hemangiomas become isoattenuating on delayed scans. Peripheral centripetal fill in coupled with delayed filling and persistence of enhancement constitute the diagnostic triad of hemangiomas by single level dynamic CT.[16]

Multiple Phase Imaging

Hanafusa et al[17] have described the appearance of hemangioma at multiple phase imaging (axial liver imaging at 30 and 55 sec. following 120 ml of contrast at 3 ml/sec). Sixty-two percent of hemangiomas in their study showed a typical appearance of low peripheral nodular

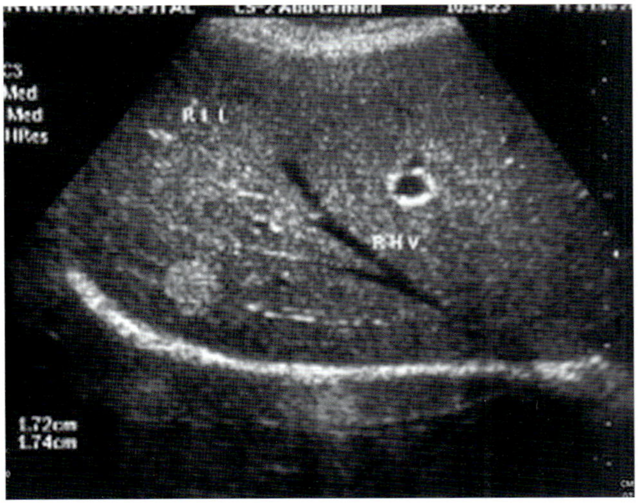

Fig. 13.6: US shows a well-circumscribed homogeneous hyperechoic lesion in the posterior segment of the right lobe of the liver—hemangioma

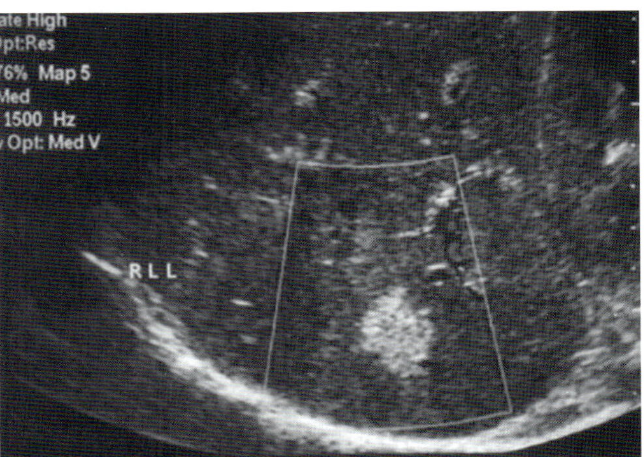

Fig. 13.7: Color flow imaging showing lack of internal vascularity in a hemangioma *(For color version see plate 3)*

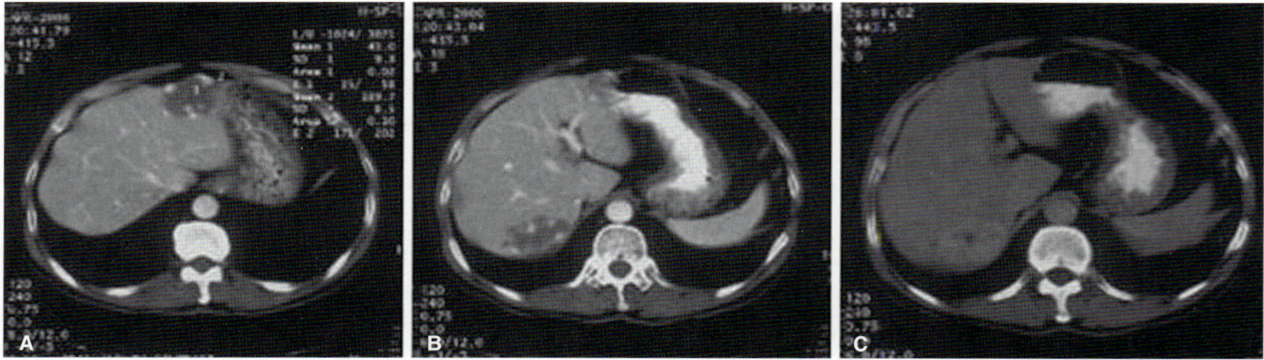

Figs 13.8A to C: (A and B) Early phase CT (within 30 seconds) showing peripheral nodular enhancement in the hemangiomas (C) Delayed phase enhancement 20 minutes later show complete fill in of one hemangioma with a central fibrous scar seen in the larger one

enhancement at 30 sec progressing to high homogeneous attenuation at 55 sec. Atypical enhancement pattern included low-(89%), high - iso (14%) or high–high (16%) enhancement on 30 and 55 second scans respectively. Atypical enhancement patterns are most common with small hemangiomas less than 15 mm.

MR Imaging

MR imaging is used for the evaluation of a suspected hemangioma because of the hemangioma's characteristic appearance. As a result of the slow blood flow through the vascular channels of the lesion, on T1-weighted (T1W) images, hemangioma is hypointense to the surrounding hepatic parenchyma with smooth, well-defined, often lobulated margins. On T2-weighted (T2W) images, it becomes significantly hyperintense to normal liver, increasing in relative signal intensity to the liver with increasing TE18 (Figs 13.9A and B). Spin-echo pulse sequences of TR 2000 msec with increasing TE from 60 to 180 msec are often used. A double-echo technique of TE 60 and 120 msec minimizes the length of the examination.[16,18] The diagnosis of hemangioma by MR imaging rests not only in the signal characteristics but also in morphological features such as sharp and geographic margins, lack of peripheral halo on T2W images, lack of deformity of the liver surface in the majority of cases, superficial location, and lack of displacement of the hepatic vessels surrounding the lesion.

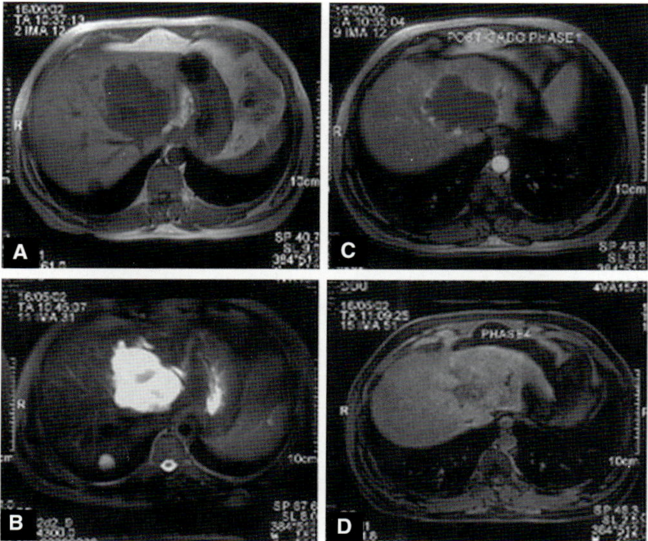

Figs 13.9A to D: (A) T_1 weighted MR image shows a well demarcated lobulated hypointense lesion in the liver, (B) T_2 weighted image reveals the lesion to be markedly hyperintense "light bulb appearance." A similar smaller lesion also seen, (C) Post-gadolinium image obtained within one minute of contrast administration shows peripheral enhancement within the lesion, (D) Delayed phase image shows centripetal fill in with a central scar—giant cavernous hemangioma

Dynamic gradient-echo MR imaging, after the intravenous injection of Gd DTPA, is useful in increasing the specificity of MR imaging for the study of hemangiomas. Gradient-echo T1W FLASH images are obtained before contrast at the level that best demonstrates the lesion on the spin-echo images. Repeated FLASH images are then obtained at that level after the injection of gadopentate dimeglumine (0.05 mmol/kg). Peripheral enhancement with centripetal fill-in similar to that demonstrated by CT is observed. Central areas lacking enhancement, especially in large tumors, correspond to areas of fibrosis that appear as low attenuation on CT. These fibrotic areas will appear hypointense on T2W images, which may be helpful in making the distinction between a large heterogeneous hemangioma containing areas of fibrosis from that of a necrotic tumor, such as hepatocellular carcinoma (HCC) or metastasis which have hyperintense necrotic area on T2W images. Dynamic Gd-DTPA-enhanced MR imaging is often useful for distinguishing hypervascular metastases from haemangioma which may not be possible simply with spin-echo imaging (Figs 13.9C and D).

MR Imaging Characteristics in Giant Hemangioma of the Liver

Giant hemangiomas commonly present distinctive features such as a heterogeneous appearance on T2-weighted images secondary to the presence of thrombus, myxoid tissue or fibrosis.[19] Some of the giant hemangiomas can reach massive dimensions and septa of fibrous tissue may confer the lesion a mutiloculated appearance. Giant hemangiomas may show irregular flame-shaped peripheral enhancement as well as central enhancement.[20] Despite these atypical features, the distinctive MR appearance with high signal intensity on T2-weighted images and discontinuous peripheral enhancement with enlargement and coalescence of the enhancing foci on serial gadolinium-enhanced gradient-echo images permits accurate diagnosis of a giant hemangioma.

Red Blood Cell Scintigraphy

Numerous studies have demonstrated that technetium–99m-labelled red blood cell (RBC) scintigraphy is an accurate technique for diagnosing cavernous hemangiomas of the liver. These lesions typically display a "hot spot" appearance on delayed labelled-RBC scans, reflecting the circulatory characteristics of these neoplasms. Because of the retarded blood flow within the vascular sinusoids, delayed scans obtained 1 to 2 hours after injection of the patient's radioistope-labelled blood reveal a progressive increase in the ratio of the blood pool activity within the haemangioma to that of surrounding normal liver. New high-resolution (triple-headed) SPECT cameras can identify hemangiomas as small as 0.5 cm. The diagnostic sensitivity of high-resolution SPECT for detecting hemangiomas 1.4 cm and larger has recently been shown to be 100%.[14]

Angiographic Findings

Angiography has long been considered the gold standard in the diagnosis of hepatic haemangioma. The classic findings consist of a normal main and feeding hepatic artery, early contrast accumulation within the lesion during the late arterial phase, and a prolonged, delayed stain that persists throughout the capillary phase and well into the late venous phase. The feeding vessels may show crowding or displacement around the lesion but are typically nondilated and have normal walls without evidence of tumor infiltration. Persistent contrast puddling within hemangiomas typically assumes a C-shaped or ring-like configuration at the periphery of the lesion. This finding reflects the presence of slow blood flow within the dilated vascular sinusoids, and usually permits a specific diagnosis to be made. Hemangiomas as small as 0.5 cm may be diagnosed when this feature is identified. Atypical angiographic features include the finding of a hypovascular mass or a dense, homogeneous hypervascular mass. The presence of arterial-portal venous shunting is extremely rare but has been encountered in both adult and paediatric cases.[21]

Hepatocellular Adenoma (HA)

Hepatocellular adenoma (HA) is an uncommon solid primary liver tumor. These are usually solitary greater than 10 cm in size. Rarely multiple adenomas may be seen involving both hepatic lobes and this is termed multiple hepatocellular adenomatosis.[22] Adenomas consist of slightly atypical hepatocytes containing areas of bile stasis and focal hemorrhage or necrosis. Unlike, focal nodular hyperplasia, they do not contain bile ducts or Kupffer cells. This tumor is usually discovered incidentally during abdominal imaging studies. Rarely patients may present with right upper abdominal mass or pain after spontaneous intra-abdominal hemorrhage of the tumor. The development of most hepatocellular adenomas is related to the use of oral contraceptives in women and of anabolic steroids in men. These may also occur in association with glycogen storage disease where there is a 8% incidence. In type I disease, the incidence is as high as 40%. In Von Gierke's disease, the overall liver texture is abnormal with an increase in size and reflectivity due to fatty and glycogen infiltration. Against this background adenomas stand out with a variable appearance ranging from low to high reflectivity.

Imaging Features

US

HA is usually seen as a heterogeneous but primarily echogenic hepatic mass, the echogenicity being due to the intratumoral fat and glycogen. Anechoic areas correspond to areas of hemorrhage and scar tissue.

Contrast enhanced US – intense rapid enhancement is seen during the arterial phase. Discrete perilesional feeding arteries manifest as enhancement around the tumor capsule, such enhancement is never seen in HCC. Heterogenous enhancement with perfusion defects corresponding to hemorhagic areas is present in larger masses. More or less rapid washout is seen during the portal and sinusoidal phase with initial hypervascularity followed by isovascularity. A hypoechoic appearance like HCC is never seen.[23]

CT

On non-contrast scans, adenomas are predominantly isodense with liver but may appear hypodense due to excessive steatosis. They may be heterogeneous where areas of hyperdensity or increased attenuation on non–contrast scans correspond to areas of intratumoral hemorrhage.[24] On contrast administration, adenomas demonstrate rapid, early and transient enhancement owing to hepatic artery hypervascularity of these tumors.[25] There is rapid wash in and washout of the contrast agent that renders the tumors isodense to liver during the portal venous phase when normal liver tissue is maximally enhanced.

Triphasic Study

During the arterial phase (15-25 sec after bolus injection of contrast material) there is dense enhancement and the lesion becomes hyperdense relative to the normal liver which has enhanced minimally at this time. Subsequently tumoral enhancement diminishes rapidly and the tumors become isodense to normal liver during the portal venous phase (45-180 sec after contrast injection) and even slightly hypodense during the equilibrium phase (3-5 min. after contrast injection).

Radionuclide Scintigraphy

Owing to the absence of Kupffer cells, most (80%) of HA appear cold on sulphur colloid scintigraphy. On hepatobiliary scintigrams, HAs usually show uptake of the tracer. Because of the lack of bile ductules, the tracer is not excreted and delayed scans therefore depict HAs as areas of markedly increased activity.

MRI

The high fat or glycogen content or both render these tumors isointense or even hyperintense on T1 images. When present, a hypointense capsule can be identified on T1 images. Blood degradation products can be seen as hyperintense regions on T1 and hypointense on T2 images. Immediate enhancement is seen on the arterial phase images after IV gadolinium chetate but rapidly fades to near isointensity on all subsequent images.

Enhancement of these tumors has been noted with the use of hepatobiliary contrast agents such as manganese DPDP.[26]

Angiograms

Has appear as hypervascular tumors with large peripheral vessels and centripetal flow. Usually there is no AV shunting/vascular invasion.

Focal Nodular Hyperplasia (FNH)

It is the second most common benign lesion of the liver after hemangioma and contains hepatocytes, bile duct elements, Kupffer cells and fibrous tissue. It is usually found incidentally on abdominal imaging studies, although about one-third of tumors are discovered because of clinical symptoms. Its aetiology is unknown but it is postulated that a congenital vascular malformation may trigger the development of hepatocyte hyperplasia because pathologic studies have shown the existence of anomalous arterial branches unaccompanied by portal venous branches feeding the numerous small lobules comprising FNH. A hormonal influence may also be the aetiologic factor because FNH is more common in women in their 3rd-5th decades.

Pathology

FNH is well-circumscribed, non-encapsulated and usually solitary (95%) mass that is characterized by a centrally located scar surrounded by nodules of hyperplastic hepatocytes.[27] Histologically, it is characterized by the presence of normal hepatocytes, with a malformed biliary system that leads to slowing of biliary excretion. It is often present on the liver surface or it may be pedunculated. The majority of lesions are smaller than 5 cm having a mean diameter of 3 cm. Occasionally FNH may replace an entire lobe of liver when it is known as lobar FNH.

IMAGING FEATURES

US

FNHs appear homogeneous and isoechoic to normal liver and may be visible only because of the mass effect they exert on adjacent hepatic vessels.[28] In some cases, FNH appears as an inhomogeneous mass containing hypoechoic and hyperechoic areas. An echo complex corresponding to the central fibrous scar, although classical, is infrequently demonstrated.

Color Doppler

FNHs are hypervascular tumors. Numerous scattered arterial and venous Doppler signals may be seen throughout the tumor exhibiting a 'comet tail' appearance.

Contrast Enhanced US

FNH manifests as a hypervascular liver mass during the arterial phase of contrast enhanced US. FNH shows a stellate lesion and a central non-enhancing scar. On the portal venous phase the lesion remains isoechoic to the liver with a central non-enhancing scar. On further delayed images there is accumulation of contrast within the scar. Portal venous phase imaging is critical to confident confirmation of the diagnosis. As apposed to HCC, in which rapid washout is generally seen FNH is isoechoic to the liver parenchyma into the portal venous phase and beyond.[29]

Focal Nodular Hyperplasia and Hepatic Adenoma: Differentiation with Low Index Contrast Enhanced Sonography

Recent advances in contrast enhanced sonography using a low mechanical index (< 0.2) and perfluorocarbon contrast agents enable real time imaging of perfusion and vascularity in liver tumors. FNH is predicted on the basis of arterial phase centrifugal filling as opposed to the centripetal filling seen in adenomas. Stellate linear or plicated non enhancing area suggests the diagnosis of FNH. Also sustained portal phase enhancement is more common in FNH than in adenoma.[30]

CT

Non-contrast CT of FNH demonstrates a non- specific low density lesion, often located adjacent to the liver capsule. They may deform the liver contours or possess a prominent stellate-shaped central scar which is seen as a central low density area. FNH is a hypervascular lesion with a prominent arterial blood supply. There is rapid enhancement of FNH appearing hyperdense relative to liver in the arterial phase (approx first 30 seconds) with a steady decrease in attenuation during the portal phase during which it appears relatively isodense to hypodense to the normal liver tissue and the central scar remains of low density. On delayed images there is accumulation of contrast within the scar which appears hyperdense. This sign is highly indicative of FNH.

Hemodynamic Characterization of Focal Nodular Hyperplasia

Focal nodular hyperplasia is supplied by an enlarged anomalous hepatic artery and its drainage is always into the hepatic veins.[31] Multiphasic multidetector CT allows greater spatial and hemodynamic characterization of focal hepatic lesions. The three-dimensional (3D) multidetector CT angiography using volume rendering displays the hemodynamics and angioarchitecture of focal nodular hyperplasia, features that help in distinguishing these lesions from malignant masses.[32]

Nuclear Scintigraphy

On sulphur colloid scan 60% of FNH lesions will have uptake of radiotracer indicating intratumoral Kupffer cell. This is infrequent with adenomas. Using trimethyl bromoimino diacetic acid (TBIDA) hepatobiliary scanning, the sensitivity of scintigraphy for FNH has been reported to be 92%.

Angiography reveals a hypervascular mass possessing a centrifugal or spoke wheel pattern of vascular supply.

MRI FNH is mostly slightly hypointense on T1-weighted images and hyperintense on T2-weighted images. MRI may demonstrate FNH by its mass effect and displacement of hepatic vessels as well as by subtle differences in signal intensity compared with adjacent liver. FNH often contains a central scar which is hyperintense on T2 due to presence of oedema and hypointense on T1 weighted images.[33] This is because the scar is composed of vascular and myxoid tissue, both of which are rich in free water. (D/D fibrolamellar HCC– central scar is of low signal on both T1 and T2-weighted images). On administration of IV Gadolinium FNH frequently shows a homogeneous tumor blush with rapid washout to isointensity with surrounding liver tissue. Contrast enhanced 3D GRE MR imaging demonstrates characteristic enhancement patterns that are helpful in the characterization. Three dimensional GRE imaging have several advantages over two dimensional dynamic imaging. 3D images can be reformatted in any plane, high quality thin sections with no gaps can be obtained and the detection and localization of small hepatic lesions is superior . In addition the small data set can be used to generate high quality images depicting the vasculature.[34] Dynamic post-gadolinium images frequently depict the central scar not seen on unenhanced images. The scar shows a delayed and persistent enhancement after administration of Gd. Contrast agents with hepato-specific properties have been shown to increase the sensitivity of MR imaging for the detection of focal hepatic lesions, though the role of these agents is to be fully elucidated. Gadobenate- dimeglumine (Gd-BOPTA) is a gadolinium based contrast agent in common with other gadolinium agents, has a vascular interstitial distribution in the first few minutes after injection. Thereafter, some 2-4% of the administered dose is taken up by functioning hepatocytes and contrast is excreted in the bile, while the remaining dose undergoes renal excretion. The fraction taken up by the hepatocytes brings about a marked hyperintensity of the liver that persists for at least 120 minutes (3 hrs) after the injection. Gd BOPTA accumulates selectively in hepatocytes.[35] In FNH, there is prolonged and excessive accumulation of this contrast agent because FNH lacks a well-formed canalicular system to permit normal excretion. There is much less enhancement of the hepatocellular adenoma on dynamic phase MR images and a markedly hypointense appearance on delayed images as compared to FNH. Although adenomas have functioning hepatocytes they lack bile ducts. Altered hepatocellular metabolism may inhibit the uptake of Gd-BOPTA in the adenoma thereby accounting for its hypointense appearance on delayed MR images.

Hepatic Adenoma and Focal Nodular Hyperplasia: MR Findings with Superparamagnetic Iron Oxide Enhanced MRI (SPIO)

SPIO is a contrast agent that undergoes phagocytosis by the reticuloendothelial system (Kupffer cells).[36] The use of SPIO results in shortening of T2-relaxation time of lesions containing Kupffer cells causing decreased signal intensity on T2-weighted images. These properties are of use in characterizing hepatic liver lesions. The distinction between FNH and hepatocellular adenoma (HA) is important because FNH can be treated conservatively, whereas HA is often resected because of its propensity for hemorrhage. On T2W SPIO enhanced MRI, FNH shows a dramatic decrease in signal intensity (60 to 70%). SPIO uptake is expected in FNH as the lesion contains Kupffer cells and has an excellent vascular supply. The uptake of SPIO in hepatic adenomas is poor compared to FNH.[37] Only 20% of signal loss on T2W is usually seen in adenomas. Tumor heterogeneity, T1 hyperintensity and only slight uptake of SPIO are MR features suggestive of adenomas while tumor homogeneity, T1 isointensity presence of central scar and the pronounced uptake of SPIO are highly suggestive of FNH.

Nodular Regenerative Hyperplasia (NRH)

It is defined as diffuse, multiple regenerative nodules not associated with fibrosis. It is also known as diffuse nodular hyperplasia and non-cirrhotic nodular hyperplasia. The nodules consist of cells resembling normal hepatocytes. The absence of fibrosis is an important distinction between NRH and regenerating nodules of cirrhosis.

NRH is a rare condition that is discovered incidentally or during the evaluation of portal hypertension.[38] Several drugs including steroids and antineoplastic drugs as well as multiple systemic conditions and collagen vascular disorders have been associated with NRH. The CT appearance of NRH may range from that of a normal liver to that of focal liver nodules of predominantly low attenuation. Multiple diffuse bulging nodules are present on the liver surface, varying in size from a few millimetres to several centimetres in diameter. Hemorrhage may occur resulting in a complex mass of mixed density.

Adenomatous Hyperplastic Nodule (AHN)

Also known as adenomatoid hyperplasia and macroregenerative nodule. AHN is a benign but premalignant lesion that appears in cirrhotic livers.[39] These are found in approximately 10-14% of patients with chronic liver disease such as advanced cirrhosis. They may also arise following massive hepatic necrosis. These are also known as dysplastic nodules. Dysplastic nodules that accumulate iron appear to have greater malignant potential than other nodules. This may result from the tumor enhancing effects of iron or to the rapid growth associated with regeneration.[40] On MR, these dysplastic nodules usually appear hyperintense on T1 and hypointense on T2-weighted images. High signal intensity on T2-weighted images should be considered highly suspicious for HCC. Dysplatic nodules are supplied primarily by the portal vein similar to the normal liver whereas HCCs are supplied almost exclusively by the hepatic artery. Hence, arterial portography is useful in differentiating between AHN and HCC. The finding of a nodule within a nodule on gradient echo and T2 W images consisting of a large low intensity nodule containing a smaller nodule of isointensity or hyperintensity relative to liver has been shown to indicate a small HCC developing within a hyperplastic nodule.

Differentiation of benign and malignant liver lesions on the basis of contrast enhanced pulse inversion sonography.

Pulse inversion is a technique that suppresses echoes from tissue in favor of those from bubbles. When used at a low mechanical index pulse inversion imaging does not cause disruption of microbubbles and preserves their integrity. A major requirement for determination of malignancy or benignancy was the appearance of the mass in the portal venous phase relative to the liver. A mass that appeared more enhanced or of greater echogenicity was interpreted as showing sustained enhancement, commonly encountered with benign lesions. Malignant lesions, in comparison, tend to show washout or hypoechogenicity relative to the enhanced liver.[41]

Lipomatous Tumors

These include lipomas, angiomyolipomas and myelolipomas depending on the variable fat, myeloid and vascular cellular composition. These tumors have no malignant potential. Hepatic lipomatous tumors may occur in approximately 10% of patients with tuberous sclerosis and renal angiolipomas. However, solitary liver lipomas may present without other lesion. Most are found incidentally and are asymptomatic but may occasionally bleed causing abdominal pain. On ultrasound, fat containing tumors are highly echogenic. Posterior acoustic enhancement can be seen with homogeneous appearing tumors, specifically lipomas.

CT

Benign lipomatous tumors of the liver have the characteristic appearance on CT scans of a lesion composed of radiolucent fat (Fig. 13.10). Enhancement ranges from none (pure lipomas) to significant (angiomyolipomas).

MRI

Fat containing tumors show a characteristic high signal intensity on T1 and T2 images and this is comparable to the signal intensity of subcutaneous or retroperitoneal fat on these images. Chemical shift imaging (CSI) may allow lipomas to be distinguished from tumors with mixed cellularity such as angiomyolipomas and myelolipomas.

Although the presence of fat can be documented with CT or US, MR imaging is the most specific imaging technique for demonstrating both microscopic and macroscopic fat.[42]

Pediatric Liver Tumors

Mesenchymal Hamartoma

Accounts for 8% of childhood liver masses, is usually asymptomatic seen in children below 2 years with a male predominance. It is a benign cystic developmental lesion consisting of gelatinous mesenchymal tissue with cyst formation and remnants of normal hepatic parenchyma. It is a large well-defined encapsulated or pedunculated

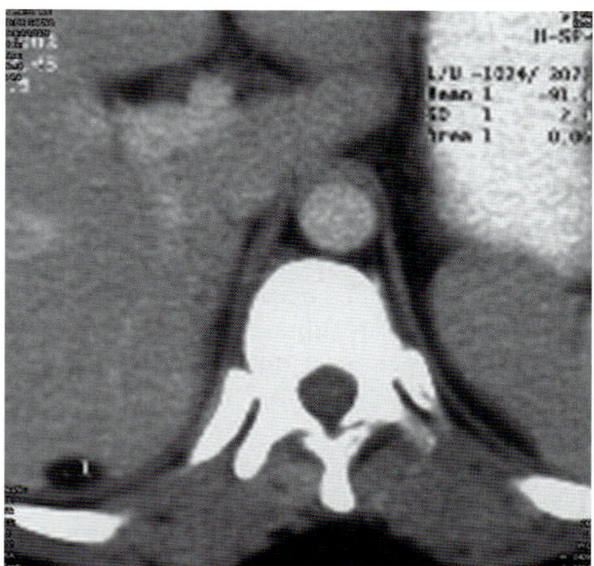

Fig. 13.10: CT image shows a small hypo-attenuating lesion with fat attenuation value within the right lobe of liver—lipoma

tumor[43] usually 15 cm or more in diameter at diagnosis. Cysts are present in 80% cases.[44] Mesenchymal hamartoma may have either mesenchymal predominance with a solid appearance or cystic predominance appearing as a multiloculated cystic mass.

US

Well-circumscribed multilocular mass with anechoic spaces separated by echogenic septa.[45] The mass may appear solid if the cystic spaces are small. Typically the lesion is located in the right lobe of the liver.

CT

Seen as a well-defined mass with central areas of low density and internal septa.[45] After administration of contrast material the central areas do not enhance but the central septa become more dense.

MRI

The MR appearance is dependent on its mesenchymal (stromal) or cystic predominance. Those with cystic component are significantly hyperintense on T2 W images because of cyst contents while those with mesenchymal predominance have lower signal intensity than normal liver on T1W images because of their fibrotic tissue component. Multiple septa are best seen on T2W imaging which demonstrates the complex nature of the cystic mass.[46]

Infantile Hemangioendothelioma (IHE)

Accounts for 12% of all childhood liver tumors with females being affected more often than males. It is a benign vascular tumor consisting of vascular channels formed by proliferating endothelial cells. On gross examination, a hemangioendothelioma is composed of multiple, round discrete nodules ranging from 2-15 cm in diameter. These nodules may become fibrotic with age.[47] Microscopically two histologic types have been described.

Type 1 consists of vascular channels lined by endothelial cells that are supported by reticular fibres.

Type 2 has larger, more irregular branching spaces lined by immature pleomorphic cells. This form has some malignant potential and rare cases of metastases have been described.

Ninety per cent of IHEs occur during the first 6 months of life. Presenting signs consist of high output congestive heart failure due to arteriovenous shunting within the lesion, asymptomatic hepatomegaly or an abdominal mass. Occasionally, patients with these lesions are seen because of thrombocytopenia due to platelet sequestration (Kasabach-Meritt syndrome) or massive hemoperitoneum due to spontaneous rupture. Cutaneous hemangiomas may be associated with the multinodular form of IHE (occurring in about 40% of patients) and may involve other organs. Although IHE may grow to a large size with resulting hemodynamic compromise, spontaneous involution will occur if the child survives.

US

The US appearances of these lesions are variable and range from highly echogenic relative to normal parenchyma to hypoechoic or anechoic with echogenic septa (Fig. 13.11A). The increased echogenicity is related to the multiple interfaces that exist between the walls of the vascular spaces and the blood within them. Doppler demonstrates high velocity and disturbed blood flow through the mass.[48] The diagnosis is often made by demonstrating changes in the hepatic veins and arteries: The coeliac axis and common hepatic artery are dilated and the calibre of the abdominal aorta reduces below the origin of the coeliac axis while the hepatic veins draining the lesion may be prominent. These findings are highly suggestive of a benign vascular tumor as these vascular abnormalities do not occur with malignant lesions of the liver.

CT

These are seen as hypodense, well-defined homogeneous lesions on precontrast scan. Calcifications within the tumor are found in about 40% of hemangioendotheliomas. After contrast administraton, peripheral enhancement occurs and on delayed CT scans, a variable degree of centripetal enhancement is seen with prolonged and persistent enhancement similar to that seen with hemangioma (Figs 13.11B and C).

Red blood cell scintigraphy demonstrates increased activity in the blood pool phase and on delayed imaging. Single photon emission CT (SPECT) may be required to detect small lesions under 3 cm.

MR

MR imaging demonstrates a heterogeneous appearance on both T1 and T2 W images because of the presence of hemorrhage, necrosis and fibrosis. High signal intensity is seen on T2 W images, which is attributed to the vascular nature of the lesion.[49] Peripheral enhancement and central fill in is noted after administration of gadolinium DTPA.

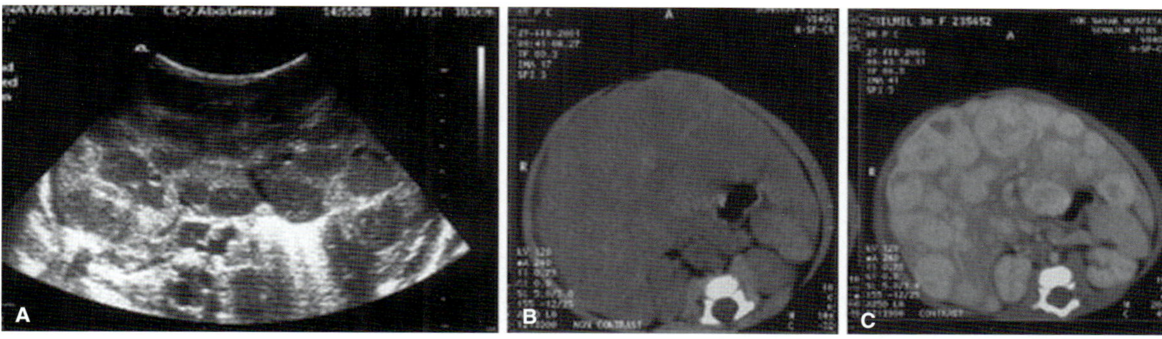

Figs 13.11A to C: (A) US scan shows multiple hypoechoic lesions within the liver, (B) Non-contrast CT scan showing the liver to be enlarged with multiple hypodense lesions within (C) Contrast enhanced CT reveals peripheral and centripetal enhancement of the lesions – infantile hemangioendothelioma

Hepatic Arteriography

Useful in those cases where definitive information about the tumor blood supply is required preoperatively or for therapeutic embolization.

Focal Inflammatory Lesions of Liver

Bacterial (Pyogenic) Liver Abscess

Liver abscess remains a serious and even lifethreatening condition despite advances in imaging and treatment.

Pathology

Bacterial abscess of the liver may develop from several routes most commonly via the biliary tree, because of ascending cholangitis from benign or malignant biliary obstructions. Other sources include portal vein or superior mesenteric vein, phlebitis secondary to appendicitis, pancreatitis, diverticulitis or other gastrointestinal infections, arterial septicemia as a result of endocarditis, pneumonitis or osteomyelitis, direct extension from contiguous organs such as perforated ulcer, pneumonia or pyelonephritis, post-traumatic and iatrogenic causes. In patients with diabetes mellitus, a cryptogenic abscess may occur with no identifiable source. Metastases may also become infected.

Anaerobic or mixed anaerobic and aerobic organisms account for the majority of bacterial liver abscesses. Facultative gram-negative enteric bacilli, anaerobic gram negative bacilli and microaerophilic streptococci are often the responsible organisms. In adults, *Escherichia coli* and in children *Staphylococcus* are the most commonly isolated[50] organisms.

Abscesses of biliary origin are often multiple, involving both hepatic lobes in 90% of cases. Abscesses from portal vein source are often solitary with 65% occurring in the right lobe, 12% in the left lobe and 23% in both lobes. This distribution has been attributed to the pattern of mesenteric blood flow in the portal vein.

IMAGING FEATURES

Plain Film Findings

Chest X-ray may show elevation of the right hemidiaphragm, right lower lobe atelectasis, right pleural effusion or infiltrates.

Abdominal radiographs may show hepatomegaly, intrahepatic gas or an air fluid level.

US

The ultrasound features of pyogenic liver abscesses are varied. Frankly purulent abscesses appear cystic with fluid ranging from echo free to highly echogenic (Fig. 13.12). Regions of early suppuration may appear solid and echogenic, related to the presence of necrotic hepatocytes. Occasionally gas-producing organisms give rise to echogenic foci with a posterior reverberation artifact. Fluid interfaces, internal septations and debris may also be seen. The abscess wall can vary from well defined to irregular and thick. Differential diagnosis includes amoebic or echinococcal infection, infected cyst, hematoma and necrotic or cystic neoplasm.

ERCP

Cholangiography may define the level and cause of biliary obstruction.[51]

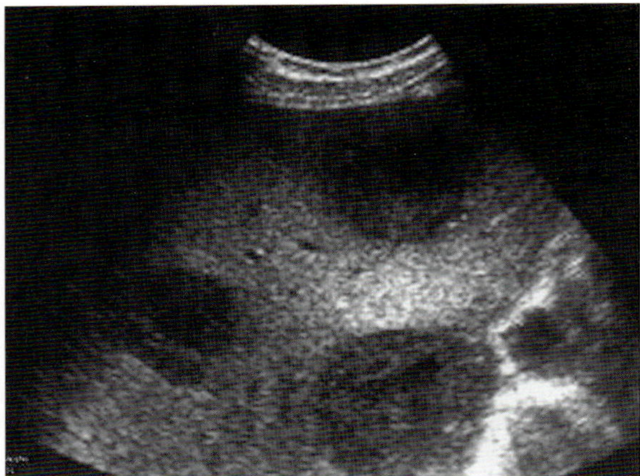

Fig. 13.12: US scan showing three lesions in the liver with well-defined walls and echoes within giving a solid appearance—pyogenic liver abscesses

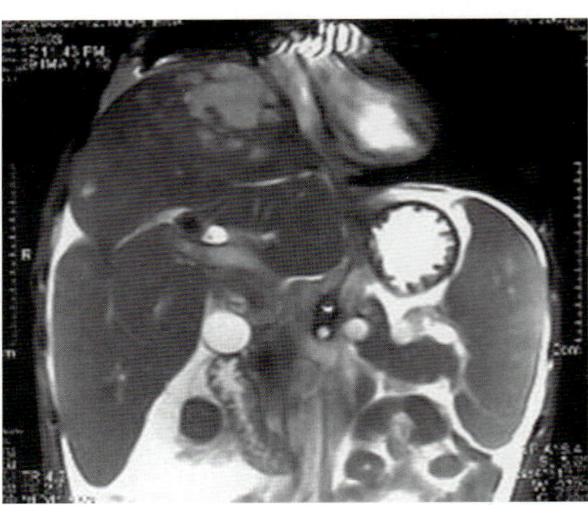

Fig. 13.14: MR image showing multiple small abscesses coalescing into a single cavity—"the cluster sign" – pyogenic liver abscesses

Nuclear scintigraphy: Appear as cold area on 99mTc sulphur colloid and hepatobiliary scintiscans.

CT and MR Imaging

CT has greater than 90% sensitivity for the detection of hepatic abscesses which appear as low attenuation rounded masses on both non-contrast and contrast-enhanced scans.[52] On administration of IV contrast, most abscesses have an enhancing peripheral rim (Figs 13.13A and B). Some abscesses have a lobulated contour or circumferential transition zones of intermediate attenuation.

The "cluster sign" may also be seen with small less than 2 cm diameter lesions clustering together with apparent coalescence into a large abscess[53] (Fig. 13.14). Perilesional oedema described as a "double target sign" is a characteristic feature (Fig. 13.15).

Gas bubbles or an air fluid level are specific signs but are seen in less than 20% of cases and may indicate the formation of an enteric communication with the abscess.

The abscess cavities are seen as hypointense signal on T1 and hyperintense on T2-weighted images (Figs 13.16A and B). Some are seen as signal void due to the presence of gas. Early intensely enhancing abscess walls which persist in thickness and intensity over time and prominent peri-lesional enhancement are distinctive characteristics observed on gadolinium enhanced images.[54]

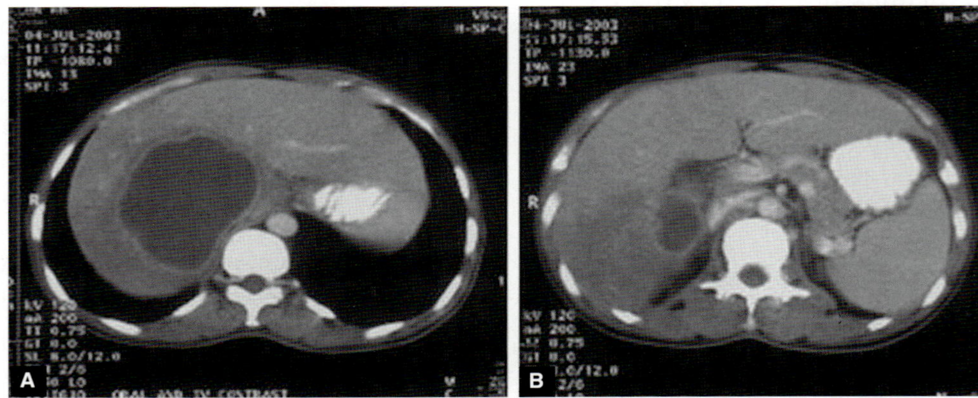

Figs 13.13A and B: Contrast enhanced CT showing irregular hypodense lesions in the liver with enhancing rim–pyogenic liver abscesses

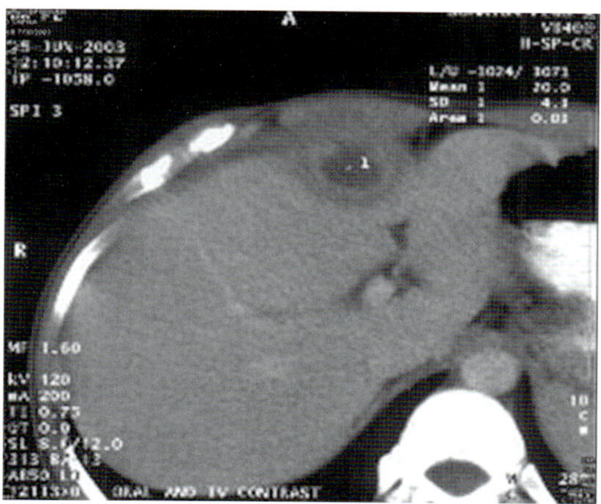

Fig. 13.15: Contrast enhanced CT showing a hypodense lesion with perilesional edema giving a 'double target sign'—pyogenic liver abscess

Amoebic Abscess

Amoebiasis occurs most often in the tropical and subtropical zones of the world. It is caused by the protozoan entamoeba histolytica. Amoebic liver abscess is the most common extraintestinal manifestation of amoebiasis. The protozoan reaches the liver by penetrating through the colon, invading the mesenteric venules and entering the portalvein. It may reach via lymphatics or directly extends into the liver from the hepatic flexure.[55]

Pathology

The cavitary amoebic abscess occurs as the liver tissue is frankly destroyed. Initially, the lesion contains necrotic tissue including the viable organism. As the lesion becomes larger, central cavitation is apparent and the active organism lies in the necrotic tissue lining the cavity. Surrounding this layer is an inflammatory zone of hepatic parenchyma invaded by the organisms. Centrally the cavity is often filled by a thick fluid that resembles "anchovy paste". Frequently solitary, the abscess is most commonly located in the right lobe. This is related to the venous drainage from the usually infected right colon, via the superior mesenteric vein to the portal vein preferentially flowing into the right lobe of the liver.

IMAGING FEATURES

Plain Film Findings

Chest and abdominal radiographs may show findings similar to that of pyogenic abscess.

Nuclear Scintigrams

Appear as cold defects on sulphur colloid scans often with "rim enhancement" occurring due to inflammation of the adjacent parenchyma. A cold lesion with a hot periphery is suggestive of the diagnosis.

US

Sonographic features include a round or oval lesion, absence of a prominent abscess wall, hypoechogenicity compared to normal liver, fine low level internal echoes,[56] distal sonic enhancement and continuity with the diaphragm (Figs 13.17A and B).

Two sonographic patterns have been found to be significantly more prevalent in amoebic abscesses.

1. Round or oval shapes in 82 versus 60% of pyogenic abscess.

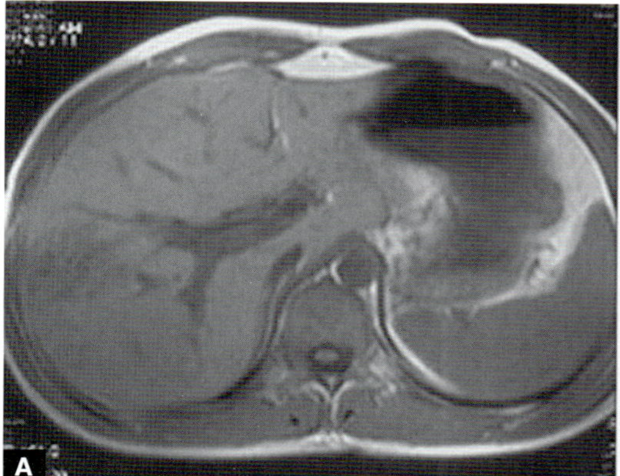

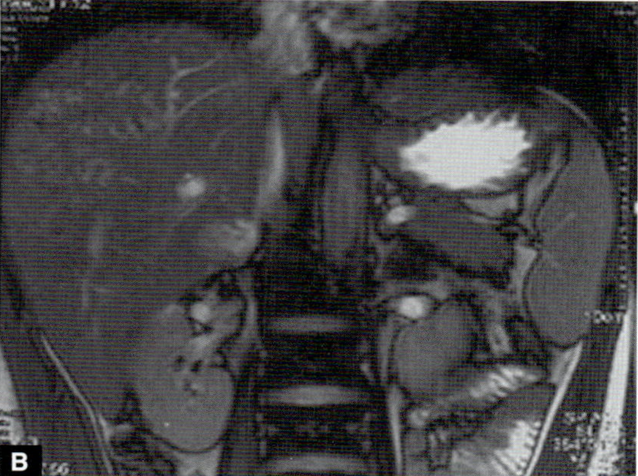

Figs. 13.16A and B: (A) T_1 weighted MR image showing an ill defined area hypointense in signal in the right lobe of liver, (B) T_2 weighted image showing the area to have a high signal with multiple small lesions clustering together—liver abscess

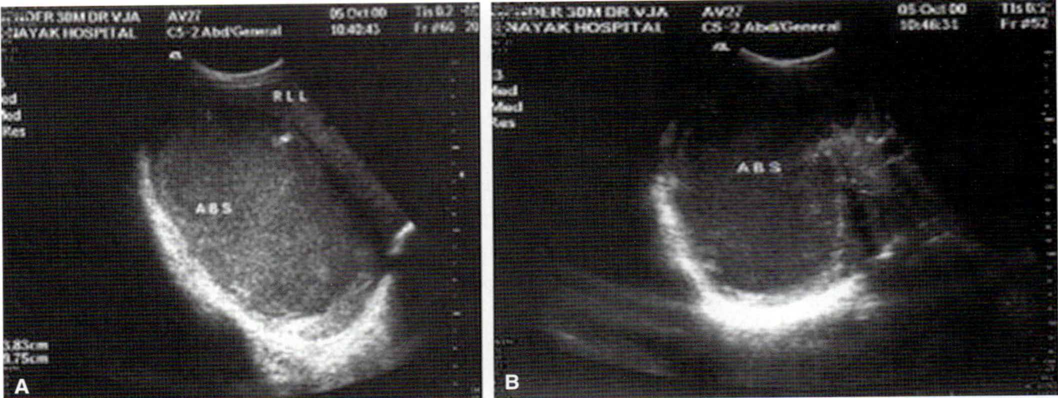

Figs. 13.17A and B: US showing a round hypoechoic lesion with low internal echoes within with absence of a well-defined abscess wall—amoebic liver abscess

2. Hypoechoic appearance with fine internal echoes at high gain in 58 versus 36% of pyogenic abscesses.

CT

On CT scans, amoebic abscesses of the liver appear as low attenuation lesions, with the density of the lesion dependent on its stage of development and internal contents.[57] Lesions that are early in development may have an appearance similar to that of solid tumors. Older abscesses are more cystic in appearance. The zone of inflammation, of variable thickness and density, is isodense to hypodense on unenhanced CT scans and usually enhances after contrast administration. A thin outer rim of lower attenuation may surround the enhancing layer giving the lesion a target appearance, and defines the outer boundary of the inflamed hepatic parenchyma.

MRI

On T1 images, the central cavity is usually of decreased signal intensity relative to liver and has increased signal intensity on T2-weighted images, the central cavity is often surrounded by a ring of higher signal intensity that corresponds to the reactive zone. After Gd-DTPA the hyperemic reactive zone demonstrates enhancement.

Complications

Pleuropulmonary amoebiasis is the most frequent complication of amoebic liver abscess,[58] occurring in 20-35% of patients. This may manifest as pulmonary consolidation, abscess, serous effusion, empyema or hepatobronchial fistula (Figs 13.18A to C).

Intraperitoneal rupture occurs in 2-7.5% of patients with amoebic liver abscess (Figs 13.19A and B). Rupture

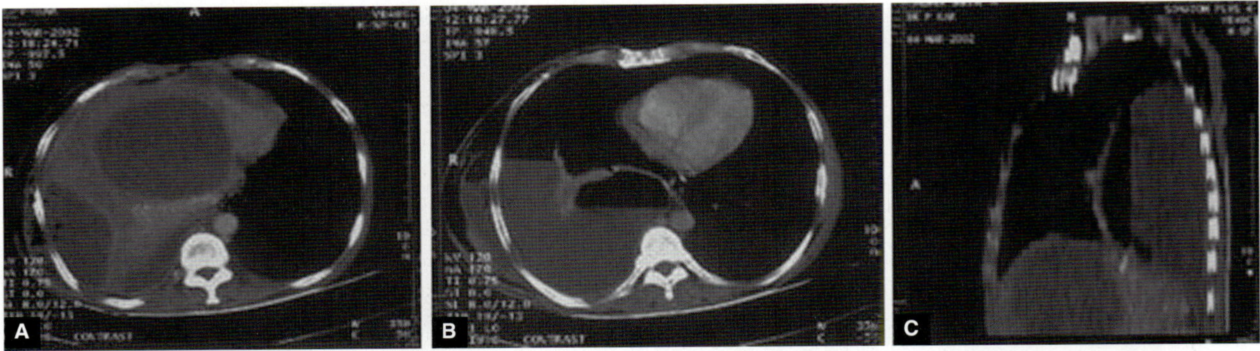

Figs. 13.18A to C: (A) Contrast enhanced CT showing two abscesses in the liver with one of lesions showing air loculi and indistinct margins, (B) A large hydropneumothorax is seen in the right pleural cavity, (C) Multiplanar reconstruction showing the communication between the abscess and the right hydropneumothorax–ruptured liver abscess

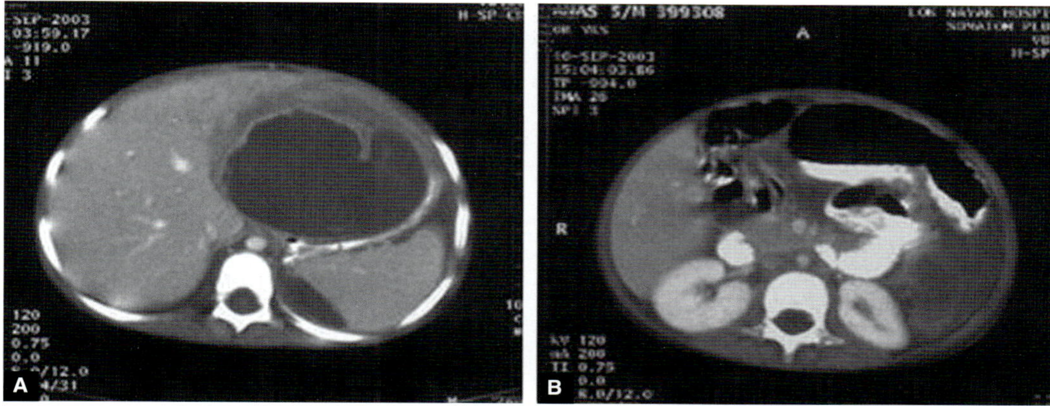

Figs 13.19A and B: (A) Contrast enhanced CT showing a large hypodense lesion with enhancing rim in the left lobe of liver. Perilesonal oedema is noted. Fluid seen in the perihepatic and perisplenic region, (B) Fluid seen in the peritoneal cavity—intraperitoneal rupture of abscess

into the pericardium is the most serious complication of amoebic liver abscess, because it can lead to progressive tamponade or sudden development of shock. Most abscesses responsible for this complication are located in the left hepatic lobe.

Abscess biliary communication is another complication in larger abscesses.

Fungal Hepatic Abscesses

Fungal abscess of liver, in general being uncommon, are seen in immunocompromised hosts, those receiving intensive chemotherapy and in patients with AIDS, lymphoma or acute leukemia.

Liver is frequently involved secondary to hematogenous spread of mycotic infections in other organs, most commonly in the lungs.

Of the various fungi, **candida** is the most common responsible agent.

Imaging Features

Sonographically, four major patterns of hepatic candidiasis are seen: (i) "Wheel within a wheel", in which a peripheral zone surrounds an inner echogenic wheel, which, in turn surrounds a central hypoechoic nidus, (ii) "Bull's eye", a lesion with a hyperechoic centre surrounded by hypoechoic rim, (iii) "Uniformly hypoechoic", the most common appearance, and (iv) "Echogenic", caused by scar formation.

On CT scan, the most common pattern is multiple small, rounded areas of decreased attenuation. Areas of scattered increased attenuation representing calcification can be seen on NCCT. Periportal areas of increased attenuation, correlating with fibrosis, may also be seen.[59]

Candida microabscesses have been reported as cold lesions on both sulphur colloid and gallium scans. On MR, these lesions show increased signal intensity on T1-weighted images and STIR sequences.

Hydatid Disease

Hydatid disease is prevalent throughout the world and the two main forms that affect humans are echinococcus granulosus and echinococcus multilocularis. Echinococcus alveolaris is less common but more aggressive form of echinococcal infection. Humans may become intermediate hosts through contact with a definitive host (usually a domesticated dog) or ingestion of contaminated water or vegetables. Once in the human liver, cysts grow to 1 cm during the first 6 months and 2-3 cm annually thereafter, depending on host tissue resistance.

Hydatid Cyst Structure

The hydatid cyst has three layers:

a. The outer pericyst, composed of modified host cells that form a dense and fibrous protective zone.
b. The middle laminated which is also referred to as ectocyst allows passage of nutrients.
c. The inner germinal layer, where the scolices (the larval stage of the parasite) and the laminated membrane are produced. This inner most or germinal layer forms the true wall of the cyst.

Daughter vesicles (brood capsules) are small spheres that contain the protoscolices and are formed from rest of the germinal layer. At gross examination, the vesicles resemble a bunch of grapes. Cyst fluid secreted by the germinal fluid, is antigenic and may also contain scolices.

When vesicles rupture within the cyst, scolices pass into the cyst fluid and may form a white sediment known as hydatid sand.

Hepatic Hydatid Disease

Once the parasite passes through the intestinal wall to reach the portal venous system or lymphatic system, the liver acts as the first line of defense and is, therefore, the most frequently involved organ. In humans, hydatid disease involves the liver in approximately 75% of cases. The right lobe is most frequently involved portion of the liver.

Imaging Features

These depend on the stage of the cyst growth, i.e. whether the cyst is unilocular, contains daughter vesicles (Fig. 13.20), partially calcified or completely calcified signifying dead parasite.

Plain Film Findings\

Calcification is seen at radiography in 20-30% of hydatid cysts and usually manifests as a curvilinear or ring like pattern representing calcification of the pericyst.[60] During the natural evolution towards healing, dense calcification of all components of the cyst occurs. Although the death of the parasite is not necessarily indicated by calcification of the pericyst it is indicated by complete calcification.

The ultrasonographic appearance of hydatid cysts vary with the stage of evolution and maturity.

i. There may be a well-defined anechoic cyst.
ii. A well-defined anechoic cyst except for hydatid sand. Multiple echogenic foci due to hydatid sand may be seen within the lesion by repositioning the patient. The echogenic foci quickly fall to the most dependent portion of the cavity without forming visible strata. This finding has been referred to as the "snowstorm sign".[61]
iii. Detachment of the endocyst from pericyst is probably related to decreasing intracystic pressure, degeneration, host response, trauma or response to therapy (Fig. 13.21). The cyst may appear as well-defined fluid collection with a localized split in the wall and "floating membranes" within the cavity (Fig. 13.22). Complete detachment of the membranes inside the cyst has been referred to as the "US water lily" sign because of its resemblance to the radiographic water lily sign in pulmonary cysts.[60,61]
iv. The development of daughter cysts from the lining germinal membrane produces a characteristic appearance of cysts enclosed within a cyst (Fig. 13.23). This appearance is extremely characteristic producing a honeycomb pattern with multiple septa representing the walls of daughter cysts. When daughter cysts are separated by hydatid matrix (a material with mixed ehogenicity) they demonstrate a "wheel spoke" pattern. The matrix

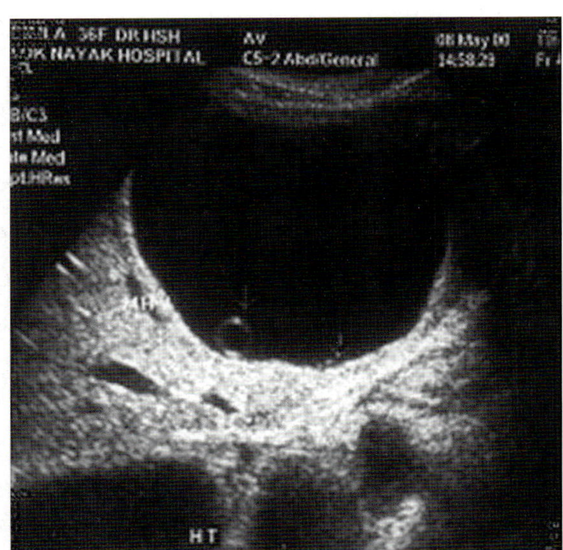

Fig. 13.20: US scan showing a well-defined anechoic cyst with a small cyst within—hydatid cyst

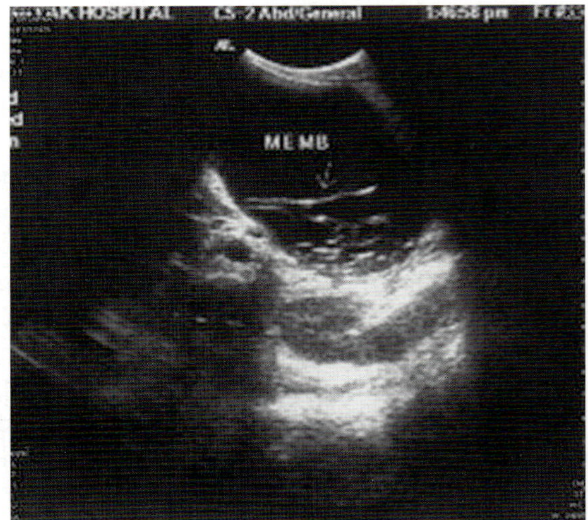

Fig. 13.21: US scan showing membranes as serpentine linear structures floating within a hydatid cyst

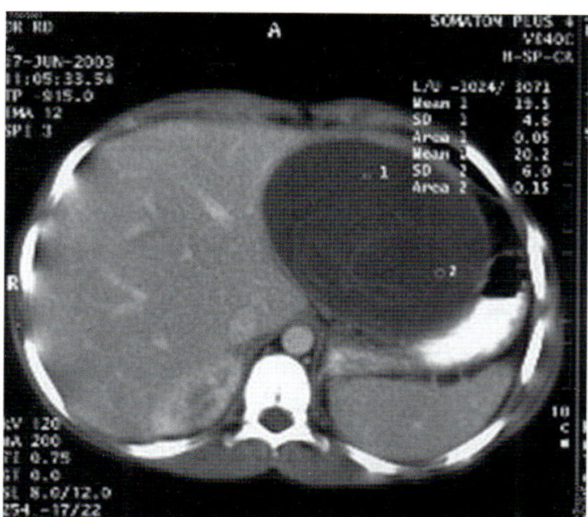

Fig. 13.22: Contrast enhanced CT scan (CECT) showing detachment of the laminated membrane from the pericyst seen as linear areas of increased attenuation within the hydatid cyst

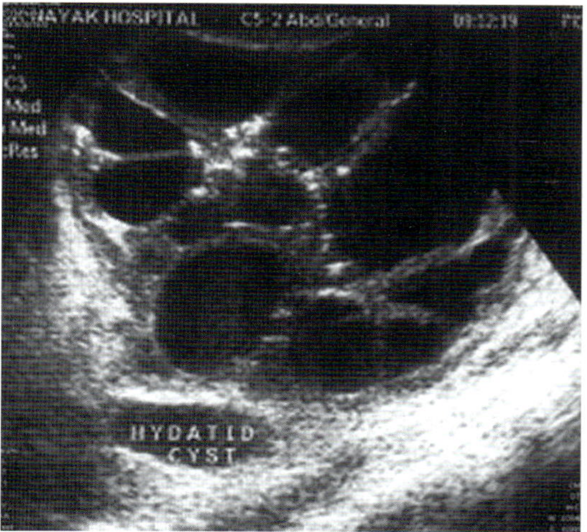

Fig. 13.23: US scan showing a characteristic appearance of cysts enclosed within a cyst giving rise to honeycomb pattern seen in a hydatid cyst

represents hydatid fluid containing membranes of broken daughter vesicles, scolices and hydatid sand. Membranes may appear within the matrix as serpentine linear structures, a finding that is highly specific for hydatid disease.[62]

v. Cyst calcification usually occurs in the cyst wall although internal calcification in the matrix may also be seen. US demonstrates a hyperechoic contour with a cone-shaped acoustic shadow. When the cyst wall is heavily calcified, only the anterior portion of the wall is visualized and appears as a thick arch with posterior concavity. Partial calcification of the cyst does not always indicate the death of the parasite, nevertheless, densely calcified cysts may be assumed to be inactive. When hydatid cysts become infected they lose their characteristic sonographic appearance and may become diffusely hyperechoic.

Nuclear Scintigraphy

These are cold on sulphur colloid scans and may demonstrate a rim of increased activity on gallium scans.

CT

CT has a high sensitivity and specificity for hepatic hydatid disease.[63] Echinococcal cyst of the liver appears on CT scans as a well- defined, round or oval cystic mass of the liver having a density near that of water where they appear hyperdense compared to normal hepatic parenchyma. Daughter cysts, indicating viability, give the lesions a multilocular appearance (Fig. 13.24). The daughter cysts usually contain fluid with a lower attenuation than that of the fluid in the mother cyst. Daughter cysts can also float free in the lumen of the mother cyst, so altering the patient's position may change the position of these cysts, confirming the diagnosis of echinococcal disease. Detachment of the laminated membrane from the pericyst can be visualized as linear areas of increased attenuation within the cyst. Postcontrast scan shows enhancement of internal septation. Calcification of the cyst wall or internal septa are easily detected at CT.

MRI

Hepatic hydatid cysts appear hypointense on T1 and hyperintense on T2-weighted images. The pericyst usually has low signal on T1 and T2-weighted images because it is rich in collagen.[64] This finding of low signal intensity rim on T2-weighted images has been proposed as a

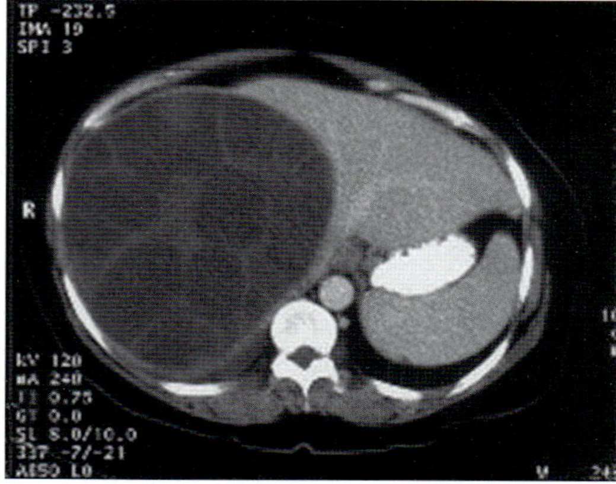

Fig. 13.24: CT scan showing the honeycomb pattern in a hydatid cyst with the multiple septa representing the walls of daughter cysts

characteristic sign of hydatid disease. The internal architecture is well demonstrated by MR imaging with the daughter cysts being hypointense to isointense on T1 imaging and isointense on T2W imaging relative to hyperintense hydatid fluid and sand of the mother cyst (Figs 13.25A and B). The floating membranes seen in a cyst undergoing degeneration appear as low intensity structures. Intraparenchymal rupture of the cyst appears as a defect in the low intensity rim. Calcifications, when present, are not as well demonstrated by MR imaging as by CT but when thick may produce a signal void.[65]

Local Complications

Intrahepatic Complications

Intrahepatic complications of hydatid cysts include cyst rupture and infection. Cyst rupture can be contained, communicating and direct.[66] Contained ruptures occur when the endocyst ruptures but the pericyst remains intact. Contained rupture may be related to degeneration, trauma or response to therapy. Communicating rupture implies passage of the cyst contents into the biliary radicals that have been incorporated into the pericyst. Direct rupture occurs when both the pericyst and the endocyst rupture, allowing free spillage of hydatid material into the peritoneal or pleural cavity, hollow viscera or abdominal wall (Figs 13.26A to C). Both US and CT may demonstrate a cyst wall defect and passage of the cyst contents through the defect, particularly in direct communication. MR imaging may demonstrate interruption in the low signal intensity rim of the cyst wall as well as extrusion of contents through the defect.

Infection occurs only after rupture of both the pericyst and endocyst leading to communicating and direct rupture which allows bacteria to pass easily into the cyst (5-8% cases). Findings that suggest infection include a solid appearance, a mixed pattern produced by solid and fluid elements, internal echogenic foci and air or air-fluid levels within the cyst (Fig. 13.27).

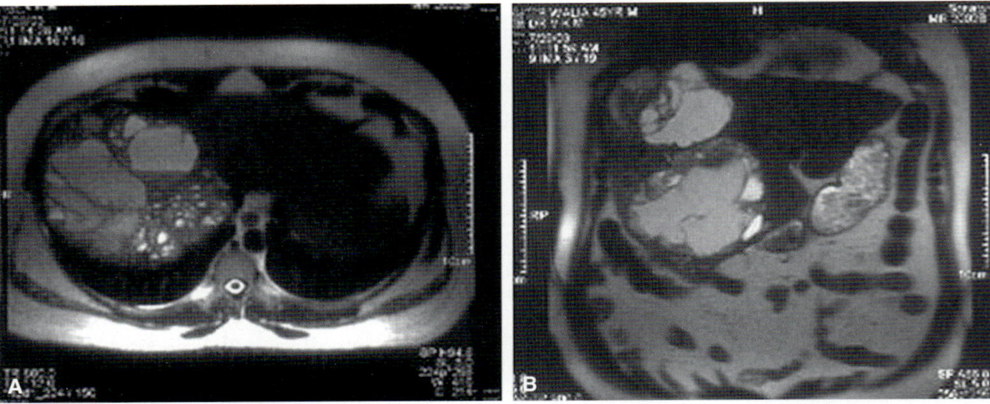

Figs 13.25A and B: Axial (A) and Coronal (B) MR images showing hepatic hydatids with multiple daughter cysts within appearing hyperintense on the T_2-weighted images

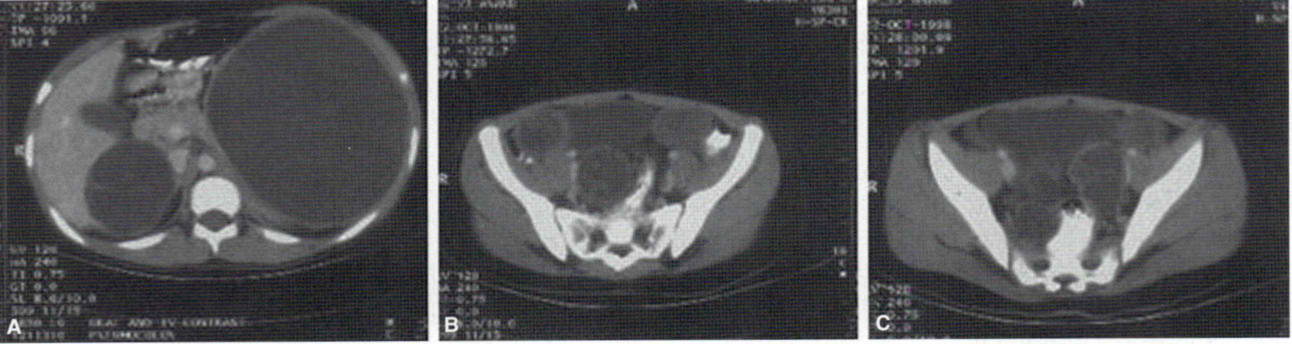

Figs 13.26A to C: (A) CT scan showing hydatid cysts in the liver and spleen, (B and C) Multiple cysts of varying sizes seen in the peritoneal cavity–peritoneal seeding of hydatid cysts

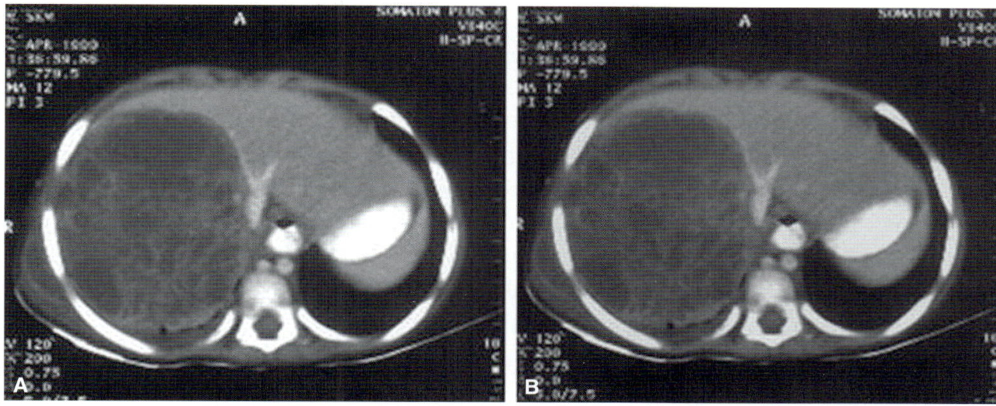

Figs. 13.27A and B: CT scan showing a solid appearance of the hydatid with enhancing sepata within-Infected hydatid

Exophytic Growth

Hydatid cysts may use the natural routes provided by the liver capsule, ligaments, and peritoneum to progress beyond the boundaries of the liver. The two most common routes of exophytic growth are the bare area of the liver and the gastrohepatic ligament.

Transdiaphragmatic Thoracic Involvement

The bare area of the liver is by far the most common route of transdiaphragmatic involvement occurring in 0.6-16% of cases of hepatic hydatid.Transdiaphragmatic migration varies from simple adherence to the diaphragm to rupture into the pleural cavity, seeding in the pulmonary parenchyma, and chronic bronchial fistula.[67]

US can help confirm the presence of hepatic hydatid disease and demonstrate pleural effusion, although the diaphragmatic defect is rarely seen. CT is valuable for demonstrating transdiaphragmatic migration of hydatid disease and evaluating the thoracic component.

Sagittal and coronal MR imaging is also very useful in demonstrating the migration of the cyst through the diaphragm and allows accurate presurgical diagnosis.

Perforation into Hollow Viscera

Spontaneous rupture of the cyst into hollow viscera is an extremely rare complication with an estimated frequency of 0.5%. This complication may be accompanied by clinical findings of hydatidemesia or hydatidorrhoea. Typically, the communication is not discovered until surgery, although in some cases it is found at radiology.[68] CT may demonstrate a cyst with an air-fluid level or orally administered contrast material inside the cavity. Barium-enhanced CT can be used to demonstrate the fistula between the cyst and the hollow viscus.

Peritoneal Seeding

Peritoneal echinococcosis is almost always secondary to hepatic disease, although some unusual cases of primary peritoneal involvement have been described.[69] The overall frequency of peritoneal disease in cases of echinococcosis involving the abdomen is approximately 13%. Peritoneal echinococcosis usually goes undetected until cysts are large enough to produce symptoms.

CT is the modality of choice in affected patients because it allows imaging of the entire abdomen and pelvis. Cysts may be multiple and located anywhere in the peritoneal cavity. Imaging findings are similar to those in hepatic disease. Peritoneal hydatid disease may grow and occupy the entire peritoneal cavity, simulating a multiloculated mass. This pathologic condition has been referred to as encysted peritoneal hydatidosis.

Biliary Communication

Communication of hydatid disease with the biliary tree has been described in up to 90% of hepatic cysts. This can be explained by the fact that during cyst growth, small biliary radicles are incorporated into the pericyst. However, frank rupture into the biliary tree occurs in only 5-15% of cases. Communicating rupture of a cyst into the biliary system may occur through small fissures or bile-cyst fistulas or through a wide perforation that allows access to a main biliary branch.

The only direct sign of rupture into the biliary tree is the visualization of the cyst wall defect or of a communication between the cyst and a biliary radicle. In some instances, the passage of hydatid material through the defect and subsequent filling of the biliary radicles or common bile duct may be seen. In such cases, US demonstrates anechoic, rounded or echogenic linear structures without posterior acoustic shadowing in the biliary tract. CT can demonstrate high-attenuation material passing through the cyst wall defect and filling the biliary radicles or common bile duct. CT is superior to US in depicting hydatid cyst content in the distal segment of the common bile duct. Endoscopic retrograde cholangiopancreatography and percutaneous transhepatic cholangiography can demonstrate the communication in more detail.

Indirect signs of biliary communication include increased echogenicity at US and fluid levels and signal intensity changes at MR imaging. An air-fluid level within the cyst, previously described as a sign of infection, is considered to be a sign either of rupture into the biliary tree or a hollow viscus or of a bronchopleural fistula. Lipid material that forms a fat-fluid level within the cyst has also been described as an indirect sign of biliary communication.[70]

Portal Vein Involvement

Compression of the portal vein and thrombosis with secondary cavernomatosis are rare and are caused by cysts located in the caudate lobe and hepatic bifurcation.[71] Direct portal invasion by hydatid cyst contents is a very unusual complication.

Abdominal Wall Invasion

Cysts may invade the right anterolateral abdominal wall from the right hepatic lobe and the anterior abdominal wall from the left hepatic lobe. Cysts usually pass through a small orifice, adopting an hourglass configuration. Imaging reveals a cystic mass within the abdominal wall that is similar to and in communication with the hepatic component of the hydatid cyst.

The alveolar form of echinococcal disease is distinct from the cystic form in several aspects.[72] This disease, in contrast to the expansile cysts of E. granulosus, is characterized by the formation of one or more infiltrative liver lesions that stimulate a granulomatous reaction. Internal necrosis, cavitation, and calcification may be seen within the lesion. The CT and MR imaging appearance of the predominately solid lesion of E. multilocularis is indistinguishable from that of primary or secondary malignant liver neoplasm. Atrophy of a lobe or segment of the liver may occur when the lesion is located centrally in the liver. Serologic testing and percutaneous biopsy may be useful for diagnosis when alveolar echinococcal disease is suspected. It should be included in the differential of hepatic lesions in patients who live in or have travelled to endemic regions of the world.

HEPATIC TUBERCULOSIS

Hepatic tuberculosis is a distinct clinical entity and is said to be found in 50-80% of all cases dying from pulmonary tuberculosis. The majority of hepatic tuberculosis fall within the 11-50 years age group.

Pathology

Usually tuberculous involvement of the liver is as a part of generalized miliary tuberculosis. Localized tuberculosis of the liver producing large abscesses or nodules is exceedingly rare, even in areas where tuberculosis is relatively common. Usual histology of hepatic tuberculosis is that of a granuloma with caseation necrosis.[73]

IMAGING FEATURES

Plain Film Findings

Chest X-ray abnormalities are found in approximately 65% of patients in the form of minimal to far advanced pulmonary tuberculosis of miliary tuberculosis.

Plain abdominal radiographs may show evidence of liver enlargement in 75% and hepatic calcification in 49% of cases. The calcification consists of numerous rounded calcific densities with ill-defined margins diffusely distributed throughout the liver. Abdominal scout film may also show evidence of splenomegaly.

PTC and ERCP may demonstrate evidence of biliary obstruction usually at the level of porta hepatis caused by enlarged lymph nodes.

Nuclear Scintigraphy

Hepatobiliary scintigraphy shows cold spot similar to neoplasm in hepatic tuberculosis.

US

Ultrasound features are non-specific. US may show mass lesion of mixed echogenicity with abnormal echoes due to calcification. Enlarged lymph nodes may be sent at porta hepatis which cause biliary obstruction leading to dilatation of intrahepatic biliary radicles, hepatic and bile duct.

CT

When involvement is focal, usually the lesion appears as hypodense mass with or without presence of calcification. Biliary obstruction may also be seen caused by enlarged lymphnodes located at the hepatoduodenal ligament and port hepatis.

HEPATIC SCHISTOSOMIASIS

Schistosomiasis is one of the most common and serious parasitic infection of the humans. Liver can be involved by any of S. Japonicum, S. mansoni or S. haematobium infection.

Schistosomiasis is an insidious and chronic disease. Because heptocellular necrosis occurs late in its course, patients may seek medical attention for portal hypertension and variceal bleeding. Patients with S. hematobium infection, which affects the liver less severely, typically present with haematuria resulting from urinary tract involvement.

IMAGING FEATURES

Plain Film Findings

Plain abdominal radiograph commonly shows splenomegaly. Calcification in the liver is too faint to be appreciated.

US

In severe hepatic involvement portal triads are replaced by thick, densely echogenic bands, radiating from the porta hepatis to the periphery. Initially the liver is enlarged, but as periportal fibrosis progresses, it becomes contracted and the features of portal hypertension (varices, splenomegaly, ascites) become more apparent.

CT

Peripheral hepatic or capsular calcification is the hallmark of *S. japonicum* infection. There is gross pseudoseptation within liver with geographic bands of calcification and notches in the liver margin. Prominent periportal low density areas may also be present. Increased incidence of hepatocellular carcinoma (HCC) is also found in these livers.

S. mansoni infection manifests as low-density, rounded foci with linear branching bands that encompass the portal tracts. These fibrotic bands sometimes show enhancement with contrast material but usually do not calcify.

MRI

The morphological changes of the liver and stigmata of portal hypertension are well seen on MR. Curvilinear low signal intensity areas corresponding to regions of fibrosis and calcification may also be seen.

HEPATIC PNEUMOCYSTIS CARINII INFECTION

Pneumocystis carinii is the commonest opportunistic infection in patients with AIDS. Nearly 80% of AIDS patients are affected, and extrapulmonary dissemination is becoming increasingly common.

Sonographically, P. carinii infection of the liver can manifest as diffuse, tiny, non-shadowing echogenic foci or extensive replacement of normal liver parenchyma by echogenic clumps of dense calcification. On CT scan, these regions are first hypodense but then become characteristically calcified.

Miscellaneous Lesions

Fatty Infiltration

Fatty infiltration of the liver is a common occurrence resulting from increased deposition of triglyceride in hepatocytes. This arises from a variety of nutritional disturbances or toxic insults to the liver. These include obesity, nutritional deficiencies, diabetes mellitus, pregnancy, steroids, hepatotoxic drugs and alcoholism. The development of fatty infiltration is a dynamic process and changes may be seen a few weeks of an insult and may regress within days. Most characteristically, the fatty involvement is uniform or geographic in distribution. However, occasionally it may be nodular or multifocal when it is indistinguishable from other focal hepatic lesions. Features suggesting the true nature of the process are sharp angular boundaries to the lesions and no evidence of displacement or effacement of venous structures.

Another well-recognised variant is focal sparing of small areas of normal liver in a more generalised fatty infiltration. The spared area appears as an echo-poor focal mass. A characteristic location for the spared area is the quadrate lobe anterior to the portal vein bifurcation or related to the gallbladder bed. The shape of the spared area or pseudomass is typically ovoid. Its location has led to the suggestion that the sparing relates to alteration of blood flow in this area.

Hematoma

Surgery and trauma are the two most common causes of hepatic bleeding. Hemorrhage within a solid liver neoplasm, especially a hepatocellular adenoma, is a third well-known mechanism by which intra-or perhepatic hematoma can be induced. Symptomatic manifestations depend on the severity of the bleeding, the location, and the time frame during which the hemorrhage occurred.

At CT, the appearance of an intrahepatic hemorrhage depends on the cause of the bleeding and the lag time between the traumatic event and the imaging procedure. In an acute or subacute setting, hemorrhage has a higher attenuation value than pure fluid due to the presence of aggregated fibrin components. In chronic cases, a hematoma has attenuation identical to that or pure fluid. Frequently, the cause of the hemorrhage can be detected on CT. In post-traumatic cases, coexistent features such as hepatic lacerations, rib fractures, or perihepatic fluid will be present. In hemorrhage induced by surgery, the locations of the hematoma (along the surgical plane) will often be a clue to the diagnosis. The presence of a perihepatic hematoma in combination with a hemorrhagic mass is highly suggestive of hepatocellular adenoma. Because of the paramagnetic effect of methaemoglobin, MR imaging is even more suitable than CT for detection and characterization of hemorrhage. A subacute hematoma appears as a heterogeneous mass with pathognomonic high signal intensity on T1-weighted and T2-weighted images.

Biloma

Bilomas result from rupture of the biliary system, which can be spontaneous, traumatic, or iatrogenic following surgery or interventional procedures. Bilomas can be intrahepatic or perihepatic. Extravasation of bile into the liver parenchyma generates an intense inflammatory reaction, thereby inducing formation of a well-defined pseudocapsule. Clinical manifestations depend on the location and size of the biloma. At both CT and MR imaging, a biloma usually appears as a well-defined or slightly irregular cystic mass without septa or calcifications. The pseudocapsule is usually not readily identifiable (Fig. 13.28A and B). This imaging appearance, in combination with the clinical history and location, should enable correct diagnosis.

REFERENCES

1. Ata Soy C, Akyar S. Multidetector CT contributions in liver imaging. Eur Radiol 2004;52:2-17.
2. Winterer JT, Kotter E, Ghanem M. Detection and characterization of bengin focal liver lesions with multislice CT. Eur Radiol 2006;16:2427-43.
3. Ros PR. Focal liver masses other than metastases. In categorical course on gastrointestinal radiology. Oak Brook III, RSNA Publications, 1999.
4. Van Sonnenberg E, Wroblicka JT, D' Agostino HB, et al. Symptomatic hepatic cysts: Percutaneous drainage and sclerosis radiology 1994;190:387-92.

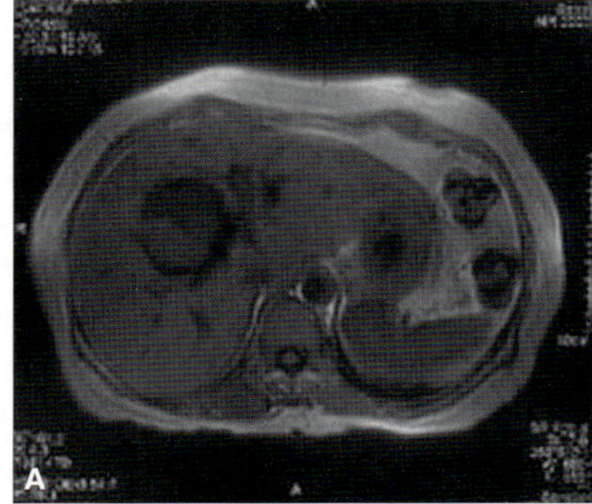

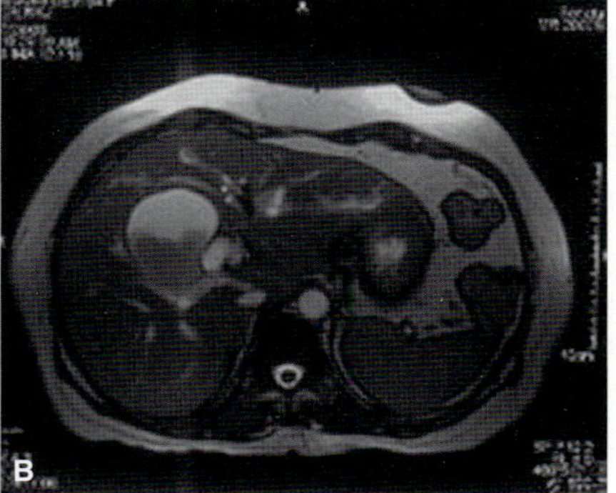

Figs 13.28A and B: (A) MR image in a post cholecystectomy patient showing a well-defined hypointense lesion in the gallbladder fossa s/o biloma, (B) T_2 weighted MR images shows a hyperintense signal in the cyst with a fluid – fluid level (due to inspissated bile/sludge)

5. Dewbury KC: Benign focal liver lesions. In, Meire H, Cosgrove D, Dewbery K, et al (Eds). Abdominal and General Ultrasound (2nd edition) Churchill Livingstone, 2001.
6. Blumke DA, Fishman EK. Spiral CT of liver tumors. In Fishman EK, Jeffrey RB (Eds) Spiral CT Principles, Techniques and Clinical Application (2nd edition) Lippincott Raven, 1998.
7. Mathieu D, Vilgrain V, Mahfouz A, et al. Benign liver tumors. Mag Reson Imaging Clin N Am 1997;5:255-88.
8. Kairaluome M, Leinonen A, Stahlberg MM, et al. Percutaneous aspiration and alcohol sclerotherapy for symptomatic hepatic cysts. Ann Surg 1989;210:208-15.
9. Oto A, Tamm EP, Szklaruk J. Multidetector Row CT of the Liver Radiol Clin N Am 2005;43:827-48.
10. Palacois E, Shannon M, Solomon C, et al. Biliary cystadenoma: Ultrasound, CT and MRI. Gastrointest Radiol 1990;15:313-16.
11. Buetow PC, Midkiff RB. Primary malignant neoplasms in the adult. Mag Reson Imaging Clin North Am 1997;5:289-318.
12. Wei SC, Huang GT, Cheu CH et al. Bile duct hamartomas. Clin Radiol 1992;45:203-05.
13. Semelka RC, Hussain SM, Marcos HB, et al. Biliary hamartomas: Solitary and multiple lesions shown on current MR techniques including Gadolinium enhancement. J Mag Resonance Imaging 1999;l10:196-201.
14. Birnbaum BA. Benign tumors of the liver: Hepatic haemangiomas. In Margulis Burhennes (Eds) Alimentary Tract Radiology (5th edition), 1994.
15. Brannigan M, Burns PN, Wilson SR. Blood flow patterns in focal liver lesions at Microbubble enhanced US. Radiographics 2004;24:921-35.
16. Powers C, Ros PR. Hepatic mass lesions. In Haaga JR, Kanzieri CF, Gilkeson RC (Eds) CT and MR Imaging of the Whole Body (4th edition) Mosby, 2003.
17. Hanfusa K, Ohashi I, Himenso Y, et al. Hepatic haemangioma: Findings with two phase CT. Radiology 1995; 196:465.
18. Yu JS, Kim MJ, Kim KW, et al. Hepatic cavernous haemangioma: Sonographic pattern and speed of contrast enhancement on multiphase Dynamic MR Imaging AJR 1998;71:1021-25.
19. Counbaras M, Weudum D, Cholley LM, et al. CT and MR Imaging features of pathologically prov Atypical Giant Haemangiomas of the liver. AJR 2002;179:1457-63.
20. Danet IM, Semelka RC, Braga L, et al. Giant haemangioma of the liver: MR imaging characteristics in 24 patients. Magnetic Resonance Imaging 2003;21:95-101.
21. Kassarjian A, Dubois J, Burrows PE. Angiographic classification of hepatic haemangiomas in infants. Radiology 2002;222:693-98.
22. Grazioli L, Federle MP, Ichikawa T, et al. Liver adenomatosis: Clinical, histopathologic, and imaging findings in 15 patients. Radiology 2000;216:395-402.
23. Catalano O, Nunziata A, LobiancoR, Siani A. Real time Harmonic Contrast material specific US of focal liver lesions. Radiographics 2005;25:333-349.
24. Horton KM, Blumke DA, Hruban RH, et al. CT and MR imaging of benign hepatic and biliary tumors. Radiographics 1999;19:431-51.
25. Tajima T, Honda H, Kuroiwa T, et al. Radiologic features of intrahepatic bile duct Adenoma: A look at the surface of the liver. J Comput Assist Tomography 1999;23(5): 690-95.
26. King LJ, Burkill GJC, Scurr ED, et al. Mn DPDP enhanced magnetic resonance imaging of focal liver lesions. Clinical Radiology 2002;57:1047-57.
27. Bartolozzi C, Cioni D, Donati F, et al. Focal liver lesions: MR imaging—Pathologic correlation. Eur Radiol 2001;11:1374-88.
28. Harvey CJ, Albrecht T: Ultrasound of focal liver lesions. Eur Radiol 2001;11:1578-93.
29. Wilson SR, Jang HJ, Kim TK, Burns PN. Diagnosis of focal liver masses on ultrasonography: comparison of unenhanced and contrast enhanced scans. J Ultrasound Med 2007;26:775-787.
30. Kim TK, Jang HJ, Burns PN, Lavallee JM, Wilson SR. Focal Nodular hyperplasia and hepatic adenoma: differentiation with low mechanical index contrast enhanced sonography. Am J Rentgenol 2008;190:58-66.
31. Rangheard AS, Vilgrain V, Audet P, et al. Focal nodular hyperplasia inducing hepatic vein obstruction. AJR 2002;179:759-62.
32. Brancatelli G, Federle MP, Katyal S, et al. Haemodynamic characterization of focal nodular Hyperplasia using three dimensional volume rendered multidetector CT angiography. AJR 2002;179:81-85.
33. Macky MD, Frazer C, deBoer WB. Magnetic resonance features of focal nodular hyperplasia of the liver. Australasian Radiology 1999;43:315-20.
34. Elsayes KM, Narra VR, Yin et al. Focal hepatic lesions: Diagnostic value of enhancement pattern approach with contrast enhanced 3D gradient Echo MR imaging. Radiographics 2005;25:1299-1320.
35. Grazioli L, Morana G, Federle M, et al. Focal nodular hyperplasia: Morphologic and functional information from MR Imaging with Gadobenate Dimeglumine. Radiology 2001;221:731-39.
36. Ba Ssalamah A, Schima W, Schmook MT, et al. Atypical focal nodular hyperplasia of the liver: Imaging features of nonspecific and liver specific MR contrast agents. AJR 2002;179:1447-56.
37. Beets Tan RGH, Van Engelshoven JMA, Greve JWM. Hepatic adenoma and focal nodular hyperplasia: MR findings with superparamagnetic iron oxide enhanced MRI. Clin Imaging 1998;22:211-15.
38. Rha SE, Lee MG, Lee YS, et al. Nodular regenerative hyperplasia of the liver in Budd—Chiari Syndrome: CT and MR features. Abdom Imaging 2000;25:255-58.
39. Quglia A, Tibballs J, Grasso A, et al. Focal nodular hyperplasia like areas in cirrhosis. Histopathology 2003;42:14-21.
40. Krinsky GA, Lee VS, Nguyen MT et al. Siderotic nodules at MR Imaging: Regenerative or Dysplastic J Comput Assist Tomography 2000;24:773-76.

41. Wilson SR, Burns PN. An algorithm for the diagnosis of focal liver masses using microbubble contrast enhanced pulse inversion sonography. Am J Roentgenol 2006; 186:1401-1412.
42. Prasad SR, Wang H, Rosas H et al. Fat containing lesions of the liver: radiologic – pathologic correlation. Radiographics 2005;25:321-331.
43. Ros PR, Goodman ZD, Ishak KG, et al. Mesenchymal hamartoma of the liver: Radiologic pathologic correlation. Radiology 1986;158:619-24.
44. Ishak KG, Kabin L. Benign tumors of the liver. Med Clin North Am 1975;59:995-1013.
45. Stanley P, Hall TR, Woolley MM et al. Mesenchymal hamartomas of the liver in childhood: Sonographic and CT findings. AJR 1986;147:1035-39.
46. O'Neil J, Ros PR. Knowing hepatic pathology aids MRI of liver tumors. Diagn Imaging 1989;11:58-65.
47. Ros PR, Rasmussew JF, Li KCP. Radiology of malignant and benign liver tumors. Curr Probl Diagn Radiol 1989;18:95-155.
48. Srivastava DN, Mahajan A, Berry M, et al. Colour Doppler flow imaging of focal hepatic lesions. Australasian Radiology 2000;44:285-89.
49. Keslar PJ, Buck JL, Selky DM. Infantile haemangioendothelioma of the liver revisited. Radiographics 1993;13:657-70.
50. Brandborg LL, Goldman IS. Bacterial and miscellaneous infections of the liver. In, Zakim D, Boyer TD (Eds): Hepathology Philadelphia: WB Saunders, 1990.
51. Lam Y-h, Wong S, Lee D et al. ERCP and pyogenic liver abscess. GI Endoscopy 1999;50:340-44.
52. Halvovsen RA, Korobkin M, Foster WL, et al. The variable CT appearance of hepatic abscesses. AJR 1984;141: 941-46.
53. Jeffrey RB, Tolentino CS, Chang FC, et al. CT of small pyogenic hepatic abscesses: The cluster sign. AJR 1988;151:487-89.
54. Balci NC, Semelhar RC, Noone TC et al. Pyogenic hepatic abscesses: MRI findings on T1 and T2 weighted and serial Gadolinuim Enhanced Gradient Echo Images. J Magn Reson Imaging 1999;9:285-90.
55. Gupta RK. Amoebic liver abscess: A report of 1000 cases. Int Surg 1984;69:261-64.
56. Philips RL. Computed tomography and ultrasound in the diagnosis and treatment of liver abscesses. Australasian Radiology 1994;38:165-69.
57. Radin DR, Ralls PW, Colletti PM et al. CT of amoebic liver abscess. AJR 1988;150:1297-1301.
58. Juimo AG, Gervez F, Angwafo FF. Extraintestinal amoebiasis. Radiology 1992;182:181.
59. Shirkhoda A. CT findings in hepatosplenic and renal candidiasis. J Comput Assist Tomogr 1987;11:795-98.
60. Beggs I. The radiology of hydatid disease. AJR 1985; 145:639-48.
61. Marti–Bonmati L, Menor Serrano F. Complications of hepatic hydatid cysts. Ultrasound, computed tomography and magnetic resonance diagnosis. Gastrointest Radiol 1990;15:119-25.
62. Von Sinner WN. New diagnostic sign in hydatid disease: Radiography, ultrasound, CT and MRI correlated to pathology. Eur J Radiol 1990;12:150-59.
63. Pedroza I, Saiz A, Arrazola J, et al. Hydatid disease; Radiologic and pathologic features and complications. Radiographics 2000;20:795-817.
64. Davolio SA, Canossi GC, Nicoli FA, et al. Hydatid disease: MR imaging study. Radiology 1990;175:701-06.
65. Agildere AM, Aytekin C, Coskun M, et al. MRI of hydatid disease of the Liver: A variety of sequences J. Comput Assist Tomography 1998;22(5):718-24.
66. De Diego J, Lecumberri FJ, Franquet T, et al. Computed tomography in hepatic echinococcosis. AJR 1982;139: 699-702.
67. Gomez R, Moreno E, Loinaz C, et al. Diaphragmatic or transdiaphragmatic thoracic involvement in hepatic hydatid disease surgical trends and classification. World J Surg 1995;19:714-19.
68. Jain R, Sawhney S, Berry M. Hydatid disease: CT demonstration and follow up of a cystogastric fistula. AJR 1992;158:212.
69. Karavias DD, Vagianos CE, Kakkos SK, et al. Peritoneal echinococcosis. World J Surg 1996;20:337-40.
70. Mendez JV, Arrazola J, Lopej J, et al. Fat – fluid level in hepatic hydatid cyst: A new sign of rupture into the biliary tree AJR 1996;167:91-94.
71. Gil – Egea MJ, Alameda F, Girvent M, et al: Hydatid cyst in the hepatic hilum causing a cavernous transformation in the portal vein. Gastroenterol Hepatol 1998;21:227-29.
72. Choji K, Fujita N, Chen M, et al. Alveolar hydatid disease of the liver: Computed tomography and transabdominal ultrasound with histopathological correlation. Clin Radiology 1992;46:97-103.
73. Balci NC, Tunaci A, Akincil A, et al. Granulomatous hepatitis: MRI findings. Magnetic Resonance Imaging 2001;19:1107-11.

Chapter Fourteen

Malignant Focal Lesions of the Liver

Raju Sharma, Madhusudhan KS

INTRODUCTION

Imaging of the liver has undergone dramatic changes during the last decade due to significant advances in technology. This has led to greater understanding and better management of many diseases which affect the liver. The advent of color Doppler flow imaging, helical CT followed by multi-detector CT and MRI have increased the sensitivity for detection and accuracy for characterization of liver lesions.[1,2] Clinical information continues to be of paramount importance as it helps to tailor the imaging technique and narrows the differential diagnosis.

Malignant focal lesions of the liver can broadly be classified as under:

Primary

Hepatocellular Tumors

- Hepatocellular carcinoma (HCC)
- Fibrolamellar hepatocellular carcinoma
- Clear cell carcinoma
- Carcinosarcoma
- Sclerosing hepatic carcinoma
- Hepatoblastoma

Cholangiocellular Tumors

- Cholangiocarcinoma
- Cystadenocarcinoma

Mesenchymal Tumors

- Angiosarcoma
- Epithelioid hemangioendothelioma (EHE)
- Leiomyosarcoma
- Malignant fibrous histiocytoma
- Lymphoma

Secondary

- Metastatic deposits
- Lymphoma

Metastasis to the liver from an extrahepatic malignancy is by far the commonest cause of a malignant hepatic neoplasm. Hepatic metastases are particularly common from primary malignancies of the gastrointestinal tract, breast and lung.

PRIMARY MALIGNANT FOCAL LESIONS

Hepatocellular Carcinoma (HCC)

HCC is the most common malignant neoplasm of the liver worldwide. The incidence varies, being more common in Africa and the far east. Etiology also varies among different population groups and the risk factors include hepatitis B and C infection, alcoholic cirrhosis, primary hemochromatosis, and exposure to carcinogens like aflatoxin. The 5-year cumulative HCC risk is 21% in hemochromatosis, 10% in hepatitis B virus infection, 8% in alcoholic cirrhosis and 5% in biliary cirrhosis.[3] Presence of multiple factors significantly increases the risk of HCC.[2] Any patient with chronic liver disease is at risk for the development of HCC and 80% of HCCs occur in cirrhotic livers.[4,5]

Majority of HCCs are thought to arise in a stepwise fashion from a regenerating nodule which develops into a dysplastic nodule which finally develops a focus of HCC. Pathologically HCC may occur in three different forms: solitary, multifocal, or diffuse. In Asia, HCC usually presents as a well defined mass, either solitary or multifocal, associated with cirrhosis secondary to hepatitis B. In the west it usually presents as a diffusely infiltrating mass and has an association with alcoholic cirrhosis. Encapsulated HCCs have a better prognosis.

HCC frequently invades the portal vein (in about 40% cases) and less often the inferior vena cava and hepatic veins (15%).[1] Biliary invasion is uncommon. With various curative therapies now available (liver transplantation, hepatic resection, percutaneous ablative techniques, chemotherapy, immunotherapy), 5-year-survival rate is about 40-75%.[2]

Clinical Presentation

The clinical signs and symptoms are often obscured by the debilitating effects of cirrhosis. Upper abdominal pain, malaise, fever, weight loss, palpable mass and rapid deterioration of liver function in patients with chronic cirrhosis are possible indicators.

Alfa-fetoprotein (AFP) is a useful serum marker and is elevated in 50-70% cases, and levels above 1000 ng/mL are strongly suggestive of HCC.

IMAGING IN HCC

Imaging in HCC is a challenge as early diagnosis is critical for successful treatment. Lesions larger than 2 cm usually do not pose a problem. However, nodules smaller than 2 cm often have non-specific imaging features and create difficulties in diagnosis.[6] MRI outperforms CT in detection of small HCCs in cirrhotic liver. The sensitivity of MRI and CT scan for HCC detection is 81% and 68% respectively. Also differentiation of regenerative and dysplastic nodules from HCC, in cirrhosis, is vital for proper management.

Ultrasonography (USG)

Ultrasonography being inexpensive and widely available is frequently used as the initial modality in the work-up of focal hepatic lesions. Recent advances in USG like tissue harmonic imaging and ultrasound contrast agents have increased its importance. The sensitivity of USG for detection of HCC ranges between 75-94% in various studies. However, sensitivity of USG for detection of HCC in the end stage cirrhotic liver is only about 50%, though the specificity has been reported to be as high as 98%. Most countries recommend a combination of USG and AFP every 6 months for HCC screening in high-risk patients.[7] Thus, any sonographically detected lesion in a cirrhotic liver should be considered malignant until proven otherwise.[1,4]

HCC has variable morphological presentations. Tumors can be solitary (Fig. 14.1A), multifocal or diffusely infiltrating. The most common finding is a discrete lesion, either solitary or multiple. These lesions are usually hypoechoic, but are sometimes isoechoic and detected chiefly by virtue of a thin hypoechoic halo which corresponds to the tumor capsule. Encapsulated HCCs are more commonly seen in the Asian and Japanese population as compared to the west. Twenty-five percent of HCCs are echogenic.

The echo pattern has been shown to correlate with tumor morphology. Solid tumors without necrosis are hypoechoic (Fig. 14.1A) whereas hyperechoic appearance is attributable to fatty metamorphosis, fibrosis, or sinusoidal dilatation. The majority of small HCCs (< 2 cm) are hypoechoic, whereas the larger HCCs are hyperechoic or of heterogeneous echo texture.

A less common pattern of HCC is diffuse parenchymal involvement with disorganization of the normal echo pattern. Multiple areas of decreased and increased echogenicity are present throughout the distorted liver without any distinct masses.

HCC has a propensity to invade the portal vein, hepatic vein or both, and this is depicted as echoes either partially or completely filling the lumen (Fig. 14.1B). Color Doppler flow imaging is a useful adjunct for detection of vascular invasion. The presence of arterial waveform within the thrombus indicates that it is neoplastic rather than bland thrombus. This distinction is vital because it has been shown that the presence of malignant portal vein thrombosis is the worst prognostic factor in predicting recurrence of HCC following surgical resection or liver transplantation. Color Doppler may also demonstrate intra-lesional vascularity in the form of a tangle of vessels within the tumor indicating hypervascularity (Fig. 14.1C) and arterio-venous shunting. A

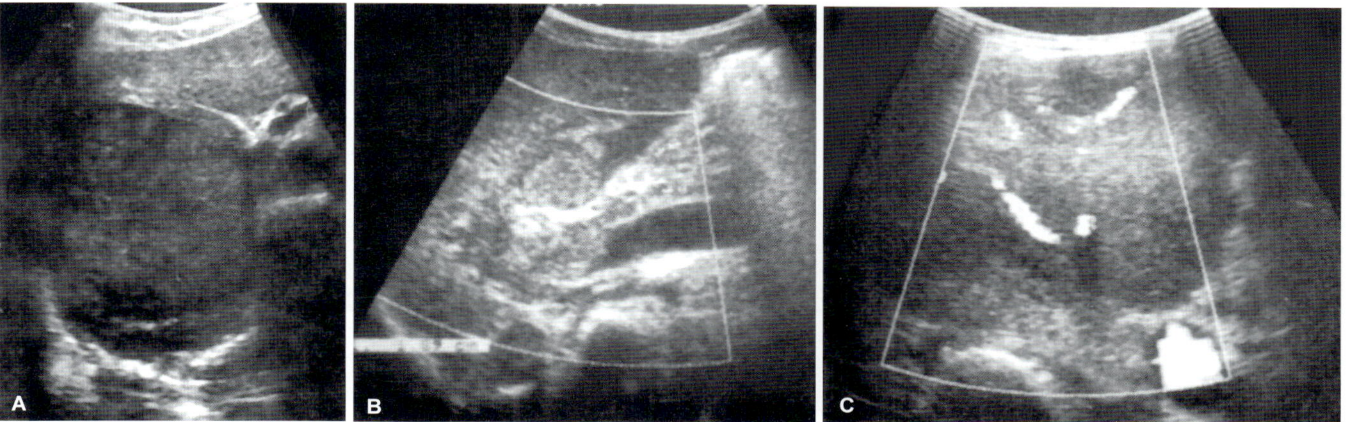

Figs 14.1A to C: HCC Ultrasound scan showing a well encapsulated hypoechoic mass in the right lobe of liver (A) echogenic thrombus in the portal vein, (B) and a hypoechoic mass with intratumoral vascularity on color Doppler (C)

basket pattern of intralesional vessels, indicating internal vascularity and shunting, may be seen in up to 15% of cases.[8] However, there is a lot of overlap in Doppler patterns. Contrast enhanced USG shows early hyper-perfusion of HCC with washout in portal venous phase.[9]

COMPUTED TOMOGRAPHY

The advent of helical CT made it possible to perform multi-phasic examination of the liver in the arterial and portal venous phase with the same bolus of contrast. This has had a major impact on the detection and characterization of hypervascular lesions like HCC. Multidetector CT (MDCT) has allowed faster scanning of liver, thus reducing respiration artifacts and has greatly increased spatial resolution leading to improvement in the characterization of smaller lesions. Also, with MDCT, good quality multiplanar reconstructions and CT angiographic images can be obtained. The latter enables proper planning of surgical resection or transplantation.

The liver receives 75-80% of its blood supply from the portal vein and 20-25% from the hepatic artery. On the other hand most liver tumors receive the majority of their blood supply from the hepatic artery. HCCs have a rich arterial supply and are better visualized on the arterial phase. It has been reported that up to 11% of lesions may be seen only on the arterial phase as they become isodense on the portal venous phase. In addition, arterial phase imaging is useful in demonstrating arterial-portal shunting (early enhancement of intra-hepatic portal venous branches) and enhancement of portal venous thrombus confirming it to be tumor thrombus.[4,10]

The CT features are variable depending on the size, vascularity and growth pattern. The multiphasic CT scan includes a non-contrast phase, followed by arterial, venous and delayed phases. On unenhanced CT, most HCCs present as solitary or multiple low attenuating lesions. Areas of fat density may be seen. In a fatty liver HCC may be seen as a hyperdense lesion. On arterial phase images the hypervascular tumor shows intense enhancement throughout the tumor (Figs 14.2A to C). The lesions are frequently encapsulated and the capsule is seen as a hypodense rim. Larger tumors are often heterogeneous due to necrosis and hemorrhage (Figs 14.3A to C). Arterial phase images may also demonstrate the

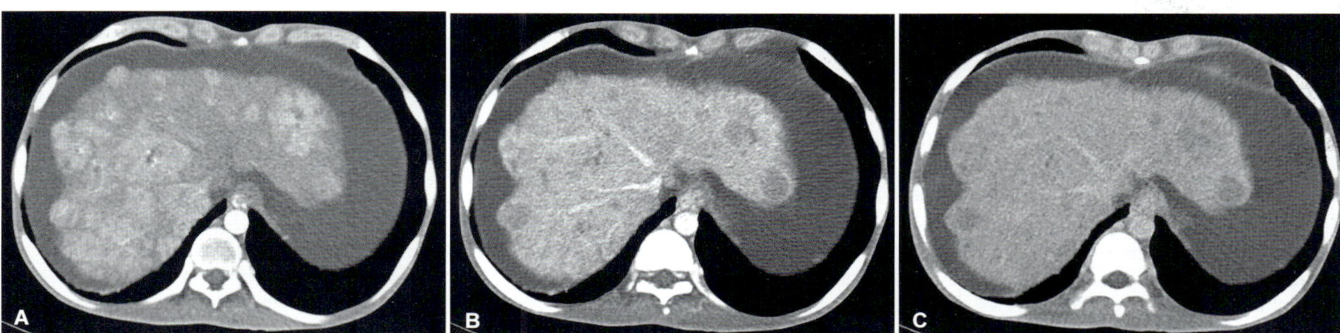

Figs 14.2A to C: Multifocal HCC. The arterial phase (A) image shows multiple hypervascular focal lesions with evidence of cirrhosis. These lesions show wash out in the portal venous phase (B) and are seen as hypodense lesions in the delayed phase (C)

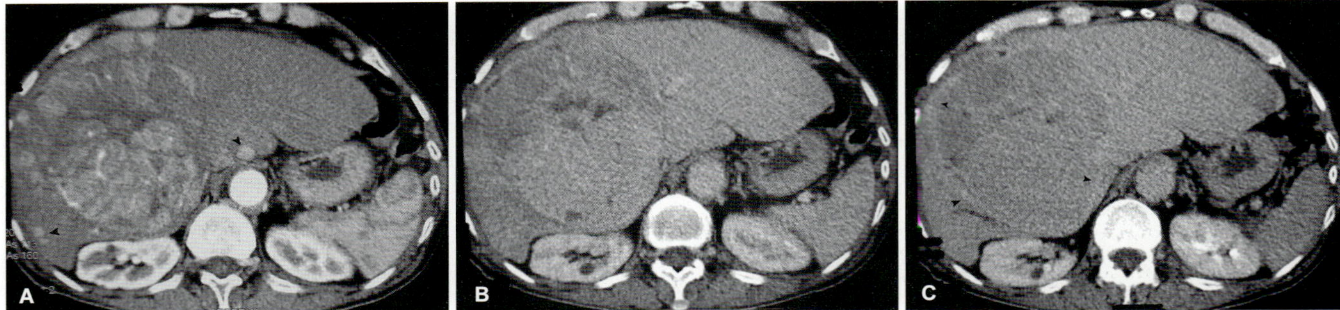

Figs 14.3A to C: HCC: The arterial phase image (A) shows a large mass in the right lobe with arterial enhancement. Two more nodules (arrow head) with similar morphology are seen in the adjacent liver. The venous phase (B) shows washout of contrast and a subtle capsule (arrow heads) is seen in the delayed phase (C)

presence of arterio-portal shunting (Fig. 14.4). During the portal venous phase there is rapid washout and the lesion becomes isodense to hypodense to normal liver (Figs 14.2B and 14.3B). On delayed phase images the capsule and fibrous septa may show prolonged enhancement (Fig. 14.3C) Vascular invasion is common with HCC. Portal vein invasion is due to portal venous drainage of HCC. A tumor thrombus in portal vein is diagnosed if the main portal vein has a diameter of $\geq$ 23 mm (bland thrombus rarely causes portal vein dilatation) and the thrombus shows enhancement in arterial phase (Figs 14.5A to C). HCCs may also extend into the hepatic veins or IVC (Fig. 14.6). HCCs may occasionally rupture and may lead to hemoperitoneum. A ruptured HCC is hypodense on arterial phase images showing only peripheral rim

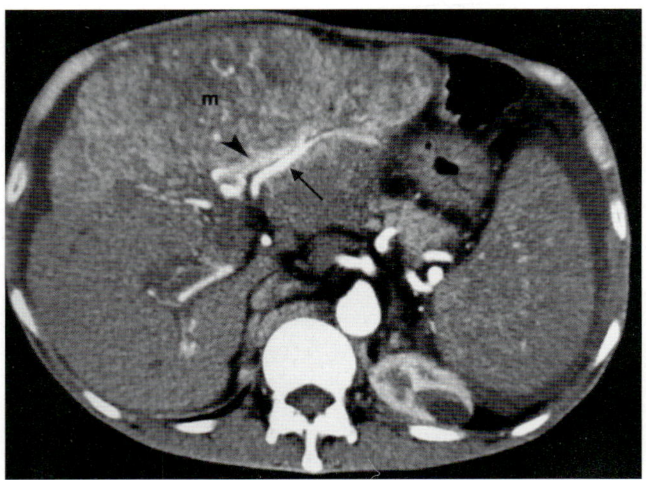

Fig. 14.4: Arterio-portal shunt: The arterial phase CT image shows a large enhancing lesion (m) in the segments 3 and 4 of liver with contrast in the left hepatic artery (arrow) and left branch of portal vein (arrow head) suggesting arterio-portal shunting

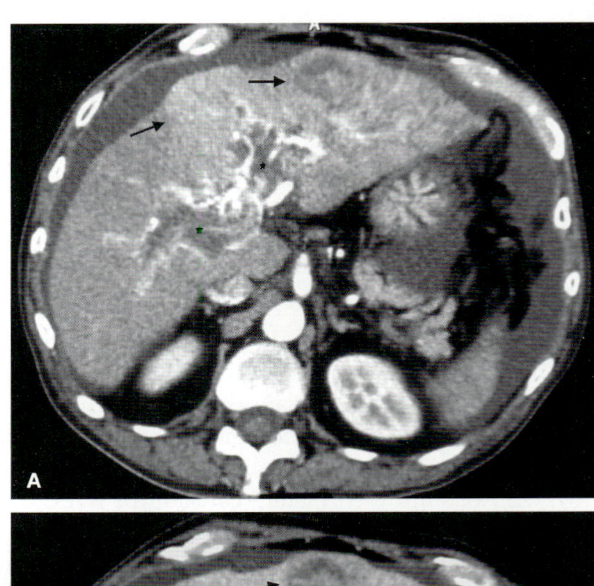

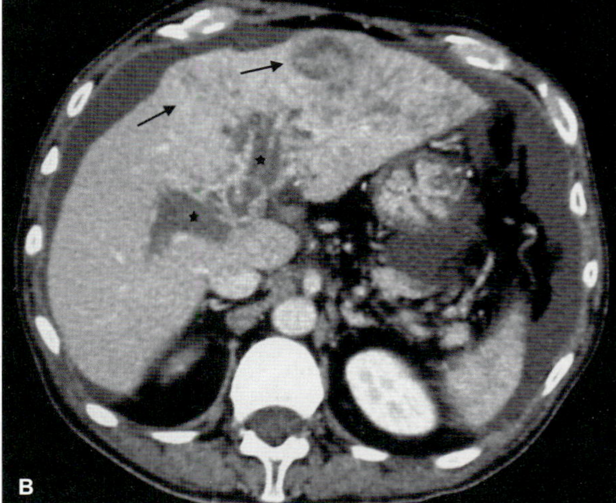

Figs 14.5A and B: Portal vein thrombus: The arterial phase CT image (A) shows two enhancing lesions (arrow) in segments 3 and 4 of liver with arterio-portal shunting. The portal vein in the venous phase image (B) shows a large filling defect (star) with 'thread and streak' pattern of enhancement suggestive of tumor thrombus

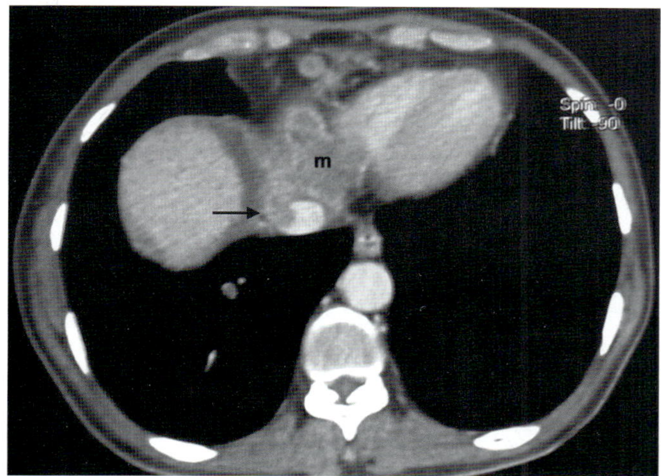

Fig. 14.6: IVC invasion: The axial CT image shows an exophytic mass (m) arising from left lobe of liver extending into the IVC (arrow)

enhancement with focal discontinuity ('enucleation sign').[2]

Imaging accuracy is often more limited in the cirrhotic liver due to architectural distortion, presence of regenerating nodules and hemodynamic alterations. Therefore, the detection of HCC in a cirrhotic liver may require several complementary imaging techniques. Since the imaging appearance of HCC can be variable it is said that any mass in a cirrhotic liver that does not fulfill criteria for a cyst or hemangioma should be considered an HCC until proved otherwise.

MAGNETIC RESONANCE IMAGING

The MR appearance depends on the type of disease (solitary, multifocal or diffuse), the degree of fibrosis, amount of fat as well as on the presence of necrosis and hemorrhage.

Usually HCC is hypointense on T1W images and mildly hyperintense on T2W images (Figs 14.7 and 14.8). The presence of fat or hemorrhage may result in increased signal intensity on T1W images (Fig. 14.7A). Encapsulated lesions have a hypointense rim on T1W images and a single or a double layered hypointense rim on T2W images. Fast gradient echo sequences allow the liver to be imaged in a breath hold and multi-phasic dynamic gadolinium enhanced MR imaging has been shown to improve detection of HCC and may be superior to dual phase CT. MRI frequently demonstrates HCCs, particularly tumors smaller than 1.5 cm, better than CT images. HCC is typically seen as a hypervascular mass with rapid washout. Tumors larger than 2 cm enhance in a heterogeneous fashion.[11]

The most sensitive sequence for detecting small HCC is the immediate post-gadolinium arterial phase on

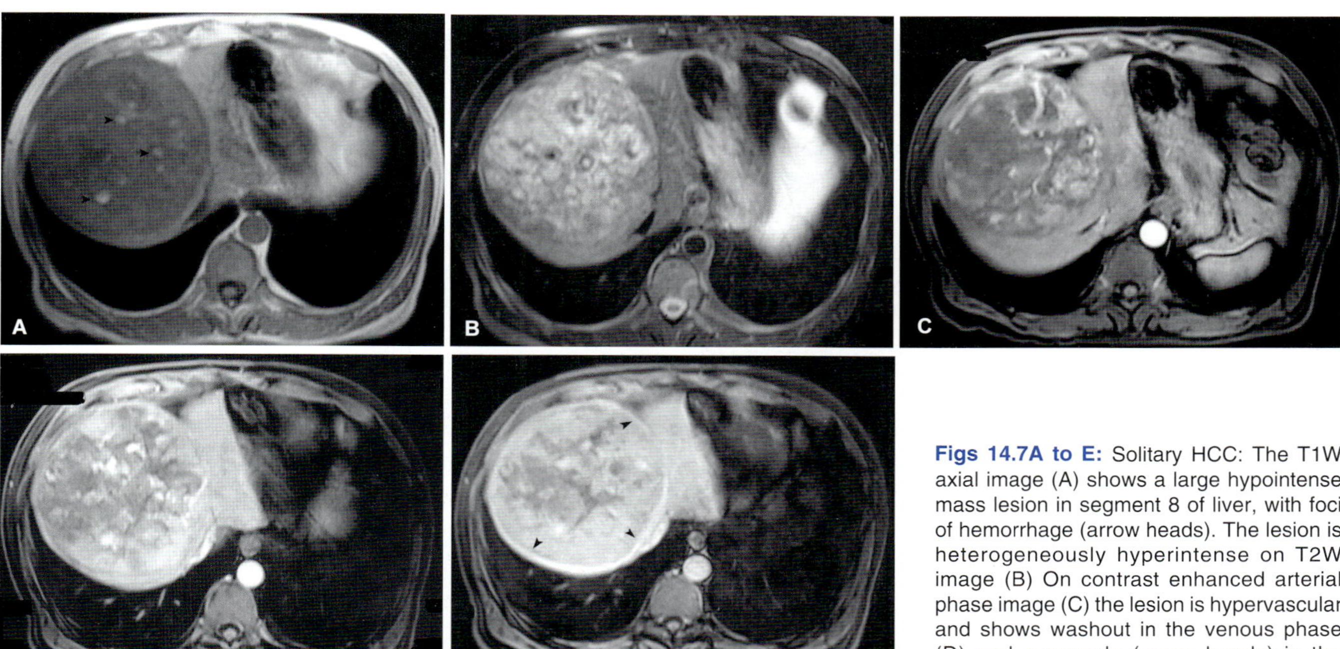

Figs 14.7A to E: Solitary HCC: The T1W axial image (A) shows a large hypointense mass lesion in segment 8 of liver, with foci of hemorrhage (arrow heads). The lesion is heterogeneously hyperintense on T2W image (B) On contrast enhanced arterial phase image (C) the lesion is hypervascular and shows washout in the venous phase (D) and a capsule (arrow heads) in the delayed phase (E)

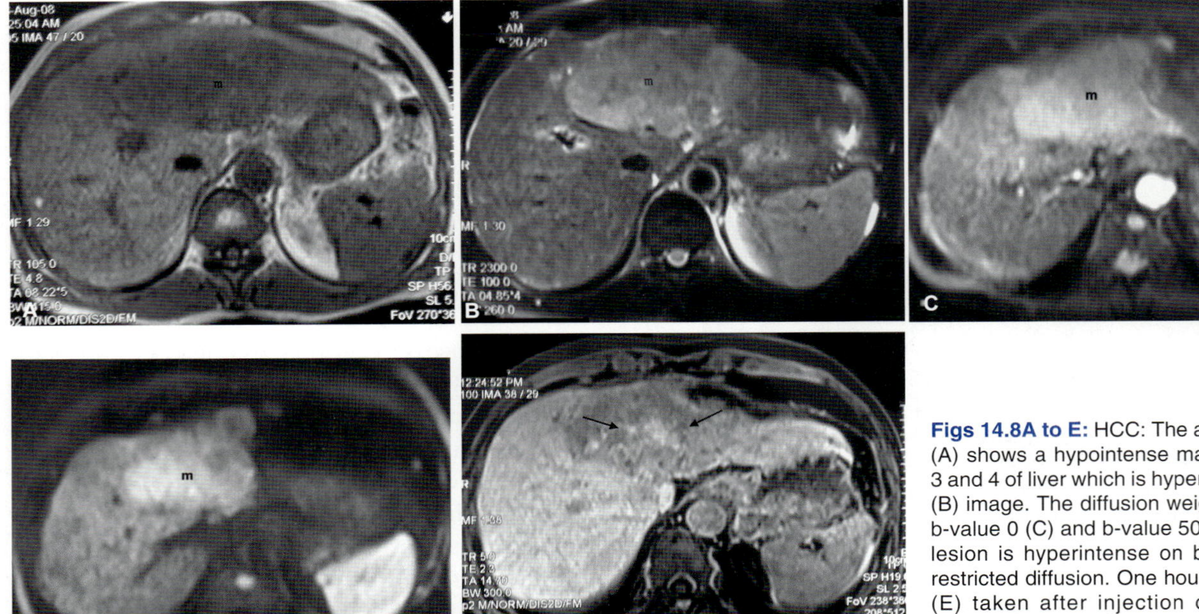

Figs 14.8A to E: HCC: The axial T1W image (A) shows a hypointense mass in segments 3 and 4 of liver which is hyperintense on T2W (B) image. The diffusion weighted images at b-value 0 (C) and b-value 500 (D) shows the lesion is hyperintense on both suggesting restricted diffusion. One hour delayed image (E) taken after injection of Gadobenate shows uptake of contrast in the central part of the lesion suggesting a hepatocellular origin

which small tumors enhance intensely. However, this feature is not specific as severely dysplastic nodules will also enhance. A more specific feature is washout of tumor below the signal of liver at 2 minutes post-contrast with late enhancement of the pseudocapsule.[11] The arterial phase also allows distinction from metastatic disease because HCCs typically demonstrate enhancing stroma through the entire tumor whereas metastases have peripheral enhancement. The degree of vascularity in HCC may vary with the majority being hypervascular but some are hypovascular.

Diffuse infiltration of liver with HCC may be subtle or simulate the appearance of chronic hepatitis or scarring. It may present as extensive hepatic parenchymal involvement with mottled punctuate high intensity on T2W images with mottled enhancement on arterial phase images. Diffuse HCC is very frequently associated with portal vein thrombosis. MRI is useful in differentiation of tumor from bland portal vein thrombus. The hyperintense signal on T2W sequence is highly suggestive of tumor thrombus.[6] Other features favoring malignant thrombus include dilatation of the vein and contrast enhancement.

Liver specific MR contrast agents such as superparamagnetic iron oxide (SPIO) and Mangafodipir have also been tried for detection and characterization of HCC.[2,4] SPIO increases the sensitivity of MRI in HCC detection and is useful in detection of small HCCs in cirrhotic liver. Gadobenate dimeglumine (Gd-BOPTA) has the advantage of being both intravascular and hepatobiliary contrast agent.[12] Although it is mainly excreted by the kidneys, about 5% is excreted in the biliary tree, which is prominently seen 60-120 minutes after intravenous injection. Gadobenate, thus can be routinely used as a contrast agent for dynamic CEMR with an additional delayed scan taken at 1-2 hours after injection. This late hepatobiliary phase improves detection of the lesion, which remains hypointense compared to the enhancing normal liver parenchyma. However, well differentiated HCCs may show uptake of the agent (Fig. 14.8E). Diffusion weighted imaging (DWI) is increasingly being used in abdomen. It has important role in differentiation of benign from malignant lesions. HCCs, being malignant, show restriction of diffusion (Figs 14.8C and D) and may help in distinguishing it from other benign arterially enhancing lesions.[13] SPIO enhanced MRI is currently considered the imaging gold standard for the diagnosis of HCC.

In a cirrhotic liver, regenerative nodules and dysplastic nodules are also common and these must be differentiated from HCC.[6] Regenerative nodules are usually isointense on both T1W and T2W images as they contain normal liver cells. They may be hyperintense on T1W (Fig. 14.9) images, which is due to the presence of protein, fat and copper. Siderotic nodules are hypointense on both T1W and T2W images, due to the presence of iron and fibrous content. They predominantly have portal venous blood supply and thus are isointense to normal liver on all three phases of CEMR. Dysplastic nodules, which are the precursors of HCC, are usually hyperintense on T1W and hypointense on T2W images. These too mostly (but not always) receive blood supply from portal veins and remain isointense on CEMR. A 'nodule within a nodule' appearance on T2W images (hyperintense focus in a hypointense nodule) is suggestive of HCC in a dysplastic nodule.[14] In doubtful cases, the features favoring HCC are size > 2 cm, hyperintense T2W appearance, delayed washout, delayed enhancement of the capsule and rapid interval growth.

Other conditions which should be differentiated from HCC include nodular regenerative hyperplasia (NRH), focal confluent fibrosis and nontumorous arterioportal shunt.[6] NRH is a non-neoplastic disease consisting of diffusely distributed regenerative nodules without associated fibrosis, occurring in non-cirrhotic conditions like Budd-Chiari syndrome. These nodules are hyperintense on T1W images, hypo- to iso-intense on T2W images and often contain a central scar. They show arterial phase enhancement and differentiation from HCC is at times difficult. Focal confluent fibrosis may some times simulate tumors. It is often located in the anterior and medial segments of liver, and is wedge shaped with base towards the liver capsule. It typically shows delayed enhancement, but occasionally arterial enhancement may be seen. The location of the lesion, shape and presence of atrophy with capsular retraction differentiate confluent fibrosis from HCC. Nontumorous arterioportal shunts are often seen in a cirrhotic liver. They are subcapsular, wedge shaped and do not produce mass effect. They are isointense on T1W and T2W scans, and show intense enhancement on arterial phase images, but become iso-intense on portal venous and delayed phase.

ANGIOGRAPHY

With the advent of dual phase CT and dynamic MRI, angiography is now seldom used for the diagnosis of HCC. It is now performed to provide a vascular road map to the surgeon or to perform chemoembolization of the tumor. Classically HCC is seen as a hypervascular mass with tumor angioneogenesis, enlarged feeding arteries and early draining veins, and a marked tumor blush. Abnormal vascular spaces and arterio-portal shunting are frequently present. Tumor thrombus can be detected in the venous phase, showing 'threads and streaks' sign.[2] About 5-10% HCCs are hypo or avascular.

The implementation of the screening programs has resulted in detection of HCC at an earlier stage. Imaging is vital for the diagnosis and biopsy is no longer performed.[15] The American Association for the study of liver diseases (AALD) recommends that if a mass > 2 cm shows typical imaging features (arterial phase enhancement and washout in venous phase) on one modality (either CECT or CEMR) a diagnosis of HCC can be made.

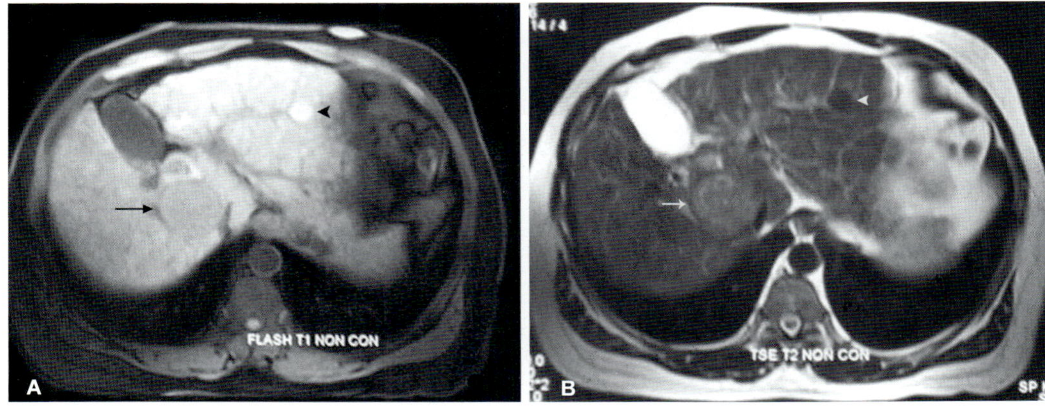

Fig. 14.9: Regenerative nodule. Axial T1W image (A) shows a small hyperintense nodule (arrow head) in left lobe which is hypointense on T2W image (B) suggestive of a regenerative nodule. In contrast to this, the segment 8 lesion (arrow) is hypointense on T1W image and mildly hyperintense on T2W image suggestive of HCC

For lesions 1-2 cm, a diagnosis of HCC requires imaging appearances to be demonstrated on two modalities.[15] Follow-up imaging is a must in all patients after treatment as recurrence rates are as high as 70% and most occur in the initial 3 years. This is done at 3-monthly intervals.

FIBROLAMELLAR HEPATOCELLULAR CARCINOMA (FLC)

This is an unusual liver tumor found in young adults with a mean age of 23 years. Patients do not have underlying cirrhosis nor are there any predisposing risk factors. It is frequently resectable and has a better prognosis than the usual HCC. The 5-year survival for FLC is 60% as compared to 30% for typical HCC. Serum AFP levels are typically normal. They usually present as a solitary large circumscribed mass that is partly or completely encapsulated. Satellite nodules are often seen. The major radiological clue to the diagnosis is the presence of central fibrous scar and central stellate calcification. Portal vein invasion, necrosis and hemorrhage are much less common than in typical HCC.[1,2]

On sonography, FLC is usually seen as a lobulated predominantly hyperechoic mass, although hypo and isoechoic forms have also been described (Fig. 14.10A). Central hyperechoic areas with foci of shadowing correlate with the central scar and calcification within the scar. On unenhanced CT, FLC is a well defined, lobulated and hypodense lesion. The central stellate calcification (Fig. 14.10B) has been reported as a distinctive radiological feature and occurs in a high proportion (up to 55%) of these lesions. After intravenous contrast, FLC shows heterogeneous enhancement in arterial and venous phases (Fig. 14.10C and D). The scar does not show early enhancement but may enhance on delayed images.[2,4] On MRI, FLC is hypo- to iso-intense on T1W images and hyperintense on T2W images. The scar because of its fibrous nature, remains hypointense on T1- and T2-weighted images. The enhancement pattern on CEMR is similar to that seen on CT scans.

The most important differential diagnosis of FLC is focal nodular hyperplasia (FNH). The central scar is hyperintense on T2W scans in FNH, but hypointense in FLC. Also, the scar of FLC shows calcification, but this is seen in < 1.5% of cases of FNH. The differentiation

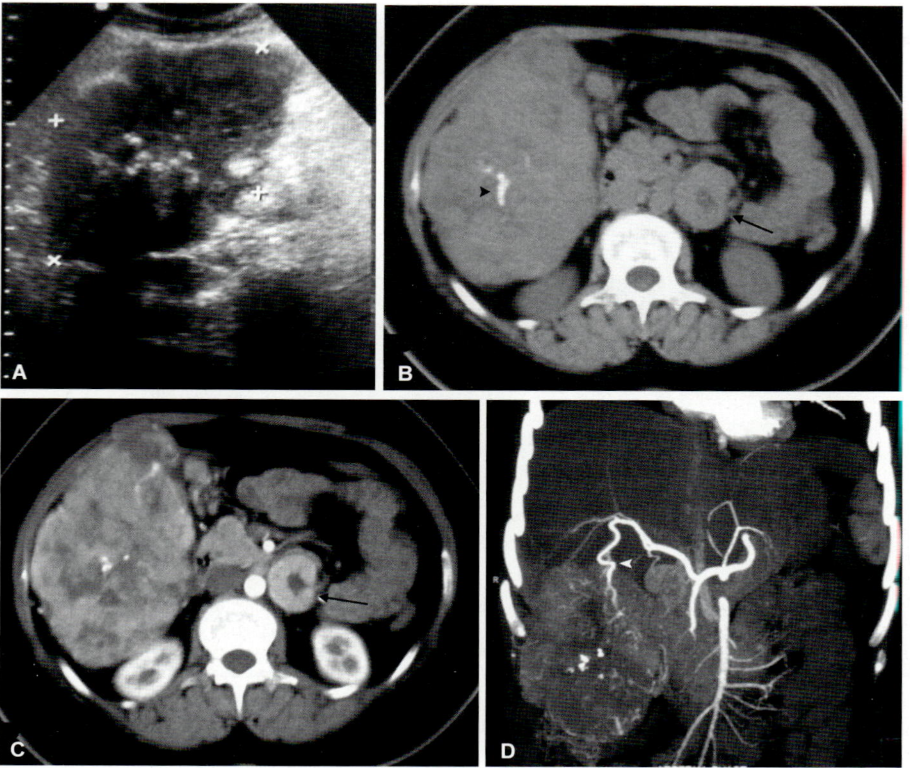

Figs 14.10A to D: Fibrolamellar carcinoma: Ultrasonography (A) shows a hypoechoic mass in segment 6 of liver showing central calcification. Non contrast CT scan (B) shows hypodense mass in the liver with central calcification (arrow head) and left para-aortic lymphadenopathy (arrow). Contrast enhanced arterial phase CT image (C) shows heterogeneous enhancement with central scar showing calcification. The para-aortic node is showing intense enhancement (arrow). The CT maximum intensity projection image (D) shows a prominent feeder arising from the right hepatic artery (arrowhead)

between the two is important as FNH is managed conservatively but FLC is surgically treated. Biopsy provides the diagnosis in difficult cases.[2]

Interventional Techniques

Many methods have been developed for the non-surgical management of HCC employing angiographic and percutaneous techniques. These include hepatic arterial infusion chemotherapy and embolization and percutaneous techniques like ethanol ablation, and radiofrequency ablation. The details of these techniques are discussed in the chapter on hepatic intervention.

INTRAHEPATIC CHOLANGIOCARCINOMA (ICCA)

It is the second most common primary malignant hepatic tumor. It accounts for 10% of all cholangiocarcinomas and arises in small intrahepatic ducts. It has an increased incidence in patients with Caroli's disease, sclerosing cholangitis, intrahepatic calculi and inflammatory bowel disease. Cholangiocarcinoma typically produces extensive desmoplastic reaction.[2]

Patients present clinically with abdominal pain, anorexia and weight loss. Jaundice occurs only if major ducts are obstructed. A normal serum AFP may be helpful in suggesting ICCA rather than HCC.

IMAGING

There are no specific imaging features of intrahepatic cholangiocarcinoma that truly distinguish it from HCC and metastatic disease. However, cholangiocarcinoma is more likely to be associated with dilated ducts than HCC or metastases.[2,4]

Sonographically, one or more hyperechoic, iso- or hypoechoic masses may be seen. Homogeneous hypoechoic pattern is more common. On Doppler USG most of them show internal vascularity. Dilated intrahepatic bile ducts distal to the mass may also be seen. On unenhanced CT it is seen as a well-defined round to oval, hypodense mass and on contrast enhanced CT scan it typically shows early peripheral enhancement. A delayed central enhancement is often seen which may take 5-15 minutes.[2] Capsule retraction and biliary dilatation adjacent to the mass are highly suggestive of ICCA (as these are rarely seen with HCC).[16] MR imaging also does not show any characteristic features and these lesions are hypointense on T1W and hyperintense on T2W images (Figs 14.11A and B). On CEMR, smaller lesions (2-4 cm) enhance homogeneously but those > 4 cm show thick peripheral enhancement with centripetal progression (Figs 14.11C to E). This is akin to a hemangioma. However, presence of satellite nodules, portal vein invasion and dilated bile ducts favor a diagnosis of ICCA. In addition, DWI shows restriction of diffusion unlike hemangioma.

The primary angiographic finding in cholangiocarcinoma is serrated or serpiginous arterial infiltration. Large tumors may be mildly vascular but in small tumors arterial encasement is the only abnormality.

HEPATOBLASTOMA

Hepatoblastoma is the most common primary liver tumor of childhood. It most commonly occurs in the first 3 years of life, whereas hepatocellular malignancies in children older than five years tend to be morphologically similar to those found in adults.

The most common presentation is a painless abdominal mass, however anorexia, weight loss, pain and jaundice can occur. Serum AFP levels are elevated in over 90% of patients.

Pathologically hepatoblastoma tends to be well defined, pseudoencapsulated, large, unifocal lesion. Less commonly multiple nodules or diffuse liver involvement may be seen. Calcification may be seen in up to one-third of patients.[2,4]

IMAGING

The sonographic appearance of hepatoblastoma is of a large, inhomogeneous echogenic mass sometimes with calcification (Fig. 14.12A). Anechoic foci due to necrosis and a lobular pattern caused by septation may be seen.

CT scan most commonly demonstrates a well-defined hypodense mass with mild enhancement (Figs 14.12B and C). Involvement of portal vein and IVC can be demonstrated. Three-dimensional reconstruction provides important information about vascular invasion. If this shows portal vein invasion, initial preoperative chemotherapy is given to shrink the tumor away from portal vein and then surgical excision is done.[17] Lung metastasis is common at presentation and CT scan of the chest is routinely performed before treatment. On MRI

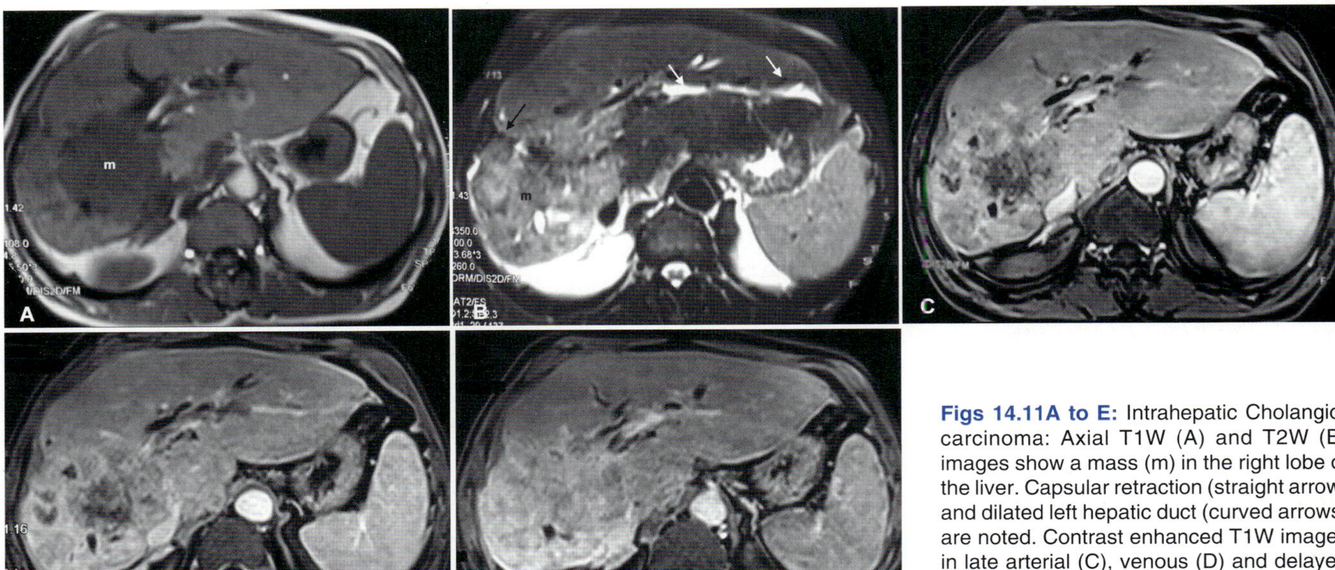

Figs 14.11A to E: Intrahepatic Cholangiocarcinoma: Axial T1W (A) and T2W (B) images show a mass (m) in the right lobe of the liver. Capsular retraction (straight arrow) and dilated left hepatic duct (curved arrows) are noted. Contrast enhanced T1W images in late arterial (C), venous (D) and delayed (E) phases show early peripheral enhancement with gradual centripetal filling in of contrast in delayed phase

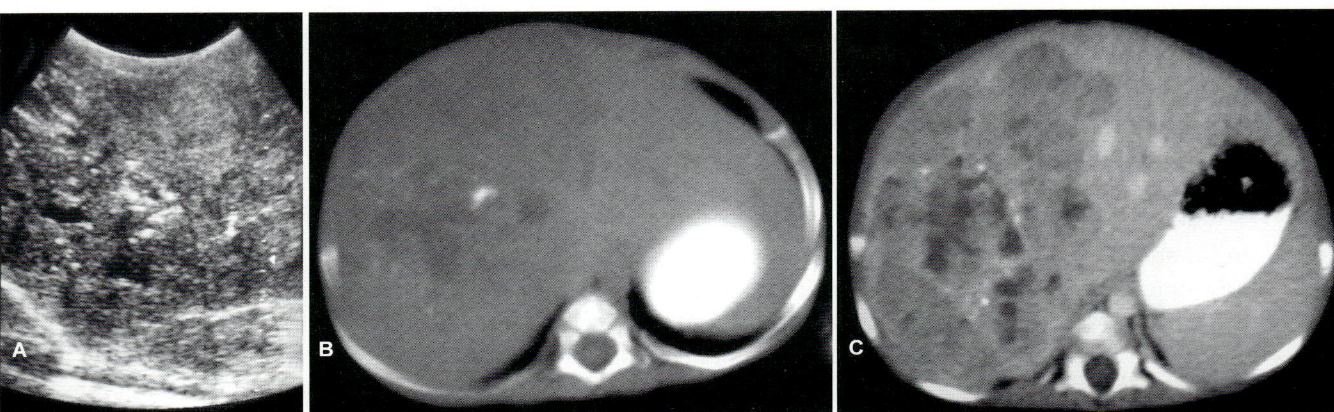

Figs 14.12A to C: Hepatoblastoma: The ultrasonography image (A) shows a heteroechoic mass in the right lobe of liver. The non contrast CT image (B) shows a hypodense lesion with foci of calcification in segments 7 and 8. Contrast enhanced CT (C) shows heterogeneous pattern of enhancement

hepatoblastoma is seen as a lobulated mass that is hypointense on T1W and hyperintense on T2W scans. Internal septa are seen as bands of low signal intensity. On CEMR, immediate diffuse enhancement followed by washout is noted. On angiography the tumor is usually hypervascular.

EPITHELIOID HEMANGIOENDOTHELIOMA

It is a rare tumor of vascular origin which develops almost exclusively in adults, with slight female predominance. Pathologically multiple tumors are usually present that tend to grow and coalesce to form confluent masses. They are typically distributed in the periphery of the liver. They have better prognosis than angiosarcoma. Metastasis is seen in about 30% cases. Adjacent capsular retraction and calcification are frequently seen.[18,19]

IMAGING

Sonographically, hemangioendothelioma (EHE) usually presents as multiple peripheral hypoechoic masses. Hyperechoic and heterogeneous appearance has also been described. On unenhanced CT scan, multiple peripheral low attenuation lesions are noted. Calcification is infrequently present (Figs 14.13A and B). After intravenous contrast it shows peripheral enhancement surrounding the low attenuation fibrous core. Retraction of the overlying capsule is a common, though non-specific, finding and should raise the possibility of this diagnosis. Large tumors are often associated with compensatory hypertrophy of the uninvolved lobes due to slow growth of these masses.[2] On MRI the lesion is hypointense on T1W images (Fig. 14.13C) with a thin peripheral dark rim. T2W images show heterogeneously hyperintense lesion (Fig. 14.13D) with or without low signal intensity peripheral rim. Moderate peripheral and delayed central enhancement may be seen on CEMR. MRI is better than CT scan in characterization of EHE.

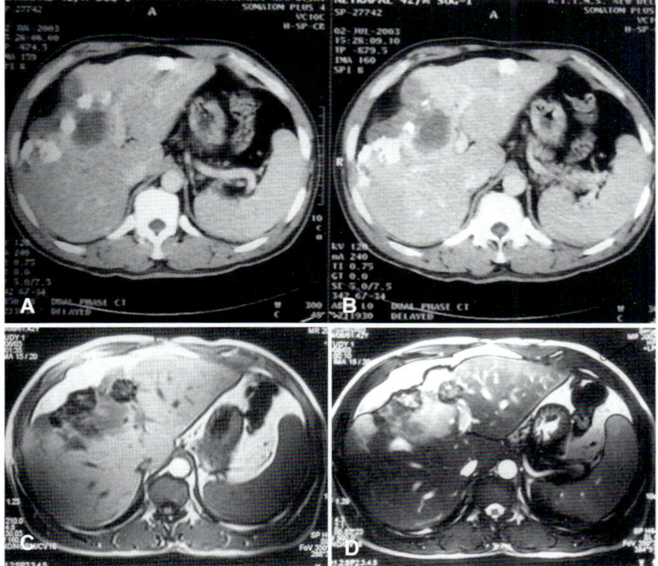

Figs 14.13A to D: Epithelioid hemangioendothelioma (A and B) CECT showing a hypodense mass in segments IVA and VIII with capsular retraction on the surface. Foci of calcification are seen in the lesion as well as another focus in the left lobe (C) Axial gradient echo T1W scan shows that the mass is hypointense. The foci of calcification are markedly hypointense (D) Axial T2W scan shows the mass is hyperintense with hypointense foci suggestive of calcification

ANGIOSARCOMA

It is a rare tumor usually seen in adults in the fifth to seventh decade and is more common in males. The risk factors include exposure to thorotrast, vinyl chloride, arsenic and steroids. Most of the angiosarcomas are multiple. Solitary lesions are unencapsulated and may contain blood-filled cystic areas. Clinical presentation is with weakness, loss of weight and appetite and abdominal pain. Thrombocytopenia may develop due to sequestration of platelets in large tumors.[2]

Sonography shows multiple or single hyperechoic masses. Anechoic areas due to necrosis and hyperechoic areas due to fresh hemorrhage may be seen. On unenhanced CT angiosarcoma has a non-specific low attenuation appearance. When the aetiology is thorotrast exposure, background of high density reticular thorotrast laden parenchyma is seen. Marked peripheral enhancement is noted after administration of contrast. The enhancement may show a peripheral spread, usually with inhomogeneity on delayed scans. Differentiation from hemangioma may be difficult.[2,4] Presence of focal enhancing areas with attenuation less than aorta and peripheral ring-like enhancement (instead of globular) suggests angiosarcoma. Angiosarcoma is hypointense on T1W and heterogeneously hyperintense on T2W MRI.[20] Fluid levels may be present representing internal hemorrhage. Dynamic CEMR shows an enhancement pattern similar to that of hemangioma. However, heterogenous appearance on T2W images is unusual for hemangiomas.

Hepatic arteries supplying an angiosarcoma are of normal size and may show displacement but not encasement. A tumor stain appears at the periphery of the tumor and persists for a prolonged period.

SECONDARY MALIGNANCIES

Metastatic Disease

The liver is second only to regional lymph nodes as a site for metastatic disease. It is far more common than primary liver cancer. The colon, stomach, pancreas, and breast are the common primary sites. Metastases are more common in the right lobe of the liver. Although the presence of liver metastases is a poor prognostic factor, the use of aggressive regimes in some subgroups can result in a better outcome. Over the past decade there has been increasing acceptance of liver resection as the best treatment for colorectal metastases. Successful outcome depends on knowledge of the size, number and location of the tumor burden and accurate radiological assessment is essential to identify the subset of patients who would benefit from aggressive management.[2,21,22]

Many patients have hepatomegaly. Ascites, jaundice and varices may also be present. Liver function tests are normal in up to half of the patients and thus are unreliable for metastasis detection or follow-up. Thus imaging is vital for diagnosis and follow-up of patients with liver secondaries.

Ultrasonography

This is a very sensitive technique for detecting metastases. Drawbacks include operator dependence, poor results in obese patients and in detecting small lesions near the dome and on the liver surface. Advances like harmonic imaging have improved the results in obese patients.

Hepatic metastases may be hypoechoic, hyperechoic (Fig. 14.14A), cystic or mixed echogenicity. The most common pattern is hypoechoic with no distal shadowing or enhancement. This is produced by highly cellular and hypovascular lesions. Hyperechoic metastases are often seen with colonic and gastrointestinal malignancies and with vascular metastases from islet cell tumors, carcinoid, choriocarcinoma and renal cell carcinoma. They may be surrounded by a hypoechoic halo (Fig. 14.14B) producing the bull's eye or target appearance (Fig. 14.14C). Presence of halo indicates an aggressive tumor and is commonly seen with bronchogenic carcinoma.[2] Calcification may be seen in mucinous metastases from colon and ovary.[21] Cystic metastases are seen with adenocarcinoma of pancreas, ovary and colon.

On color Doppler imaging, metastases usually do not show intra-tumoral signal but a 'detour' pattern with a dilated portal vein meandering around the tumor nodules has been described.

Intraoperative sonography is a very useful adjunct in patients who are candidates for surgical resection of metastases. It may show additional lesions in comparison with preoperative USG, CT and even CT arterial portography (CTAP).

Computed Tomography

The advent of helical and multi-detector CT has led to a lot of flexibility but has also added complexity to the imaging protocols for liver evaluation. Advantages include significant reduction in scan time, elimination of respiratory misregistration, improved Z axis resolution, better multiplanar and 3D reformats and it allows a more precise timing for evaluation of liver in different phases of contrast enhancement. It also helps in demonstration of a vein close to a lesion as this determines the response to radiofrequency ablation. Lesions in proximity to a vessel have higher chances of recurrence.

Since most metastases are hypovascular (Figs 14.15A and B) the usual protocol is to scan in the portal venous phase of enhancement. Dual phase scanning may be useful for detection of metastases from hypervascular primaries such as renal cell carcinoma and islet cell tumors (Figs 14.16A and B). Although breast carcinoma metastases can be hypervascular, studies have not shown any added benefit of biphasic CT over portal phase CT for this indication.[2,21]

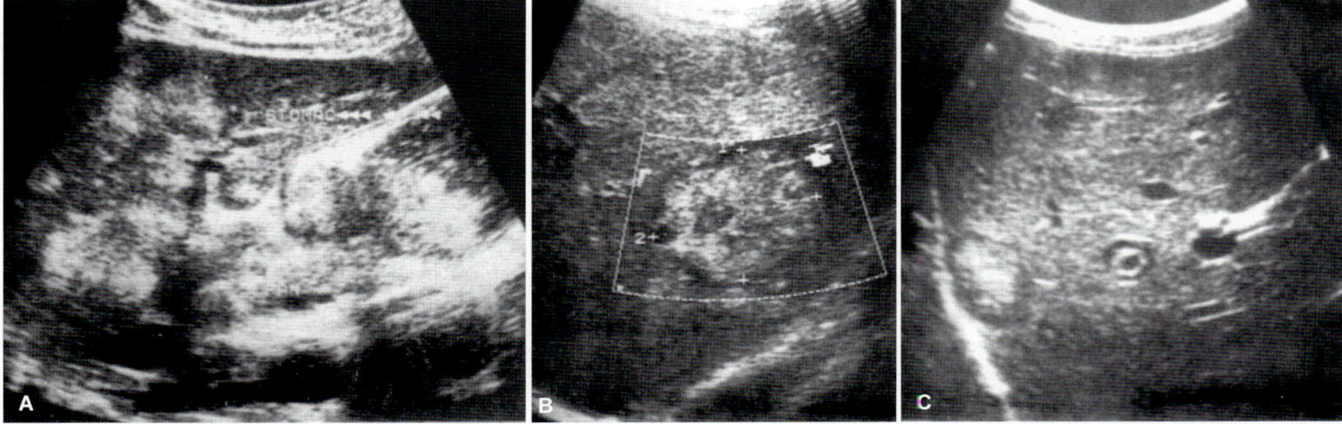

Figs 14.14A to C: (A) Ultrasound scan showing multiple echogenic metastatic deposits (B) Ultrasound scan showing an echogenic lesion with a hypoechoic halo and no internal vascularity. Biopsy—Metastatic adenocarcinoma (C) Ultrasound scan showing a lesion with target morphology and another echogenic lesion with halo. Biopsy—Metastatic adenocarcinoma

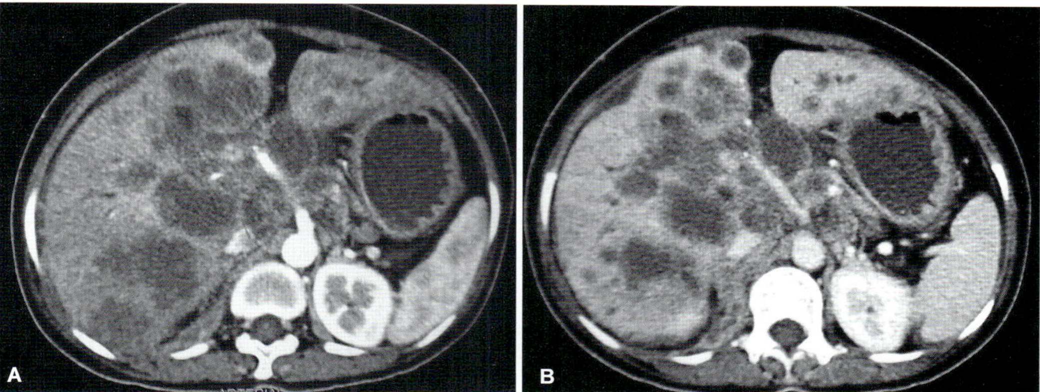

Figs 14.15A and B: Hypovascular metastases: The contrast enhanced arterial phase (A) and venous phase image (B) shows multiple hypodense lesions involving all segments of liver. The lesions do not show any enhancement in either of the phases

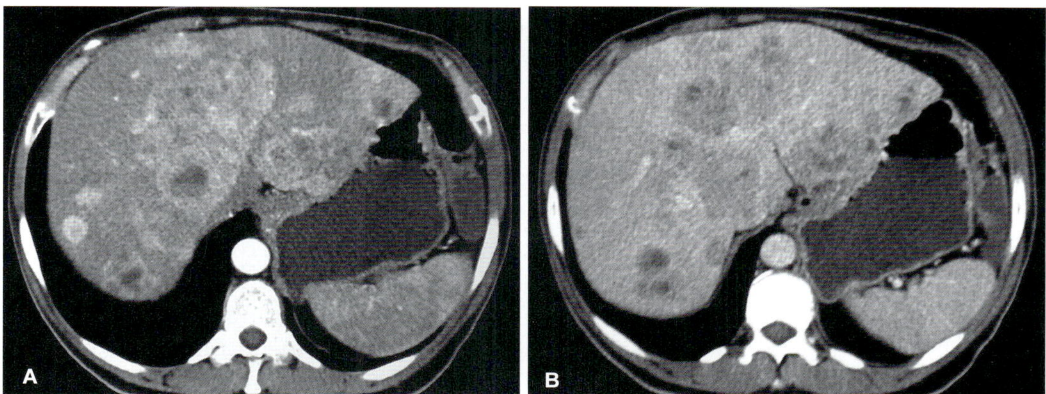

Figs 14.16A and B: Hypervascular metastases: The contrast enhanced arterial phase image (A) shows multiple intensely enhancing lesions in both lobes of a non-cirrhotic liver with wash out seen in the venous phase (B)

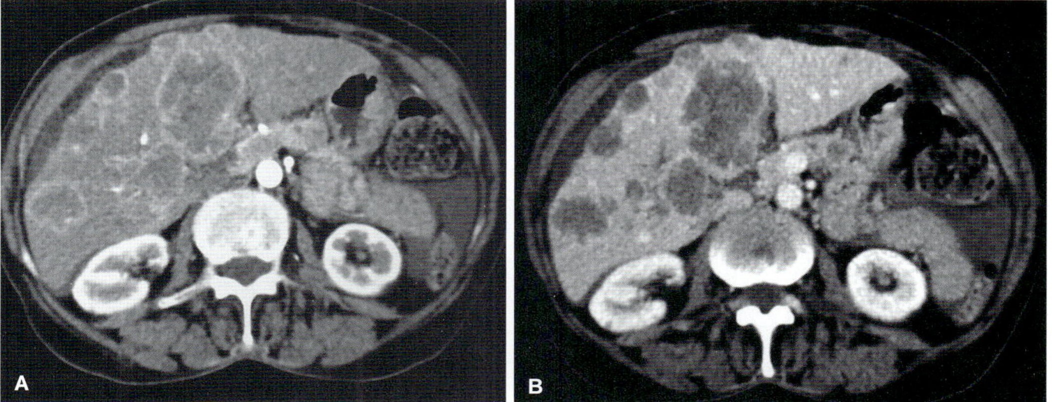

Figs 14.17A and B: Rim enhancing metastases: The contrast enhanced arterial phase image (A) shows multiple rim enhancing lesions with wash out seen in the venous phase image (B)

On unenhanced CT most metastases are hypodense to the liver parenchyma, whereas some are indistinguishable from normal liver. Small lesions are nodular and homogeneous, while larger lesions are more irregular, heterogeneous and with ill-defined margins. Calcification is common in mucinous GI tract carcinomas and in chemotherapeutically treated hypervascular lesions (e.g. carcinoid). After contrast administration, metastases from hypovascular tumors may have an enhancing rim (Figs 14.17A and B) that can be seen during arterial phase and occasionally during portal phase. Lesions that do not have an enhancing rim show little if any enhancement during the arterial phase and become hypoattenuating during the portal phase.

Hypervascular metastases show moderate to intense enhancement during the arterial phase that may persist during the portal phase. However, most show a rapid washout and become iso- or hypo-dense to surrounding liver.

MAGNETIC RESONANCE IMAGING

Liver metastases like most other liver lesions are hypointense to normal liver on T1W images and hyper-intense on T2W images (Figs 14.18A to C). The use of fat suppression on T2W sequences, particularly fast spin echo T2W scans, is important as it improves the detection of subcapsular lesions. Morphological features have been shown to be useful in differentiating metastatic lesions from common benign lesions such as hemangioma and cysts. Heterogeneous signal intensity and irregular or indistinct margins, smooth or irregular areas of high signal intensity surrounded by a ring of relatively lower signal intensity are said to be suggestive of metastatic disease. The acquisition of at least one sequence in the coronal plane is useful to evaluate the superior and inferior margins of the liver.

Six appearances of liver metastasis have been described on MRI.[2] Doughnut shape is usually seen with larger lesions, where the lesion is of low signal intensity on T1W images with central necrosis which has even lower signal. These lesions have target appearance on T2W image. Amorphous appearance is seen with heterogenous masses with ill-defined margins. Peripheral halo is seen with some metastasis and represents either tumor infiltration or surrounding edema. Light bulb morphology, where the lesion is hyperintense on T2W images, is seen with cystic and hypervascular metastasis. Cauliflower appearance is typically seen with colorectal metastasis. Here the lesion has scalloped margins with enhancing periphery and internal septae.

Hypervascular metastases such as those from islet cell tumors, carcinoid and renal cell carcinoma are generally high in signal intensity on T2W images and show intense peripheral ring of enhancement immediately after gadolinium administration. This appearance may mimic hemangiomas. Dynamic serial gadolinium enhanced MR is very helpful in differentiating these metastases from hemangiomas. Hemangiomas typically show early discrete nodular enhancement which shows a centripetal progression on delayed scans. Metastases often show a transient enhancement of the periphery with a peripheral washout on delayed scans. Enhancement of hypervascular metastases is better shown on MR than on CT images because of the higher sensitivity of MR to gadolinium chelates and the more compact bolus of contrast delivered to the hepatic parenchyma.[2,21] Hypovascular metastasis may show enhancing rim in arterial phase, with incomplete centripetal filling-in in delayed phase but remain hypointense in all the phases.

State of the art MRI has a higher diagnostic accuracy and greater effect on patient management than spiral CTAP and it is also less expensive. Liver specific contrast agents such as superparamagnetic iron oxide (SPIO) have been found to better than unenhanced MRI and CECT and was comparable to CTAP in detection of the number of metastatic deposits prior to surgical resection. On a SPIO-enhanced scan, metastases are hyperintense against

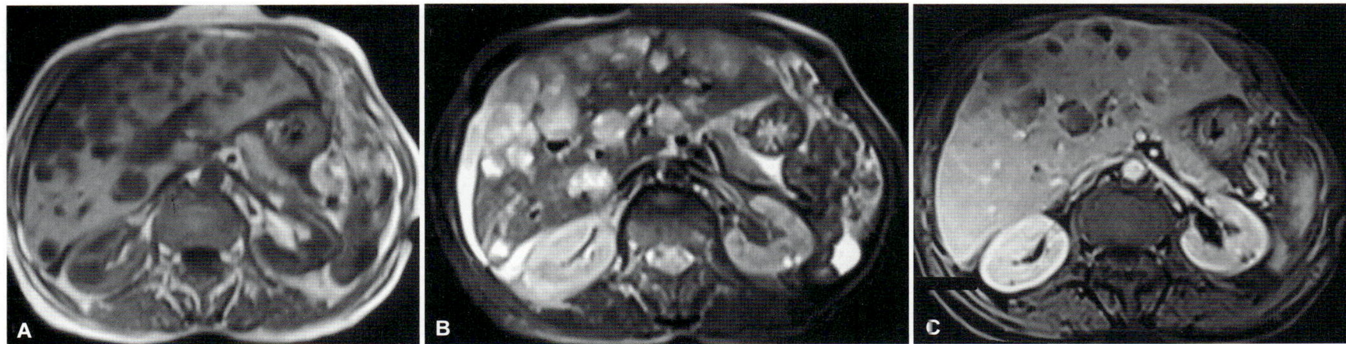

Figs 14.18A to C: Metastases: The axial T1W image (A) shows multiple hypointense lesions in both lobes of liver which are hyperintense on T2W image (B) The lesions show minimal peripheral enhancement in the contrast enhanced T1W image (C)

the hypointense enhancing liver parenchyma.[2] These agents are presently not available in India. Gadobenate, a hepatobiliary contrast agent, is also useful in evaluation of liver metastasis.

Despite the marked improvement in the accuracy of detection and characterization of metastatic disease, a significant number of lesions are found at surgery that goes undetected on preoperative imaging. These include subcentimeter and subcapsular lesions.

IMAGE GUIDED BIOPSY

Histological proof of metastatic disease can be obtained through percutaneous biopsy guided by USG or CT. Although aspiration cytology is usually sufficient, tissue cores can be obtained using rapid-firing cutting needles.

LYMPHOMA

Primary hepatic lymphoma is rare and most often of Non-Hodgkin's (diffuse histiocytic) type. Primary hepatic lymphoma is much more common in organ transplant recipients treated with cyclosporine and patients with AIDS. The most common appearance is that of a solitary large mass, which is hypodense on unenhanced CT and does not enhance significantly after intravenous contrast. Tumors are moderately low in signal intensity on T1W scans and mild to moderately hyperintense on T2W scans and show mild heterogeneous enhancement on immediate postgadolinium images.[2,4]

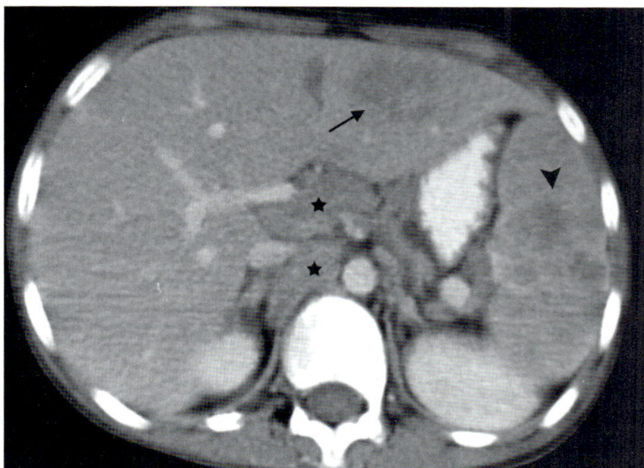

Fig. 14.19: Lymphoma: The contrast enhanced CT scan of a patient with non-Hodgkin's lymphoma shows a focal hypodense lesion (arrow) in segment 3 of liver. Multiple hypodense lesions in the spleen (arrow head) and periportal and inter aortico-caval lymph nodes (star) are also noted

Secondary liver involvement in lymphoma is more common than primary lymphoma and occurs both in Hodgkin's disease and in Non-Hodgkin's lymphoma. Diffuse infiltration is more common in Hodgkin's disease, whereas diffuse and nodular hepatic involvement is equally frequent in Non-Hodgkin's lymphoma (Fig. 14.19). Imaging findings are non-specific and cannot be differentiated from other space occupying lesions.

REFERENCES

1. Gazelle SG, Saini S, Mueller P. Hepatobiliary and Pancreatic Radiology Imaging and Intervention. Thieme 1998.
2. Ros PR, Erturk SM. Malignant tumors of the liver. In Gore RM, Levine MS (Eds): Text book of gastrointestinal radiology. Philadelphia, Saunders 2008;1623-62.
3. Fattovich G, Stroffolini T, Zagni I, Donato F. Hepatocellular carcinoma in cirrhosis: Incidence and risk factors. Gastroenterology 2004;127:S35-S50.
4. Fernandez MP, Redvanly RD. Primary hepatic malignant neoplasms. Hepatic Imaging. Radiol Clin N Am 1998; 36:2:333-48.
5. Llovet JM, Burroughs A, Bruix J. Hepatocellular carcinoma. Lancet 2003;362:1907-17.
6. Willatt JM, Hussain HK, Adusumilli S, Marrero JA. MR imaging of hepatocellular carcinoma in the cirrhotic liver: Challenges and controversies. Radiology 2008;247: 311-30.
7. Daniele B, Bencivenga A, Megna AS, et al. Alphafetoprotein and ultrasonography screening for hepatocellular carcinoma. Gastroenterology 2004;127:S108-S112.
8. Brannigan M, Burns PN, Wilson SR. Blood flow patterns in focal liver lesions at microbubble-enhanced US. Radiographics 2004;24:921-35.
9. Yu SC, Yeung DT, So NM. Imaging features of hepatocellular carcinoma. Clin Radiol 2004;59:145-56.
10. Baron RL, Oliver JH III, Dodd GD III, et al. Hepato–cellular carcinoma: Evaluation with biphasic contrast enhanced, helical CT. Radiology 1996;199:505-11.
11. Semelka RC. Abdominal-Pelvic MRI. Wiley-less, 2002.
12. Balci NC, Semelka RC. Contrast agents for MR imaging of the liver. Radiol Clin N Am 2005;43:887-98.
13. Glockner JF. Hepatobiliary MRI: Current Concepts and controversies. J Magn Reson Imaging 2007;25:681-95.
14. Goshima S, Kanematsu M, Matsuo M, et al. Nodule-in-nodule appearance of hepatocellular carcinoma: Comparison of gadolinium-enhanced and ferumoxides-enhanced magnetic resonance imaging. J Magn Reson Imaging 2004;20:250-55.
15. Bruix J, Sherman M. Practice guidelines committee, American association for the study of liver diseases. Management of hepatocellular carcinoma. Hepatology 2005;42:1208-36.

16. Choi BI, Lee JM, Han JK. Imaging of intrahepatic and hilar cholangiocarcinoma. Abdom Imaging 2004;29: 548-57.
17. Lu M, Greer ML. Hypervascular multifocal hepatoblastoma: Dynamic gadolinium-enhanced MRI findings indistinguishable from infantile hemangioendothelioma. Pediatr Radiol 2007;37:587-91.
18. Miller WJ, Dodd GD III, Federle MP, et al. Epithelioid hemangioendothelioma of the liver. Imaging findings with pathological correlation. Am J Roentgenol 1992; 159:53-57.
19. Garcia-Botella A, Diez-Valladares L, Martin-Antona E, et al. Epithelioid hemangioendothelioma of the liver. J Hepatobiliary Pancreat Surg 2006;13:167-71.
20. Buetow PC, Buck JL, Ros PR, et al. Malignant vascular tumors of the liver: Radiologic-pathologic correlation. Radiographics 1994;14:153-66.
21. Paley MR, Ros PR. Hepatic metastases. Hepatic Imaging. Radiol Clin N Am 1998;6(2):349-64.
22. Baker ME, Pelley R. Hepatic metastases: Basic principles and implications for radiologists. Radiology 1995;197: 329-37.

Chapter Fifteen

Diffuse Liver Diseases

Ashu Seith Bhalla, Harsh Kandpal, Sanjay Thulkar

INTRODUCTION

Diffuse liver diseases can have diverse etiology. Diagnosis based on imaging alone is generally more difficult to make than in focal liver lesions, as their effect on normal liver architecture may be minimal. However, imaging can help in assessing the severity and extent of the diffuse liver diseases and to demonstrate its sequela such as portal hypertension and neoplasia. The following conditions are included under the term diffuse liver diseases:

- Hepatic steatosis
- Hepatitis: Viral, alcoholic, radiation induced
- Hemosiderosis and hemochromatosis
- Amyloidosis
- Wilson's disease
- Granulomatous diseases
- Cirrhosis

FATTY LIVER (HEPATIC STEATOSIS)

Fatty liver (hepatic steatosis) refers to an excessive accumulation of triglycerides in the form of small or large vacuoles within the hepatocytes. The common causes are alcoholism, diabetes mellitus and obesity. Malnutrition, chronic illnesses, ileal bypass, drugs and toxins, total parenteral nutrition, inflammatory bowel disease, severe hepatitis, steroid intake, acquired immune deficiency syndrome and congestive heart failure can also result in fatty liver. Excess fat deposition in the liver can result from excess synthesis, decreased utilization, impaired release of hepatic lipoproteins and excess mobilization from fatty tissue. One-third of asymptomatic alcoholic patients and upto 50% of patients with diabetes mellitus develop fatty liver. [1]

With increasing prevalence of obesity, hepatic steatosis has become a major source of liver dysfunction even though in most cases fatty liver is asymptomatic and has normal liver function tests. Radiologist is frequently the first to suggest the diagnosis. Mild hepatomegaly with or without vague right upper abdominal pain can be present in symptomatic patients. In acute fatty liver associated with pregnancy or alcoholic binge, patients may present with jaundice, acute hepatic failure or even encephalopathy. Histologic spectrum of fatty infiltration of liver includes macrovesicular fatty liver; non-alcoholic steatohepatitis (NASH); steatohepatitis with fibrosis; and cirrhosis.[1]

Ultrasonography (US)

Ultrasonography reveals hepatomegaly, increased parenchymal echogenicity with impaired visualization of normally echogenic walls of intrahepatic portal venous branches. There is increased attenuation and poor penetration of the sound beam resulting in poor visualization of the deeper portion of liver, the diaphragm, hepatic and portal veins (Fig. 15. 1). Echogenicity of the liver can be compared with that of adjacent kidney. The degree of echogenicity is roughly proportional to the degree of steatosis and tends to parallel biochemical and clinical dysfunction. Hepatic steatosis and fibrosis often coexist and produce similar US findings. Focal fat infiltration may produce single or multiple hyperechoic lesions, while areas of focal fat sparing appear hypoechoic

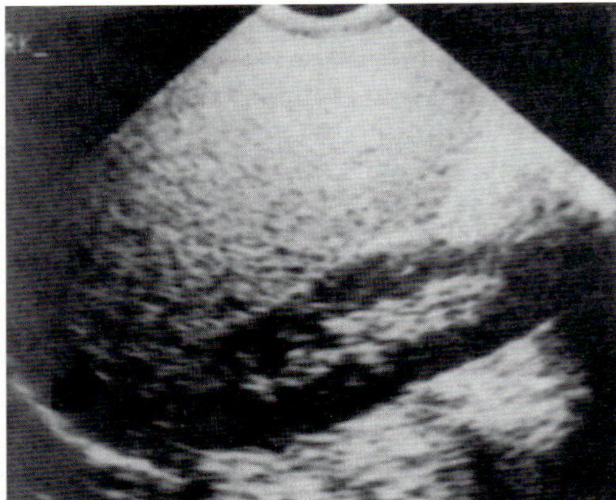

Fig. 15.1: Fatty liver: Increased echogenicity of the liver is seen on ultrasound. Note the poor depiction of diaphragm (↑) and gross difference in the echogenicity of the liver and the kidney

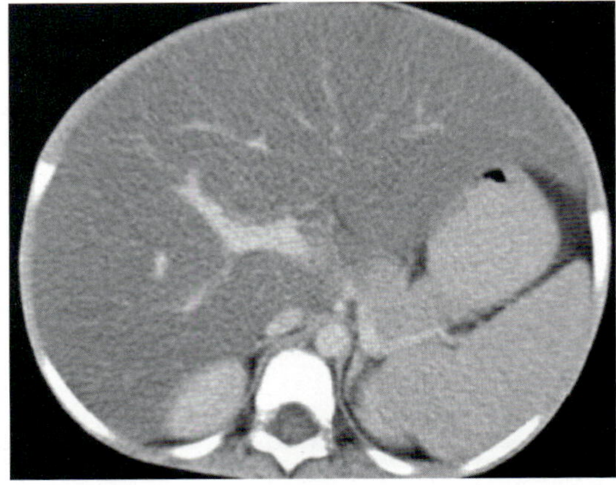

Fig. 15.3: Fatty liver: Contrast-enhanced CT reveals diffuse decrease in attenuation of the liver parenchyma.

in an otherwise hyperechoic liver. In the presence of fatty liver, hepatic hemangiomas may appear hypoechoic necessitating MR or CT for their differentiation (Figs 15. 2A to C).

Computed Tomography (CT)

There exists an excellent correlation between the CT attenuation of liver and the amount of fat deposition as determined on liver biopsy specimens.[2] Fatty liver is seen as reduced attenuation of the liver parenchyma (Fig. 15. 3) Normal liver attenuation on unenhanced scans is 8-10 HU more than spleen due to its glycogen content.[2] This relationship is reversed in fatty liver. The attenuation is often reduced below that of the normal portal vein and IVC so that these structures stand out prominently simulating contrast-enhanced image of the liver.[3] Decreased attenuation in fatty liver can hamper detection of hypodense liver lesions like abscess or neoplasms. Unlike unenhanced scans, contrast enhanced CT is less reliable in the diagnosis of fatty liver. A confident CT diagnosis of focal fat infiltration can be made when it is lobar, segmental or wedge shaped. In such cases the area of decreased attenuation typically extends to the liver capsule, without causing contour bulge and typically has a straight margin. Nodular areas of fat deposition or fat sparing can however mimic true lesions and may require MRI for differentiation.

Magnetic Resonance Imaging (MRI)

Opposed phase GRE (chemical shift imaging) MR imaging is the investigation of choice in cases with focal nodular or multifocal fat deposition/sparing that may be confused

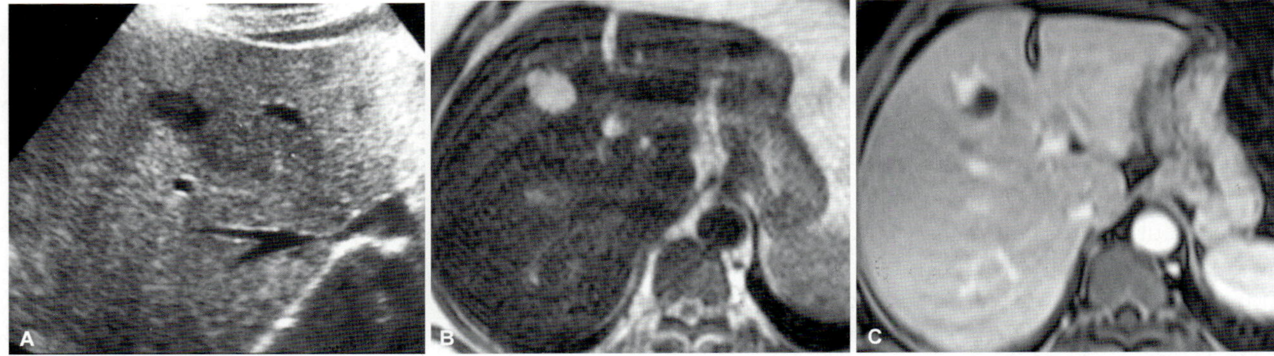

Figs 15.2A to C: Fatty liver with hypoechoic hemangioma: (A) Transverse US of the liver shows a small hypoechoic focal lesion against a background of diffusely increased echogenicity of fatty liver (B) The lesion is hyperintense on T2W image, with (C) typical peripheral nodular enhancement, suggestive of hemangioma

with liver metastases on US or CT. Loss of signal on the opposed phase image when compared with the in phase image readily identifies excess fat containing areas in the liver. Although fatty infiltration may demonstrate increased signal intensity of liver on T1- and T2-weighted spin echo images, this increase in signal may not be apparent even with massive fat deposition in liver.[4] MR spectroscopy can be used for quantitative assessment of fatty liver. In steatosis, there is an increase in the lipid peak amplitude.

On cross sectional imaging fat deposition is most often diffuse. Focal fat deposition and focal fat sparing are less common patterns that typically occur adjacent to the falciform ligament, fissure for ligamentum venosum, porta hepatis, gallbladder fossa and in the subcapsular portions of the liver. Their characteristic locations, geographic/ wedge shape configuration with angulated margins, lack of mass effect, presence of normal blood vessels coursing through them and enhancement similar to normal liver help differentiate these from true lesions. When multifocal or nodular these may however simulate true masses and may require chemical shift MRI for their confirmation (Figs 15.4A to E).

VIRAL HEPATITIS

Hepatitis is diffuse inflammation of the liver that can be divided into acute and chronic forms. The later is in turn, subdivided into persistent and chronic active categories. Imaging is relatively non-specific but can help to exclude biliary obstruction in acute hepatitis. In chronic hepatitis, imaging is useful in monitoring the progression of the disease, development of portal venous hypertension and complications such as HCC.

US

In acute viral hepatitis, liver and spleen are frequently enlarged. Severe acute hepatitis may result in decreased parenchymal echogenicity against which the portal vein branches appear brighter than normal.[1] This pattern is seen in upto 60% of patients with acute viral hepatitis and is best appreciated in thin patients.[5] Gallbladder wall thickening or contraction or both are other non-specific findings seen in patients with hepatitis. Severe chronic hepatitis causes coarsening of parenchymal echotexture and increased echogenicity resulting in poor visualization of portal venous branches. This finding, however, is non-specific and it is also seen in fatty infiltration and cirrhosis. Periportal lymphadenopathy may be seen in hepatitis.

CT

CT attenuation of liver is generally not altered in hepatitis unless fatty infiltration is present. Hepatomegaly, gall-bladder wall thickening, and periportal hypodensity can be seen in acute hepatitis and periportal lymphadenopathy is commonly seen in chronic active hepatitis.

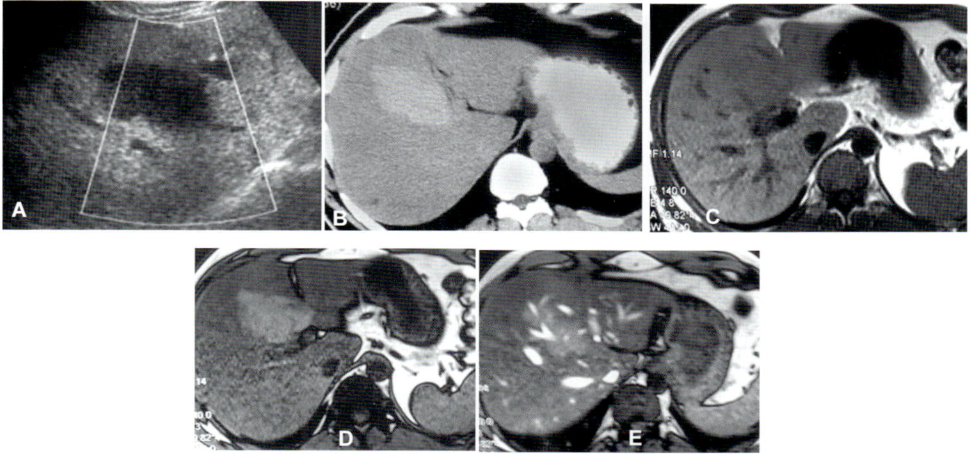

Figs 15.4A to E: Fatty liver with focal fat sparing: US (A) reveals diffuse increase in liver echogenicity with a geographic hypoechoic area. NCCT (B) focal fat sparing seen as an area of increased attenuation against a background of diffusely hypodense liver. The focal area is located adjacent to the fissure for ligamentum teres. MR T1W in phase (C), opposed phase (D) images: The fatty liver parenchyma shows drop in signal intensity in the opposed phase image unlike the area of fat sparing which appears relatively hyperintense on the opposed phase image. True-FISP MR image (E) illustrates normal vessels coursing through the area of fat sparing

MRI

On MRI, the edematous liver in acute hepatitis may appear heterogeneous especially on T2 weighted images and early postcontrast images. Periportal T2 hyperintense signal can also be seen. Likewise heterogeneous contrast enhancement and T2 hyperintensity signify severe ongoing inflammation in chronic hepatitis, while absence of patchy enhancement suggests low inflammatory reaction.[6] Progressive enhancement in the delayed phase suggests the presence of liver fibrosis in patients with chronic hepatitis.[7]

ALCOHOLIC HEPATITIS

Alcoholic liver disease manifests as three distinct but overlapping entities: fatty liver, alcoholic hepatitis and cirrhosis. Unlike acute viral hepatitis, liver echogenicity is increased in acute alcoholic hepatitis due to presence of concomitant fatty infiltration.

RADIATION HEPATITIS

In acute radiation hepatitis, CT shows a sharply defined, hypodense area in the liver corresponding to the radiation ports. This represents edema or fatty infiltration of the involved area. Clinically, onset is 2-6 weeks after therapy and is generally seen in patients receiving dose of more than 35 Gy to the liver. The CT changes may be seen several weeks after the initiation of the therapy and resolve by 3-5 months. Radiation hepatitis on MR imaging is seen as geographic areas of edema on T1 and T2-weighted images.[8]

HEMOCHROMATOSIS AND HEMOSIDEROSIS

Hepatic iron overload can be divided into parenchymal iron deposition (hemochromatosis) and reticuloendothelial iron deposition (hemosiderosis). In hemosiderosis the excess iron (body iron stores 10-20 gm) is derived from red blood cells typically due to repeated blood transfusions or hemolytic anemia. Because such iron is deposited primarily in the reticuloendothelial system (liver, spleen, lymph nodes, bone marrow) organ function is generally preserved.

Hemochromatosis on the other hand is a more severe form of iron accumulation (body iron stores upto 50-60 gm) that adversely affects organ function. Hemochromatosis may be primary or secondary. Primary hemochromatosis is an autosomal recessive metabolic disorder of excessive iron absorption in duodenum/ jejunum. The causes of secondary hemochromatosis include excess iron intake, anemia due to ineffective erythropoiesis requiring multiple blood transfusions, congenital transferrin deficiency, portocaval shunts and alcoholic cirrhosis.

The excess iron in hemochromatosis is stored as ferritin and hemosiderin in various organs including liver, pancreas, myocardium, joints, endocrine glands and skin, in decreasing order of severity. Sometimes iron is deposited in spleen and kidneys. Brain and nervous tissues are spared. A fibrous tissue reaction is found wherever iron is deposited. Iron deposits are greatest in liver and pancreas where they can contain 50-100 times the normal amount of iron. The liver is the first organ to be damaged in hemochromatosis resulting in hepatomegaly in 95% of symptomatic patients. Fibrosis is maximal in periportal areas resulting in micronodular pigment cirrhosis. Fatty change is unusual. Iron induced interstitial fibrosis in the pancreas affects endocrine functions to a greater extent than exocrine functions. Skin hyperpigmentation and diabetes mellitus results in so called bronze diabetes in these patients. Splenomegaly is present in approximately 50% cases, arthropathy of small joints of the hand with or without evidence of chondrocalcinosis on radiographs occurs in 20-50% and cardiac involvement is the presenting complaint in 15% cases. Diminished sexual activity, loss of body hair and testicular atrophy can be seen due to decreased production of gonadotropins.

Primary hemochromatosis usually presents in fourth to sixth decade of life. It is ten times more frequent in males. Women are generally spared due to iron loss with menstruation and pregnancy. The disease responds favorably to treatment that includes venesection/removal of blood and iron chelators. However once cirrhosis sets in, it is irreversible and is complicated by development of hepatocellular carcinoma in about one-third of patients despite adequate therapy.[9] Early diagnosis and treatment of hemochromatosis is therefore of vital importance.

US

Ultrasonography only depicts nonspecific changes of cirrhosis in patients with hemochromatosis and therefore has no role in the diagnosis.

CT

Unenhanced CT shows an overall homogeneous increase in density of hepatic parenchyma. While normal liver attenuation is between 45-65 HU, in hemochromatosis this ranges from 70 to 135 HU. The intrahepatic vessels stand out against the background of hyperdense liver. A CT value of 70 HU or more on unenhanced scan is very sensitive and fairly specific indicator of severe iron overload (Fig. 15.5),[4] although amiodarone treatment and glycogen storage disease can result in similar increased attenuation. Dual energy CT is useful in quantifying the amount of iron stored in the liver. Changing the scanning energy from 120-80 kVp will result in a change of CT value, which correlates with the amount of iron present in the liver. CT can also demonstrate increased density in spleen, pancreas, adrenal and lymph nodes. The increased background liver attenuation in hemochromatosis may hamper detection of hepatocellular carcinoma in the postcontrast images but facilitates tumor detection in unenhanced scans.

MRI

MR imaging is the most sensitive and specific imaging modality for demonstration of hepatic iron overload and also for follow-up of patients under treatment.[10] On MRI, hemochromatosis is characterized by dramatic loss of T1 and T2 signal of the liver (90%) and pancreas (20%) (Fig. 15.6). Gradient echo sequences are more sensitive than spin echo sequences. Contrary to what is seen in fatty infiltration, iron deposition results in loss of signal in the in phase image which conventionally is acquired at a longer TE than the opposed phase image (Figs15.7A and B). Decreased signal intensity in hemochromatosis is also demonstrated in pancreas and myocardium, and only occasionally in spleen. In transfusional siderosis, the signal intensity of both spleen and liver is diminished while the signal of pancreas remains unchanged as it is devoid of reticuloendothelial cells (Figs 15.8A and B). This feature helps to differentiate transfusional siderosis from hemochromatosis. MRI can be used for quantitative determination of iron overload. A liver/paraspinal muscle (L/M) signal ratio below 0. 6 on spin echo T2-weighted images is diagnostic of severe iron overload. It correlates well with the amount of iron present in the liver.[4]

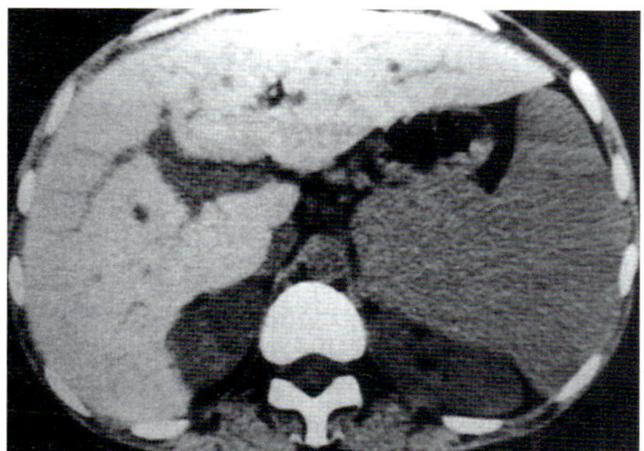

Fig. 15.5: Unenhanced CT scan of another patient with primary hemochromatosis shows diffuse highly increased attenuation of the liver

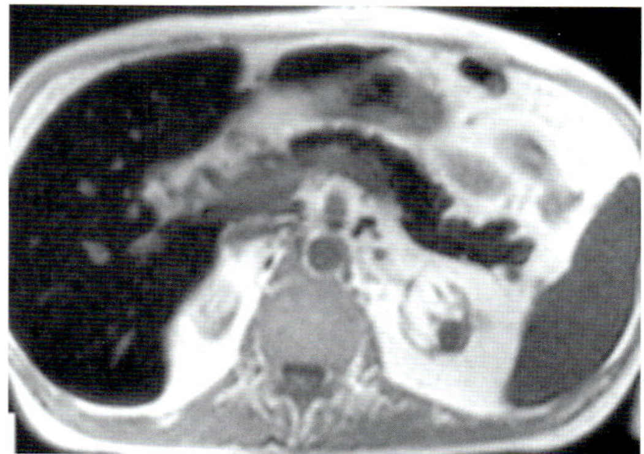

Fig. 15.6: Primary hemochromatosis: FSE T2W image reveals markedly hypointense signal of the liver and pancreas, while the spleen shows normal signal intensity

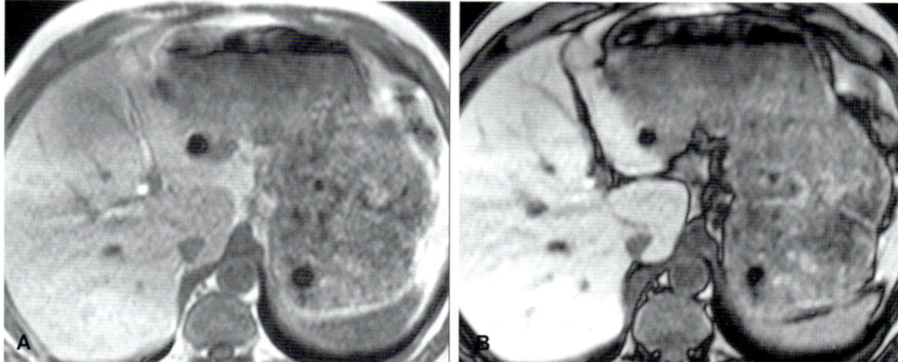

Figs 15.7A and B: Hemosiderosis secondary to repeated blood transfusions: MRI spoiled GRE T1W in phase image (A), and Opposed phase image (B) show increase in signal intensity of the liver parenchyma in the opposed phase image due to iron deposition

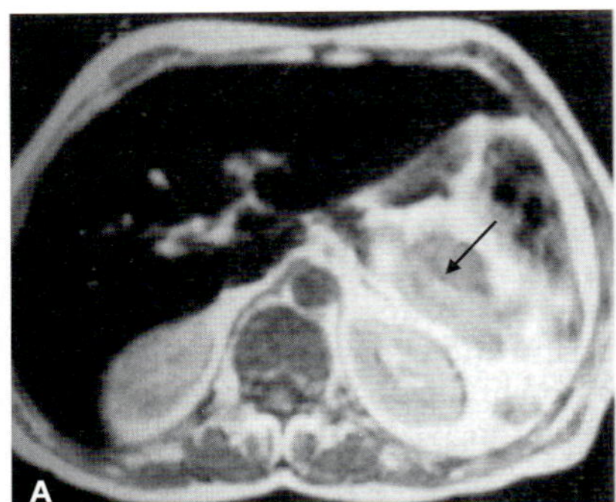

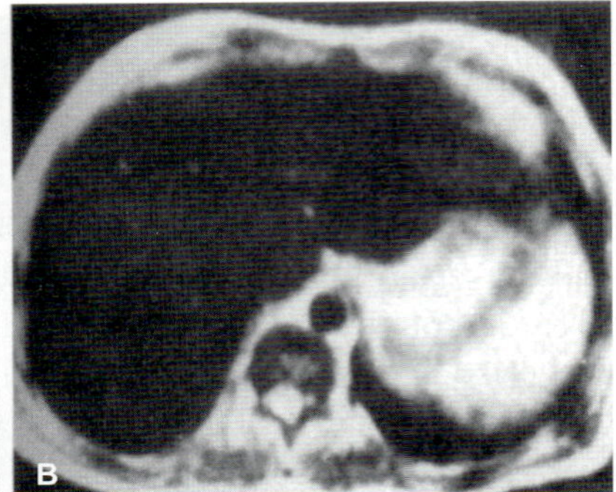

Figs 15.8A and B: Hemosiderosis: Almost no signal intensity is seen on T_1-weighted (A) and T_2-weighted axial MR images (B). Normal signal intensity of the pancreas (↑) helps in differentiation from hemochromatosis. Spleen is not seen because of previous splenectomy in this patient

AMYLOIDOSIS

Amyloidosis is characterized by the deposition of an extracellular fibrous protein in the organs. It may be primary or secondary. Primary amyloidosis is due to deposition of AL protein. It may occur without pre-existing disease or may be seen as a complication of multiple myeloma. Secondary amyloidosis is due to the deposition of AA protein and is seen with chronic infections, rheumatoid arthritis, ulcerative colitis, Crohn's disease, malignant tumors and Hodgkin's lymphoma. Clinically, there is smooth, non-tender hepatomegaly. Hepatic function is usually preserved despite massive amyloid deposition.

Ultrasound is usually normal except for presence of hepatomegaly. Rarely US reveals a heterogeneous echotexture due to non-uniform deposition. On unenhanced CT scans amyloid deposition results in hepatomegaly and generalized decreased attenuation. On contrast-enhanced scans, focal areas of decreased enhancement corresponding to the non-uniform involvement may be seen. The involved areas may show contrast enhancement in the delayed phase. Concomitant decrease in splenic enhancement may help differentiate amyloid deposition from fatty liver in appropriate settings. MR imaging has little role in the assessment of hepatic amyloidosis as there is no significant change in the T2 signal of involved liver.[11]

WILSON'S DISEASE

Wilson's disease or hepatolenticular degeneration is a rare, inherited autosomal recessive disorder of copper metabolism characterized by impaired biliary excretion of copper. Initially the excess copper accumulates in the liver. Subsequently copper deposition occurs in the basal ganglia, renal tubules, cornea, bones, joints and parathyroid glands. The spectrum of liver injury in Wilson's disease is non-specific and includes fatty infiltration, acute hepatitis, chronic active hepatitis, cirrhosis or massive liver necrosis. Development of HCC is extremely rare.

Most patients present in childhood or adolescence with liver disease before the onset of neurologic manifestations. They may have progressive jaundice, ascites or even fulminant hepatitis. Patients presenting after the age of 20 years can present with a clinical picture simulating chronic active hepatitis or with neurological symptoms like Parkinson like movement disorder and psychiatric disturbance. The Keyser-Fleischer ring is a characteristic corneal pigment that is invariably present. Early recognition is important as treatment with penicillamine and zinc can prevent toxic deposition of copper in the liver and brain. However cross sectional imaging is disappointing in making a specific diagnosis. Imaging findings of cirrhosis, fatty liver are non-specific (Figs15.9A and B). Fatty infiltration and excess copper can cancel each other out in advanced Wilson's disease so that a high CT density is usually not seen. Skeletal changes are seen in over 85% patients with Wilson's disease.[12] These include osteomalacia, chondrocalcinosis, premature osteoarthritis, anterior wedging of dorsal vertebrae, Schmorl's nodes, osteochondritis dissecans and a periosteal reaction at the trochanters.

GRANULOMATOUS DISEASES

Granulomatous diseases denote the presence of a focal inflammatory process with the histological features of granuloma. The causes include various viral, bacterial, fungal and parasitic infections, sarcoidosis, Wegener's granulomatosis and toxic reaction to drugs and chemicals.

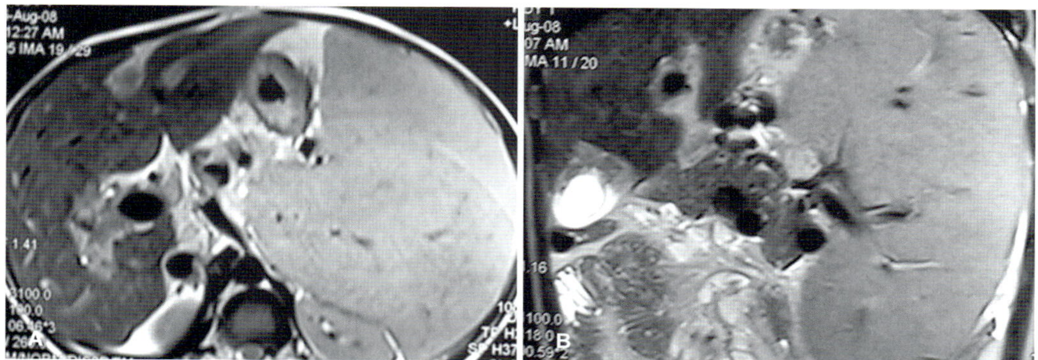

Figs 15.9A and B: Wilson's disease: Axial (A) and coronal (B) TSE T2W image of a 15-year-old boy showing non-specific changes of liver cirrhosis with a shrunken liver and massive splenomegaly

Tuberculosis: Miliary tuberculosis is the most common form of hepatic tuberculosis. Usually it is not accompanied by radiological abnormalities because of its diffuse micronodular nature. Macronodular tuberculomas are uncommon and may be solitary or multiple. These are hypoechoic on ultrasound. CT scan shows hypodense lesions with or without rim enhancement (Fig. 15.10). Tubercular cholangitis and tubercular pylephlebitis result from rupture of tubercular abscess and spread of caseous material into bile ducts and portal vein respectively. Both these conditions are extremely rare. Multiple small intrahepatic calcifications with no associated masses are seen on ultrasound and CT, and these represent old healed granulomas.[4]

Sarcoidosis: Liver involvement occurs in 24-79% patients of sarcoidosis.[13] Clinically apparent liver disease is however rare. In sarcoidosis small (< 2 mm) non-caseating granulomas are seen diffusely in the liver. Cross sectional imaging most frequently reveals hepatomegaly, often with associated splenomegaly. Occasionally granulomas are seen as nodular lesions 0.5-2 cms in size in the liver and spleen. These nodular lesions appear hypoechoic on US, hypodense on CT and hypointense on both T1 and T2-weighted images. Upper abdominal adenopathy is frequently associated in these patients. Occasionally these nodes enlarge sufficiently to cause biliary obstruction at porta hepatis.

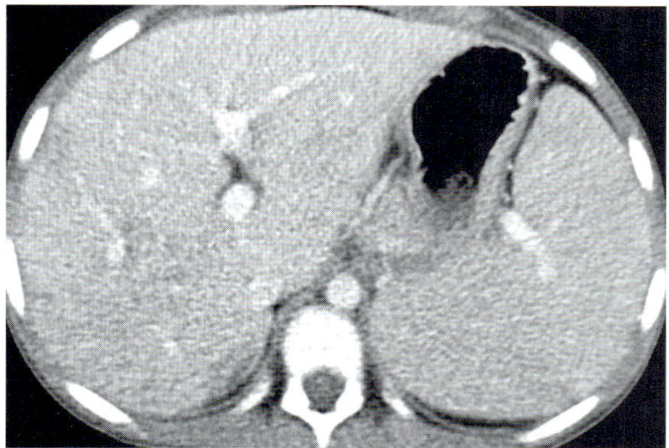

Fig. 15.10: Granulomatous disease: Contrast-enhanced CT of a young adult with disseminated tuberculosis reveals hepato-splenomegaly and ill-defined hypodense lesions in the right lobe of liver

Schistosomiasis: It is a common parasitic infestation with high prevalence in endemic areas such as Africa, South America, Middle East, China and Japan. The adult worms release ova in portal and mesenteric veins, which are embolized to liver. The host reacts to the ova with a granulomatous inflammation, which is then replaced by fibrous tissue, leading to periportal fibrosis and portal hypertension. On ultrasound, periportal fibrosis is seen in the form of thick, echogenic bands replacing the normal portal venous walls, which radiate from porta hepatis to the periphery of the liver. These bands are seen as tubular, round or oval structures depending on the plane of the section. There may be evidence of portal hypertension. On unenhanced CT scans, the bands of periportal fibrosis are hypodense and they enhance markedly after contrast administration. They produce round, linear or branching patterns depending on the plane in which they are sectioned. The portal vein may not enhance, if it is thrombosed. Hepatic calcification, if seen, is fairly characteristic and has been termed as 'turtle back'.[14] It occurs within the capsule and hepatic parenchyma, perpendicular to the capsule looking like a septum. Sometimes the calcifications may be dense enough to be seen on the plain films.

Liver fluke or fasciola hepatica: It is a trematode that infests cattle. Humans are accidental hosts. There is an acute phase of hepatic invasion that lasts for 1-3 months and a chronic phase of persistent adult flukes in the biliary tree. In hepatic fascioliasis, CT shows peripheral small, hypodense, serpentine or nodular lesions whose visibility is improved on dynamic or delayed enhanced CT. The tortuous peripheral channels correspond to the migratory tracts.[15] There are many other causes of granulomatous infections, which include brucellosis, leptospirosis, syphilis, leishmaniasis, actinomycosis, aspergillosis and cryptococcosis. These are not associated with any specific radiological features.

CIRRHOSIS

Cirrhosis is a chronic disease of the liver, which is characterized by fibrosis, and nodular regeneration of the liver in response to hepatocellular necrosis. The etiology is diverse which includes viral hepatitis, alcoholism, prolonged cholestasis, hepatic venous outflow tract obstruction, malnutrition, cryptogenic cirrhosis, metabolic causes like hemochromatosis and Wilson's disease, Indian childhood cirrhosis, various toxins and therapeutic agents. Cirrhosis is conventionally considered as an irreversibly scarred, end stage disease of the liver. Although the causes are many, the end result is same.[16] The response of the liver to the necrosis is limited, the most important are collapse of hepatic lobules, formation of diffuse fibrous septa and nodular re-growth of liver cells. The initiating hepatocyte injury leads to inflammation, structural collapse and fibrogenesis. The resulting septa cause circulatory disturbances, portal hypertension and intrahepatic cholestasis. A vicious cycle is set up whereby further hepatocyte injury is caused leading to progression of the disease. Morphologically cirrhosis is classified into micronodular and macronodular varieties. Micronodular disease is characterized by thick, regular septa, small regenerating nodules of uniform size, and involvement of every lobule. It may represent impaired capacity of re-growth as in alcoholism or malnutrition. Macronodular variety is characterized by septa and nodules of various sizes and presence of normal liver in between larger nodules. Regeneration in micronodular cirrhosis results in macronodular or mixed appearance.[16] A regenerative nodule is defined as a hepatocellular nodule containing one or more portal tracts located in a liver that is otherwise abnormal due to either cirrhosis or other severe disease. These nodules are present in all cirrhotic livers, and cirrhosis is classified on the basis of size of these on pathologic specimen as micronodular (< or = 3 mm), macronodular (> 3 mm) or mixed. A dysplastic nodule is defined as a nodule of hepatocytes of at least 1mm in diameter, with dysplasia of low or high grade but no histological criteria for malignancy. Dysplastic nodules are found in 15-25% of cirrhotic livers. Steatosis (fatty infiltration) can occur in either form, and either form may result in an enlarged or shrunken liver. Focal confluent fibrosis (or confluent hepatic fibrosis) refers to mass like fibrosis in advanced cirrhosis, associated with volume loss seen as retraction of overlying hepatic capsule or total shrinkage of segment or lobe.

Child's classification, which depends on jaundice, ascites, encephalopathy, serum albumin and nutrition, is used to determine short-term prognosis. Prothrombin time is used instead of nutritional status in Child -Pugh modification. The total score classifies patients into grade A, B or C.[16] Complications of cirrhosis include portal hypertension, variceal bleeding, spontaneous bacterial peritonitis, coagulopathies, hepatic encephalopathy, hepatorenal syndrome and hepatocellular carcinoma (HCC). Risk of development of HCC in cirrhotic liver is approximately 3% per year. Although, cirrhosis of any etiology may lead to HCC, the risk is particularly high in cirrhosis which occur secondary to viral hepatitis. Imaging studies play an important role in screening of HCC in cirrhotic patients.

US

Liver is either enlarged or normal in size in early stage of cirrhosis. A small shrunken liver is seen only in advanced cases. Criteria for sonographic diagnosis include heterogeneously increased parenchymal echogenicity, decreased beam penetration through liver and poor depiction of diaphragm and intrahepatic portal venous walls. These features are common to both fatty infiltration and fibrosis and there is poor interobserver agreement on interpreting these finding. Echogenicity largely depends on gain settings; however, it can be compared with that of adjacent organs in cases of doubt. Normally, echogenicity of liver and kidneys are almost equal or there is only a mild difference. If gross difference in echogenicity is seen, the organ with higher echogenicity is usually diseased.

Morphological changes in cirrhosis include relative hypertrophy of the caudate lobe and left lobe segments 2, 3 and atrophy of the right hepatic lobe and segment 4 of left lobe. Sonographically, a right/left lobe ratio of sagittal diameters in midclavicular line and midline respectively of 1. 3 or less can differentiate cirrhosis from normal liver with 93% accuracy, while a ratio of 1. 4 or more excludes cirrhosis.[17] In advanced case of cirrhosis, accentuation of fissures, contour indentations, nodularity and occasionally regenerating nodules are seen. Regenerating nodules vary in size from 2 mm to 2 cm. These may be visible on US as hypoechoic nodules with echogenic border and are difficult to differentiate from small HCC on US. US scanning with a high frequency probe can depict a nodular liver contour even in early cirrhosis.[18] Atrophy of the liver, along with heterogeneous echotexture and poor beam penetration, however, limits the sonographic detection of small focal lesions in advanced cirrhotic liver. Sonography has a poor sensitivity in detection of HCC; it detects only 14% of lesions smaller than 2 cm[19] and its sensitivity for detecting HCC during screening of cirrhotic patients is only 50%.[1]

Doppler evaluation is valuable as it provides the hemodynamic information. Portal hypertension can be seen in the form of enlarged portal vein, diminution or reversal of portal venous flow and presence of porto-systemic collaterals. Hepatic venous evaluation by Doppler is also helpful. Normal hepatic venous waveform is triphasic with a short phase of reversed flow. The fibrosis and decreased compliance of liver parenchyma leads to decreased amplitude of the phasic variations with loss of reversed flow. Alternatively, there may be a completely flat waveform. These features may be seen even in early stages of cirrhosis.[20] As the liver atrophies in end stage cirrhosis, hepatic veins may become attenuated and difficult to visualize. This can cause difficulties when the diagnosis of hepatic venous occlusion is being considered.[3]

CT

Fatty liver is the most common CT feature of early cirrhosis. Morphological changes in advanced cirrhosis include an overall decrease in liver volume accompanied by atrophy of the right lobe and hypertrophy of left and caudate lobes. The dual arterial supply and shorter intrahepatic course of vessels supplying the caudate lobe along with the fact that caudate vein drains directly into the inferior vena cava permits better oxygenation/relative preservation of its function resulting in compensatory hypertrophy.[21] On the other hand it is postulated that alcohol and other toxins in the portal vein stream preferentially to the right hepatic lobe. Caudate lobe to right lobe size ratio has been proposed as an objective means of diagnosing cirrhosis. Three lines are drawn: Line 1 is parasagittal through the right lateral wall of main portal vein just caudal to its bifurcation, line 2 is parallel to line 1 through the medial margin of caudate lobe, and line 3 is perpendicular to these lines drawn midway between portal vein and IVC. The distances are measured on line 3. The distance between right abdominal wall and line 1 is right lobe size and distance between line 1 and line 2 is caudate lobe size (Fig. 15.11). If the caudate lobe to right lobe ratio exceeds 0. 65, cirrhosis is most likely present and certainly if it exceeds 0. 73.[22] The hepatic fissure, gallbladder fossa and porta hepatis are wider than usual because of parenchymal atrophy (Fig. 15.12). These morphological changes are by and large similar irrespective of the underlying etiology of cirrhosis. However patients with biliary cirrhosis/sclerosing cholangitis tend to have marked caudate lobe hypertrophy and often have atrophy of lateral segments of the left hepatic lobe in addition to atrophy of right lobe.

Cirrhotic liver often appears heterogeneous on both unenhanced and enhanced CT scans due to underlying fibrosis, iron accumulation and regeneration and altered portal venous flow.[3] Irregular enhancement of fibrosis can sometimes mimic tumor. Regenerating nodules and

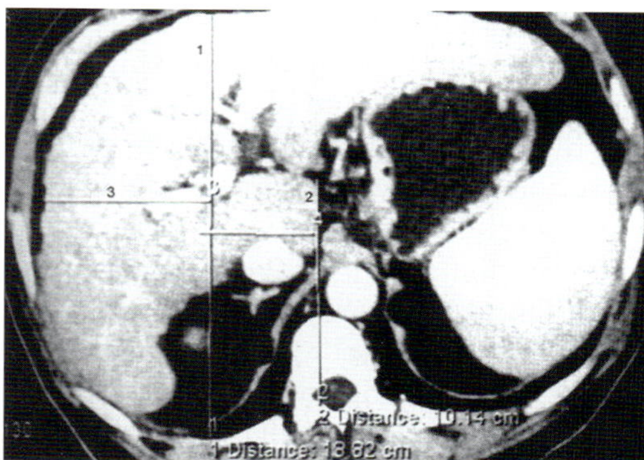

Fig. 15.11: CT scan shows method measurements of right and caudate lobes. The diameters of right and caudate lobes are measured on line 3 as shown

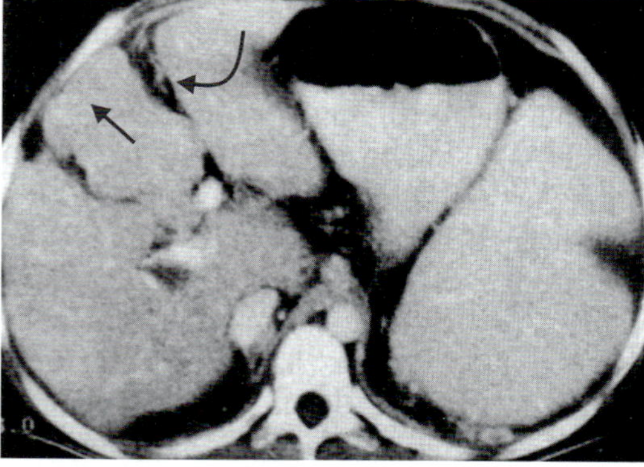

Fig. 15.12: Cirrhosis: Atrophy of the right lobe and hypertrophy of the caudate lobe with splenomegaly is seen on CT. Widened hepatic fissure (curved arrow), porta and nodularity of the contour of the liver (straight arrow) are also seen

atrophy cause nodularity of liver contour. Ancillary CT features in cirrhosis include ascites, splenomegaly, enlargement of the hepatic artery, evidence of porto-systemic collaterals, pericaval fat collection that may appear intraluminal on axial CT scans and increased attenuation of the mesenteric/retroperitoneal fat.

Although regenerating nodules are present at histopathology in all cases, these are infrequently demonstrated on CT as they are usually isoattenuating to liver parenchyma on both unenhanced and contrast enhanced CT. CT therefore is unable to depict or differentiate evolution from regenerative nodules to dysplastic nodules. Siderotic nodules however appear dense on unenhanced CT but even these become isodense to liver parenchyma following contrast administration. Dual phase multi detector CT of liver is however sensitive in detection of HCC occurring in cirrhotic liver. Uncommonly, when regenerating nodules are seen, these appear as hypodense lesions on contrast enhanced CT mimicking HCC.

Focal confluent fibrosis that is seen in 30% of patients with advanced cirrhosis can also simulate tumor appearing hypodense on unenhanced CT and isodense to slightly hypodense in contrast-enhanced CT. However typical associated features including wedge shaped lesion radiating from the porta hepatis, characteristic location in the anterior segments of right lobe and segment 4 and focal retraction of the overlying liver capsule can help differentiate these form tumor. Similar to hepatitis, patients with cirrhosis can have enlarged upper abdominal lymph nodes and this finding is particularly common in patients with biliary cirrhosis/sclerosing cholangitis.

MRI

MR imaging can often detect cirrhosis at an earlier stage than US or CT.[1] In early cirrhosis, MRI demonstrates fine strands of fibrosis, which are seen as lace like hypointense fine network on heavily T2- weighted images. Out of phase spoiled gradient echo images are very sensitive in this regard. These fine fibrotic strands show progressive enhancement following intravenous gadolinium. Enlargement of hilar periportal space, which is a space anterior to right branch of portal vein, is considered as an early manifestation of cirrhosis. It is caused by atrophy of segment 4. Early detection of cirrhosis by MRI is of clinical importance as these patients may benefit from newer treatment options now available.[10] As cirrhosis progresses, MRI demonstrates all features which are seen on CT, including contour nodularity, relative right lobe atrophy and left/caudate lobe hypertrophy, splanchnic vessels enlargement, hepatic arterial enlargement, collaterals, splenomegaly and ascites. Expansion and widening of interlobar fissure is also seen.

MR imaging can demonstrate regenerating nodules with greater sensitivity than any other modality. While only approximately 25% of regenerating nodules are seen on CT mainly due to their iron content, MR can demonstrate 50% regenerative nodules.[1] MR imaging can also characterize focal hepatic masses better than CT/US. Regenerating nodules are hypointense on T1-weighted images (occasionally T1 hyperintense) and hypointense on T2-weighted images (Figs 15.13A and B). Gradient echo sequences are useful for their demonstration. Following gadolinium administration, these nodules show low signal intensity than rest of the normal liver parenchyma. Iron deposition may be found in 25% of the regenerating nodules and this account for low intensity on T2-weighted spin echo and gradient echo images.

Dysplastic nodules (previously called adenomatous hyperplastic nodules) represent premalignant intermediary phase in pathway of hepatocellular carcinogenesis. Unlike regenerative nodules which are usually

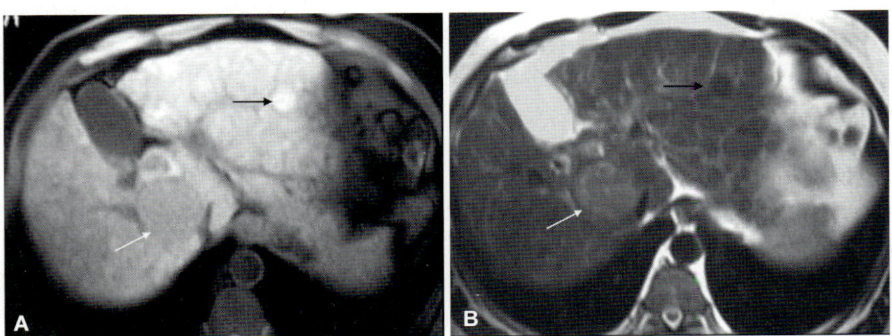

Figs 15.13A and B: Cirrhosis with regenerative nodule and HCC: Axial T1W (A) and T2W (B) MR images shows a well defined focal lesion in segment VIII of liver (white arrow) which is hypointense on T1 and hyperintense on T2W images suggestive of HCC. A regenerative nodule is also seen in segment II (black arrow) which appears hyperintense on T1 and hypointense on T2W images

T1 hypointense and only occasionally show hyperintense signal on T1-weighted images, dysplastic nodules are usually hyperintense on T1-weighted images. Regenerative siderotic nodules however cannot be differentiated from dysplastic siderotic nodules on MR images. In contrast to most HCC that are hyperintense on T2-weighted images, dysplastic nodules are hypointense on T2-weighted images (Fig. 15.13). The presence of bright focal area within a low intensity nodule on T2-weighted image (nodule within nodule) is therefore highly suspicious for HCC occurring within a dysplastic/siderotic nodule.

Focal confluent fibrosis has T1 and T2 signal similar to HCC: i. e. hypointense on T1 and hyperintense on T2-weighted images. As with CT, differentiation therefore rests mainly on identifying the characteristic location and associated capsular retraction.

Abnormal hepatic periportal intensity, which is seen as hyperintense rings or track marks surrounding the portal vein branches on T2-weighted images, can be seen in cirrhosis. It is a non-specific finding and also seen in many biliary or hepatocellular diseases. Gamma Gandy bodies in spleen are seen as multiple, small, low intensity spots on gradient echo images. These represent hemosiderin deposits in collagen bundles and may be the result of small hemorrhages.

MR imaging is useful in differentiating viral from alcoholic cirrhosis. Larger caudate lobe volume, presence of a notch in the outline of right posterior segment of liver and smaller size of regenerating nodules favors the diagnosis of alcoholic cirrhosis over virus induced cirrhosis.[23] Recently MR elastography has shown promising results in assessing the degree of hepatic fibrosis.[24]

MALIGNANT DIFFUSE LIVER DISEASES

Occasionally, a malignant process may diffusely involve the liver. Metastases, particularly from breast cancer, may give rise to diffusely increased heterogeneous echotexture on ultrasound. HCC, lymphoma and leukemia can also be seen as diffusely altered echotexture of the liver. Diagnosis is difficult in such situations and may require biopsy in appropriate clinical context.[3]

REFERENCES

1. Gore RM. Diffuse Liver disease. In Gore RM, Levine MS (eds): Textbook of Gastrointestinal Radiology 3rd ed. Saunders Elsevier: Philadelphia 2008;1685-1729.
2. Park SH, Kim PN, Kim KW, et al. Macrovesicular hepatic steatosis in living liver donors: Use of CT for quantitative and qualitative assessment. Radiology 2006;239:105-12.
3. Lomas DJ. The liver. In Grainger RG, Allison D, Adam A, Dixon AK (Eds): Diagnostic Radiology 4th ed. Churchill Livingstone: London 2001;1237-76.
4. Venbrux AC, Freidman AC. Diffuse hepatocellular diseases. In: Friedman AC, Aachman AH (Eds): Radiology of the Liver, Biliary Tract and Pancreas. Mosby year book: St Luis 1994;49-167.
5. Tchelepi H, Ralls PW, Radin R. Grant E. Sonography of diffuse liver disease. J Ultrasound Med. 2002;21:1023-32.
6. Danet IM, Semelka RC, Braga L. MR imaging of diffuse liver disease. Radiol Clin North Am 2003;41:67-87.
7. Martin DR, Semelka RC. Magnetic resonance imaging of the liver: review of techniques and approach to common diseases. Semin Ultrasound CT MR 2005;26:116-31.
8. Semelka RC, Braga L. Armao D: Liver. In Semelka RC (ed): Abdominal Pelvic MRI. New York, Wiley-Liss, 2002;33-318.
9. Kauffman JM, Grace ND. Hemochromatosis. In Weinstein WM, Hawkey CJ, Bosch J (eds): Clinical Gastroenterology and Hepatology. Philadelphia, Elsevier-Mosby 2005; 659-64.
10. Danet IM, Semelka RC, Braga L. MR imaging of diffuse liver diseases. Radiol Clin N Am 2003;41:67-87.
11. Georgiades CS, Neyman EG, Fishman EK. Cross-sectional imaging of amyloidosis: an organ system-based approach. J Comput Assist Tomogr 2002;26:1035-41.
12. Gitlin JD: Wilson's disease. In Zakim D, Boyer TD (eds): Hepatology: A textbook of liver disease. Philadelphia, Saunders 2003;1273-88.
13. Karagiannidis A, Karavalaki M, Koulaouzidis A. Hepatic sarcoidosis. Ann Hepatol 2006;5:251-56.
14. Fataar S, Bassiony H, Satyanatus P: CT of hepatic schistosomiasis. AJR 1985;145:63-66.
15. Serrano MAP, Vega A, Oretega E, et al. CT of hepatic fascioliasis. J Comput Assist Tomogr 1987;11:269-72.
16. Sherlock S, Dooley J. Hepatic cirrhosis. In Sherlock S, Dooley J (Eds): Diseases of the Liver and Biliary System. 11th edn. Blackwell Science: Oxford 2002;365-80.
17. Goyal AK, Pokhrana DS, Sharma SK. Ultrasonic diagnosis of cirrhosis-reference to quantitative measurement of hepatic dimensions. Gastro Radio 1990;15:32-34.
18. DeLeio A, Cestari C, Lomazz A, et al. Cirrhosis with sonographic study of the liver. Radiology 1989;172:389-92.
19. Liu WC, Lim JH, Park CK, et al. Poor sensitivity of sonography in detection of hepatocellular carcinoma in advanced liver cirrhosis. Eur Radiol 2003;13:1693-98.
20. Kemla A, Mural O, Umit C, et al. Hepatic vein Doppler waveform changes in early (child Pugh A) chronic parenchymal liver diseases. J Clin Ultrasound 1997;25:15-19.
21. Dodds WS, Erickson SJ, Lawson T, et al. Caudate lobe of liver - anatomy, embryology and pathology. AJR 1990;154:87-93.
22. Giorgio A, Amoroso P, Lettieri G, et al. Value of caudate to right lobe ratio in diagnosis with US. Radiology, 1986;161:443-45.
23. Okazaki H, Ito K, Fujita T, Koike S, Takano K. Matsunaga N. Discrimination of alcoholic from virus-induced cirrhosis on MR imaging. AJR Am J Roentgenol 2000;175:1677-81.
24. Rouvière O, Yin M, Dresner MA, et al. MR elastography of the liver: preliminary results. Radiology 2006;240:440-48.

Chapter Sixteen

Imaging of Obstructive Biliopathy

Raju Sharma, Harsh Kandpal

INTRODUCTION

Evaluation of biliary tract obstruction is a common but challenging radiological problem. Continuing advances in ultrasonography (US), computed tomography (CT) and magnetic resonance imaging (MRI) have enhanced our ability to evaluate the biliary tract. The aim of imaging is to diagnose biliary obstruction, delineate the level and if possible the cause of obstruction. Sonography is the initial modality for the detection of biliary obstruction. Other imaging modalities include CT, MRI, MRCP, endoscopic ultrasound and endoscopic retrograde cholangio-pancreatography (ERCP) and percutaneous cholangiography (PTC).[1] There have been encouraging reports on the role of 3D cholangiography and intravenous cholangiography with helical CT.[2, 3]

ULTRASONOGRAPHY

Ultrasonography is a useful and accurate screening modality to diagnose biliary obstruction and determine the level of obstruction. The common bile duct (CBD) diameter of up to 6-7 mm is considered normal in adults.[4] With high-resolution ultrasound equipments, normal intrahepatic biliary ducts may be seen, but these should not measure more than 2 mm and should not be greater than 40% of the diameter of the accompanying portal veins. Dilated intrahepatic biliary ducts appear as "too many tubes" or give "Swiss cheese" appearance.

ENDOSCOPIC ULTRASONOGRAPHY (EUS)

Endoscopic ultrasonography first introduced as a research tool has emerged as a significant advance in gastro-intestinal endoscopy, and allows high resolution images of pancreaticobiliary system.[5]

Two types of echoendoscopes are used - radial and linear, at frequencies ranging between 5-20 MHz. The high frequencies provide superb resolution but limited penetration. The linear echoendoscope can track the path of a needle and hence is used for EUS guided FNAC. EUS is a very sensitive technique for detecting small pancreatic and bile duct malignancy and accurately perform local staging of these tumors.

COMPUTED TOMOGRAPHY

In addition to US, CT is often performed for the evaluation of biliary obstruction. Both these modalities can accurately define the level and cause of obstruction in more than 90% patients. On CT, the upper limit of normal for the common hepatic duct diameter is considered to be 6 mm and the common bile duct 9 mm, although higher values are accepted in postcholecystectomy patients. Intrahepatic ducts more than 2-3 mm diameter or ducts that become confluent rather than scattered, is considered abnormal. Advances in CT technology including the development of multidetector row CT (MDCT) scanners and the development of better post processing software have significantly improved the ability of CT to image patients with obstructive biliopathy. Dynamic contrast enhanced CT; superior off axial reformats, volume rendering, maximum intensity projection (MIP) and minimum intensity projection (MinIP) provide useful display of the vascular map and/or biliary tract.

HEPATOBILIARY SCINTIGRAPHY

Hepatobiliary scintigraphy generally does not compare favorably with sonography and CT. However scintigraphy has some distinct advantages in the work-up of a jaundiced patient, particularly in the postoperative setting. The agents routinely used for hepatobiliary imaging are iminodiacetic acid (IDA) derivatives, which are accumulated by hepatocytes and secreted into the bile and subsequently into the small bowel.

MAGNETIC RESONANCE IMAGING

At the time of initial clinical application of MR cholangiopancreatography (MRCP), over a decade ago, MRCP was regarded a new technique with questionable potential for imaging the biliary tract and pancreatic duct.[6] Since that time, however, MRCP has been shown to have a wide range of clinical applications and has virtually replaced diagnostic ERCPs.[1] The acceptance of MR is related to technical refinements such as advances in hardware and software which have greatly improved image quality and shortened examination times. The technical refinements include development of breathing independent sequences that suppress artifacts associated with surgical clips, stents and bowel gas and allow image acquisition at section thickness of 2-5 mm.

MRCP is performed with heavily T2-weighted sequence that image fluid in the biliary tree while suppressing background signal from nonfluid structures. Single shot fast spin echo sequences are a robust method for doing this with a short acquisition time and relatively high spatial resolution. Disadvantages include image blurring induced by long echo train length, and flow artifacts within biliary tree which can occasionally simulate calculi. A relatively more recent approach is the use of 3D fast recovery fast spin echo sequences which can be breath hold or respiratory triggered. It provides volumetric acquisition with thin sections and isotropic resolution that can be reformatted in any plane. Parallel imaging is frequently used with MRCP techniques to reduce acquisition times or improve resolution. The combination of high field systems like 3Tesla with parallel imaging also offers the scope of improving image quality of MRCP and the future holds a lot of promise.

An alternative to heavily T2 weighted MRCP is the use of contrast agents with biliary excretion coupled with gradient echo T1 weighted sequence. The contrast agents that can be used include Mangafodipir sodium, gadobenate dimeglumine and gadolinium-EOB-DTPA. Advantages of contrast enhanced T1 weighted MRCP include possibility of more functional information, delineation of biliary leaks and the fact that background suppression of ascites and bowel fluid is less problematic.

MRCP offers a number of advantages compared with ERCP/PTC. MRCP being noninvasive is devoid of ERCP related complications like pancreatitis, gastrointestinal tract perforation and hemorrhage that occur in upto 5% of all ERCP examinations.[7] Unlike ERCP; MRCP does not expose patients to ionizing radiation or iodinated contrast material. In contrast to ERCP, it can depict ducts proximal to a high grade obstruction, which is vital for planning surgical procedures as well as any endoscopic or percutneous intervention. MRCP is also useful in the evaluation of patients with incomplete or failed ERCP and also in evaluation of patients in whom ERCP is technically difficult or not possible due to surgical alterations of the gastrointestinal tract. When MRCP is performed along with conventional MR study and if required MR angiography, it can provide detailed information regarding the solid organs and vessels, thus helping to stage malignancies that cause obstructive biliopathy. The major disadvantage of MRCP is that it is entirely diagnostic in contrast to ERCP, which provides diagnostic information as well as access for therapeutic interventions.

ENDOSCOPIC RETROGRADE CHOLANGIOPANCREATOGRAPHY

Endoscopic retrograde cholangiopancreatography is the gold standard for evaluation of pancreatic and biliary duct. However, due to a large number of advantages which MRCP offers vis a vis ERCP, it has replaced ERCP to a great extent as a means of identifying diseases of the bile and pancreatic ducts.

However, ERCP is still useful in clarifying complex ductal anatomy, providing information in the setting of an equivocal or nondiagnostic MRCP and identifying the bile duct and cystic duct leaks. Once disease has been detected with MRCP, patients may then be selected appropriately for therapy with ERCP, surgery or other radiological interventions. Both benign and malignant causes of obstructive biliopathy are discussed in this chapter.

BENIGN LESIONS CAUSING OBSTRUCTIVE BILIOPATHY

- Choledocholithiasis
- Benign strictures
- Choledochal cyst

- Primary sclerosing cholangitis
- Primary biliary cirrhosis
- Parasitic diseases
- Infections
- Ampullary stenosis
- Choledochal varices
- Hemobilia
- Benign biliary tract tumors

CHOLEDOCHOLITHIASIS

Choledocholithiasis is found in about 7-20% of patients undergoing cholecystectomy.[8] The majority of bile duct calculi are secondary calculi that originate in the gallbladder and then migrate via the cystic duct or through cholecystocholedochal fistula. Primary calculi that form de novo in the bile duct are less common and develop in the setting of bile stasis and colonization of bile with enteric organisms.

Ultrasonography is the initial screening modality due to its low cost and easy availability. While US can detect gallstones accurately in approximately 90-100% of cases,[9] its ability to detect CBD stones is less impressive. The reported diagnostic accuracy varies from as low as 13% to as high as 82%.[10,11] US sensitivity is limited by its inability to visualize the entire length of CBD especially distal CBD due to interposed bowel gas. Factors known to increase the diagnostic accuracy of US include meticulous technique, presence of dilated common bile duct, proximal position and larger size of the calculus. [11] Typically, the proximal bile duct is best seen in the parasagittal/ longitudinal plane with patient in right anterior oblique (RAO) position, and distal CBD is best visualized in the transverse plane. Distal CBD stones are most likely to be overlooked and their detection can be facilitated by scanning in the right lateral position which minimizes gas in the gastric antrum and duodenum. Positioning the patient in a semi erect or erect position also affords better visualisation as the left lobe of the liver descends over the region of interest, providing an acoustic window for sound wave transmission. Typical US appearance of CBD calculus is an echogenic nodule with acoustic shadowing seen in a dilated CBD (Fig. 16.1). Acoustic shadowing is not seen if the CBD is minimally dilated or of normal caliber. Nonshadowing stones in the CBD can mimic sludge or soft tissue masses.

CT: The reported sensitivity of CT in detecting CBD stones varies from 45-90%.[12] Similar to gallstones, bile duct calculi depending on their composition, may appear

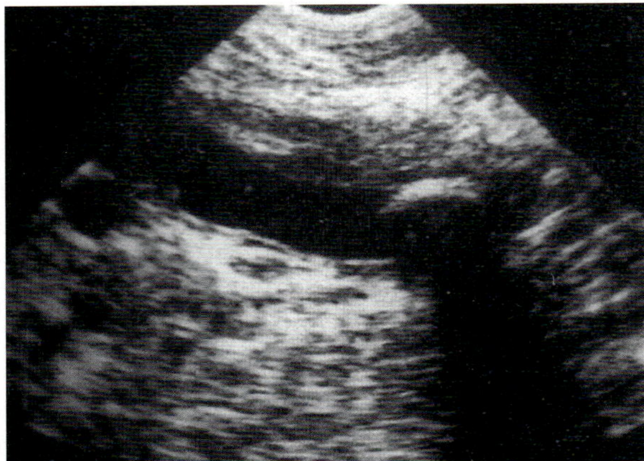

Fig. 16.1: Choledocholithiasis: A. Dilated CBD with calculus seen in longitudinal US scan

calcified, of soft tissue density, isodense or hypodense with respect to bile. Unenhanced CT is better for their detection as most calculi are slightly hyperdense. High attenuation calculi can easily be seen on CT; contrasted against the lower attenuation of bile or that of ampullary soft tissue (Fig. 16.2). Bile duct calculi may reveal a faint hyperdense rim with a central low density area (rim sign). Even impacted stone with no surrounding bile can be detected by noting that the visualized calcific nodule (stone) lies in the course of the CBD. The duct wall may be thickened at the level of CBD calculus, often because of an associated inflammatory stricture. Approximately 50% of the bile duct calculi are of faint attenuation only slightly greater than the surrounding bile or are isoattenuating of adjacent pancreas. Detection of these stones is facilitated by looking for a rim or crescent of bile that outlines these subtle intraluminal densities. Adjusting the window level

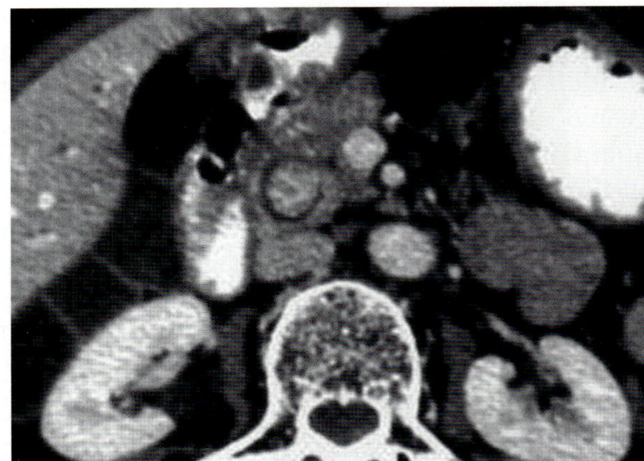

Fig. 16.2: Choledocholithiasis. CT scan shows a rounded hyperdense calculus in the distal CBD surrounded by a crescent of bile

setting to the attenuation of CBD and window width to 150 HU improves visualization of non calcified stones by creating better contrast between the bile and soft tissues [13] Abrupt termination of dilated CBD in absence of any direct evidence of calculus is an indirect sign of choledocholithiasis. This finding is however nonspecific and is more often due to a malignant etiology .[14]

When a strong suspicion of CBD stone exists, water should be used to opacify bowel. Positive oral contrast should be withheld as it may obscure stones impacted at the ampulla of Vater. CT visualisation of bile duct calculi is optimized with the thin collimation isotropic MDCT scanners. MDCT has revived interest in CT cholangiography. This technique can be performed in two ways: using oral or IV cholangiographic agents that are excreted into and opacify the bile ducts or by utilizing natural contrast of bile accentuated by minimum intensity projection display. CT cholangiography using cholangiographic agents was shown to provide excellent visualization of the biliary anatomy with 95% sensitivity for choledocholithiasis.[15] Use of high kilovoltage technique makes stones more conspicuous on CT images.

Magnetic Resonance cholangiopancreatography: MRCP is an excellent modality for the detection of bile duct stones with sensitivity/specificity of 90-100% being similar to or exceeding that of ERCP.[16-18] MRCP reveals calculi as low signal intensity filling defects in the biliary tract (Fig. 16.3A) and is capable of detecting even tiny calculi as small as 2 mm.[19] Common diagnostic pitfalls that can mimic or obscure stones at MRCP include pneumobilia, intraluminal sludge/blood clots, signal loss due to surgical clips (Fig. 16.3B) or due to pulsatile compression by the right hepatic artery and artifacts due to flowing bile. [20, 21]

On cholangiography, calculi within the bile ducts are seen as round or faceted filling defects within the contrast column. These defects are usually mobile. When impacted, a typical convex border of the contrast column in the distal CBD is seen outlining the proximal stone margin and obstruction to flow of contrast is noted. Air-bubbles are a common problem at cholangiography, but can usually be differentiated by their smooth, round appearance and their tendency to group together and rise to the non-dependent surface as compared to stones which are usually faceted or elliptical and tend to fall at the dependent portion of the biliary tree.

BENIGN STRICTURES

Benign strictures of the biliary tree can be due to surgical and other trauma, chronic pancreatitis, gallstones and duodenal ulcer.

POSTOPERATIVE BILIARY STRICTURES

Benign strictures are most often a sequel of direct injury or ischemic injury to bile ducts during biliary tract surgery. The incidence of postoperative bile duct strictures has increased with the growing popularity of laparoscopic cholecystectomy.[22] These strictures are sometimes recognized months to years after surgery with cholangitis as the most common presenting symptom. In patients

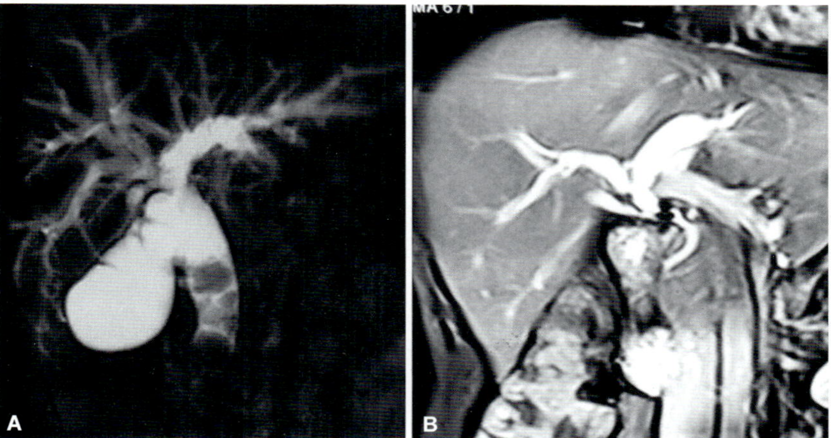

Figs 16.3A and B: Choledocholithiasis (A) Coronal thick slab projectional MRCP reveals a hypointense calculus in the distal CBD forming a meniscus and causing dilatation of proximal biliary tree. Additional calculi are seen in the mid CBD. (B) Coronal T2-weighted image reveals a hypointensity in the region of CBD due to surgical clip

suspected of postoperative CBD strictures, US should be carried out as a screening procedure. In the presence of proximal dilatation of CBD with smooth tapering stenosis or sudden cut off of CBD (Fig. 16.4), no further investigation is required.[21] If US findings are equivocal or normal despite strong clinical suspicion of CBD stricture, MRCP and if required ERCP/PTC should be performed. MRCP can accurately diagnose and anatomically classify biliary strictures that can assist in planning corrective surgery. ERCP and PTC are established modalities in the evaluation of CBD strictures that in addition to depicting the presence, precise site and length of stricture, can also provide biliary drainage. Bismuth H[22] classified postoperative benign bile duct strictures into five types:

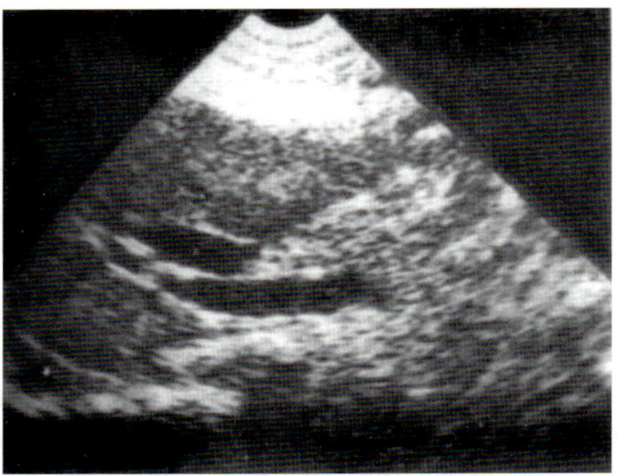

Fig. 16.4: Postoperative CBD stricture—US showing dilated proximal part of the CBD with sudden cut off

Type I: Low common hepatic duct strictures, the hepatic duct stump being longer than 2 cm (Fig. 16.5).

Type II: Middle common hepatic duct stricture, the hepatic duct stump being less than 2 cm (Fig. 16.6).

Type III: High stricture or hilar stricture, with preservation of the biliary confluence but no communication with the common hepatic duct.

Type IV: Hilar stricture interrupting the confluence, communication between right and left ducts no longer demonstrable (Fig. 16.7).

Type V: Stricture involving an anomalous distribution of the segmental branches. (Fig. 16.8).

Patients with post-cholecystectomy strictures are treated with biliary enteric anastomosis such as hepatico-jejunostomy. These surgical anastomosis may also undergo narrowing with time. In this setting ERCP is not feasible due to the altered anatomy and sonography is hampered by the presence of pneumobilia. MRCP is the modality of choice to depict these strictures (Figs 16.9A to C).

POST-INFLAMMATORY STRICTURES

Post-inflammatory strictures can be caused by cholangitis, chronic pancreatitis, gallstones and penetrating or perforating duodenal ulcer. In chronic pancreatitis, strictures occur in less than half of the patients. The most frequent configuration on cholangiography is about 3

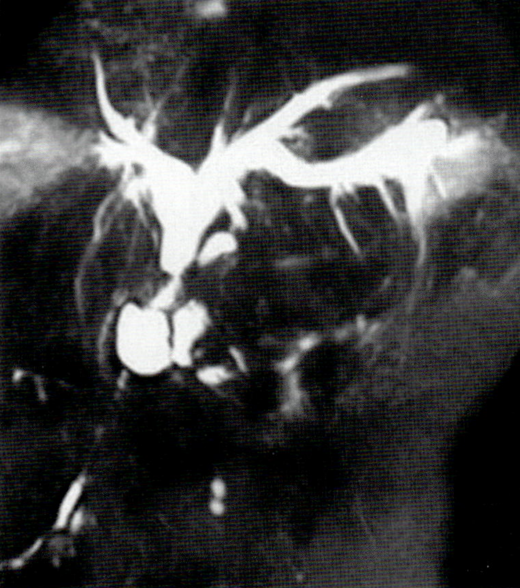

Fig. 16.5: Post-Cholecystectomy Benign Biliary Stricture (Type 1). Coronal thick slab projectional MRCP reveals stricture of the CBD more than two cms beyond the confluence

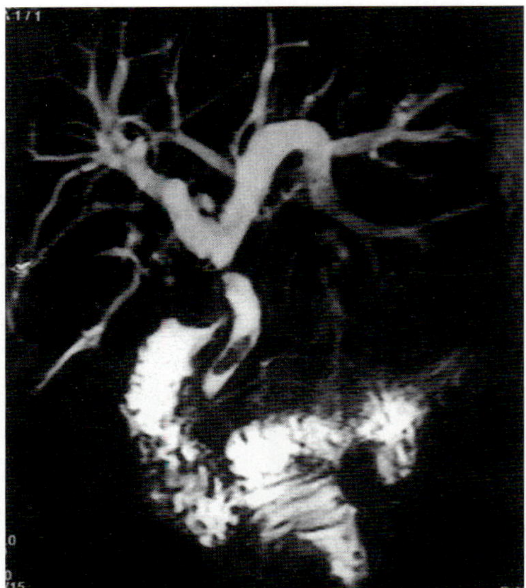

Fig. 16.6: Middle common hepatic duct stricture, the hepatic duct stump less than 2 cm (Type II) seen on MRCP

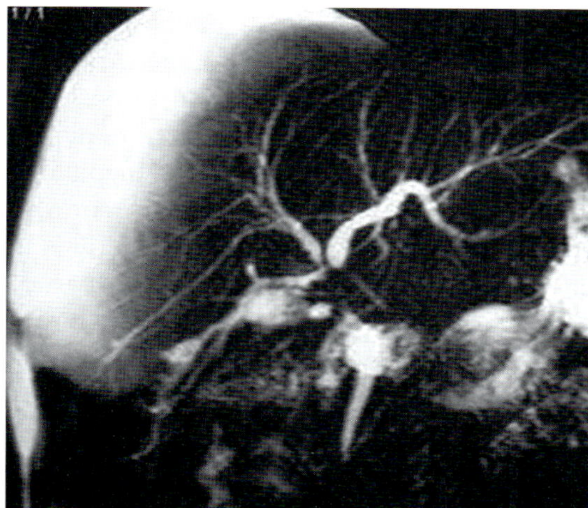

Fig. 16.7: Post-Cholecystectomy Benign Biliary Stricture (Type 4). Coronal thick slab HASTE image shows block at the level of primary confluence

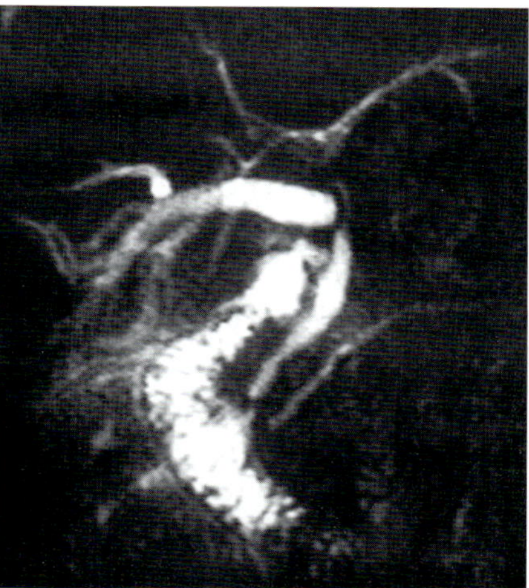

Fig. 16.8: Post-Cholecystectomy Benign Biliary Stricture (Type 5) Coronal T2W thick slab image shows isolated dilatation of the aberrant right posterior sectoral duct at its site of junction with the CBD

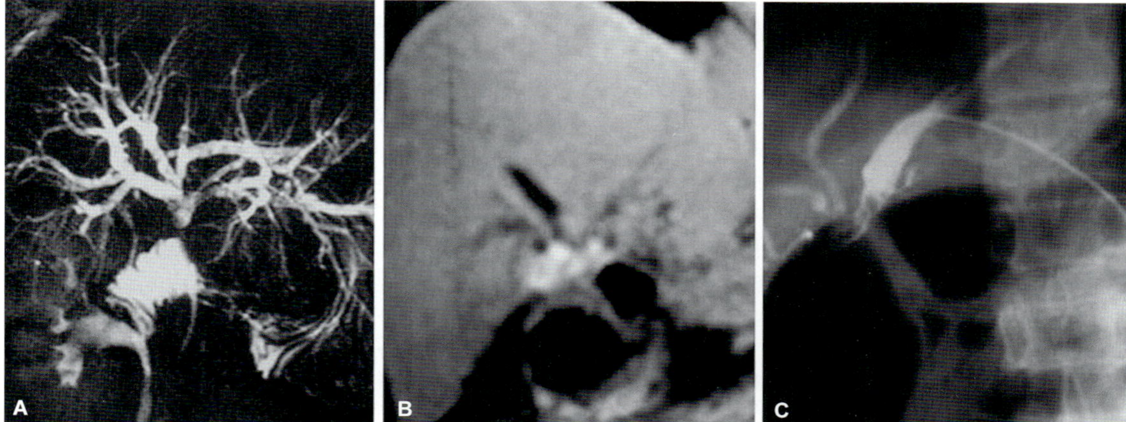

Figs 16.9A to C: Hepaticojejunostomy Stricture. (A) T2W coronal thick slab image shows dilated IHBR and narrowing at the anastamotic site. (B,C) Gd-BOPTA enhanced T1W MRCP shows pooling of contrast proximal to the site of narrowing, confirmed on PTC (C)

to 5 cm, smooth, concentric, often tapered narrowing of the intrapancreatic portion of the CBD (Fig. 16.10). An hour-glass configuration or deviation by a pseudocyst may also be seen. Strictures associated with gallstones are often short and sometimes web like. These may be single or multiple and may involve any portion of the biliary tree. Common duct stricture may result from fibrosis secondary to an adjacent inflamed gallbladder. US, CT and MRI primarily demonstrate biliary dilatation but may also reflect the primary pathology leading to strictures e. g. pancreatitis, gallstones or CBD stones.

BILE DUCT FISTULA

Bile duct fistula can be classified as internal (fistula with another organ) or external (to the skin).

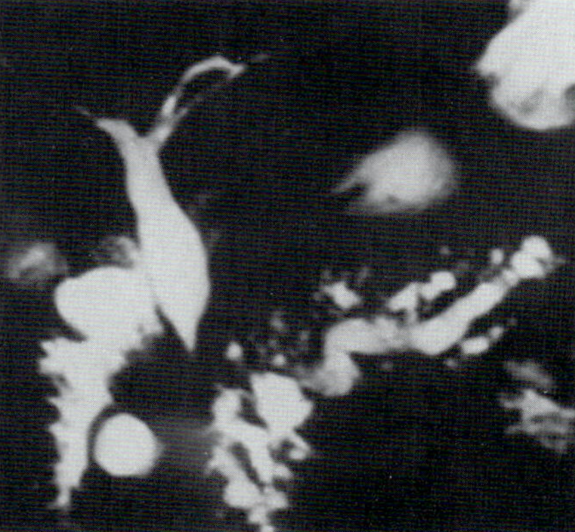

Fig. 16.10: Chronic pancreatitis with Benign Biliary Stricture. Coronal T2W thick slab image shows smooth gradual tapering of distal CBD. The MPD and its side branches are dilated

Choledochoduodenal fistula is the most common bile duct fistula. The communication usually forms between the first part of the duodenum and CBD as it passes behind the duodenum. Penetrating duodenal ulcer is the most common cause of this type of fistula. An eroding common duct stone is an uncommon cause. A biliary enteric fistula may be evidenced by penumobilia on radiograph; US or CT. Barium contrast studies are definitive in identifying a choledochoduodenal fistula in majority of the patients. Cholangiography can also demonstrate the fistula.

Bronchobiliary fistula may result from pyogenic, amoebic or echinococcal intrahepatic abscess that erodes through the diaphragm into the pleural space, lung and bronchi. Biliary vascular fistulae once exceedingly rare are also seen more frequently now due to trauma and interventional procedures. External biliary fistulae are uncommon. When a postoperative biliary cutaneous fistula is preceded by jaundice, bile duct occlusion is suggested. Liver injuries may be associated with a bile leak which may result in external fistula via a surgical or percutaneous drain.

MIRIZZI SYNDROME

Mirizzi syndrome is an uncommon complication of long standing cholelithiasis characterized by common hepatic duct or CBD obstruction due to extrinsic compression from an impacted gallstone in the cystic duct or gallbladder neck or from associated inflammatory changes. It may be complicated by fistula formation between the gallbladder and common hepatic duct/common bile duct secondary to an eroding stone. Preoperative diagnosis is important so as to forewarn the surgeon regarding increased risk of extrahepatic bile duct injury due to dense fibrosis around the hepatoduodenal ligament. The hallmark imaging features include cholelithiasis with intrahepatic biliary dilatation and dilated common duct till the porta hepatis beyond which the CBD is normal in caliber (Figs 16.11A and B).[23] Multiplanar reformatted images are particularly useful in depicting the extrinsic nature of the obstruction. Definite diagnosis of internal biliary fistula can be established by ERCP/PTC.

CHOLEDOCHAL CYSTS

Choledochal cyst is an uncommon congenital cystic dilatation of the bile duct. The underlying etiology is believed to be an anomalous junction of the pancreatic duct and CBD that allows free reflux of pancreatic enzymes into the CBD weakening its wall. Most patients present in childhood although no age is exempt. The triad of jaundice, right upper quadrant pain and a palpable subcostal mass is diagnostic but is not seen in all cases. Choledochal cysts can be associated with biliary atresia, congenital hepatic fibrosis and cystic disease of the kidney especially renal tubular ectasia, sometimes combined with cortical and medullary cysts. Reported complications of choledochal cysts include secondary calculus formation, pancreatitis, biliary cirrhosis, cyst rupture with bile peritonitis, cholangitis, intrahepatic abscess, portal vein thrombosis and malignant transformation into cholangiocarcinoma (Figs 16.12A and B).

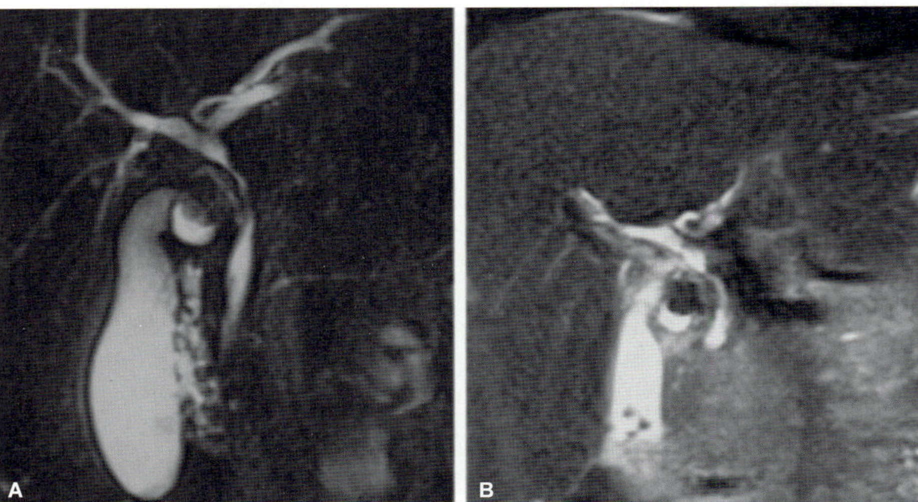

Figs 16.11A and B: Mirizzi syndrome. (A,B) T2W coronal thick slab image (A) and thin slice (B) MRCP images show a calculus at the neck of gallbladder causing extrinsic narrowing of the common hepatic duct

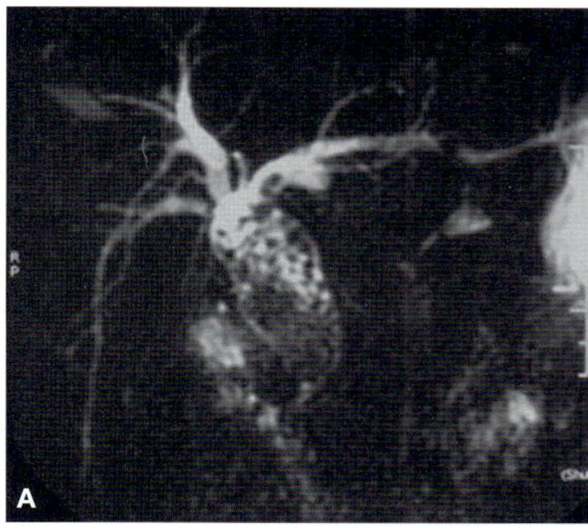

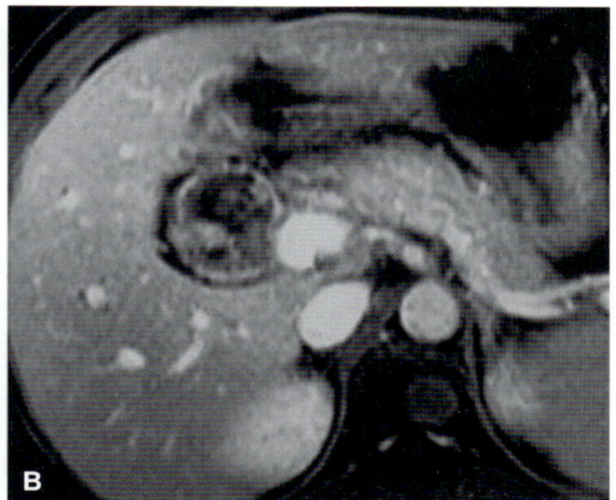

Figs 16.12A and B: Choledochal cyst type 1 with calculi and cholangiocarcinoma. (A) T2W thick slab MRCP shows fusiform dilatation o0f CBD with multiple calculi, (B) Post-Gadolinium T1W axial image reveals a nodular enhancing mass within the dilated duct

Todani et al [24] have classified choledochal cysts into five types:

- Type I: Fusiform cystic dilatation of extrahepatic CBD (Figs 16. 13A and B).
- Type II: Eccentric fluid-filled cyst (diverticulum)
- Type III: Localised cystic dilatation of distal intramural segment of CBD
- Type IVA: Multiple intrahepatic and extrahepatic bile duct cysts (Fig. 16.14).
- Type IVB: Multiple extrahepatic bile duct cysts
- Type V: Multifocal saccular dilatation of IHBR (Caroli's disease) (Figs 16.15A and B).

Ultrasonography is preferred for initial evaluation. It reveals an anechoic cystic structure separate from the gall bladder that communicates with the hepatic ducts.[25, 26] Differential diagnoses on US include other fluid filled structures in this region namely pancreatic pseudocyst, large right renal cyst, enteric duplication cyst and hepatic artery aneurysm. Hepatobiliary scintigraphy can confirm the diagnosis by showing late accumulation of radioisotope in the cystic structure.

Type II choledochal cysts may appear separate from the CBD as its neck may be narrow. Type III choledochal cysts (choledochocele) are rare and difficult to diagnose on US and CT but MRCP and cholangiography can reveal the typical cobra head appearance bulging into the duodenum. In patients with type 5 choledochal cyst (Caroli's disease), imaging reveals multiple cystic areas in the liver and tiny enhancing portal venous radicals can be seen within the bile ducts. MRCP and in particular cholangiography are best to show the communication of these cystic areas with the biliary tree.

CT, MRI and cholangiography can accurately diagnose and classify choledochal cyst. MRCP is equivalent

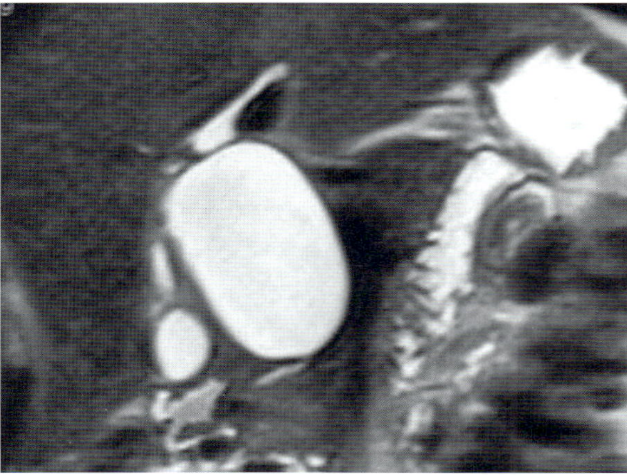

Fig. 16.13: Choledochal cyst type 1. T2W coronal MRCP image shows globular dilatation of the CBD

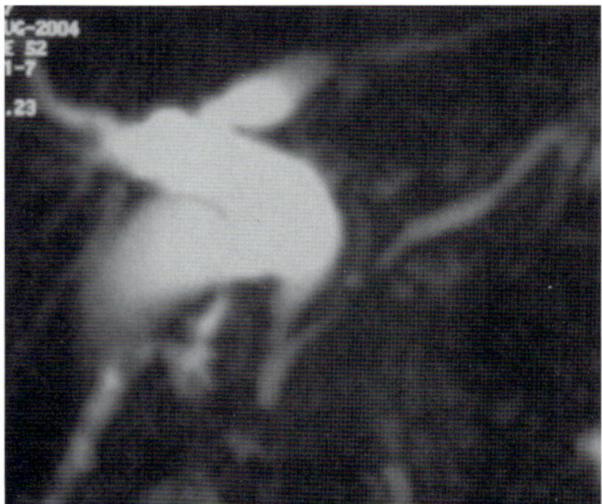

Fig. 16.14: Choledochal cyst type IV A. T2W coronal MRCP image shows dilated CBD and intrahepatic ducts with anomalous pancreatico-biliary junction

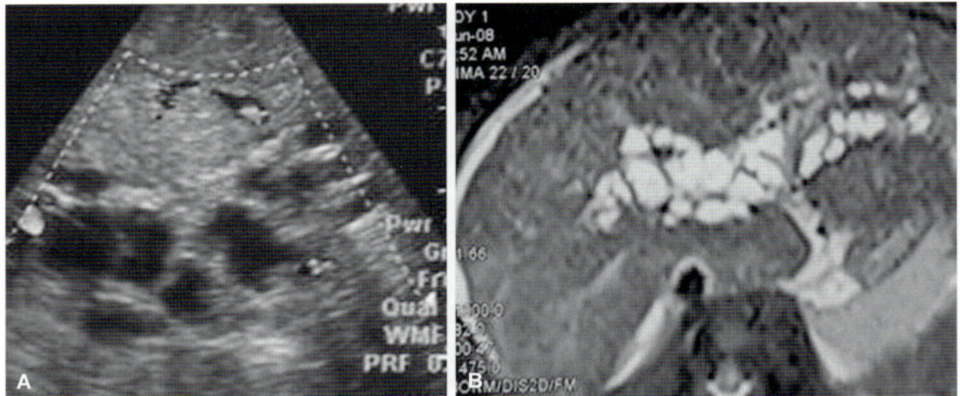

Figs 16.15A and B: Choledochal cyst type V: Caroli's Disease. Ultrasound (A) and axial T2W MR image (B) shows saccular dilatation of the intra-hepatic biliary ducts

to ERCP in detecting and defining the morphology of choledochal cysts and in detecting the presence of anomalous union of the pancreatic and bile ducts. [27] Preoperative knowledge of the type and extent of choledochal cyst is important for surgical planning which in most cases involves excision of the choledochal cyst and biliary drainage by Roux-en-Y hepaticojejunostomy. Caroli's disease when localized to one hepatic lobe can be treated with hepatectomy, while diffuse involvement may necessitate liver transplantation.

PRIMARY SCLEROSING CHOLANGITIS

Primary sclerosing cholangitis (PSC) is a chronic progressive cholestatic disease of unknown etiology that occurs more commonly (70%) in males and has a median age of onset of 40 years.[1] Nearly 70% patients with PSC have associated ulcerative colitis (UC) and conversely 3-7% of all patients with UC develop PSC. Other less consistently reported associations of PSC include Riedel's struma, orbital pseudotumor, retroperitoneal fibrosis and mediastinal fibrosis Cholangiocarcinoma can complicate PSC in 15% cases. PSC pursues a progressive downhill course with a median survival of 11.9 years. Liver transplantation is the only available treatment. Radiology plays a crucial role in the diagnosis of PSC as clinical features are nonspecific, there is no specific serological marker and histology alone is not diagnostic.

Cholangiography is the most definitive imaging modality for the diagnosis of PSC. In most cases ERCP is sufficient and PTC is performed only if certain segments of the biliary tract are not opacified at ERCP. Diffuse, multifocal, short (1-2 cm in length) strictures in both intrahepatic and extrahepatic bile ducts are the hallmark of PSC. Strictures alternate with normal or mildly dilated intervening duct resulting in a beaded duct appearance (Figs 16.16A and B). Other manifestations of PSC are

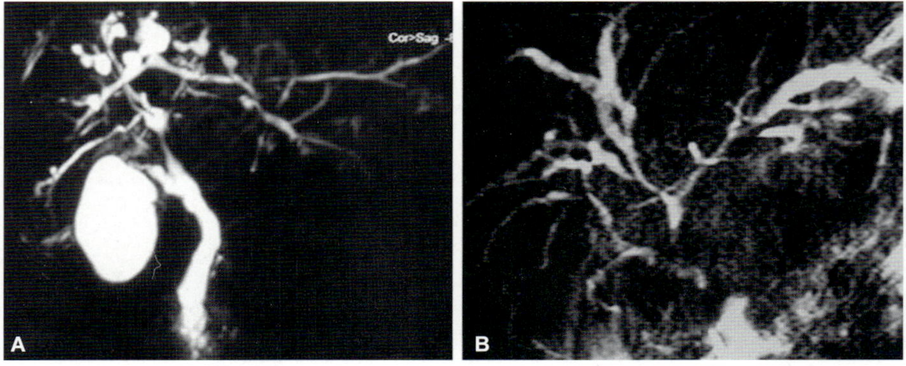

Figs 16.16A and B: Primary Sclerosing Cholangitis. T2W coronal MRCP images of two different patients show diffuse multifocal short strictures in intra and extra-hepatic ducts with intervening dilated segments (beaded appearance)

shorter (1-2 mm) band-like strictures and small diverticulum-like outpouchings (1mm to 1 cm), seen most frequently in the extrahepatic bile ducts and also intraluminal webs.[28] Fibrous obliteration of peripheral bile ducts can result in "pruned-tree" appearance. In approximately 50% patients with PSC bile duct irregularity is seen as subtle brush-border like appearance to coarse, shaggy or frankly nodular appearance. PSC can involve both large bile ducts that are visible at cholangiography and small intrahepatic ducts seen only at microscopy. On cholangiography CBD, CHD and distal 1 cm of right and left hepatic ducts are involved in almost all cases.

Cross sectional imaging in PSC reveals thickening and dilatation of bile ducts. US diagnosis is however difficult because bile duct dilatation in PSC is minimal due to surrounding fibrotic reaction. Thickening of either intra or extrahepatic bile duct walls are also nonspecific findings that may be seen in other conditions like suppurative cholangitis and cholangiocarcinoma. Intraluminal webs have also been reported on US in patients with PSC.[29]

Duct wall thickening often with marked contrast enhancement, skip dilatations and stenosis and mural webs have also been demonstrated on CT as well. Intrahepatic bile duct calculi can be seen as faint foci of high attenuation. Upper abdominal lymphadenopathy is frequently seen in patients with PSC and does not necessarily indicate development of cholangiocarcinoma. PSC induced cirrhosis induces unique morphological changes in the liver. There occurs atrophy of the lateral segments of the left lobe of liver in addition to atrophy of posterior segments of the right hepatic lobe and marked hypertrophy of the caudate lobe. The liver appears rounded with a lobulated contour. Other evidence of cirrhosis and portal hypertension can also be seen.

There is a good correlation between ERCP and MRCP in the diagnosis of PSC; although ERCP may still be required to diagnose early stages of the disease. MRCP findings are similar to those already described in ERCP. Additional findings seen on MRI include duct wall thickening and enhancement and morphological changes as seen on CT. Randomly distributed T1-hyperintense areas, reticular or peripheral wedge shaped T2 hyperintense areas and large (> 3 cm) nodular lesions (isointense on T1 and hypointense on T2) predominantly in the central portion of the liver are other reported MRI findings. PSC results in atrophy of peripheral wedge shaped areas in the liver which appear hypointense on T1, hyperintense on T2 and show delayed enhancement. It is often difficult to diagnose cholangiocarcinoma coexisting with PSC. Marked ductal dilatation, progressive stricture and the presence of an intraluminal polypoidal mass 1 cm. or more in diameter suggest the possibility of cholangiocarcinoma.

PRIMARY BILIARY CIRRHOSIS

Primary biliary cirrhosis is a chronic progressive cholestatic syndrome of unknown etiology characterized by inflammation and destruction of small intrahepatic bile ducts. Clinicopathological features can differentiate PBC from PSC. Unlike primary sclerosing cholangitis, primary biliary cirrhosis occurs predominantly (90%) in females, frequently shows high titers of antimitochondrial antibody and is associated with collagen vascular diseases but not with ulcerative colitis. Imaging plays a minor role in diagnosis as bile duct abnormalities are much less severe in PBC (compared to PSC) and often confined to small intrahepatic ducts. Cholangiograms are normal in most cases or may show nonspecific changes of tortuous and attenuated bile ducts due to cirrhosis. Diagnosis is made primarily on clinical features and typical laboratory findings. Cross sectional imaging shows findings of cirrhosis and portal hypertension in advanced cases. Periportal and portocaval lymphadenopathy is seen in the majority (80-90%) of patients with PBC.

RECURRENT PYOGENIC CHOLANGITIS

Recurrent pyogenic cholangitis (also known as oriental cholangiohepatitis) is endemic in certain Asian populations. These patients have a propensity to form pigment stones in the extrahepatic and intrahepatic bile ducts accompanied by recurrent episodes of gram negative bacterial cholangitis. Recurrent nature of the disease leads to progressive biliary strictures with marked ductal dilatation and stone formation. The disease often progresses to biliary cirrhosis. The combination of marked extrahepatic bile duct dilatation (often up to 3-4 cm in diameter), intrahepatic duct dilatation limited to segmental branches often most pronounced in the lateral segments of left lobe, peripheral tapering of ducts with numerous stones/debris comprising nearly a cast of the biliary tree is nearly pathognomic of this disease process (Fig. 16.17). The stones are composed mostly of bile pigment with varying degrees of calcification. Because of the soft mud-like consistency of many stones, CT is often better able to depict stones than ultrasound.[30] Mild extrahepatic duct

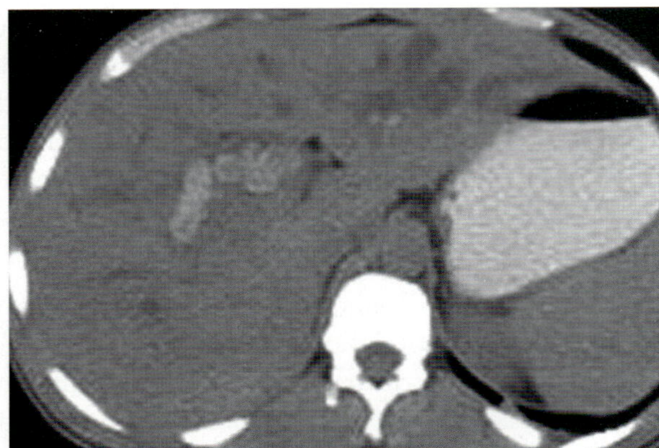

Fig. 16.17: Recurrent Pyogenic Cholangitis. CT scan shows dilated IHBR with hepatolithiasis and left lobe atrophy

wall thickening and enhancement, parenchymal atrophy, fatty change in liver, segmental parenchymal enhancement, hepatic abscess, pneumobilia and bilioma are additional cross sectional imaging findings.

BACTERIAL CHOLANGITIS AND AIDS RELATED BILIARY ABNORMALITIES

Bacterial cholangitis is nearly always associated with biliary tract obstruction. Benign causes of biliary obstruction are much more likely to be complicated by cholangitis than malignant causes. *E coli* is the most common infecting organism although the infection is polymicrobial in most cases. Echogenic/high density debris within the bile ducts on US/CT and filling defects on cholangiography due is suggestive of cholangitis in the clinical setting of sepsis. Complication such as cholangitic abscess which communicate with the biliary tree may also be seen (Figs 16.18A and B). Chronic obstructive cholangitis with repeated episodes of infection can lead to bile duct strictures and biliary cirrhosis simulating PSC.

Patients with AIDS can develop a secondary cholangitis possibly due to opportunistic infection by Cryptosporidium and/or CMV. This entity is characterized by irregularities and strictures of both intrahepatic and extrahepatic bile ducts with ductal dilatation closely resembling PSC. Gallbladder and bile duct wall thickening, papillary stenosis, hyperechoic nodule at the distal end of CBD due to edema of papilla of Vater and ERCP demonstration of polypoidal intraluminal filling defects due to granulation tissue are other reported biliary tract changes seen in AIDS patients.

PARASITIC DISEASES

Although many parasites of the gastrointestinal tract may traverse the biliary tract, clinically significant infestation is seen most commonly with Ascaris lumbricoides, Clonorchis sinensis and Echinococcus granulosus.

Ascaris lumbricoides: Ascaris lumbricoides is the most prevalent human helminth worldwide that inhabits the small intestine. These have a propensity to migrate from small intestine through the ampulla of Vater to lodge in the gallbladder and biliary tract. Ultrasound is the most valuable diagnostic tool that reveals the worms as tubular, nonshadowing, echogenic structures in the dilated biliary ducts. When alive the worms can be seen to move. Sonolucent inner tube within the echogenic tubular structure is often seen and this represents the alimentary

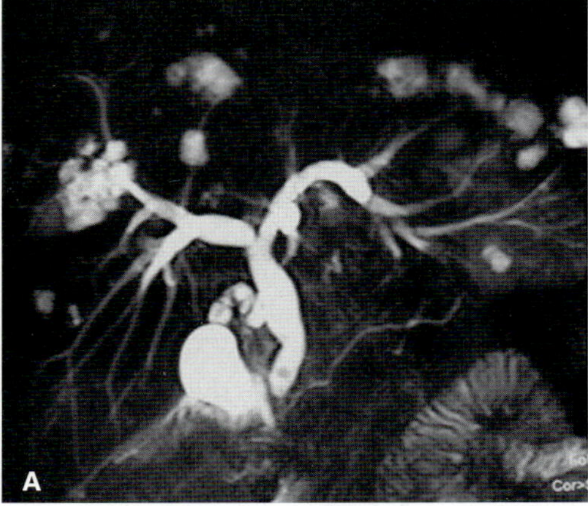

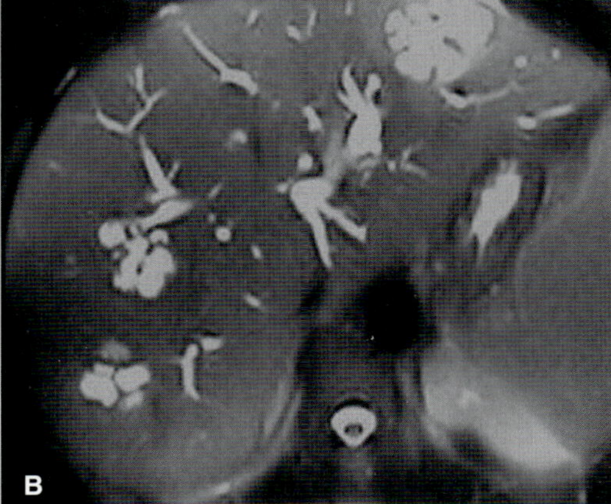

Figs 16.18A and B: Cholangiolar Abscesses. T2W coronal and axial images show dilated biliary radicles and multiple cholangiolar abscesses. A calculus is noted in the distal CBD

canal of the worm (Figs 16.19A and B). On unenhanced CT, they appear as hyperattenuating tubular structures surrounded by less attenuated bile. In transverse sections on both US and CT, a "bull's eye" image may be seen caused by the worm inside a dilated bile duct. Ultrasound and CT may also reveal hepatic abscesses complicating biliary ascariasis. On cholangiography, the worms may be seen as smooth cylindrical filling defects.

Clonorchis sinensis: Clonorchis sinensis is the most important among liver flukes. The disease is endemic in Asia. Humans are the definitive host. Adult worm resides in the intrahepatic bile ducts where it causes biliary obstruction, incites an inflammatory response with recurrent pyogenic cholangitis and in later stages causes periductal fibrosis. These worms appear as small short and curvilinear leaf like filling defects (2 to 10 mm in length) on cholangiograms. The flukes tend to concentrate in the peripheral bile ducts. Cross sectional imaging is therefore characterized by the presence of dilatation of small (peripheral) intrahepatic bile ducts with concomitant thickening of the duct wall and periductal tissues. The extrahepatic bile ducts are typically spared. CT reveals branching low attenuation structures in the liver due to bile duct dilatation and associated periductal fibrosis. Complications of clonorchiasis include: development of cholangiocarcinoma which also tend to be peripheral in this setting, intraductal calculi formation, cholangiohepatitis and liver abscess formation.

Hydatid cyst: Hydatid disease can affect any organ of the body; most commonly the liver. The cyst may rupture into the biliary system, peritoneal cavity and thorax. In patients with rupture into the biliary system, daughter cysts and membranes pass into the common bile duct producing surgical obstructive jaundice.[31] Accurate preoperative diagnosis of biliary communication of hydatid disease is possible on US, CT, MRI and cholangiography (Figs 16.20A and B). Doyle et al [32] described three different patterns of intraductal filling defects on ERCP :(i) filiform linear material in the CBD due to laminated hydatid membranes, (ii) rounded filling defects due to hydatid daughter cysts, and (iii) amorphous debris in the CBD due to a mixture of hydatid membranes and daughter cysts. MRCP and nuclear scan (HIDA) have also been found to be valuable in diagnosis of intrabiliary rupture of hydatid cyst.[33]

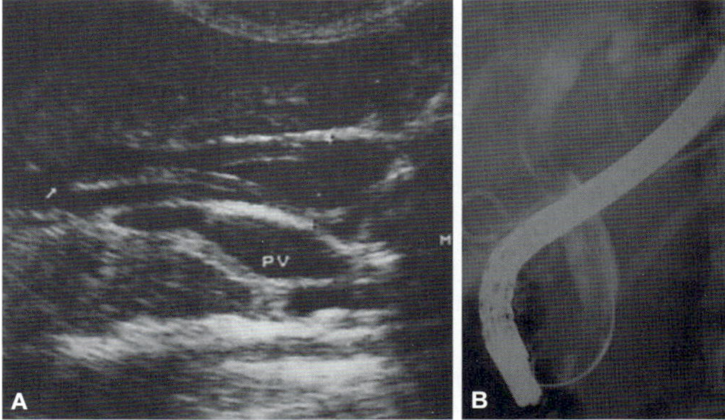

Figs 16.19A andB: Biliary Ascariasis. US scan (A) showing linear echogenic lesion in the dilated CBD. (B) ERCP confirms the same finding

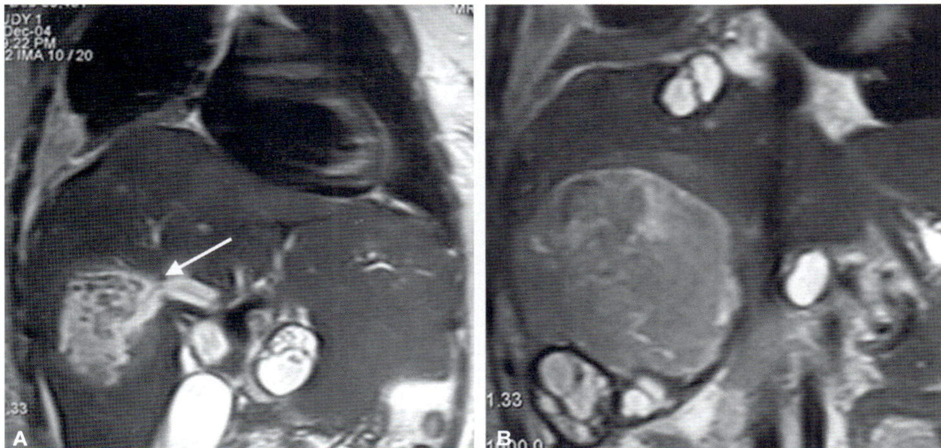

Figs 16.20A and B: Complicated Liver Hydatid Cyst. Coronal (A,B) T2W MR scan showing a hyperintense lesion in the right lobe of liver with internal membranes suggestive of hydatid cyst. Lesion shows biliary communication (arrow). Transdiaphragmatic migration giving rise to right pleural effusion is noted in (B)

RARE INFECTIONS

Tuberculosis: Hepatobiliary tuberculosis is a rare cause of biliary strictures, predominantly seen in underdeveloped countries. The most common involvement is at porta hepatis and less frequently distal common bile duct. Cholangiographic findings include irregular strictures, extrinsic impression and marked proximal dilatation or in less severe cases minimal wall irregularity or narrowing of the common hepatic duct. Dense chalky liver calcification and periportal or periductal nodal calcification suggests the possibility of tuberculosis.[34] Periportal tubercular adenitis causing biliary obstruction has been demonstrated by US and CT.[35] Other uncommon infections with Cryptococcus, Candida and Trichosporon, may lead to common duct stricture and obstruction.

AMPULLARY STENOSIS

Biliary obstruction may be caused by morphologic stenosis of the ampulla of Vater or sphincter of Oddi. Although unclear, probable causes include passage of gallstones and pancreatitis. Imaging studies are frequently abnormal but not always conclusive. On US, CT and cholangiography (ERCP/MRCP) bile duct and sometimes pancreatic duct dilatation may be seen. Ultrasound may show partial obstruction by demonstrating an increase in CBD diameter following a fatty meal. Hepatobiliary scintigraphy is also useful in the diagnosis. ERCP is the most valuable study for assessing the diagnosis of papillary stenosis, where direct endoscopic inspection of the papilla is possible. Tumors of the papilla or surrounding duodenum may be identified, if present. Cholangiographic findings of common bile duct dilatation, an elongated or rigid ampullary segment and failure of the common duct to empty contrast material in 45 minutes are suggestive of ampullary stenosis. For distinguishing morphologic stenosis from functional spasm or dyskinesia, cholecystokinin or glucagon may be required which will relieve the spasm in functional dyskinesia.

PORTAL BILIOPATHY

In portal hypertension, specially due to extrahepatic portal venous obstruction, varices of the paracholedochal veins of Petren and epicholedochal venous plexus of Saint may occur.[36] Smooth, extrinsic, nodular, spiral or stenotic appearing duct abnormalities and extrahepatic bile duct obstruction caused by portal collaterals may be seen at cholangiography (Figs 16.21A and B). Some of these changes are reversible after porto-systemic shunt surgery whereas some strictures are ischemic in etiology and do not improve. MRCP is currently the modality of choice for the diagnosis of this entity.

HEMOBILIA

Hemobilia or bleeding into the biliary tree has many causes, most frequent being trauma. Other causes include cholangitis, gallstones, tumors, hepatic artery aneurysms, coagulopathy and interventional procedures. Definite diagnosis rests with either direct endoscopic observation of blood entering the duodenum from the ampulla of Vater or angiographic demonstration of the bleeding site in the liver, gallbladder or biliary tract. Cholangiography

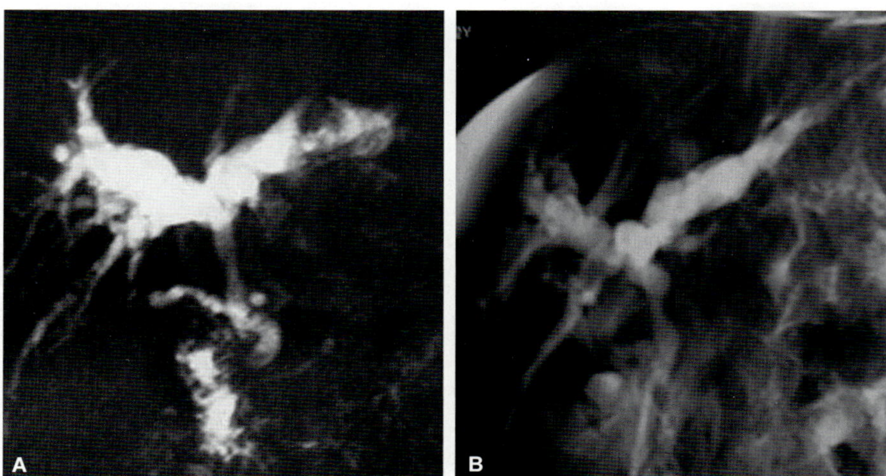

Figs 16.21A and B: Portal Biliopathy. Coronal (A,B) T2W MR scan of two different patients showing multiple extrinsic impressions on the CBD and intrahepatic ducts giving a stretched out nodular appearance

(ERCP/MRCP) may show clotted blood as a cast-like filling defect in the bile ducts and may reveal a bile duct leak or a biliary vascular communication. Blood may be seen as echogenic material in gallbladder or CBD on US. On CT, blood is seen as high attenuating area (> 50 HU) in the gallbladder or bile ducts. Liver laceration, hematoma or other sources of blood may be detected. Hemobilia may be demonstrated by 99m Technetium labeled red blood cells. Selective hepatic arteriography may demonstrate extravasation of contrast material in the biliary tract or a pseudoaneurysm which can be occluded by embolization.

BENIGN TUMORS OF THE BILE DUCT

Benign bile duct tumours are very rare. Adenomas are the most common type. Other benign tumors include fibroma, granular cell tumor, myeloblastoma, neurofibroma, hamartoma, lipoma and leiomyoma. Benign tumors are most frequently found in the periampullary region or in the common bile duct and are quite uncommon in the common hepatic or intrahepatic ducts. Most adenomas are asymptomatic and detected incidentally at the time of surgery. Sonographically they are moderately echogenic nonshadowing filling defects. The lack of shadowing and relatively low echogenicity suggests a tumor rather than a stone. On CT, these are seen as soft tissue masses indistinguishable from noncalcified stones. Cholangiographically the tumors usually present as round or oval filling defect with smooth borders which do not change their position. Papillary adenomas can be multiple.

MALIGNANT LESIONS CAUSING OBSTRUCTIVE BILIOPATHY

- Carcinoma gallbladder
- Cholangiocarcinoma
- Carcinoma head of the pancreas

Carcinoma Gallbladder

Carcinoma gallbladder (Ca GB) is the most common biliary tract malignancy and the incidence is particularly high in some geographic areas including India. Risk factors include cholelithiasis (seen in 75% patients of Ca GB), anomalous pancreaticobiliary ductal union, chronic typhoid infection, porcelain gallbladder and exposure to carcinogenic chemicals.[37] Carcinoma gallbladder is two to three times more common in females and most cases present after 50 years of age. Pain in right upper abdomen is the most common symptom. Nausea, vomiting, weight loss and jaundice can also be seen. Histologically most (90%) Ca GB are adenocarcinomas (papillary, tubular, mucinous or signet cell type).[37] Approximately 60% arise in the fundus 30% in the body and 10% in the neck of gallbladder. Most tumors are inoperable at the time of diagnosis with an average survival of 6 months after the first symptom appears. Long term survival is seen only in patients in whom the tumor is found incidentally at the time of cholecystectomy for gallstones.

Gallbladder carcinoma spreads most commonly via direct invasion of the liver parenchyma. Invasion of the duodenum, stomach, colon and pancreas is seen less often. The rich lymphatic drainage of gallbladder allows rapid spread to lymph nodes most commonly at the porta-hepatis, peripancreatic and paraaortic region (Fig. 16.22). Hematogenous metastases to the liver and peritoneal dissemination can also occur. Biliary obstruction is seen in approximately 50% patients at the time of presentation typically due to direct tumor invasion of the hepatoduodenal ligament, often at the porta hepatis or compression of CBD by lymphadenopathy and infrequently due to intraductal tumor growth or choledocholithiasis.

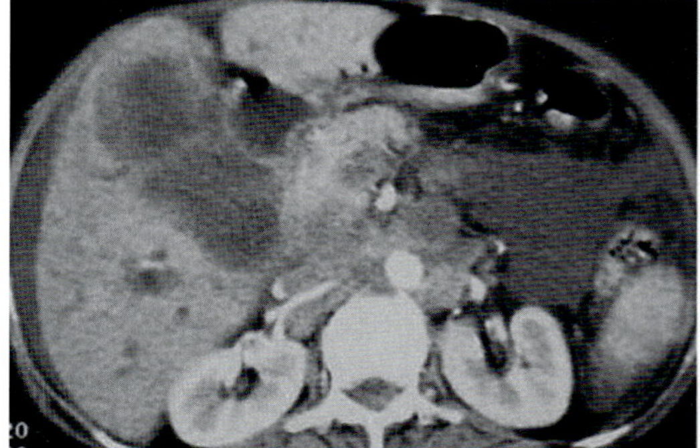

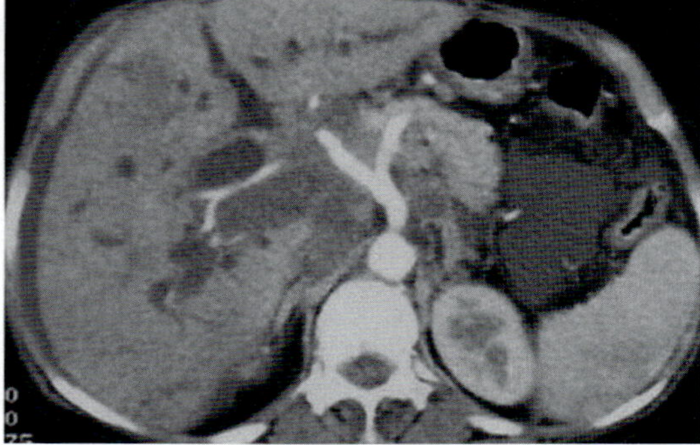

Fig. 16.22: Carcinoma GB. Contrast enhanced CT shows a mass replacing the gallbladder with extensive adenopathy encasing hepatic artery and causing biliary obstruction

The diagnostic accuracy of US in Ca GB exceeds 80%, but it has limitations in tumor staging.[38] Endoscopic US can depict the depth of tumor invasion and can characterize polypoidal lesions.[39] Dynamic contrast-enhanced CT or MRI with MRCP are useful in staging. MRCP depicts biliary involvement better than US or CT and can differentiate adenomyomatosis or chronic cholecystitis from Ca GB.

On imaging Ca GB can appear as focal or diffuse mural thickening or irregularity, as a mass replacing the gall-bladder fossa or as polypoidal mass (Fig. 16.23) or as a combination of these.[40]

A large mass replacing the gallbladder is the most common presentation of Ca GB (42-70%). The mass appears complex with areas of necrosis and typically shows irregular contrast enhancement. These lesions are hypointense on T1-weighted images and heterogeneously hyperintense on T2-weighted images. Early enhancement is a recognized feature on dynamic contrast enhanced MRI. The differential diagnosis includes hepatocellular carcinoma, cholangiocarcinoma or metastasis close to gall bladder fossa.

Focal or diffuse mural thickening is the least common form of Ca GB that is most difficult to diagnose especially in early stages when the tumor can be flat or only slightly elevated. Gallbladder wall thickening is also a nonspecific finding of Ca GB that can be seen in cholecystitis, xanthogranulomatous cholecystitis, adenomyomatosis, portal hypertension, hepatitis, hypoalbuminemia and hepatic, cardiac or renal failure. Gallbladder wall thickening more than 1 cm, focal or asymmetric thickening and mucosal irregularity are suspicious for malignancy. CT is inferior to US in evaluating mural thickening/irregularity. A low attenuation intrahepatic halo around the gallbladder is considered a fairly specific sign of complicated cholecystitis on CT.[41] Xanthogranulomatous cholecystitis results from intramural extravasation of bile caused by rupture of Rokitansky-Aschoff sinuses. CT/US can reveal hypodense or hypoechoic nodules in the GB wall. Xanthogranulomatous cholecystitis may be associated with lymphadenopathy and can be locally invasive thereby closely mimicking Ca GB. Adenomyomatosis results in focal or diffuse GB wall thickening and can mimic Ca GB on CT. MRI however can provide specific diagnosis by revealing T2 hyperintense foci in the GB wall.

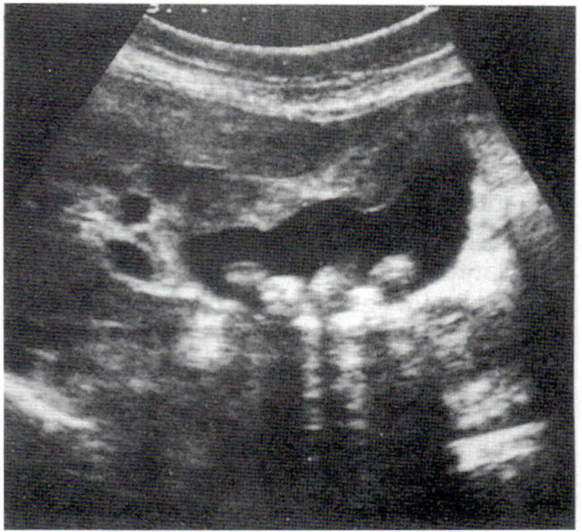

Fig. 16.23: CaGB: A polypoid intraluminal mass is seen along the anterior wall of GB on ultrasound. Gallstones are also seen

The polypoidal form of Ca GB is seen in one fourth cases and is more likely to be confined to the gallbladder at the time of diagnosis. These tumors are usually homogenous, hyperechoic, isoechoic or hypoechoic relative to the liver and do not cast an acoustic shadow. Necrosis or calcification is uncommon and the tumor shows homogenous enhancement. Small polypoidal Ca GB can be indistinguishable from cholesterol polyp, adherent non calcified stone, adenoma, tumefactive sludge or blood clot. Polyps should be removed surgically if the size exceeds one cm, associated calculi are present, age of the patient is more than 50 years and the patient is symptomatic. Sludge is usually mobile when patient's position is changed, is more echogenic than tumor and does not show vascularity unlike tumor.[42]

Ancillary findings that can be seen in all these types include gallstones, gallbladder wall calcification, dilated biliary radicals, hepatic metastases, lymphadenopathy, ascites, and peritoneal deposits and extension into stomach, duodenum, colon or pancreas. The lymph nodes may show necrotic center.

Cholangiocarcinoma

Cholangiocarcinoma is an uncommon tumor with increased prevalence in the Far East and South East Asia where liver fluke infection and choledocholithiasis are common. Other risk factors are primary sclerosing cholangitis, Caroli's disease, choledochal cysts, familial polyposis, congenital hepatic fibrosis, biliary enteric anastomosis and history of exposure to thorotrast.[37]

Incidence peaks in sixth or seventh decade and is slightly more common in males. More than 95% are adenocarcinomas of bile duct epithelium and have abundant fibrous stroma.

Anatomically cholangiocarcinoma are classified as:[43]

- Intrahepatic peripheral cholangiocarcinoma (10%): Arises peripheral to secondary biliary confluence
- Hilar cholangiocarcinoma (25%): Arises from right or left hepatic ducts or from primary biliary confluence
- Extrahepatic cholangiocarcinoma (65%)

Morphologically these tumors are classified as:

- Mass forming cholangiocarcinoma
- Periductal infiltrating cholangiocarcinoma
- Intraductal cholangiocarcinoma

Patients with hilar or extrahepatic cholangiocarcinoma usually present early with painless jaundice while intrahepatic cholangiocarcinoma remains asymptomatic till late. Cholangiocarcinoma is slow growing and metastasizes late so that survival is long if jaundice can be relieved. Patients usually die of hepatocellular failure and infection secondary to biliary obstruction. Local and distant metastases are uncommon even at autopsy. Distally placed tumors are more likely to be resectable than those at the hilum. Ultrasonography is used for initial evaluation and can quickly establish the presence and level of biliary obstruction. CT, MRI and MRCP are required for staging and treatment planning. Cholangiography (ERCP/PTC) is often used to assess the extent of biliary involvement and for palliation.

Intrahepatic (Peripheral) Cholangiocarcinoma

Peripheral intrahepatic cholangiocarcinoma are usually large (mass forming) at presentation because symptoms occur late. Ultrasonography reveals a hypoechoic, isoechoic or hyperechoic mass, which may be homogenous or heterogeneous. Unenhanced CT reveals a hypodense solitary mass that may have satellite lesions. On enhanced CT/MRI, the tumor shows thin rim or thick band of peripheral and patchy enhancement. The central area of the tumor, which contains fibrous tissue, does not enhance during early phase but becomes hyperdense during the delayed phase, 4-20 minutes after injection, a feature which may help to differentiate it from HCC.[44] The delayed enhancement may be bright enough to simulate hemangioma. Focal intrahepatic biliary ductal dilatation and atrophy of the segment of the liver drained by these ducts with retraction of overlying liver capsule may also be seen. On MRI, intrahepatic cholangiocarcinoma is seen as irregular, heterogeneous mass hypointense on T1-weighted images and hyperintense on T2-weighted images.[45] Peripheral cholangiocarcinoma can also be of periductal infiltrating type or intraductal polypoidal type and these may cause segmental bile duct dilatation and lobar atrophy. Polypoidal (papillary) variant can occasionally produce abundant mucin similar to IPMT of the pancreas. This can result in gross dilatation of the bile duct. Demonstration of direct continuity of tumor with bile ducts helps differentiate this entity from biliary cystadenocarcinoma.

Hilar Cholangiocarcinoma (Klatskin Tumor)

Hilar cholangiocarcinoma are usually periductal infiltrating type and most often arise at the primary confluence or in the proximal common hepatic duct (Fig. 16.24). Sonographic findings include intrahepatic bile ductal dilatation with or without isolation of right and left sided ducts and lobar atrophy. Definite mass is rarely seen on US and demonstration of dilated intrahepatic ducts without any evidence of extrahepatic dilatation alone should raise the suspicion of hilar cholangiocarcinoma. Uncommonly the tumor may be seen on US as bile duct wall thickening and less commonly as a polypoidal lesion. The tumors are moderately echogenic, reflecting the fibrous nature of the tumor.

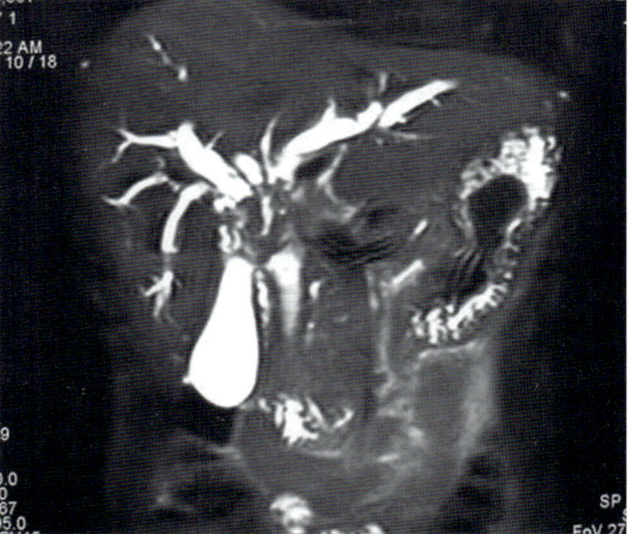

Fig. 16.24: Cholangicarcinoma. Coronal T2W images shows an infiltrating mass at the confluence

CT (particularly MDCT) are superior to US in identification of these small tumors.[46] Although the tumor appears hypodense to liver in both unenhanced and enhanced CT scans, the focally thickened bile duct wall due to infiltrating tumor may appear hyperdense to the liver in the arterial and portal venous phase. In keeping with their fibrous rich stroma, delayed enhancement can be seen 8-15 minutes after contrast injection on CT/MRI.[47] Cholangiocarcinoma are isointense/hypointense on T1-weghted images while T2 signal varies from markedly hyperintense to only mildly increased signal relative to liver in fibrous rich tumors. Lobar hepatic atrophy is seen in one fourth of patients with cholangiocarcinoma and this finding coupled with biliary dilatation is strongly suggestive of cholangiocarcinoma. Atrophy results from long standing biliary obstruction or portal venous involvement and results in crowding of dilated bile ducts and volume loss most often affecting the left lobe of liver.[45] Contiguous invasion of the liver parenchyma and hepatoduodenal ligament is frequent in Klatskin tumors. Lymph nodal metastases can be seen in periportal and peripancreatic regions. Retroperitoneal adenopathy, proximal intestinal obstruction and peritoneal dissemination occur in advanced stages.

Diagnostic PTC and ERCP are now less commonly employed for cholangiocarcinoma. The involved ducts appear stenosed with smooth shouldering or irregular tapering on cholangiography/MRCP. CT and cholangiography provide complimentary information as superficial (mucosal) involvement is better assessed on direct cholangiography while submucosal/extramucosal involvement and areas not opacified on cholangiography are better seen on CT. MRCP coupled with contrast enhanced MRI can provide most comprehensive tumor staging. [48] Imaging is essential to select operable patients. Hilar cholangiocarcinoma are unresectable if they involve bilateral secondary confluence or main portal vein or hepatic artery or bilateral vascular involvement or vascular involvement on one side and extensive bile duct involvement on the other side.

Hilar Cholangiocarcinoma are Graded according to Bismuth Classification.[49]

Type I: Involves common hepatic duct only, confluence patent (Fig. 16.25)

Type II: Involves primary confluence. (Fig. 16.26).

Type III: Involves primary and either right/left side secondary confluence (Fig. 16.27).

Type IV: Involves bilateral secondary confluence

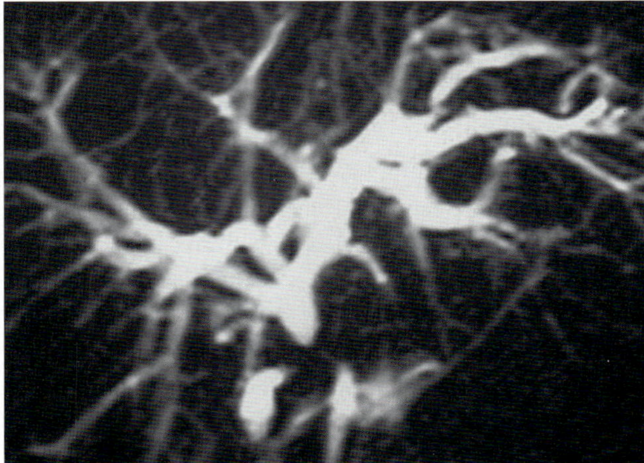

Fig. 16.25: Malignant Biliary Stricture Type 1. Coronal T2W coronal thick slab image shows an abrupt stricture of the common hepatic duct

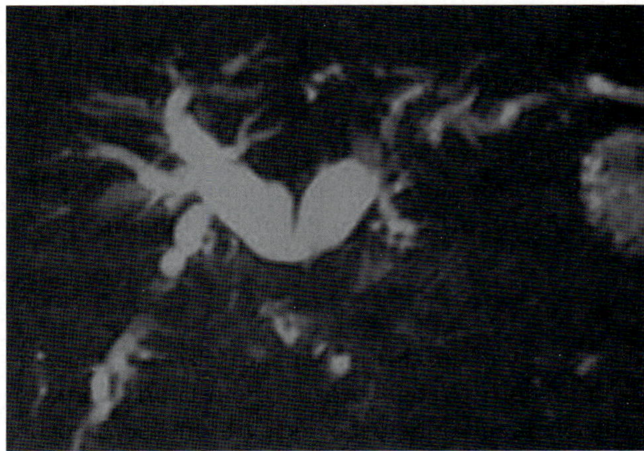

Fig. 16.26: Malignant Biliary Stricture Type 2. Coronal T2W coronal thick slab image shows an abrupt stricture at the confluence

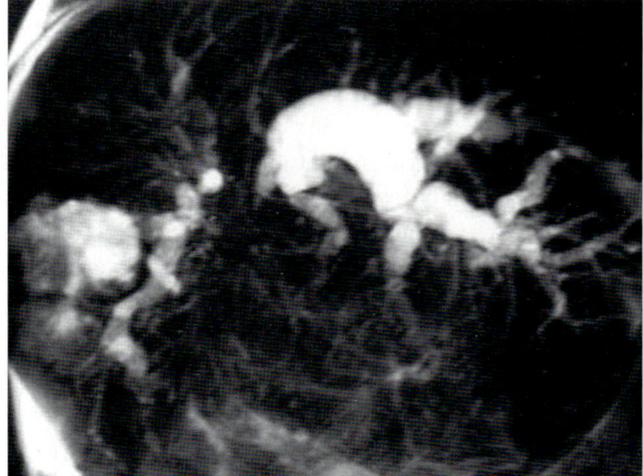

Fig. 16.27: Malignant Biliary Stricture Type 3. Coronal T2W coronal thick slab image shows an abrupt stricture involving the primary and right secondary confluence. A metastatic lesion is noted in the right lobe of liver

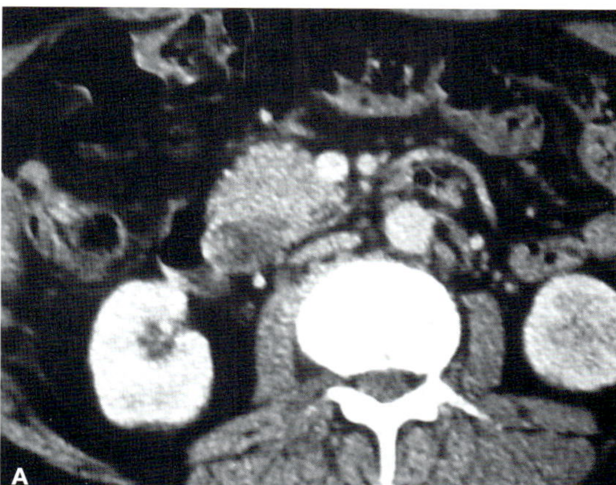

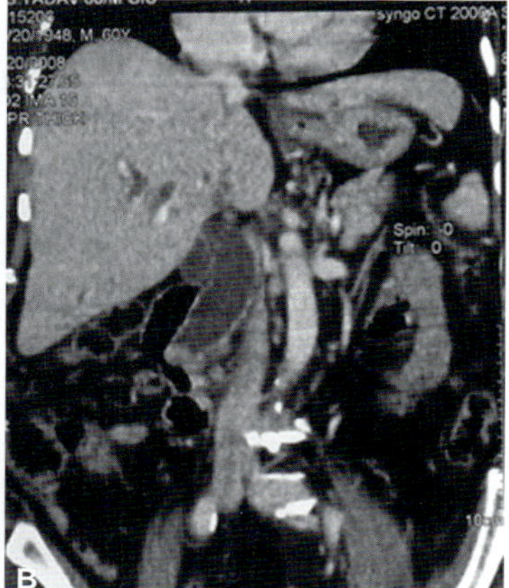

Figs 16.28A and B: Periampullary Carcinoma. Contrast enhanced axial CT (A) and coronal reformatted image (B) shows an enhancing polypoidal mass at the lower end of CBD causing biliary obstruction

Extrahepatic Cholangiocarcinoma

Extrahepatic cholangiocarcinoma are usually small and have better prognosis tha Klatskin tumors. Fifty to 75% occur in the proximal third, 10-30% in middle third and 10-20% arise in the distal third of the extrahepatic duct. Ultrasound demonstrates biliary dilatation proximal to an abrupt obstruction. Site of the lesion will determine the GB distention. Demonstration of mass is rare, so that differentiation from benign strictures may be difficult. In the absence of history of previous surgery, cholangiocarcinoma should be suspected when abrupt obstruction of distal duct is seen without visualisation of a mass or calculus and the pancreas is normal. If the mass is seen near head of the pancreas, carcinoma of the pancreas is more likely.[45] The bile duct at the level of obstruction in cholangiocarcinoma is narrowed if the process is primarily desmoplastic and widened if there is an obstructing intraluminal mass. Demonstration of the lesion in the form of wall thickening, persistent intraluminal echoes or an obstructing mass largely depends on the skill of the radiologist and resolution of the ultrasound equipment. CT manifestations of cholangiocarcinoma include biliary dilatation till the level of obstruction and less commonly, demonstration of a mass. The diagnosis is suggested by abrupt cut-off without a mass or calculus. Diffuse, enhancing wall thickening may be seen. If a mass is seen, it is hypodense in nonenhanced scans and shows delayed enhancement. Rarely, a peripheral ring enhancement pattern is seen.[50]

Cholangiography reveals a short stricture which appears as U or V shaped occlusion having nipple, rat tail, smooth or irregular termination with prestenotic dilatation. Polypoidal lesions are less common and are seen as nodular or polypoidal intraluminal filling defects attached to the wall. The diffuse sclerosing type of cholangiocarcinoma causes widespread strictures of both intra and extrahepatic ducts resembling sclerosing cholangitis. Clues for the correct diagnosis of cholangiocarcinoma include absence of diverticuli, more severe disease in extrahepatic ducts and prominent dilatation of the ducts.

Periampullary carcinoma is the term used to describe tumours that arise from or within 1 cm of the papilla of Vater. These include pancreatic, bile duct, ampullary and duodenal cancers. Histologic examination is often not able to differentiate these tumors. Because of their strategic location, jaundice occurs early and hence tumors are detected when very small. Periampullary tumors tend to be polypoidal and lower in grade than more proximal biliary neoplasm (Figs 16.28A and B). Consequently, these tumours have much better prognosis. On imaging, the biliary obstruction is seen till the level of ampulla, with or without dilatation of pancreatic duct is seen. Liver metastases and lymphadenopathy is present in only a minority of cases.

Carcinoma Head of the Pancreas

Carcinoma of the head of the pancreas is an important cause of biliary obstruction. It is described in detail in the chapter on pancreas.

OTHER MALIGNANT TUMORS OF BILIARY TRACT

Biliary cystadenoma and cystadenocarcinoma: These are rare biliary tract tumors that arise from intrahepatic bile ducts and are lined by mucin secreting columnar epithelium Majority occur in middle - aged women. The tumor appears as a unilocular or multilocular cystic mass with mural nodularity. Each loculus may have a different CT density and fluid -fluid levels may be seen.[45] CT is superior to US in showing tumor extent while US reveals internal morphology better. Cystadenomas can have papillary growths, mural nodules and occasionally fine septal calcifications. Thick, coarse mural and septal calcifications and solid areas are seen more often in cystadenocarcinomas. These tumors generally do not communicate with large intrahepatic ducts. Differential diagnosis includes hepatic cysts, hydatid cyst, liver abscess, hematoma, cystic metastases, choledochal cyst and intraductal mucin secreting cholangiocarcinoma. In adults cholangiocarcinoma and cystadenocarcinoma account for most malignant tumors of the biliary tree. Lymphoma, Leiomyosarcoma, carcinoid tumors and metastases rarely occur in the bile ducts. Embryonal rhabdomyosarcoma (Sarcoma botryoides) is the second most common cause of obstructive jaundice in children beyond infancy; first being choledochal cyst. Average age of onset is four years with rapid progression and death. It grows along the wall of CBD beneath the mucosa resulting in polypoidal intraluminal projections. US and CT show dilated intrahepatic ducts and a soft tissue mass in the region of CBD. On cholangiography, grape like filling defects are seen in dilated CBD.

REFERENCES

1. Fulcher AS, Turner MA. MR Cholangiopancreatography RCNA 2002;40:1363-76.
2. Kwon M, Uetsuji S, Boku T, et al. Three-dimensional cholangiography with spiral CT for analysis of the biliary tract - preliminary report. Nippon Geka Gakkai Zasshi 1993;94:658.
3. Slockberger SM, Wass JL, Sherman S, et al. Intravenous cholangiography with helical CT- comparison with endoscopic retrograde cholangiography. Radiology 1994;192:675-80.
4. Niederau C, Muller J, Sonnenberg A, et al. Extrahepatic bile ducts in healthy subjects, in patients with cholelithiasis and in post cholecystectomy patients: A prospective ultrasonic study. J Clin Ultrasound 1983;11:23-27.
5. Mallery S, Dam JV. Current status of diagnostic and therapeutic endoscopic ultrasonography. RCNA 2001;39:449-63.
6. Wallner BK, Schumacher KA, Weidenmaier W, et al. Dilated biliary tract: Evaluation with MR cholangiography with a T2 weighted contrast enhanced fast sequence Radiology 1991;181:805-08.
7. Masci E, Toli G, Mariani A, et al. Complications of diagnostic and therapeutic ERCP: A prospective multicenter study. Am J Gastroentrol 2001;96:417-23.
8. Raraty MG, Finch M, Neoptolemos JP. Acute cholangitis and pancreatitis secondary to common duct stones: Management update. World J Surg 1998;22:1155-61.
9. Berk RN, Leopold GR. The present status of imaging of the gallbladder. Invest Radio 1978;13:477-89.
10. Koenigsberg M, Weiner SN, Salzer A. The accuracy of sonography in the differential diagnosis of obstructive jaundice-A comparison with cholangiography. Radiology 1979;133:157-65.
11. Bhargava S, Vashisht S, Kakaria A, et al. Choledocholithiasis-An ultrasonic study with comparative evaluation with ERCP/PTC. Australas Radiol 1988;32: 220-26.
12. Pedrosa CS, Casanova R, Lezana AH, et al. Computed tomography in obstructive jaundice, Part II-The cause of obstruction . Radiology 1981;139:635-45.
13. Genevieve L Bennet. Cholelithiasis, Cholecystitis, Choledocholithiasis and Hyperplastic cholecystoses. In Richard M Gore and Marc S Levine (Editors): Textbook of Gastrointestinal Radiology. (Third Edition) Saunders Elsevier 2008.
14. Baron RL. Common bile duct stones: Reassessment of criteria for CT diagnosis. Radiology 1987;162:419-424
15. Cabadas Giadas T, Sarria Octavia de Toledo L, Martinez-Berganza Asensio MT, et al. Helical CT cholangiography in the evaluation of the biliary tract: Application to the diagnosis of choledocholithiasis. Abdominal Imaging 2002;27: 61-70.
16. Fulcher AS, Turner MA, Capps GW, et al. Half Fourier RARE: MR Cholangiopancreatography in 300 subjects. Radiology 199;207:21-328.
17. Reinhold C, Taourel P, Bret P et al. Choledocholelithiasis: Evaluation of MR cholangiography for diagnosis Radiology 1998;209:435-42.
18. Soto JA, Barish MA, Alvarez O, et al. Detection of choledocholithiasis with MR cholangiography: Comparison of three-dimensional fast spin-echo and single and multisection half fourier rapid acquisition with relaxation enhancement sequences. Radiology 2000;215:737-45.
19. Hartman EM, Barish MA. MR cholangiography. Magn Reson Imaging Clin N Am 2001;4:841-55.
20. Lillemoe KD: Benign post-operative bile duct strictures. Baillieres Clin Gastroenterol 1997;11:749-79
21. Vashisht S, Tandon RK, Berry M. Postoperative bile duct strictures-Ultrasound and endoscopic retrograde cholangiopancreatography/percutaneous transhepatic cholangiography evaluation. Australas Radiol 1993;37: 325-28.
22. Bismuth H. The biliary tract-post-operative strictures of the bile duct. In Blumgart LII (Ed): Clinic Surgery International Edinburgh: Churchill Livingstone 1982;5: 209-18.
23. Mishra MC, Vashisht S, Tandon RK. Biliobiliary fistula-preoperative diagnosis and management implications. Surgery 1990;108:835-39.

24. Todani T, Watanabe Y, Narusue M, et al. Congenital bile duct cysts-Classification, operative procedures, and review of thirty-seven cases including cancer arising from choledochal cysts. Am J Surg 1977;134:263-69.
25. Renter K, Raptopoulos VD, Cantelmo N, et al. The diagnosis of a choledochal cyst by ultrasound. Radiology 1980;136: 437-38.
26. Aggarwal S, Tandon RK, Vashisht S. Radiologic approach to choledochal cysts. Ind J Gastroenterol 1989;8:107-08.
27. Matos C, Nicaise N, Deviere J, et al. Choledochal cysts: Comparison of findings at MR cholangiopancreatography and endoscopic retrograde cholangiopancreatography in eight patients. Radiology 1998;209:443-48.
28. Gulliver DJ, Baker ME, Putnam W, et al. Bile duct diverticulae and Webs-nonspecific cholangiographic features of primary sclerosing cholangitis. AJR 1991;157: 281-85.
29. Sharma R, Vashisht S, Singh SP, et al. Sonographic features of sclerosing cholangitis. Ind J Radiol Imag 1994;4:153-56.
30. Federle MP, Cello JP, Laing FC, et al. Recurrent pyogenic cholangitis in Asian immigrants-use of ultrasonography, computed tomography and cholangiography. Radiology 1982;143:151-56.
31. Kumar A, Lal BK, Vashisht S, et al. Hydatid jaundice: A case report and review of literature. Indian Practitioner 1992;65:321-24.
32. Doyle TCA, Roberts-Thomson IC, Dudley FJ. Demonstration of intrabiliary rupture of hepatic hydatid cyst by retrograde cholangiography. Australas Radiol 1988;32: 92-97
33. Kumar R, Reddy SN, Thulkar S. Intrabiliary rupture of hydatid cyst: Diagnosis with MRI and hepatobiliary isotope study (A case report) Br J Radiology 2002;75: 271-74.
34. Maglinte DDT, Alvarez SZ, et al. Patterns of calcification and cholangiographic findings in hepatobiliary tuberculosis. Gastrointestinal Radiol 1988;13: 331.
35. Pombo F, Soler R, Arrojo L, et al. US and CT findings in biliary obstruction due to tubercular adenitis in the periportal areas-2 cases. Eur J Radiol 1989;9:71.
36. Baron RL, Campbell WL. Non-neoplastic diseases of the bile ducts. In Freeney PC, Stevenson GW (Eds): Margulis and Burchnne's Alimentary Tract Radiology. St. Louis: Mosby Year Book 1994;1294-1324.
37. Sherlock S, Dooley J. Tumours of the gallbladder and bile ducts. In Sherlock S, Dooley J (Ed) Diseases of the liver and biliary system. Blackwell science. 11th edition, Oxford 2002;647-56.
38. Bach AM, Loring LA, Hann LE, et al. Gall bladder cancer: Can ultrasonography evaluate extent of disease? J Ultrasound Med 1998;17:303-09.
39. Soyer P, Gouhiri M, Boudiaf M, et al. Carcinoma of the gall bladder: Imaging features with surgical correlation. AJR 1997;169:781-84.
40. Kumar A, Aggarwal S, Berry M, et al. Ultrasonography of the carcinoma of the gallbladder: an analysis of 80 cases. J Clin Ultrasound 1990;18:715-20.
41. Schwartz LH, Black J, Fong Y, et al.Gal bladder carcinoma: Findings at MR imaging with MR cholangiopancreatography. J Comput Assist Tomogr 2002;26:405-10.
42. Wilbur AC, Sagieddy PB, Aizenstein RL. Carcinoma of the gallbladder: Colour Doppler ultrasound and CT findings. Abdom Imaging 1997;22:187-89.
43. Baron RL, Tublin ME, Peterson MS: Imaging the spectrum of biliary tract disease. RCNA 2002;40: 1325-54.
44. Loyer FM, Chin H, DuBrow RA, et al. Hepatocellular carcinoma and intrahepatic peripheral cholangiocarcinoma. Enhancement patterns with quadruple phase helical CT. Radiology 1999;212:866-71.
45. Choi IB, Han KJ, Kim TK. Benign and malignant tumours of the biliary tract. In Gazelle GC, Saini S, Meuller PR (Eds) Hepatobiliary and pancreatic radiology. New York, 1st edition, Thieme 1998;630-76.
46. Choi BI, Lee JH, Han MC: Hilar cholangiocarcinoma. Comparative study with sonography and CT. Radiology 1989;172:689-92.
47. Motohara T, Semelka RC, Bidar TR. MR cholangiopancreatography. RCNA 2003;41:89-96.
48. Yeh TS, Jan YY, Tseng JH, et al. Malignant perihilar biliary obstruction: MRCP findings. Am J Gastroenterol 2000;95: 432-40.
49. Bismuth H, Corlette MB: Intrahepatic cholangioenteric anastomosis in carcinoma of the hilus of the liver. Surg Gynecol Obstet 1975;140:170-78.
50. Takayusu K, Ikeya S, Mukai K, et al. CT of hilar cholangiocarcinoma-Late contrast enhancement in six patients. AJR 1996;154:1203-06.

Chapter Seventeen

Clinical Aspects of Liver Cirrhosis: A Perspective for the Radiologist

Shashi Bala Paul, Shivanand R Gamanagatti,
Arun Kumar Gupta, Subrat Kumar Acharya

INTRODUCTION

Cirrhosis is defined as the histological development of regenerative nodules surrounded by fibrous bands in response to chronic liver injury, which leads to portal hypertension and end-stage liver disease.[1] Diagnosis of cirrhosis is histological and role of imaging in determining the presence of cirrhosis is limited. On the contrary, it plays a vital role in the detection and treatment of complications of this end stage liver disease, in particular, portal hypertension and hepatocellular carcinoma (HCC). Imaging also has a key role in the screening of this "at risk" population and the therapeutic manoeuvres required for complicated cases of cirrhosis. It is therefore imperative for the radiologists to understand the clinical aspects and natural course of this disease.

Epidemiology

Precise prevalence of cirrhosis worldwide is difficult to ascertain and is unknown. It is estimated to be 0.15% in USA.[1] Similar burden has been reported from Europe, whereas higher figures are noted in Asia and Africa on account of higher prevalence of chronic viral infections of Hepatitis B or C. These figures are most likely an underestimate because compensated cirrhosis invariably remains undetected due to lack of overt symptomatology. Additionally, in countries where problems of non-alcoholic steatohepatitis and hepatitis C exist, there is a high prevalence of undiagnosed cirrhosis in these patients. It is estimated that upto 1% of the population could have histological cirrhosis.[1]

In India, the exact burden of this disease is not known. However, HBV infection is of intermediate endemicity with nearly 4% of the population being chronic HBV carriers.[2] Frequency of HCV infections is just about 0.87% in the community.[3]

Pathology

Cirrhosis is always preceded by several reversible pathologic changes, including steatosis and inflammation, before irreversible changes set in. Fibrosis causes architectural distortion and results in the development of a spectrum of nodules ranging from benign regenerating nodules to hepatocellular carcinoma (HCC).[4] In assessing the stage, the degree of fibrosis is used as a quantitative measure. The amount of fibrosis is staged on a 0–4+ (histology activity index) or 0–6+ (Ishak scale).[5]

The nodular lesions are classified as regenerative, dysplastic or neoplastic according to the international nomenclature of hepatocellular nodules proposed in 1994.[6] Regenerative nodules represent a region of hepatic parenchyma that enlarges in response to necrosis and is surrounded by fibrous septa. The regenerative nodules are classified as micronodular (< 3 mm), macronodular (> 3 mm), or mixed forms. Macronodules rarely exceed 20 mm in size. When regenerative nodules contain iron, they are called siderotic nodules. Dysplastic nodules are classified as low or high grade on the basis of a spectrum of pathologic changes that include HCC. One such change is the appearance of a new vascular supply to the nodule, which becomes the dominant blood supply in large dysplastic nodules and the small HCC.[7]

Causes and Risk Factors of Cirrhosis

Multiple causes of cirrhosis are known (Table 17.1).[8] These can invariably be identified by patient's history combined with serological and histological investigations. In North America, approximately 75% of patients with cirrhosis are chronic alcoholics. Viral hepatitis and other identifiable causes are seen in about 15% of patients; the remaining 10% of cases are of idiopathic (cryptogenic) cirrhosis. In Asia and Africa, cirrhosis is associated predominantly with chronic viral hepatitis.[9]

In India, 50% of the chronic liver disease is due to HBV and 20% due to HCV infection.[2,10] Identification of cause of cirrhosis helps in predicting complications and planning treatment. Regular (moderate) alcohol consumption, older age (> 50 years) are important risk factors for developing cirrhosis in chronic hepatitis C infection. While, obesity, older age, insulin resistance or type 2 diabetes, hypertension and hyperlipidemia are identified in non-alcoholic steatohepatitis.[1]

Table 17.1 Main causes of cirrhosis

Etiology	*Examples*
Infectious	Hepatitis B,C,D Schistosomiasis Syphilis HIV (sclerosing cholangitis)
Metabolic/inherited	Non-alcoholic steatohepatitis (NASH) in association with the metabolic syndrome Wilson's disease Haemochromatosis Alpha-1 antitrypsin deficiency Glycogen storage disease Cystic fibrosis Tyrosinemia Galactosemia Fructose intolerance Byler's disease Mucopolysaccharidosis Abetalipoproteinemia Prophyria Wolman's disease
Biliary disease	Extrahepatic obstruction Intrahepatic obstruction
Immunological	Autoimmune hepatitis Primary biliary cirrhosis Primary sclerosing cholangitis
Vascular	Veno-occlusive disease Budd-Chiari syndrome Cardiac failure Hereditary haemorrhagic telangiectasia
Drugs and toxins	Alcohol Amiodarone Dantrolene Halothane Isoniazid Methotrexate Methyldopa Aflatoxin Diclofenac Hypervitaminosis A
Miscellaneous	Indian childhood Malnutrition Sarcoidosis Ischemia Graft vs. host disease

Natural History and Prognosis

The natural history of cirrhosis is related to its underlying etiology and the treatment. Yearly decompensation rates for hepatitis C and B are 4% and 10% respectively. The decompensation in alcoholic cirrhosis with continued alcohol use is extremely rapid. Once the decompensation sets in, the mortality (without transplant) is as high as 85% in 5 years. Mortality of HCC associated with cirrhosis is rising in most developed countries whereas mortality with cirrhosis not related to HCC is decreasing.[11]

Severity of Cirrhosis

Cirrhosis is graded on the basis of the Child Pugh Turcotte (CPT) classification[12] which takes into account the findings of serum bilirubin, serum albumin, prothrombin time, presence of ascites and encephalopathy (Table 17.2). Estimated child's score categorizes the severity of cirrhosis into CPT class A, B and C on the score of 6 and less, 7-9 and more than 10 respectively. CPT class also predicts the development of complications and response to treatment. The 1-year survival rates of CPT class A, B and C patients are 100%, 80% and 45%

Table 17.2 Child pugh classification for grading the child's score

Clinical and biochemical measurements	*Points for increasing abnormality* 1	2	3
Encephalopathy (grade)	None	I and II	III and IV
Ascites	-	Mild	Moderate
Bilirubin (mg/dl)	1-2	>2-3	>3
Albumin (g/dl)	>3.5	2.8-3.5	<2.8
Prothrombin time (seconds prolonged)	1-4	>4-6	>6

Total score 5-6 = Child's A, 7-9 = Child's B, 10 or more-Child's C respectively.[13] The model for end stage liver disease (MELD)[14] has been developed more recently, which provides better prediction of severity and short-term mortality. The model is based on creatinine, bilirubin and international normalized ratio (INR) and does not include features of portal hypertension.

Types of Cirrhosis

Morphologically, cirrhosis is classified into micronodular, macronodular and mixed forms. Micronodular form is characterized by presence of micronodular regenerative nodules of relatively uniform and small size. This pattern is seen in cirrhosis from chronic alcoholism and hepatitis C, in patients with biliary cirrhosis. In macronodular cirrhosis, the parenchymal nodules are larger, coarser, and more variable in size. The most common cause of macronodular cirrhosis is chronic hepatitis B. Mixed cirrhosis consists of both micronodular and macronodular forms in equal proportions.

Clinically, cirrhosis is divided into two types, compensated and decompensated. Compensated cirrhosis is often indolent and may progress insidiously. It is usually detected incidentally on routine clinical examination, biochemical screening, during abdominal surgery for some other ailment or on autopsy. About 30-40% of cases of cirrhosis may be asymptomatic.[15] In others, cirrhosis may be suspected when non specific symptoms like low grade fever, general deterioration, anorexia, anemia, and weight loss appear.

Decompensated cirrhosis has clinical manifestations (Table 17.3) resulting from a mix of hepatocellular insufficiency, fibrosis and distorted architecture which consists of jaundice, edema, coagulopathy, metabolic

Table 17.3 Clinical features of cirrhosis

	Description	*Cause*
Jaundice occurs	Icterus	Compromized hepatocyte excretory function, when serum bilirubin >20 mg/L
Spider angiomata	Central arteriole with tiney radiating vessels, mainly on trunk and face	Raised estradiol, decreased estradiol degradation in liver
Nodular liver	Irregular, hard surface on papation	Fibrosis, irregular regeneration
Splenomegaly	Enlarge on palpation or in ultrasound	Portal hypertension, splenic congestion
Ascites	Proteinaceous fluid in abdominal cavity, clinically detected when $\geq$1.5L	Portal hypertension
Caput medusae	Prominent veins radiating from umbilicus	Portal hypertension, reopening of umbilical vein that shunt blood from portal vein
Cruveihier-Baumgarten syndrome	Epigastric vascular murmur	Shunts from portal vein to umbilical vein branches, can be present without Caput medusae
Palmar erythema	Erythema sparing central portion of the palm	Increased estradiol, decreased estradiol degradation in liver
White nails	Horizontal white bands or proximal white nail plate	Hypoalbuminemia
Hypertrophic osteoarthropathy/ finger clubbing	Painful proliferative osteoarthropathy of long bones	Hypoxemia due to right-toleft shunting, portopulmonary hypertension
Dupuytren's contracture	Fibrosis and contraction of palmar fascia	Enhanced oxidative stress, increased inosine (alcohol exposure or diabetes)
Gynecomastia, loss of male hair pattern	Benign proliferation of glandular male breast tissue	Enhanced conversion of androstenedione to estrone and estradiol, reduced estradiol degradation in liver
Hypogonadism	Mainly in alcoholic cirrhosis and haemochromatosis	Direct toxic effect of alcohol or iron
Flapping tremor (asterixis)	Asynchronous flapping motions of dorsiflexed hands	Hepatic encephalopathy, disinhibition of motor neurons
Foetor hepaticus	Sweet, pungent smell	Volatile dimethylsulfide, espically in portosystemic shunting and liver failure
Anorexia, fatigue, weight loss, muscle wasting	Occurs in >50% of patients with cirrhosis	Catabolic metabolism by diseased liver, secondary to anorexia
Type 2 diabetes	Occurs in 15-30% of patients with cirrhosis	Distrubed glucose use or decreased insulin removal by the liver

disturbances, gastroesophageal varices, ascites, spontaneous bacterial peritonitis, splenomegaly and hepatic encephalopathy.[16]

Diagnosis of Cirrhosis

Since diagnosis of cirrhosis is based on the histological findings, therefore, liver biopsy has been regarded as the 'gold standard'. Nonetheless, it has numerable limitations. Therefore, in practical clinical terms, the diagnosis of cirrhosis is formulated on the basis of clinical, biochemical, hematological, endoscopic and radiological findings.

Clinical evaluation includes detailed history and physical examination. Investigations include complete blood count, liver function tests and serum alphafetoprotein. Viral markers for hepatitis B include HBsAg, total anti-HBc, HBeAg and HBVDNA while for hepatitis C are anti-HCV and HCV RNA. Auto immune markers are done if the markers of hepatitis B and C are found negative. Radiological work up comprises of an abdominal ultrasonogram (US), triple-phase CT (TPCT) of the liver and or contrast enhanced multiphasic MRI.

Endoscopy

Endoscopy is routinely performed in patients of cirrhosis to look for the presence of esophageal varices. The size, extent and the appearance of varices is of immense relevance clinically. Grading of varices is done since the risk of bleeding increases with the size.[17] and associated mucosal abnormalities.[18] The stomach and duodenum are evaluated for features of gastropathy due to portal hypertension and associated ulcers are also looked for.

Liver Biopsy

Liver biopsy is needed to confirm cirrhosis in patients with compensated liver function in whom imaging by US is usually normal. On the other hand if clear signs of cirrhosis are present like, shrunken liver, ascites or coagulopathy, biopsy confirmation is not necessary.[1] Additionally, sequential histological grading and staging of fibrosis can assess the risk of progression. It is important for establishing the cause of cirrhosis in upto 20% of patients with previous unknown cause. The procedure is associated with a significant level of morbidity and mortality. The sensitivity of liver biopsy is lower than 80% in detecting cirrhosis particularly in macronodular cirrhosis.[19]

The method of obtaining liver biopsy varies from blind to image guided transabdominal approach, transjugular, laparoscopic, open approach at surgery or autopsy. Studies have shown that use of ultrasound guidance reduces the complication rate and improves results in terms of quality of samples.[20,21] In patients with increased risk of hemorrhage, a transjugular liver biopsy route is preferable. The percutaneous procedure of liver biopsy is the most commonly employed route.

Aspirin and other antiplatelet drugs should be stopped one week before the scheduled procedure. Mild sedation is given prior and using local anesthesia, a 14/18 gauge needle is introduced under aseptic conditions into the last intercostal space as low and lateral, to avoid injury to the gallbladder and vascular structures. Biopsy is performed in sustained expiration to avoid penetrating the pleural space.

The contraindications to percutaneous liver biopsy are an uncooperative patient, coagulopathy, abundant ascites that can increase the risk for hemorrhage, or generalized dilatation of the intrahepatic bile ducts, with an associated risk for choleperitoneum. Only 2-35% require hospitalization for the management of complications, of which pain and hypotension are the predominant causes. A total of 60% of the complications are recorded within 2 hours of biopsy while 96% occur within 24 hours. The mortality, mainly due to severe bleeding is extremely rare. If the coagulopathy is moderate, it is possible to perform percutaneous liver biopsy with a preliminary transfusion of fresh plasma or platelets.

Imaging in Cirrhosis

Role of imaging in the evaluation of cirrhosis is primarily for characterizing the morphologic manifestations of the disease, and for the detection and quantitation of complications of cirrhosis that is, ascites, portal hypertension, hepatic vein and portal vein thrombosis and detection and characterization of hepatocellular carcinoma (HCC). It is important to highlight that normal imaging findings do not exclude compensated cirrhosis. At the same time, in some patients with clinically unsuspected disease, the morphologic characteristics of the disease may be detected incidentally during abdominal imaging as part of screening strategies.

Role of US in determining the presence of cirrhosis is limited. US is widely available, inexpensive and provides vital information pertaining to the hepatic architecture. In the early stages, the liver appears normal in majority of the cases while late changes in cirrhosis are often detected. These changes are, coarse, heterogeneous echo pattern of the liver, change of hepatic morphology, liver surface nodularity (Figs 17.1A and B) and shrunken size of the liver.

US is very useful in the detection of complications of cirrhosis (Figs 17.2A to C).[22,23] Doppler US (DU) and Colour Doppler are useful in the evaluation of vascular structures by virtue of their ability for prompt differentiation between vascular and nonvascular structures. DU is the initial technique for confirming suspected portal hypertension, differentiating benign from malignant thrombus, evaluating portal or hepatic venous system, characterizing hepatic parenchymal disease and lastly screening for complications of cirrhosis like HCC. US is the first imaging modality for suspected HCC, although its sensitivity and specificity is less than that of CT and MRI.

Conventional CT and MRI can be used to define the severity of cirrhosis Findings in cirrhosis are variable. Early parenchymal changes in cirrhosis may be subtle and not visible, while morphological changes of advanced cirrhosis are easily seen. Multiphasic contrast enhanced CT and MRI are the modalities of choice for the detection and characterization of the liver nodules in the background of a cirrhotic liver. By assessing characteristic changes in signal intensity, specific MR sequences allow for accurate detection of hepatic iron and fat content in hemochromatosis and liver steatosis.[24,25]

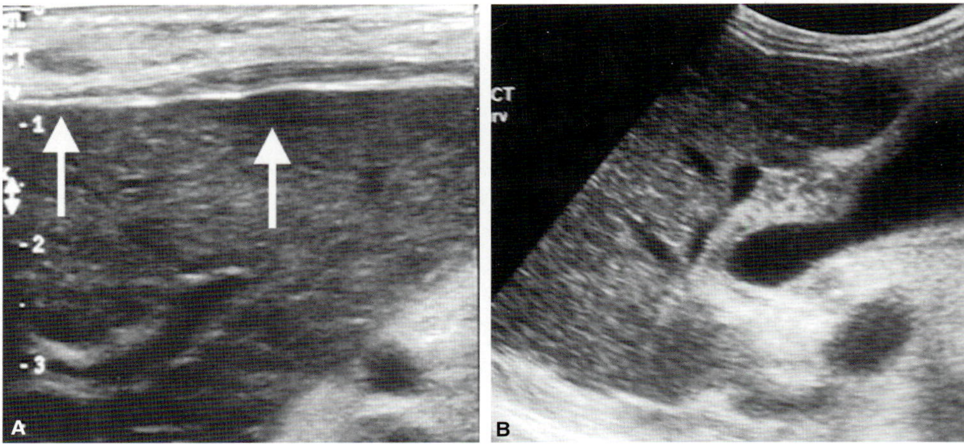

Figs 17.1A and B: (A) High frequency US showing the wavy and nodular outline of the surface of the liver in cirrhosis. The liver shows in addition coarsened echotexture in a case of cirrhosis. (B) It is particularly useful to look for nodularity of the liver adjacent to the gallbladder

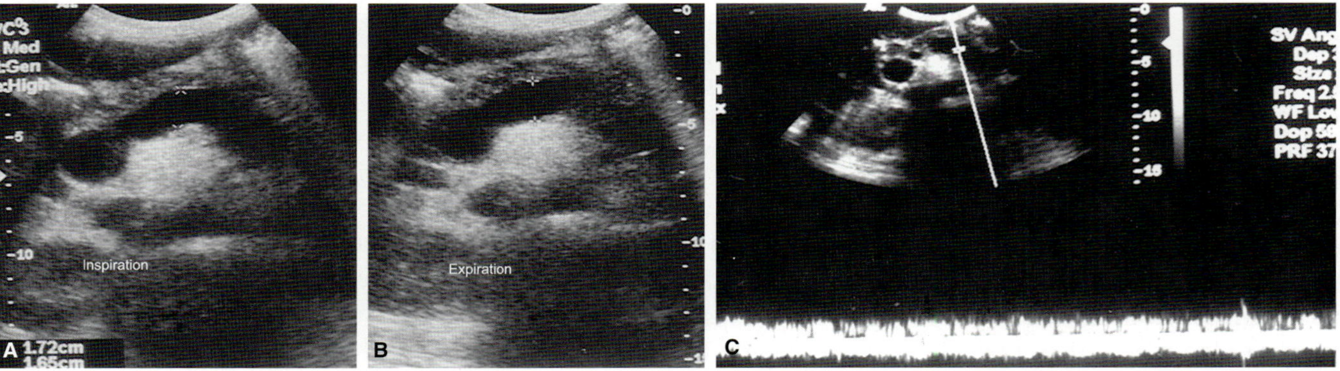

Figs 17.2A to C: (A and B) US of a known cirrhotic patient showing no appreciable change in size of the splenic vein during inspiration or expiration suggesting presence of portal hypertension. (C) Doppler of the same patient depicting dilated portal vein with continuous waveform without respiratory variation

A promising new noninvasive technique for assessment of liver fibrosis has come into existence.[26] The measurement of liver stiffness is made on the velocity of the elastic wave via the intercostally placed transmitter. The shear wave velocity is estimated by pulse ultrasound and correlates with liver fibrosis. These elastic scans represent a useful, noninvasive diagnostic test for cirrhosis.

Complications of Cirrhosis

Recent advances have focused on preventing and treating complications of cirrhosis. Major clinical challenges are the complications of portal hypertension that include ascites, hypersplenism, renal dysfunction (hepatorenal syndrome) and gastrointestinal hemorrhage. The latter occurs more frequently and is most dramatic. Prospective studies show that as large as 90% of patients of cirrhosis will develop esophageal varices and a third of these would bleed.[27] More recently, there has been an increasing understanding of cirrhosis *per se* on the myocardium resulting in cirrhotic cardiomyopathy. Sepsis is known to occur in 30-40% of hospital admissions due to cirrhosis[28] and this leads to 30% excess mortality independent of the severity of the liver disease. Haematological, endocrine, pulmonary and cardiac complications are also encountered. Gall stones and peptic ulcer are more common in these patients. However, it is the development of HCC that is the most severe and fatal complication.

Cirrhosis and HCC

More than 80% of the HCCs arise in cirrhotic liver. It is the fifth most common neoplasm in the world, and the third most common cause of cancer-related deaths.[30] Incidence of HCC ranges from 5-15 patients per 100,000 in Europe and United states, and between 27-36 patients per 100,000 in Asian countries In India, the estimated incidence is 1.6% per year.[29] It affects 5% of the asymptomatic cirrhotics and 15-20% of patients with acute decompensation in both low and high incidence areas.[30] In a recent study on screening symptomatic patients of cirrhosis at the tertiary care hospital in India, 35.5% of cirrhotics were found to have coexistent HCC at their first presentation to the hospital.[31]

Since, by and large, it is only the patients of cirrhosis who get HCC, it would be prudent to investigate patients of cirrhosis for the presence of HCC at diagnosis and periodically reinvestigate to see if they have developed HCC in order to pick up early, treatable lesions. HCC is a potential candidate for screening as it fits with the generic criteria enunciated for cancer screening.[32] These criteria include: the disease must be common with substantial morbidity and mortality, a clear cut 'at risk' population be identifiable (e.g. cirrhosis), the screening tests must have a low morbidity, high sensitivity and specificity, there must be an established treatment therapy, and the screening program must be cost effective. Surveillance of cirrhosis patients can potentially lead to diagnosis of HCC at an early stage when the tumor might be amenable to resection, liver transplantation or percutaneous ablation. Hence, it is imperative to screen these patients and treat this fatal disease at early stages.

The population at risk for HCC is relatively easy to identify. Chronic hepatitis B and C infections are the major factors increasing HCC hazard.[30] Cirrhosis is another outstanding risk factor irrespective of etiology. It should, however, be noted that 20-56% of patients with HCC have previously undiagnosed cirrhosis.[33,34] Patients with more advanced Child-Pugh scores are at higher risk of liver cancer, Child-Pugh class B/C cirrhosis were found to have a 3-8 fold increased risk respectively.[35,36] Older age, male sex and sustained high serum alanine aminotransferase (ALT) levels have been found in longitudinal studies among persons with cirrhosis of different etiologies to be associated with an increased risk and more rapid development of HCC.[37,38]

Other risk factors are, Type 2 diabetes, non- alcoholic steatohepatitis, associated alcohol abuse and coinfection with multiple viruses (hepatitis B,C and HIV) The presence of large cell change (initially called large cell dysplasia), irregular regeneration of hepatocytes and macroregenerative nodules have been evaluated as morphologic predictors of HCC in cirrhosis.[39-41]

Screening Tests

Most surveillance programs use US and AFP as screening tests. CT too has been used in addition in special situations. The tests of US and AFP are simple and safe. Suffice it is to say here, that both the tests have limitations

Alpha Feto Protein (AFP) has been used as a marker of HCC for many years. However, only 60-70% of patients of HCC in USA and Europe and 80-90% of patients in Asia have elevated serum AFP.[42] In different studies, AFP is reported to have a sensitivity of 39%-65%, a specificity of 76%-94% and a positive predictive value (PPV) of 9%-50% in diagnosing HCC.[43-49]

As patients with clinically overt disease often have high levels of AFP, the conventional diagnostic level of AFP in HCC is > 400 ng/ml.[50] AFP levels could also be elevated in the presence of chronic viral hepatitis with reactivation but without HCC. On the other hand, 'normal' serum levels of AFP (< 20 ng/ml) are not an uncommon occurrence in association with small HCCs.[51] A correlation between the level of AFP and the size of HCC masses has also been observed, larger the mass, higher the serum AFP level.[31] A high cut-off value of AFP (> 400 ng/ml) has no place if AFP is to be used as a screening test to detect early, small HCCs that invariably produce lower levels of AFP. Lower AFP cut off levels of 20 ng/ml also show a low sensitivity of 41-65% and specificity of 80–94%.[43-49] Role of AFP as a screening test has been has been studied at length in a recent study, which does not find the utility of a single cut off value in screening.[31] Accordingly, serum AFP is no longer recommended because of its poor sensitivity and specificity.[1] However, AFP has an important role in characterizing the liver mass as malignant at a diagnostic level more than 400 ng/ml, and because of this fact, it is rightly an important ingredient of the diagnostic criteria for HCC as suggested by European Association for the Study of the Liver (EASL).[52]

Ultrasound is widely used for screening patients with liver cirrhosis for detection of HCC (Figs 17.3A and B). Imaging of a cirrhotic liver poses a real challenge to the Radiologist. In advanced cirrhosis, liver is shrunken and therefore the sonographic window is usually limited. Additionally, the hepatic echotexture is heterogeneous on account of fibrosis, fatty infiltration, parenchymal necrosis and myriads of micro and macronodular cirrhotic regenerative nodules. Detection of HCC in such a background liver is a difficult task. Despite limitations, US is the first imaging modality in suspected cases of HCC. In different studies, sensitivity of US for detecting HCC in patients of cirrhosis ranges from 27–94% and specificity from 90–98%.[53-58]

Complimentary techniques like harmonic US and US contrast agents are utilized to improve detection and characterization of HCC. Sensitivity of US for detecting satellite nodules is poor and therefore underestimates the extent of disease. Besides, US is also operator-dependent and a less proficient operator can misdiagnose the disease. The sensitivity of detection of HCC is directly proportional to the size of the mass.[59] For tumours less than 2 cm and more than 2 cm, US shows a sensitivity of 31.6% and 78.6%, and CT, 59% and 94.7% respectively.

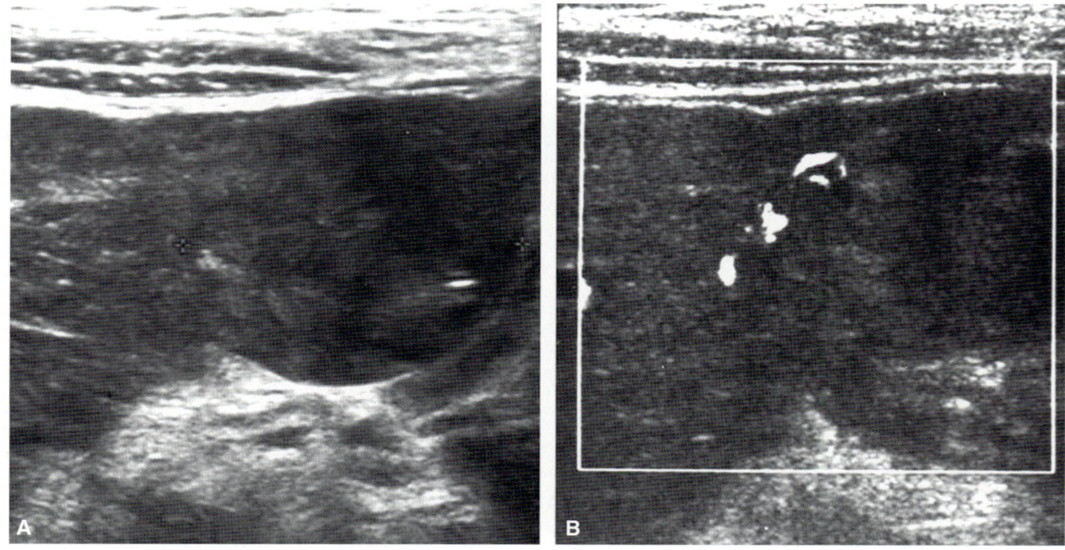

Figs 17.3A and B: (A) Screening US at one year in a patient of HCV cirrhosis showing a 2.5 cm heterogeneously hypoechoic lesion in the left lobe of liver. On power Doppler, a tortuous feeding artery is seen supplying the tumor (B)

Even though all imaging modalities show relatively poor sensitivities for detection of small HCC < 2cm in diameter, CT fares better than US and thus delineates the extent of disease better.[59]

Contrast enhanced MRI is the best tool for early detection of small malignant lesions in cirrhotic patients. MRI scores over CT in the detection of small HCC (1-2 cm).[60] However, it has a major disadvantage in terms of limited availability and cost which is of great relevance for a developing country.

Different imaging modalities have a complimentary role in the characterization of the liver tumour. HCC exhibits a variety of classical patterns on US, multiphasic CT and MRI which facilitate its diagnosis. However, Imaging does not provide any pointers towards the underlying etiology of HCC, that is, no differences in imaging profile of HBV associated HCC and HCV associated HCC have been observed.[61]

Surveillance Intervals

The optimal screening interval for HCC surveillance should depend on the knowledge of the growth rate of HCC and related premalignant lesions. According to studies performed on tumor growth, the reasonable interval is between 3-12 months.[62,63] The use of surveillance interval of 6 months allows most tumors to experience at least one doubling between surveillance intervals and would appear to allow ample opportunity to detect most tumors before they become more than 5 cm in diameter. Clearly, additional prospective studies are needed to validate this surveillance interval. Determination of this screening interval would have a direct implication on the stage of HCC detected and the cost effectiveness of the program.

Protocol for HCC Surveillance

The most widely used protocol is the one proposed by The European Association for the study of liver (EASL) expert panel (Table 17.4).[52] It proposes that only those patients of cirrhosis should be included in the surveillance in which the curative treatment can be provided. Ideally, they should be Child-Pugh class A and B patients. EASL endorsed surveillance based on the use of US and serum AFP every 6 months. In nodules smaller than 1cm, which are malignant in less than 50% of cases, reliable HCC diagnosis is difficult. Thus, close follow-up (3 monthly) is recommended while waiting for the tumor to grow. In nodules of 1-2 cm, HCC diagnosis requires positive cytopathology. However, there is a 30-40% false-negative rate with fine-needle biopsy.[64] A negative result, therefore, does not rule out malignant disease. Noninvasive diagnostic criteria need to be applied solely in patients with cirrhosis and tumors larger than 2 cm (Fig. 17.4). This noninvasive diagnostic criteria is established by the concomitant finding of two imaging techniques (CT, MRI), showing a nodule larger than 2 cm with arterial hypervascularization, or by one positive imaging technique, showing hypervasculari-zation associated with AFP in concentration higher than 400 ug/L.[52]

It is important to note whether the HCC surveillance programs improve patient outcomes This question can only be answered through randomized controlled trials.

Table 17.4 EASL Diagnostic criteria for HCC (Ref 52)

Nodules larger than 2 cm	1. Non invasive method: Any two of the following: • AFP more than 400 ng/ml • Arterialization on TPCT • Arterialization on contrast enhanced MRI Or 2. Fine needle aspiration cytology
Nodules between 1-2 cm	Cytohistology
Nodules less than 1cm	Close monitoring by US every 3 months until lesion grows to >1 cm*

*(Absence of growth on follow up does not rule out malignancy)

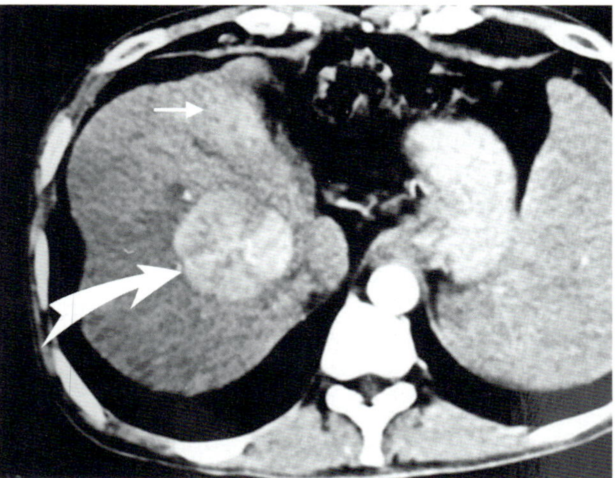

Fig. 17.4: Arterial phase CT images of a patient of HBV cirrhosis showing two enhancing focal lesions (white arrows) suggestive of HCC. AFP of this patient was 1720 ng/ml and hence the EASL noninvasive diagnostic criteria was fulfilled obviating the need for FNAC

Because, randomized controlled trials with non-screened groups are unlikely to be developed at least in the west, the survival benefit cannot be proven. The best reported survival of HCC a decade ago was 65% at 3 years for Child-Pugh class A patients who had one tumor.[65] Advances in treatment have now led to 5-year survival rates in the range of 50–70%,[30] affirming the notion that outcomes have changed with available therapies.

Cost Effectiveness

The cost effectiveness of screening cirrhotic patients depends on the incidence of HCC, efficacy of therapy and the age of the patient. In India, using the protocol of US and AFP six monthly and a yearly CT, the cost effectiveness of screening program from the patient perspective was Rs. 126,345 (US$ 2,808) for each HCC detected for local patients and Rs. 448,440 (US$ 9,965) for the outstation patients.[66] This cost per HCC case detected by the HCC surveillance program is exorbitant for low/middle income countries like India. Hence measures for reducing cost need to be looked into.

Treatment of Cirrhosis

Treatment is aimed at delaying the progression of disease and preventing the onset of complications. A multi-faceted approach is required for the management of the patients of cirrhosis which includes treatment of the presenting signs and symptoms and the underlying cause of cirrhosis. When medium and large varices are detected on endoscopy, prophylaxis with B-blocking agents is recommended.

Patients of alcoholic cirrhosis need to discontinue with the use of alcohol to prevent progression to hepatic fibrogenesis and decompensation. Alcohol has an immunosuppressive effect and liver function deteriorates in first two weeks following withdrawal.[67]

Replicating hepatitis B and C infections need specific therapies. Patients with compensated cirrhosis and with replicating hepatitis C virus benefit from interferon therapy. Viral eradication and lowered risk of decompensation can be achieved in upto 40% of patients of hepatitis C, genotype 1 and in 70% of genotype 2 or 3.[68] Long term treatment with oral nucleoside and nucleotide inhibitors of hepatitis B virus DNA polymerase might not only retard or reverse cirrhosis but also prevent complications of end stage liver disease. Additionally, drugs like lamivudine, adefovir, entecavir or telbivudine or their combinations have shown to induce low viral resistance and a different mutational profile. Liver transplantation is considered as the ultimate treatment for end stage liver disease. Survival rates following transplant at 1, 5 and 8 years are 83%, 70% and 61% respectively.[69]

Treatment of Complications

Portal hypertension and its complications are managed with various radiological intervention procedures apart from surgery. Transjugular intrahepatic portosystemic shunt (TIPS) is indicated for control of active bleed refractory to sclerotherapy, intractable ascites, and an alternative to shunt surgery in high risk patients and in cirrhosis due to Budd-Chiari Syndrome. Splenic artery embolization is considered these days for cases of hypersplenism since surgical splenectomy is associated with risk of morbidity.

HCC is the terminal, fatal complication of liver cirrhosis. Treatment of HCC is based on the Barcelona Clinic Liver Cancer (BCLC) staging classification.[70] Curative options of surgical resection and liver transplant are considered for BCLC stage 0 and stage A patients. However, most patients with cirrhosis are not found suitable for surgery. Liver transplant is considered in cases who fulfill the Milan criteria. Patients who fail to meet the criteria for surgical resection and liver transplant, locoregional therapies like percutaneous ablative procedures are considered and mostly widely used are radiofrequency ablation (RFA) or chemical ablation with ethanol (PEI) or acetic acid (PAI) (Figs 17.5A to C). Certain centers have also undertaken RFA as the first line of therapy for BCLC A stage and have shown cumulative survival rates of 95.2%, 69.5% and 58% at 1, 3 and 5 years respectively. [71] For BCLC stage B and C, palliative option of chemoembolization (TACE) is offered. These modalities can also serve as a bridge for transplantation. The current trend is to resort to the multimodality approach that is, combining regional and local therapies. This approach has been shown to produce better results than using single therapy alone.[72,73] Combinations tried are, TACE with RFA, TACE with PEI, TACE with PAI etc (Figs 17.6A to C). In advanced disease of BCLC D, the main stay of treatment is supportive therapy. However, oral chemotherapy too has been tried with little benefit.

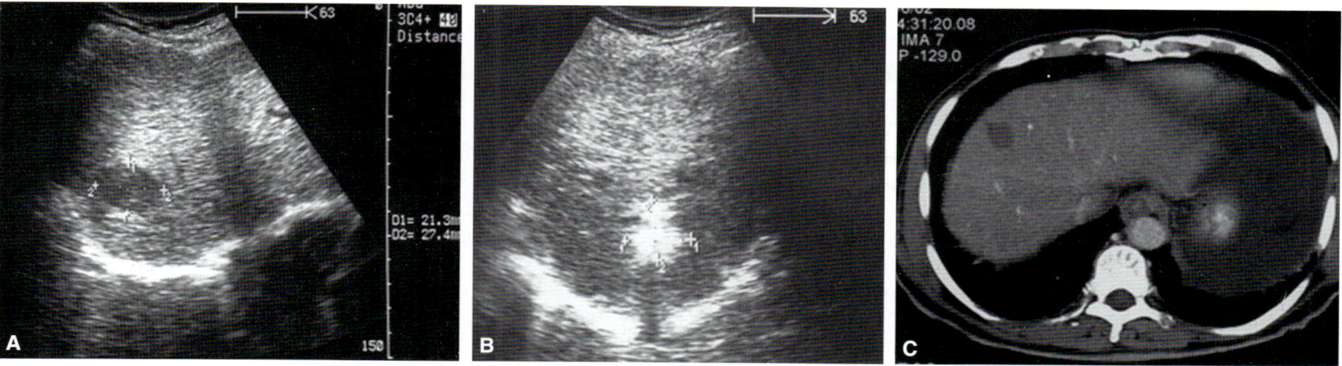

Figs 17.5A to C: Patient of HBV cirrhosis with solitary small HCC (BCLC A) showing a 2.5 cm hypoechoic lesion in the right lobe of cirrhotic liver on US (A).) On subjecting to PAI, the lesion is completely hyperechoic on US immediately following PAI (B). Follow up CT at one year later shows that the ablative area has slightly reduced in size, is sharply demarcated and shows no residual or recurrent disease on venous phase CT (C)

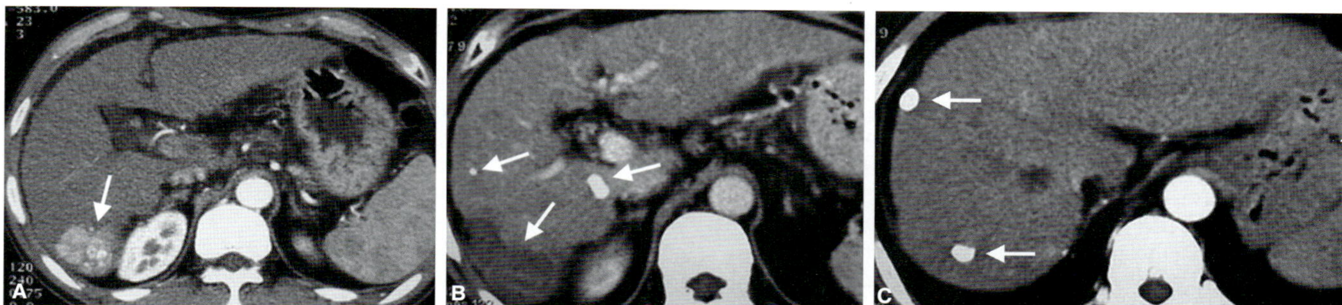

Figs 17.6A to C: Combination modalities (RFA followed by TACE) HBV cirrhosis patient found to have a small, solitary enhancing mass in segment 7 of liver on arterial phase CT (A), which was treated with RFA. At 18 months, multiple fresh lesions along with recurrence at the margin of the defect was noted and TACE was done. Post TACE CTs (B and C) show all lesions covered with lipiodol (straight arrows and curved arrow respectively)

CONCLUSION

Role of a Radiologist is vital for patients of liver cirrhosis. Careful screening, early detection of life threatening complications, and management by safe therapeutic image- guided interventions have significant impact on the outcome of the course of the disease. Hence, understanding of the clinical profile, presentation, natural history and complications of this end stage liver disease is crucial.

REFERENCES

1. Schuppan D, Afdhal NH. Liver cirrhosis. The Lancet 2008;371:838-51.
2. Tandon BN, Acharya SK, Tandon A. Epidemiology of hepatitis B virus infection in India. Gut 1996;38:S56-9.
3. Chowdhury A, Santra A, Chaudhuri S, Dhali GK, Maity SG, Naik TN, et al. Hepatitis C virus infection in the general population: A community-based study in West Bengal, India. Hepatology 2003;37:802-9.
4. Popper H. Pathological aspects of cirrhosis: A review. Am J Pathol 1977; 87:228-64
5. Ghany M, Hoofnagle JH. Liver and biliary tract disease. In Harrison's Principles of Internal Medicine.15th edition, vol 2, page 1707-11.
6. International working party: Terminology of nodular hepatocellular lesions. Hepatology 1995;22:983-93.
7. Kamel IR, Bluemke DA. Imaging evaluation of hepatocellular carcinoma. J Vasc Interven Radiol 2002;13: S173-83.
8. Guha IN, Iredale JP. Clinical Aspects and diagnostic aspects of Cirrhosis. In Text book of Hepatology. From basic science to clinical practice. 3rd edition, 1:604-19.
9. Brown JJ, Naylor MJ, Yagan N. Imaging of hepatic cirrhosis. Radiology 1997;202:1-16.
10. Panigrahi AK, Panda SK, Dixit RK, Rao KV, Acharya SK, Dasarathy S, Nanu A Magnitude of hepatitis C virus infection in India: prevalence in healthy blood donors,

acute and chronic liver diseases. J Med Virol 1997;51: 167-74.

11. Fattovich G, Stroffolini T, Zagni I, Donato F. Hepatocellular carcinoma in cirrhosis: Incidence and risk factors. Gastroenterology 2004;127(5 suppl 1):S35-50.
12. Pugh R N, Murray-Lyon IM, Dawson JL, et al. Transection of esophagus for bleeding esophageal varices. Br J Surg 1973;60:646-9.
13. Infante-Rivard C, Esnaola S, Villeneuve JP. Clinical and statistical validity of conventional prognostic factors in predicting short-term survival among cirrhotics. Hepatology 1987;7:660-64.
14. Wiesner R, Edwards E, Freeman R, et al. Model for end-stage liver disease (MELD) and allocation of donor livers. Gastroenterology 2003;124:91-96.
15. Conn HO and Atterbury CE. Cirrhosis. Diseases of the liver. In Schiff L and Schiff ER, 6th edn. Philadelphia; Lippincort 1987:725-864.
16. Chung RT, Podolsky. Cirrhosis and its complications. In: Braunwald E, Hauser SL, Fauci AS, Longo DL, Kasper DL, Jameson JL, eds. Harison's Principles of Internal Medicine. New York 2001;1754-61.
17. Lebrec D, et al. Portal hypertension, size of esophageal varices, and risk of gastrointestinal bleeding in alcoholic cirrhosis. Gastroenterology 1980;79:1139-44.
18. North Italian Endoscopic Club for the Study and Treatment of Esophageal varices. Prediction of the first variceal haemorrhage in patients with cirrhosis of the liver and esophageal varices. A prospective multicenter study. New England Journal of Medicine 1988;39:319:983-9.
19. Gaiani S, Gramantieri L, Venturoli N, et al. What is the criterion for differentiating chronic hepatitis from compensated cirrhosis? A prospective study comparing ultrasonography and percutaneous liver biopsy. J Hepatology 1997;27:979-85.
20. Caturelli E, Giacobbe A, Facciorusso D, et al. Percutaneous biopsy in diffuse liver disease: Increasing diagnostic yield and decreasing complication rate by routine ultrasound assessment of puncture site. Am J Gastroenterol 1996;91:1318-1221.
21. Farrel RJ, Smidy PF, Pilkington RM, et al. Guided versus blind liver biopsy for chronic hepatitis C: Clinical benefits and costs. J Hepatol 1999;30:580-87.
22. Larcos G, Sorokopud H, Berry G, et al. Sonographic screening for hepatocellular carcinoma in patients with chronic hepatitis or cirrhosis: An evaluation 1998;171: 433-5.
23. Zweilbel WJ. Sonographic diagnosis of diffuse liver disease. Semin Ultrasouind CT MRI 1995;16:8-15.
24. Bonkovsky HL, Rubin RB, Cable EE, et al. Hepatic iron concentration : Noninvasive estimation by means of MR imaging techniques. Radiology 1999;212:227-34.
25. Qayyum A, Goh JS, Kakar S, et al. Accuracy of liver fat quantification at MR imaging: comparision of out-of-phase gradient-echo and fat-saturated fast spin-echo techniques - initial experience. Radiology 2005;237: 507-11.
26. Ziol M, Handra-Luca A, Kettaneh A, et al. Noninvasive assessment of liver fibrosis by measurement of stiffness in patients with chronic hepatitis C. Hepatology 2005;41:48-54.
27. The North Italian Endoscopic club for the study and treatment of Esophageal varices. Predication of the first variceal hemorrhage in patients with cirrhosis of liver and esophageal varices. A prospective multicentre study. N Engl J Med 1988;319:983-9.
28. Caly WR, Strauss E. A prospective study of bacterial infections in patients of cirrhosis. J Hepatol 1993;18: 353-8.
29. Paul SB, Gulati MS, Sreenivas V, Madan K, Gupta AK, Mukhopadhyay S, Acharya SK. Incidence of Hepatocellular carcinoma among patients of cirrhosis of liver: an experience from a tertiary care centre in northern India. Indian J Gastroenterol 2007;26,274-78.
30. Llovet JM, Burroughs A, Bruix J. Hepatocelluar carcinoma. Lancet 2003;362:1907-17.
31. Paul SB, Gulati MS, Sreenivas V,Madan K, Gupta AK, Mukhopadhay S, Acharya SK. Evaluating patients with cirrhosis for Hepatocellular carcinoma: value of clinical symptomatology, Imaging and Alpha-fetoprotein. Oncology 2007;72:117-23.
32. Prorok PC. Epidemiologic approach for cancer screening. Problems in design and analysis of trials. Am J Pediatr Hematol Oncol 1992;14:117-28.
33. Liver Cancer study group of Japan, Primary Liver cancer in Japan. Clinicopathological features and results of surgical treatment. Am Surg 1990;211:277-87.
34. Zaman SN, Johnson PJ, Williams R. Silent cirrhosis in patients with hepatocellular carcinoma. Implication for screening in high incidence and low incidence areas. Cancer 1990;65:1607-10.
35. Bolondi L, Sofia S, Siringo S, et al. Surveillance programme of cirrhotic patients for early diagnosis and treatment of hepatocellular carcinoma: a cost effectiveness analysis. Gut 2001;48:251-9.
36. Tsai JF, Jeng JE, Ho MS, et al. Effect of hepatitis C and B virus infection on risk of hepatocellular carcinoma a prospectrive study. Br J Cancer 1997;76:968-74.
37. Fattovich G, Stroffolini T, Zagni I, Donato F. Hepatocellular carcinoma in cirrhosis: incidence and risk factor. Gastroenterology 2004;127;S35-50.
38. Benvegnu L, Fattovich G, Noventa F, et al. Concurrent hepatitis B and C virus infection and risk of hepatocellular carcinoma in cirrhosis. A prospective study. Cancer 1994;74:2442-8.
39. Ganne-Carrie N, Chastang C, Chapel F, et al. Predictive score for the development of hepatocellular carcinoma and additional value of liver large cell dysplasia in Western patients with cirrhosis. Hepatology 1996;23: 1112-8.
40. Shibata M, Morizane T, Uchida T, et al. Irregular regeneration of hepatocytes and risk of hepatocellular carcinoma in chronic hepatitis and cirrhosis with hepatitis-C-virus infection. Lancet 1998;351:1773-7.

41. Borzio M, Fargion S, Borzio F, et al. Impact of large regenerative, low-grade and high-grade dysplastic nodules in hepatocellular carcinoma development. J Hepatol 2003;39:208-14.
42. Matsumoto Y, Suzuki T, Asadi T, et al. Clinical classification of hepatoma in Japan according to serial changes in serum alphafetoprotein levels. Cancer 1982;49:354-6.
43. Sherman M, Peltekian KM, Lee C. Screening for hepatocellular carcinoma in chronic carriers of hepatitis B virus: incidence and prevalence of hepatocellular carcinoma in a North American urban population. Hepatology 1995;22:432-8.
44. Trevisani F, D'Intino PE, Morselli-Labate AM, et al. Serum alpha-fetoprotein for diagnosis of hepatocellular carcinoma in patients with chronic liver disease: influence of HBsAg and anti-HCV status. J Hepatol 2001;34:570-5.
45. Gambarin-Gelwan M, Wolf DC, Shapiro R, Schwartz ME, Min AD. Sensitivity of commonly available screening tests in detecting hepatocellular carcinoma in cirrhotic patients undergoing liver transplantation. Am J Gastroenterol 2000;95:1535-8.
46. Nguyen MH, Garcia RT, Simpson PW, Wright TL, Keeffe EB. Racial differences in effectiveness of alpha-fetoprotein for diagnosis of hepatocellular carcinoma in hepatitis C virus cirrhosis. Hepatology 2002;36:410-7.
47. Peng YC, Chan CS, Chen GH. The effectiveness of serum alpha-fetoprotein level in anti-HCV positive patients for screening hepatocellular carcinoma. Hepatogastroenterology 1999;46:3208-11.
48. Cedrone A, Covino M, Caturelli E, et al. Utility of alpha-fetoprotein (AFP) in the screening of patients with virus-related chronic liver disease: does different viral etiology influence AFP levels in hepatocellular carcinoma? A study in 350 western patients. Hepatogastroenterology 2000;47:1654-8.
49. Tong MJ, Blatt LM, Kao VW. Surveillance for hepatocellular carcinoma in patients with chronic viral hepatitis in the United States of America. J Gastroenterol Hepatol 2001;16:553-9.
50. Daniele B, Bencivenga A, Megna AS, Tinessa V. Alpha fetoprotein and ultrasonography screening for hepatocelluar carcinoma. Gastroenterology 2004;127:S108-12.
51. Johnson J. Tumor marker in the diagnosis and management of patients with hepatocullular carcinoma. Recent results in Cancer Research 1986;100:68.
52. Bruix J, Sherman M, Llovet JM, et al. EASL panel of experts on HCC. Clinical management of hepatocellular carcinoma. Conclusions of the Barcelona 2000 EASL conference. European Association for the study of liver. J Hepatol 2001;35:421-30.
53. Gambarin-Gelwan M, Wolf DC, Shapiro R, Schwartz ME, Min AD. Sensitivity of commonly available screening tests in detecting hepatocellular carcinoma in cirrhotic patients undergoing liver transplantation. Am J Gastroenterol 2000;95:1535-8.
54. Dodd GD III, Miller WJ, Baron RL, Skolnick ML, Campbell WL. Detection of malignant tumor in end-stage cirrhotic liver: efficacy of sonography as a screening technique. Am J Roentgenol 1992;159:727-33.
55. Rizzi PM, Kane PA, Ryder SD, et al. Accuracy of radiology in detection of hepatocellular carcinoma before liver transplantation. Gastroenterology 1994;107:1425-9.
56. Vilana R, Martinez X, Gilabert R, et al. Detection and staging of hepatocellular carcinoma with ultrasound: Analysis of 320 consecutive explanted livers. J Ultrasound Med 1998;17:119.
57. Bennett SL, Krinsky GA, Abitbol RJ, Kim SY, Theise ND, Teperman LW. Sonographic detection of hepatocellular carcinoma and dysplastic nodules in cirrhosis: correlation of pretransplantation sonography and liver explant pathology in 200 patients. Am J Roentgenol 2002;179:75-80.
58. Liu WC, Lim JH, Park CK, et al. Poor sensitivity of sonography is detection of hepatocellular carcinoma in advanced liver cirrhois: accuracy of pretransplantations sonography in 118 patients. Eur Radiol 2003;13:1693-8.
59. Rao ARW, Chui AKK, Shi LW, et al. Sensitivity of Radiological investigations in diagnosing hepatocellular carcinoma in cirrhotic liver. Transplantation proceedings 2003;35:348-9.
60. Burrel M, Llovet JM, Ayuso C, et al. MRI angiography is superior to helical CT for detection of HCC prior to liver transplantation : an explant correlation. Hepatology 2003;38:1034-42.
61. Paul SB, Gulati MS, Jain V, Sreenivas V, Mukhopadhyay S, Gupta AK and Acharya SK. Does imaging differentiate between hepatocellular carcinoma of hepatitis B or C virus origin? Hepatology International 2007;1A:174.
62. Sheu J, Sung J, Chen D, et al. Growth rates of asymptomatic hepatocellular carcinoma and its clinical implications. Gastroenterology 1985;89:259-66.
63. Barbara L, Benzi G, Gaiani S, et al. Natural history of small untreated hepatocellular carcinoma in cirrhosis: A multivariate analysis of prognostic factors of tumor growth rate and patient survival. Hepatology 1992;16: 132-36.
64. Durand F, Regimbeau JM, Belghiti J, et al. Assessment of the benefits and risk of percutaneous biopsy before surgical resection of hepatocellular carcinoma. J Hepatol 2001;35:254-8.
65. Barbara L, Benzi G, Gaiani S, et al. Natural history of small untreated hepatocellular carcinoma in cirrhosis: a multivariate analysis of prognostic factors of tumor growth rate and patient survival. Hepatology 1992;16:132-7.
66. Paul SB, Gulati MS, Sreenivas V, Madan K, Gupta AK, Mukhopadhyay S, Acharya SK. Economic evaluation of HCC surveillance program in India. Hepatology International 2008 DOI 10:1007/S 12072-008-9054-5.
67. Stickel F, Schuppan D, Hahn EG, Seitz HK. Co-carcinogenic effects of alcohol in hepatocarcinogenesis. Gut 2002;51:132-39.
68. Everson GT. Management of cirrhosis due to chronic hepatitis C. J Hepatol 2005;42:S65-74.

69. Roberts MS, Angus DC, Bryce CL, Valenta Z, Weissfeld L. Survival after liver transplantation in the United States: a disease-specific analysis of the UNOS database. Liver Transpl 2004;204;10:886-97.
70. Llovet JM, Bru C, Bruix J. Prognosis of hepatocellular carcinoma: the BCLC staging classification. Sem Liv Dis 1999;19(3):329-38.
71. Choi D, Lim HK, Rhim H, Kim YS,Lee WJ, Paik SW et al. Percutaneous Radiofrequency ablation foe early stage hepatocellular carcinoma as a first line treatment: long term results and prognostic factors in a large single-institution series. Eur Radiol 2007;17(3):684-92.
72. Yamakado K, Nakatsuka A, Ohmori S, et al. Radio-frequency ablation combined with chemoembolization in hepatocellular carcinoma treatment response based on tumor size and morphology. J Vasc Interv Radiol 2002;13:1225-32.
73. Kurokohchi K, Watanabe S, Masaki T, et al. Combined use of percutaneous ethanol injection and radiofrequency ablation for the effective treatment of hepatocellular carcinoma. Int J Oncol 2002;21:841-6.

Chapter Eighteen

Imaging and Interventions in Pancreatitis

Ashu Seith Bhalla, Chandan J Das

Pancreatitis especially in its acute form is a common disease with potentially serious outcomes. Multiple imaging modalities play a crucial role in the evaluation of the disease process and its associated complications. Understanding the pathogenesis of this disease, indications for imaging, modality and imaging protocol selection, staging systems, and the merits and demerits of various modalities can help in optimizing the patient care.

ACUTE PANCREATITIS

Acute pancreatitis is defined as an acute, mainly diffuse, inflammatory process of the pancreas that exhibits great variation in the degree of involvement of the gland, the adjacent retroperitoneal tissues and other remote organ systems.[1,2]

Gallstones and alcohol abuse are the most common causes of acute pancreatitis. Biliary pancreatitis is highest among patients who have small gallstones (less than 5 mm in diameter) or microlithiasis.[1,3] Less common causes of acute pancreatitis are hypertriglyceridemia, hypercalcemia, medications, ductal obstruction caused by tumor, trauma, endoscopic retrograde cholangiopancreaticography, and developmental abnormalities including pancreas divisum and annular pancreas. No matter what the underlying cause of acute pancreatitis, inflammation is triggered by premature activation of pancreatic enzymes with resultant autodigestion of the pancreatic parenchyma. The inflammatory process may remain localized to the pancreas or spread to regional tissues, or even involve remote organ systems resulting in multiorgan failure and occasional death. Furthermore, ischemic/reperfusion injury has been recognized increasingly as an important mechanism in the pathogenesis of acute pancreatitis, especially in patients who have severe necrotizing pancreatitis.[4]

Clinically, acute pancreatitis generally presents with upper abdominal pain and may be accompanied by vomiting, fever, tachycardia, and leukocytosis. The clinical diagnosis is supported by an elevation of the serum amylase and lipase often in excess of three times the upper limit of normal.[5]

Classification

The International Symposium on Acute Pancreatitis held in Atlanta In 1992, Georgia, established a clinically based classification system and defined and standardized certain terminologies commonly associated with acute pancreatitis.[6] Acute pancreatitis is classified as mild or severe, based on the presence of local complications and organ failure.[6,7] Organ failure is assessed best using clinical and laboratory parameters, whereas local complications are evaluated by imaging, the standard criterion being contrast enhanced CT.[6] EL Bradley III devised a clinically based classification system for acute pancreatitis.[8,9] This classification helps identify patients who have severe disease and who require close monitoring and ICU care.

Mild acute pancreatitis also known as "interstitial" or "edematous" pancreatitis is a more common and self-limiting disease with minimal organ dysfunction and an uneventful recovery. Pathologically, the mild form of acute pancreatitis is characterized by interstitial edema and, infrequently, by microscopic areas of parenchymal necrosis.[5]

Severe acute pancreatitis, also known as "necrotizing pancreatitis," occurs in 20–30% of all patients and is associated with organ failure and/or local complications such as necrosis, abscess, or pseudocyst.[5] Overall, the mortality associated with severe acute pancreatitis ranges from 10-30%.[1,9] Pathologic findings include macroscopic areas of focal or diffuse pancreatic necrosis, fat necrosis, and hemorrhage in the pancreas and peripancreatic tissues.[5] Pancreatic parenchymal necrosis usually is limited to the periphery of the gland; only rarely does necrosis involve the entire gland.[10,11]

Besides these two forms of acute pancreatitis, there are many intermediate forms as well.

Assessment of Severity

Most crucial initial step in the management of acute pancreatitis is the assessment of disease severity. Although mild pancreatitis can be managed conservatively, severe acute pancreatitis requires more aggressive approach in the intensive care unit with or without surgical or percutaneous interventions.[1]

The severity of pancreatitis can be assessed by C-reactive protein and by using scoring systems that assess inflammation, organ failure.[1,7] Several scoring systems that combine clinical and laboratory parameters have been devised in an attempt to identify patients who have severe pancreatitis.[12-17] Ranson's scoring system is used commonly and comprises five clinical criteria measured at admission (for local inflammatory effects of pancreatic enzymes) and six measured at 48 hours for (systemic effects).[12] Ranson criteria of three or more predict a severe course and increased mortality.[7] A limitation of this method is the requirement for 48 hours of observation before one can identify patients who have severe disease.[7] Among various scoring systems, the APACHE II monitoring system, which encompasses 12 physiologic measurements, has been considered the most reliable, with an accuracy of about 75% for the assessment of the severity of pancreatitis at admission.[15-17] An APACHE II threshold score greater than 8 indicates severe pancreatitis.[7] A newly introduced score system called 'Sepsis-Related Organ Failure Assessment (SOFA)-score' predicts the outcome in the first 48 hours, and provides a daily assessment of treatment response with a high positive predictive value.[14]

Role of Imaging in Patient Management

Imaging plays a pivotal role in the management of patients who have acute pancreatitis. CT and abdominal ultrasound are useful to confirm the diagnosis of acute pancreatitis and to rule out other causes of acute abdomen that can mimic acute pancreatitis. In established cases of acute pancreatitis, contrast-enhanced CT is considered the investigation of choice in the assessment of pancreatic necrosis and has become an integral part of the new classification system.[5]

Computed Tomography

Computed tomography (CT) is integral in the diagnosis and management of acute pancreatitis. MDCT permits high-quality, multiphase imaging of the pancreas in a short breathhold. This attribute is important, because often the patients being imaged are quite sick and are not able to hold their breath. CT is used to grade the severity of the disease and to detect local complications of necrosis, abscess, or pseudocyst. CT can be useful in determining the underlying cause of disease, the rest of the abdomen and pelvis can also be surveyed to study ancillary findings and related complications. Moreover, CT can also be used for performing percutaneous interventions

CT Protocol

Published study on animal suggested that the administration of intravenous contrast media may exacerbate the severity of acute pancreatitis by the impaired oxygenation of the pancreatic parenchyma. However, data from subsequent outcome studies in patients who had acute pancreatitis, and also the risk of not using imaging have now led to the routine use of CECT for this indication.[18-22] Unenhanced CT is rarely performed except in case where there is clinical suspicion of pancreatic or intraabdominal hemorrhage. For a dedicated pancreas protocol study, the administration of 900–1000 mL of neutral oral contrast (such as water) typically is encouraged. This approach facilitates better assessment of the duodenal wall and ampullary region, especially when this region is being evaluated as the possible cause of pancreatitis. In most cases of acute pancreatitis, a singlephase CT performed in the portal venous phase is sufficient. When vascular complications are suspected, an additional arterialphase scan can be added to the imaging protocol following a rapid bolus intravenous injection of a contrast agent. The image data can be acquired in a volumetric fashion; hence high-quality two-dimensional (2D) and three-dimensional (3D) images can be post processed in any desirable plane. More recently, MDCT is being used to evaluate regional pancreatic blood flow quantitatively. Preliminary data suggest that pancreatic perfusion measurements could be helpful in diagnosing pancreatic necrosis and also in assessing the severity of acute pancreatitis.[23]

CT Findings in Acute Pancreatitis

The normal pancreas is a sharply defined homogeneously enhancing organ with smooth or slightly lobulated outline. Pancreas is obliquely placed, the tail is higher at splenic hilum and head is lower and surrounded by the duodenal loop. The size of the normal pancreas is variable. Head measures about 3–4 cm, body 2–3 cm and tail 1–2 cm in A-P diameter. The pancreas can also be measured in relation to A-P diameter of the adjacent vertebral body. Pancreatic enlargement is suggested when the pancreatico vertebral ratio exceeds 1.[24] The main pancreatic duct may be seen in 50% of normal individuals (1 mm width).

MILD ACUTE PANCREATITIS OR EDEMATOUS PANCREATITIS

CT may be normal in cases with mild form of pancreatitis. In a study by Balthazar et al the reported incidence of normal CT scan is 14–28 % in mild acute pancreatitis with transitory elevation of serum amylase. In contrast to this all patients with moderate to severe acute pancreatitis exhibit CT abnormalities.[25]

The pancreas in most cases is diffusely enlarged (slight to moderate enlargement), the contour becomes shaggy and the parenchyma may become slightly heterogeneous in density. In some cases, only a portion of the gland may be involved, commonest being the head area. This form is clinically mild and is often associated with cholelithiasis. In mild acute pancreatitis, the diffusely enlarged gland may show dilatation of the main pancreatic duct both of which usually subside within days to weeks, if there is no complication. Since the pancreas does not have a well-developed fibrous capsule, commonly there is extravasation of pancreatic secretions around the gland into the retroperitoneal space.

CT findings depend upon the severity of the pathological changes. In mild-form there is mild increase in the density of the peripancreatic fat with hazy, dirty or lace-like appearance (Fig. 18.1). In more severe form, extravasation of pancreatic enzymes, inflammation, haemorrhage and fat necrosis are found. In the CT scan, moderate to extensive ill-defined areas of heterogeneous soft tissue and fluid densities are seen. Fluid collections are seen as non-encapsulated homogeneous collections of water density.

Commonest sites for extra pancreatic exudates are left anterior pararenal space and lesser sac. When large in

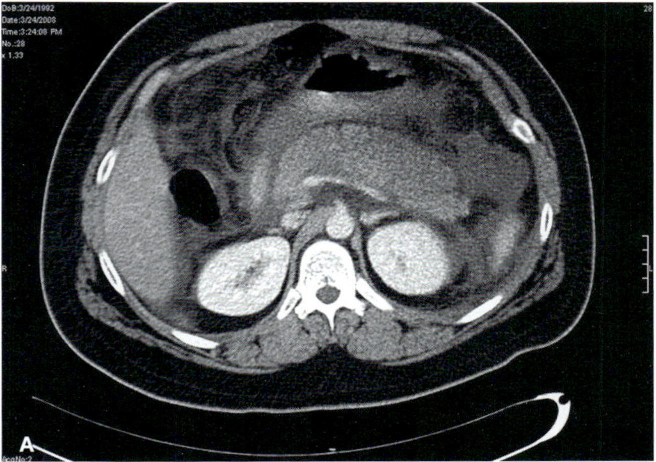

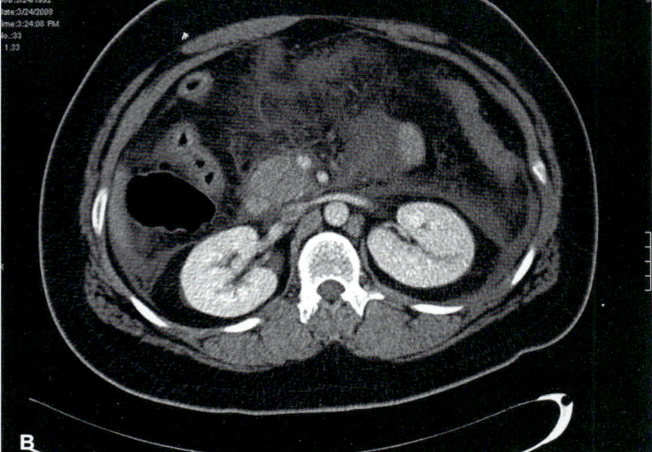

Figs 18.1A and B: Mild acute pancreatitis: CECT showing enlargement of the pancreas with blurring of its margins and streaky increase in density of peripancreatic fat.There is extension of inflammation to the anterior pararenal space and mesentry

quantity, fluid may extend inferiorly along anterior pararenal space, anterior to psoas muscles and extend into the pelvis. Exudates may invade the small bowel mesentery, transverse mesocolon, posterior pararenal space, perirenal space and the peritoneal cavity. There is alteration of the density of mesenteric fat, either in the root of the mesentery or along mesenteric border of transverse colon or small bowel (Fig. 18.2).

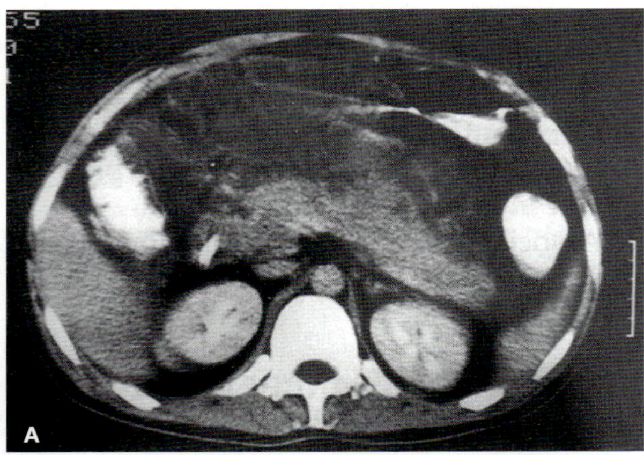

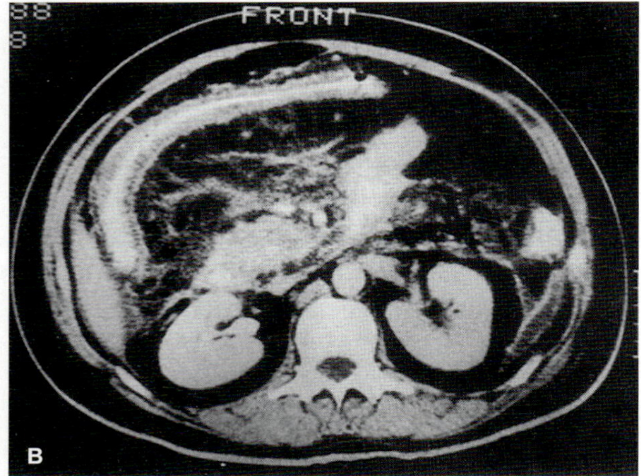

Fig 18.2: Peripancreatic spread of inflammation. CT showing bulky pancreas with spreading inflammation into mesentery (A), transverse mesocolon and bilateral pararenal spaces (B) along with thickening of bilateral Gerota's fascia

SEVERE ACUTE PANCREATITIS

In the severe form of acute pancreatitis, patchy areas of necrosis develop within the pancreas. In an enhanced scan, lack of contrast enhancement, loss of normal glandular texture and fragmentation or liquefaction of a part of the gland indicates necrosis (Fig. 18.3).

Most patients with necrotizing acute pancreatitis develop significant peripancreatic collection of fluid. These patients need follow- up repeat CT scan that may show various changes in the fluid collections. In about 50% cases, fluid resolves without further complications, most of the retroperitoneal fluid is absorbed with 2–3 weeks; smaller collections may remain for longer period.

The 1992 International Symposium on Acute Pancreatitis defined and standardized various terminologies commonly associated with acute pancreatitis;[5] these terms should be used in the radiologic report.

Acute Fluid Collections

Acute fluid collections occur early in the course of acute pancreatitis (within 48 hours) and consist of collections of enzyme-rich pancreatic juices that lack a wall of granulation or fibrous tissue. Fluid collection may involve the pancreatic, peripancreatic and distant areas. The pancreatic fluid is composed of inflammatory exudates, necrotic tissue and blood. Initially there is collection within the pancreas and appears as low density area within the pancreas in CT scan. Peripancreatic fluid can collect in various locations.

Lesser sac located anterior to the pancreas and behind the stomach is the commonest site for fluid collection. CT clearly defines fluid collection in this area. Anterior pararenal space is the second most common site for fluid collection. Perirenal space lies within the confines of the anterior and posterior renal fascia and contains the kidney and adrenal gland. Inflammatory process can involve this space directly or extend upwards from the pelvis. Multispace involvement can be caused by perforation of fascial planes by pancreatic enzymes (Figs 18.3 and 18.4).

Extrapancreatic fluid collection may spread into the mediastinum by dissecting beneath the diaphragmatic crura or through aortic or esophageal hiatus. In CT scan usually continuity can be demonstrated between mediastinal collection and peripancreatic inflammation. Associated small pleural effusion or basal atelectasis of the lungs is often seen especially on the left side.

Acute Pseudocyst

A pseudocyst is a collection of pancreatic juice enclosed by a wall of fibrous or granulation tissue. Formation of a pseudocyst requires 4 or more weeks from the onset of

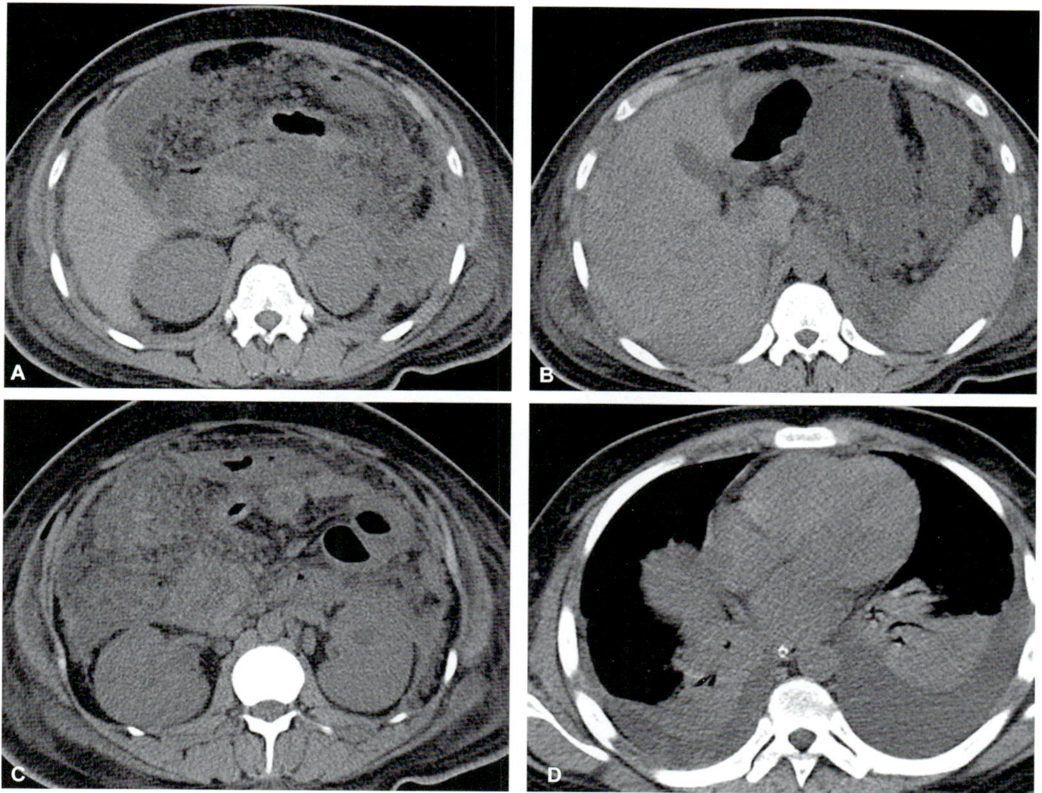

Figs 18.3A to D: Severe acute pancreatitis: Non-contrast MDCT reveals loss of normal architecture of the pancreas with multiple focal hypodense areas suggesting necrosis (A).There is spread of inflammation to the extrapancreatic tissues with fluid collections extending to the lesser sac (B), anterior pararenal space and mesentry. (C) Pleural and basal passive lung atelectasis is also present.Contrast was withheld due to deranged renal functions (D)

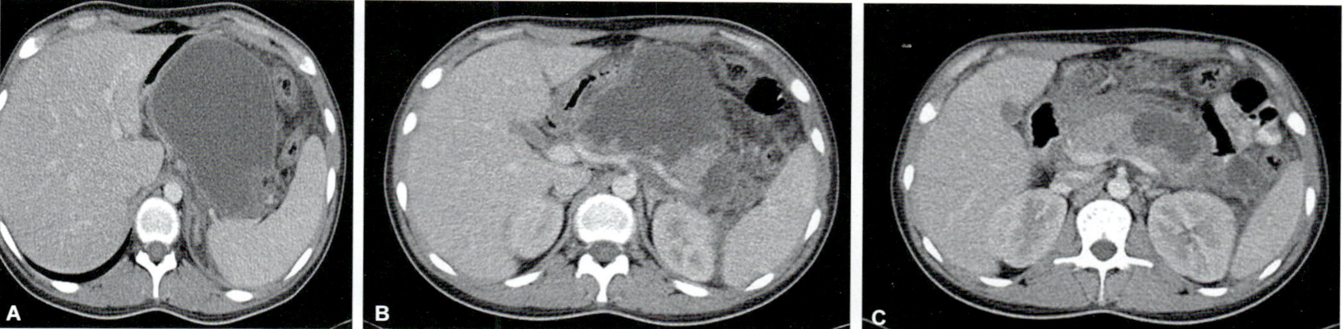

Figs 18.4A to C: Cranial to caudal, Severe acute pancreatitis with acute fluid collections: MDCT of 58 years old male obtained on day 10 shows necrotizing pancreatitis with multiple pancreatic and extrapancreatic fluid collections

acute pancreatitis.[26] On CT, a pseudocyst appears as a well-circumscribed, low-attenuation collection within or in the vicinity of the pancreas (Figs 18.5 and 18.6). Pseudocyst can occur in other locations such as the mediastinum[27] and usually are sterile (Fig. 18.7). When there is pus in a pseudocyst, it is referred to as an "abscess".

Pancreatic Abscess

These appear as ill-defined, poorly encapsulated fluid collections of varying density, often indistinguishable from noninfected fluid collection on CT. A pancreatic abscess should also be suspected when lingering, confined, low attenuation fluid collections of different sizes and shapes

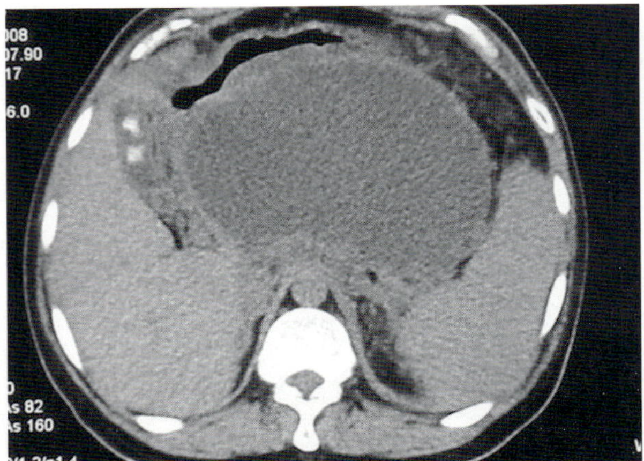

Fig. 18.5: Pseudocyst: Axial non-contrast CT showing a large pancreatic fluid collection with well defined walls and multiple gall stones

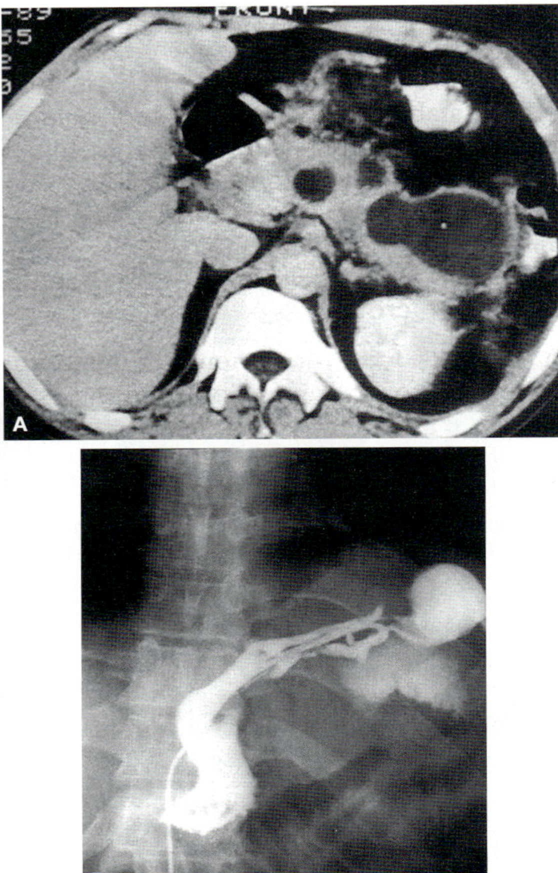

Figs 18.6A and B: Pseudocyst communicating with MPD (A) CT showing pseudocysts in the body and tail of pancreas and (B) Cystogram after pigtail catheter drainage shows communication of the pseudocyst with MPD

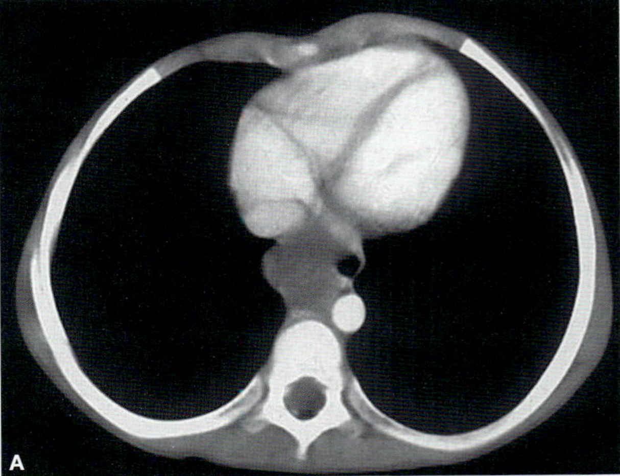

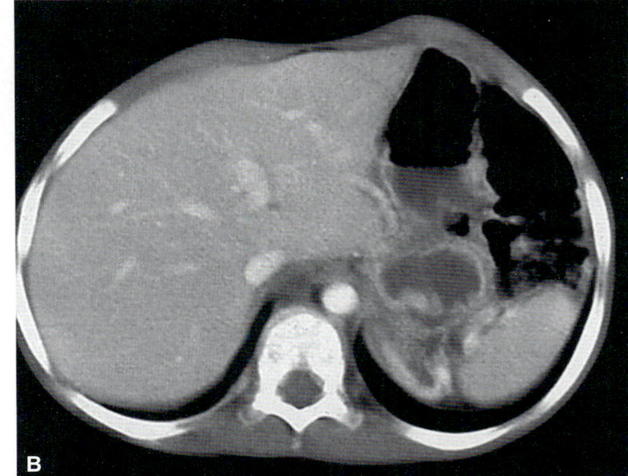

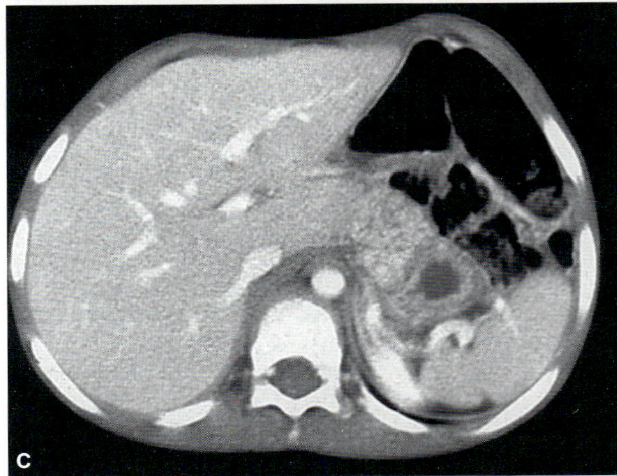

Figs 18.7A to C: Cranial to caudal: Pseudocyst with mediastinal extension:CECT of a 5 years old boy with traumatic pancreatitis reveals a pseudocyst involving the pancreatic tail region with extension into the posterior mediastinum

are depicted in septic patients with a 3-4 weeks history of acute pancreatitis. Presence of gas bubble in these collections reinforces the clinical suspicion and confirmation of CT diagnosis is by fine needle aspiration with bacteriologic examination. Percutaneous drainage under image guidance is an accepted method of treatment of pancreatic abscess (Fig. 18.8).

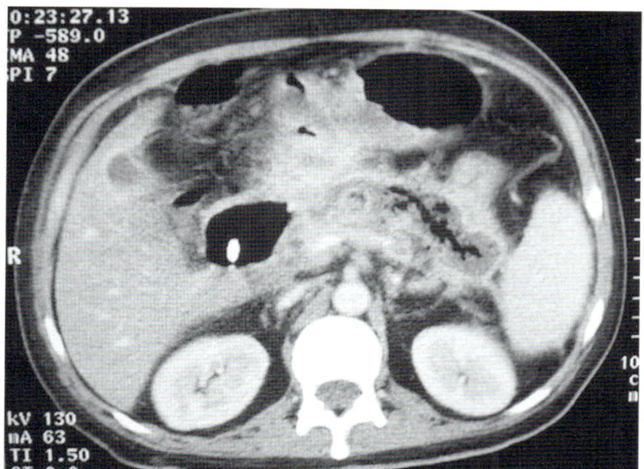

Fig. 18.8: Pancreatic abscess: CECT obtained 2 weeks after onset of acute pancreatitis shows extensive pancreatic necrosis and peripancreatic fluid collections with air bubbles within. The collection has developed well defined walls. Splenic vein thrombosis is also present

Pancreatic Necrosis

On CT pancreatic necrosis is suggested if any part of the pancreatic parenchyma does not enhance or enhances less than 30 HU when compared with a baseline enhanced scan. Sterile necrotic tissue undergoes liquefaction within first 2-3 days and CT imaging depicts a zone of decreased attenuation demarcating viable from necrotic tissue. If contamination does not occur, the liquefied collections either remain stable, evolve into pseudocyst or resolve, eventually resulting in parenchymal atrophy and scarring depending on the extent and severity of parenchymal injury (Fig. 18.9).

Necrotic pancreatic tissue serves as a good medium for infection, which occurs in approximately 20%–70% of cases, usually in the second to third week following the onset of acute pancreatitis.[28] In patients with documented pancreatic necrosis, secondary infection should be suspected if gas bubbles are seen within the necrotic tissue. Although extraluminal retroperitoneal air may be caused by intestinal fistulae and sterile production of gas in the necrotic tissue may occur (Fig. 18.10). Infected pancreatic necrosis, when diagnosed, is an indication for necrosectomy or aggressive percutaneous intervention.[29-31]

Retroperitoneal fat necrosis is seen invariably in patients who have pancreatic necrosis, but the converse is not true.[7] Because CT cannot reliably diagnose retroperitoneal fat necrosis, it has been suggested that all heterogeneous peripancreatic collections should be considered as areas of fat necrosis until proven otherwise.[7]

Vascular Complications

Vascular complications, both arterial and venous, are known to occur in patients who have severe acute pancreatitis.[32] Arterial bleeding is one of the most life-threatening complications,[33] and although virtually all peripancreatic vessels can be involved, the splenic artery is the most common because of its anatomic contiguity with the pancreas. About 5% patients of acute pancreatitis develop haemorrhage due to effect of pancreatic enzymes on small or large vessel wall. Hemorrhage may occur into fluid collections or into the peritoneal cavity. On CT, high density fluid collections with or without fluid levels and evidence of extravascular contrast extravazation are

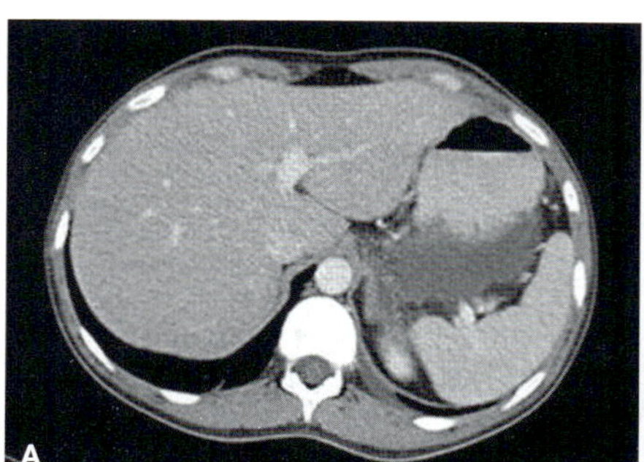

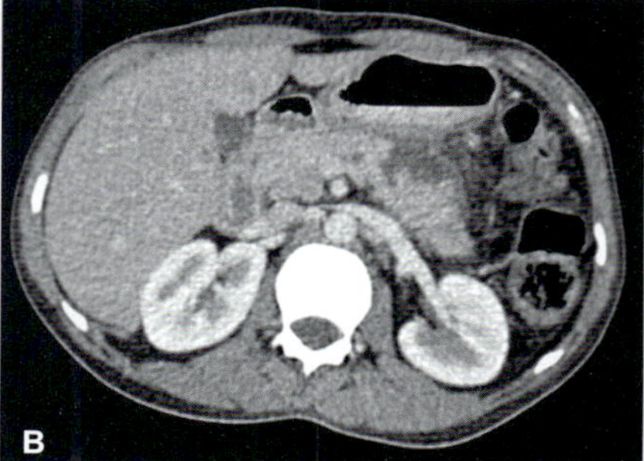

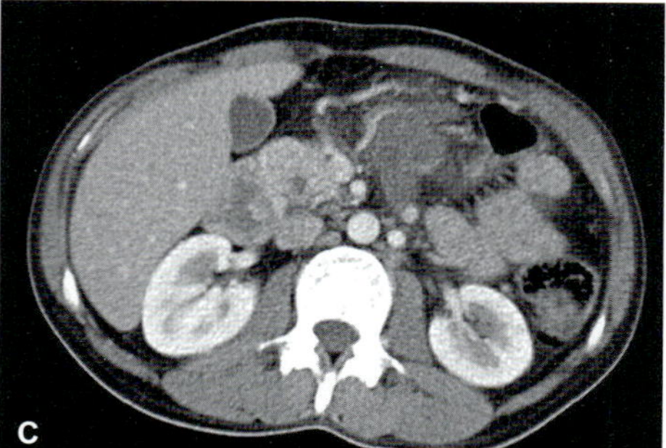

Figs 18.9A to C: Cranial to caudal, pancreatic necrosis (less than 30%): MDCT reveals an irregular non enhancing area within the pancreatic body suggesting necrosis. Fluid collections seen in the adjoining lesser sac and mesentry

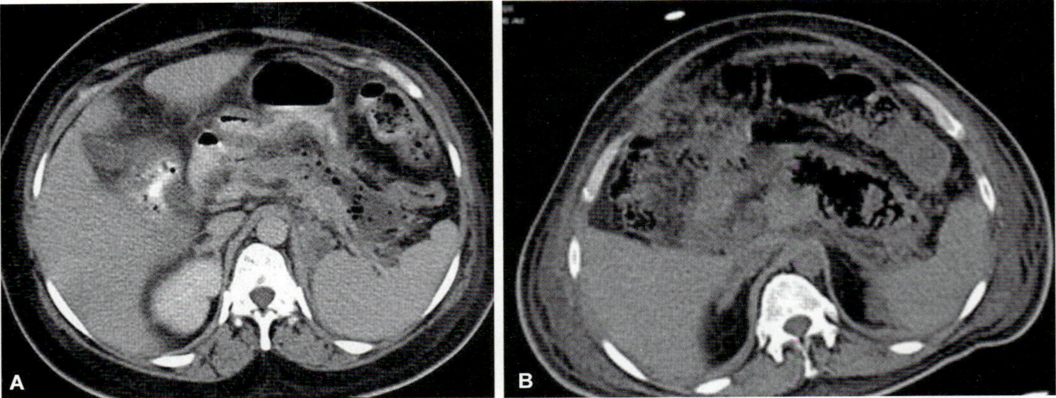

Figs 18.10A and B: Infected Necrosis: CECT at day 7 of acute pancreatitis showing ill defined margins of pancreas with pancreatic/peripancreatic collection which has air pockets within

indicators of intraabdominal hemorrhage and need urgent attention.

Extravasation of proteolytic enzyme can erode peripancreatic vessels resulting in bleeding or formation of pseudoaneurysm. Pseudoaneurysms may be located in the pancreas, adjacent retroperitoneum or within wall of pancreatic pseudocyst. Aneurysms may occur in 10% of severe acute pancreatitis mostly involving the splenic, gastroduodenal, pancreaticoduodenal and superior mesenteric arteries (Fig. 18.11). In non-enhanced CT, they appear as hyperdense pseudocysts. CT angiography or DSA should be performed when necessary. Embolization and when necessary an aggressive surgical approach should be followed. Arterial embolization has become the treatment of choice whenever feasible either as a temporizing procedure or as definite therapy to control bleeding.

Thrombosis of splenic or portal vein may occur as a late complication with non-visualization of splenic vein with or without surrounding inflammatory tissue and retroperitoneal collaterals (Fig. 18.12).

Extrapancreatic Adjacent Organ Involvement

In addition to peripancreatic fluid collections and vascular complications, inflammation may involve adjacent solid organs (e.g. liver, spleen and left kidney) and colon. Because of the close proximity of the pancreatic tail and spleen, inflammatory processes may extend along splenic vessels into the splenic hilum. Splenic involvement in pancreatitis includes intrasplenic pseudocyst, abscess, hemorrhage, and infarction (Fig. 18.13). Intrasplenic hemorrhage occurs because of the erosion of small intrasplenic vessels. Blood may collect beneath the splenic

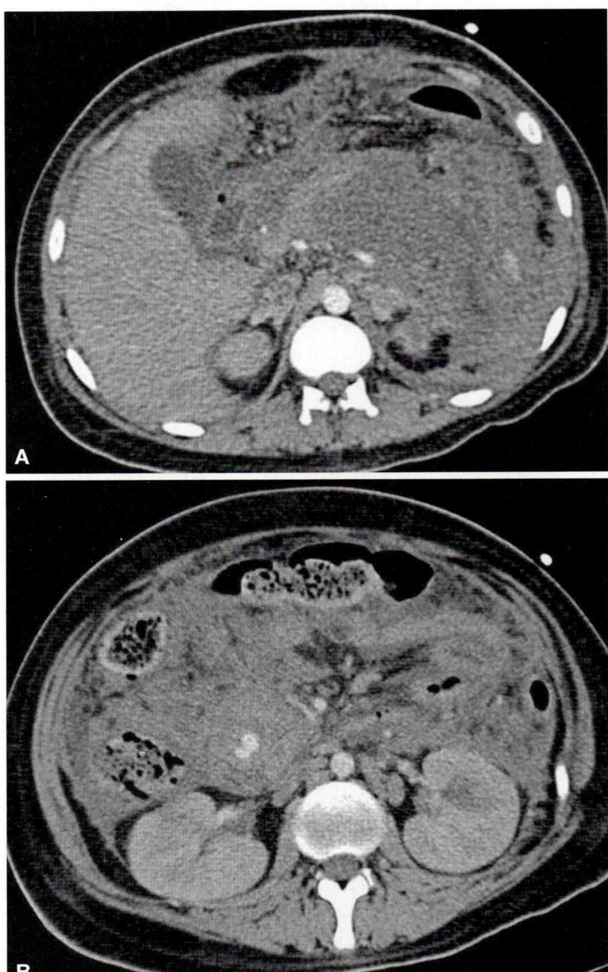

Figs 18.11A and B: Pseudoneurysm: CECT of a 19 years old boy with extensive necrotic pancreatitis (A), shows an intensely enhancing nodular structure in the region of head of pancreas paralleling the aortic enhancement (B), suggestive of a pseudo neurysm likely from gatroduodenal artery

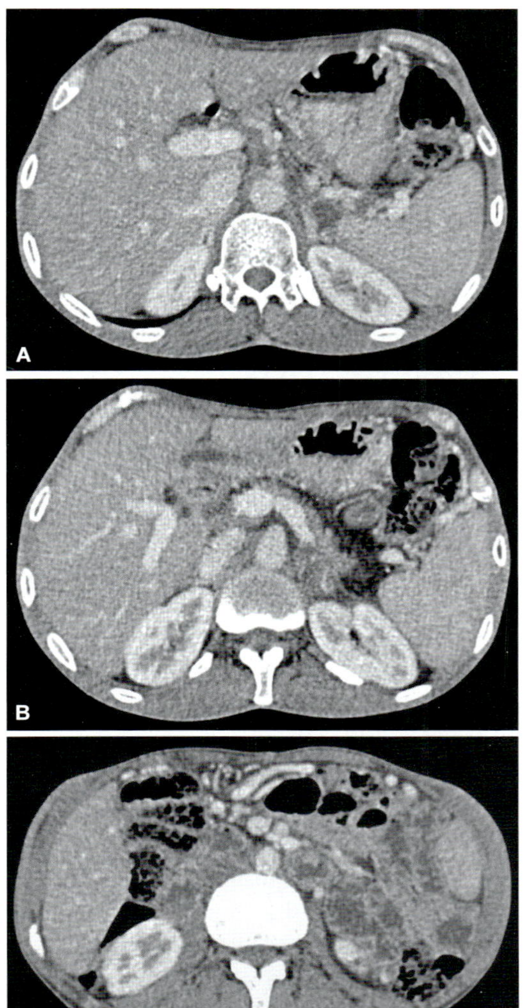
Figs 18.12A to C: Splenic vein thrombosis: CECT of a 34 years old male patient shows pancreatitis involving the pancreatic tail with spread to the pararenal space and splenic hilum. The proximal splenic vein is not visualized with perigatric, perisplenic and mesenteric collaterals

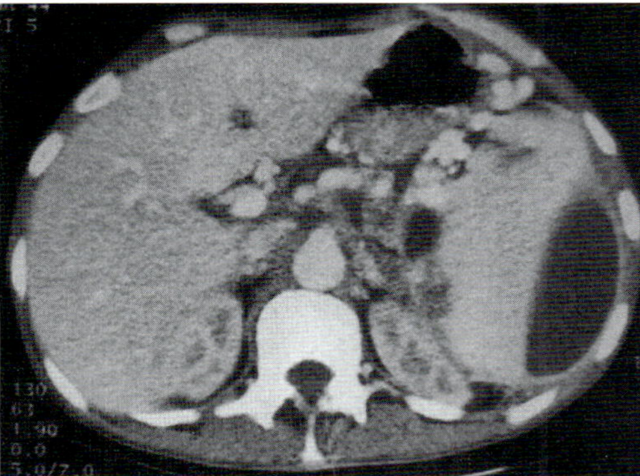
Fig. 18.13: Subcapsular splenic collection. CT showing a large subcapsular fluid collection. Multiple retroperitoneal and perisplenic collaterals are seen suggestive of splenic vein thrombosis in a patient of acute pancreatitis

capsule resulting in subcapsular hematoma. When hemorrhage is large, splenic laceration and rupture can occur and may be catastrophic. Splenic infarction can occur if inflammatory exudates compress the splenic vasculature.

In rare cases, the colon can be affected by local inflammation because of the direct contact of the pancreas with the transverse colon.[34] Direct extension of the inflammatory process or pseudocyst may compress, inflame, or erode the large bowel. There could be resultant bowel obstruction, ischemic necrosis, perforation, hemorrhage, or fistula formation. Large bowel involvement may present weeks or months after an attack of acute pancreatitis. Vascular thrombosis can lead to colonic ischemia.

Staging of Acute Pancreatitis

Staging of severity of acute pancreatitis helps to improve patient management.

Balthazar et al introduced a system of classification (Table 18.1) of patients of acute pancreatitis and indicated prognostic implication of this system based on initial CT findings.[25] They have found that most patients who have severe pancreatitis exhibit one or several fluid collections on initial CT scan. In their study, patients who had grade D or E pancreatitis had a mortality rate of 14% and a morbidity rate of 54%, compared with 0% mortality and 4% morbidity in patients who had grade A, B, or C pancreatitis.[25]

This grading system has been refined based on the extent of pancreatic necrosis seen on imaging, and the term "CT severity index" (CTSI) is now used (Table 18.2).[35] Balthazar and colleagues[35] report that patients with less than 30% necrosis seen on CT exhibit no increase in mortality, although they do show a 48% morbidity rate. Larger areas of necrosis (30–50% and > 50%) are associated with a morbidity rate of 75–100% and a mortality rate of 11–25%. The CTSI score correlates positively with morbidity and mortality. Patients who

Table 18.1 Balthazar grading system

Grade	*Description*
A	Normal-appearing pancreas
B	Focal or diffuse enlargement of the pancreas
C	Pancreatic gland abnormalities accompanied by mild peripancreatic inflammatory changes
D	Fluid collection in a single location
E	Two or more fluid collections near the pancreas or gas in or adjacent to the pancreas

Table 18.2 CT severity index

CT Grade	Score	Necrosis (%)	Score
A	0	None	0
B	1	<30%	2
C	2	30-50%	4
D	3	>50%	6
E	4		

CT severity index (maximum score 10) = CT grade (0–4) + necrosis (0–6).

have CTSI scores of 0–3 showed a 3% mortality rate and 8% morbidity rate, whereas in patients who had CTSI scores of 7 to 10, the mortality and morbidity rates were 17 and 92%, respectively.[35]

Magnetic Resonance Imaging

Magnetic Resonance (MR) imaging is comparable to CT in the depiction of morphologic changes from acute pancreatitis, including the extent of pancreatic necrosis and peripancreatic fluid collections.[36-37] MR imaging can be used as an alternative imaging modality in patients who cannot receive iodinated contrast media because of allergy or renal insufficiency. Patients who have acute pancreatitis often are young and require multiple follow-up CT examinations. In this regard, MR imaging has an advantage over CT, because exposure to excessive ionizing radiation can be avoided.

A T2-weighted fast spin-echo sequence accurately depicts fluid collections, pseudocysts, and hemorrhage. T2-weighted images are more sensitive than CT in the evaluation of a fluid collection's internal characteristics and therefore in the assessment of its drainability (Figs 18.14A to C).[38] Breath-hold, T1-weighted in-phase (TR/TE: 120/4.2) and opposed-phase (TR/TE: 120/2.1) sequences are useful to depict pancreatic and peripancreatic edema.

Dynamic gadolinium enhanced (0.1 mmol/kg body weight) MR imaging is performed using breath-hold, fat-suppressed, 3D gradient echo sequences. Images are acquired in the arterial (20-40 seconds), portal venous (70–80 seconds), and equilibrium (180 seconds) phases. Dynamic contrast-enhanced images are extremely useful for depicting viable from nonviable pancreatic parenchyma. The dynamic contrast-enhanced sequences can be used to produce excellent MR angiography images for the delineation of possible peripancreatic vascular complications.

In addition, comprehensive MR imaging of the pancreas includes MRCP, which is an excellent non-invasive technique to depict biliary and pancreatic ductal anatomy.[39] MRCP is highly sensitive and specific for diagnosing choledocholithiasis, thus limiting ERCP to those patients requiring therapeutic intervention.[39-42] In addition, MRCP accurately demonstrates pancreatic ductal abnormalities associated with pancreatitis, including ductal dilatation, disruption, or leakage.[43] The recently introduced 3D MRCP provides exceptionally high-quality images of the pancreatic and biliary ductal system.[44] Intravenous administration of gadolinium frequently suppresses the depiction of background structures and the renal pelves and therefore improves the depiction of the biliary tracts or main pancreatic duct in selected patients.[45]

Communication of a pseudocyst with the pancreatic duct can be well depicted by MRCP. In patients presenting with recurrent attacks of acute pancreatitis, MRCP is capable of identifying contributing structural anomalies

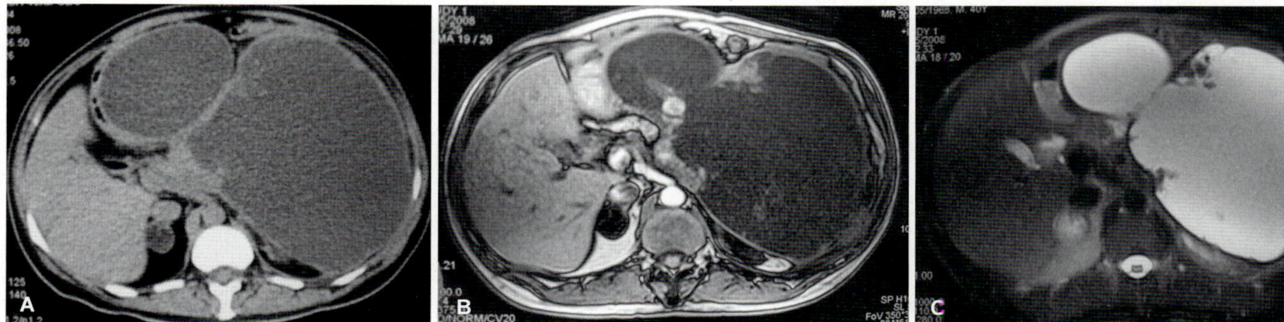

Figs 18.14A to C: Pseudocyst: CECT of a 42 year old male obtained 5 weeks after onset of acute pancreatitis, reveals a large peripancreatic fluid collection with well defined walls and thick septae. MRI (Spoiled gradient T1W and Fast spin echo T2W images) showing the large cyst with septations and isointense nondependent contents. Note is made of bilateral adrenal adenomas

such as pancreas divisum and of diagnosing pancreatic neoplasms (eg, intraductal papillary mucinous neoplasms), which can also present as recurrent disease (Fig. 18.15). Secretin-enhanced MRCP is useful in identifying structural anomalies such as pancreas divisum and has been useful in making an early diagnosis of ductal disruption.[46-48]

Ultrasound

The usefulness of transabdominal ultrasound in acute pancreatitis is limited. Early in the course of an episode of acute pancreatitis, ultrasound is used to evaluate biliary dilatation and also to determine presence of stones in the gallbladder and common bile duct. The major Limiting technical factor for ultrasound evaluation is failure to visualize the pancreas due to distended bowel loops because of paralytic ileus is common in these patients. The ultrasonographic findings in acute pancreatitis can range from a normal-appearing pancreas to a diffusely enlarged hypoechoic gland (Fig. 18.16). One should assess the presence of intrapancreatic or peripancreatic fluid collections, particularly in the lesser sac and anterior pararenal space (Fig. 18.17). Sonography cannot reliably differentiate these fluid collections from pancreatic necrosis, thus limiting its role in the assessment of disease severity. It is however useful for follow up of pseudocysts and guiding percutaneous interventions.

Although a growing body of literature supports the usefulness of endoscopic ultrasound in the evaluation of various pancreatic diseases, its role is limited in patients who have acute pancreatitis. There have been reports suggesting that endoscopic ultrasound is accurate in identifying common bile duct stones.[49-50] MRCP, however, is a highly accurate, noninvasive alternative for detecting common bile duct stones measuring more than 3 mm in diameter. The reported sensitivity of MRCP for the detection of common bile duct stones varies from 57 to 100%; specificity varies from 73 to 100%. With more refined techniques, the values for sensitivity and specificity values are toward the higher end of the spectrum.[51] In patients who have unexplained recurrent pancreatitis, endoscopic ultrasound may be useful in identifying occult pancreatic neoplasms not seen on thin-section MDCT or MR imaging. Likewise, fine-needle aspiration guided by endoscopic ultrasound may be needed to enable distinction of focal pancreatitis from a pancreatic neoplasm, a distinction that often is difficult on CT and MRI.

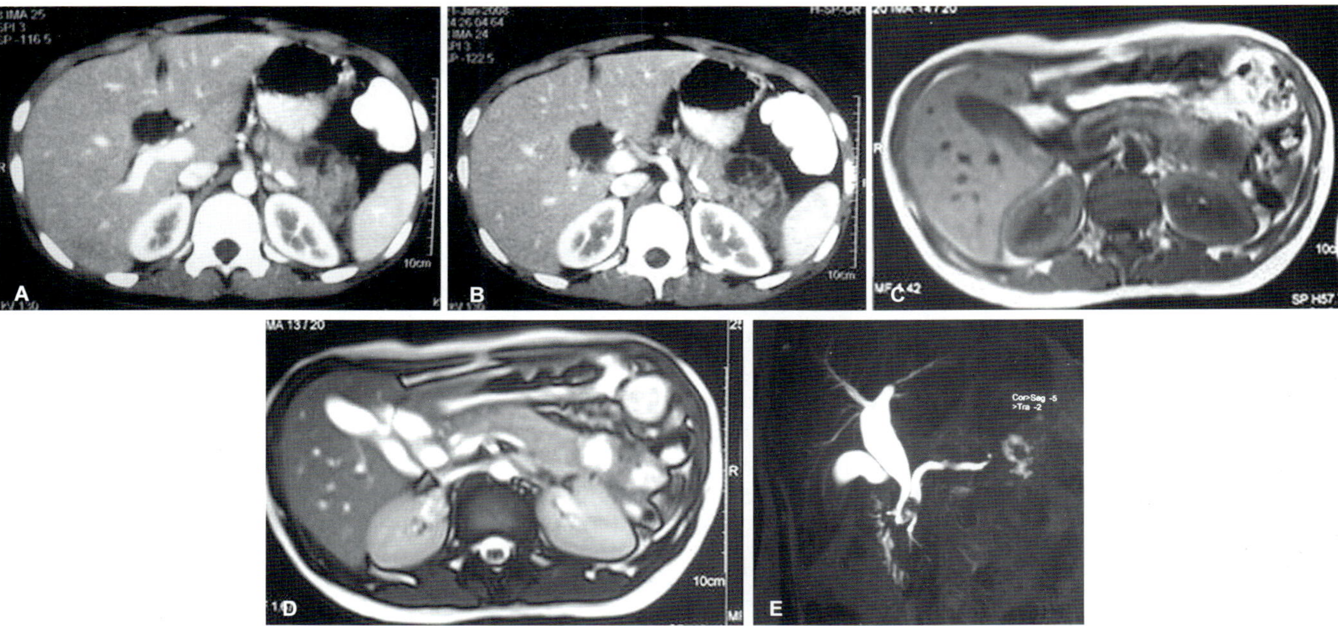

Figs 18.15A to E: Choledochal cyst with pancreatitis: CECT(A&B) of a 15 years old girl reveals a dilated common bile duct with pancreatitis involving the pancreatic body and tail regions. MRI obtained 1 week later shows reduction in the acute fluid collection which appears hypointense on Gradient echo T1W image (C) and hyperintense on FSE T2W image(D). MRCP(E) reveals fusiform dilatation of the CBD and LHD suggesting a choledochal cyst. The MPD ia also dilated with a large calculus seen in the head region.a long common channel is also present

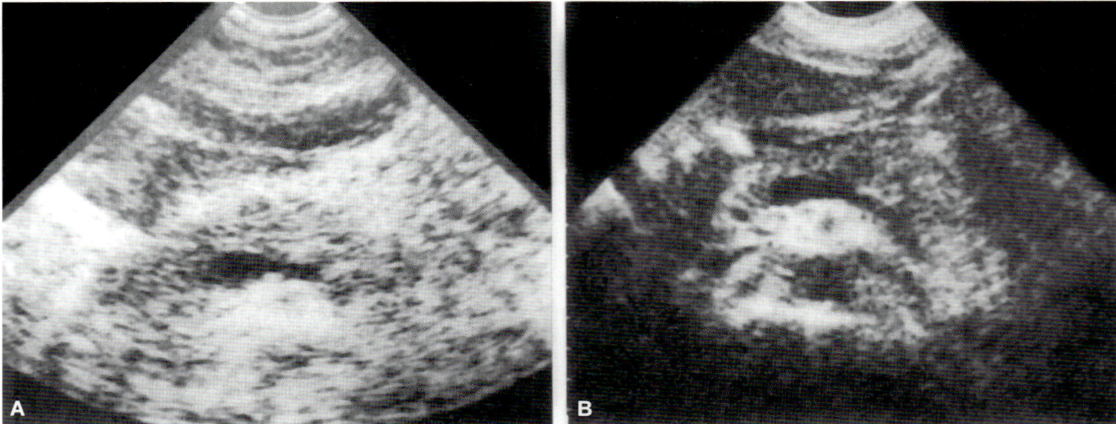

Figs 18.16A and B: Mild acute pancreatitis. US shows (A) Diffusely enlarged pancreas and (B) Enlarged body and tail of pancreas with heterogeneous echopattern

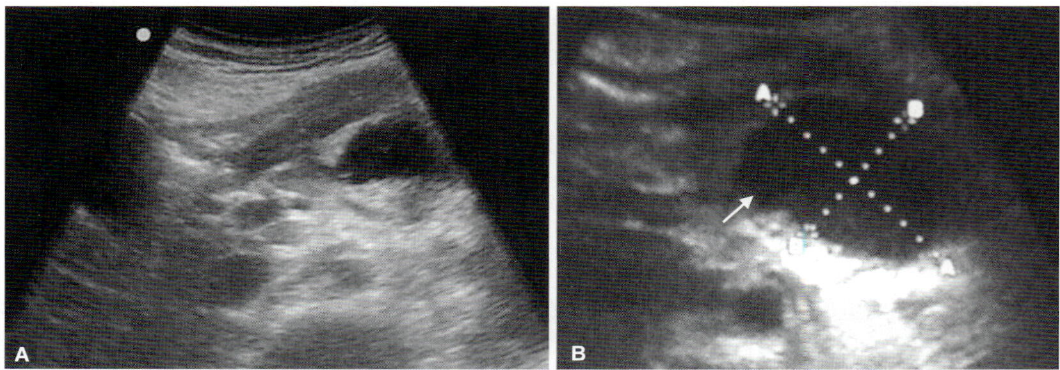

Figs 18.17A and B: Pseudocyst follow up:US of a 19-year-old boy obtained 5 weeks after episode of acute pancreatitis revals a well-defined,walled off collection involving the pancreatic body and lesser sac

Percutaneous Cross-sectional Image–guided Interventions

Both diagnostic and therapeutic percutaneous interventions are performed on a variety of collections in patients who have acute pancreatitis. Diagnostic aspiration for Gram stain and culture is performed on fluid collections, pseudocysts, or pancreatic necrosis when there is a clinical suspicion for infection. Percutaneous catheter drainage is indicated in patients who have established infection. Although most pseudocysts regress spontaneously, large (> 5 cm), unresolving (> 6 weeks), or symptomatic (pain, gastric outlet obstruction, or biliary obstruction) pseudocysts require drainage, which can be performed using percutaneous or endoscopic techniques. Pancreatic abscesses and infected necrosis often require multicatheter drainage either as definitive treatment or as a temporizing measure before surgery. Infected pancreatic necrosis, when diagnosed, is an indication for necrosectomy or aggressive percutaneous intervention.[31]

US and CT are the imaging modalities most commonly used to guide percutaneous intervention (Figs 18.18 and 18.19). MR imaging is superior to CT in determining the viscosity of pancreatic collections, including the presence of solid debris. Internal consistency may predict the success of percutaneous techniques in draining focal fluid and the size of the catheter necessary for successful drainage.[38] The presence of septations and lobulations also may guide the number of catheters needed to produce effective drainage. If an endoscopic drainage procedure such as cystogastrostomy is contemplated, CT is useful in determining the relationship of the relevant collection to the stomach or duodenum .

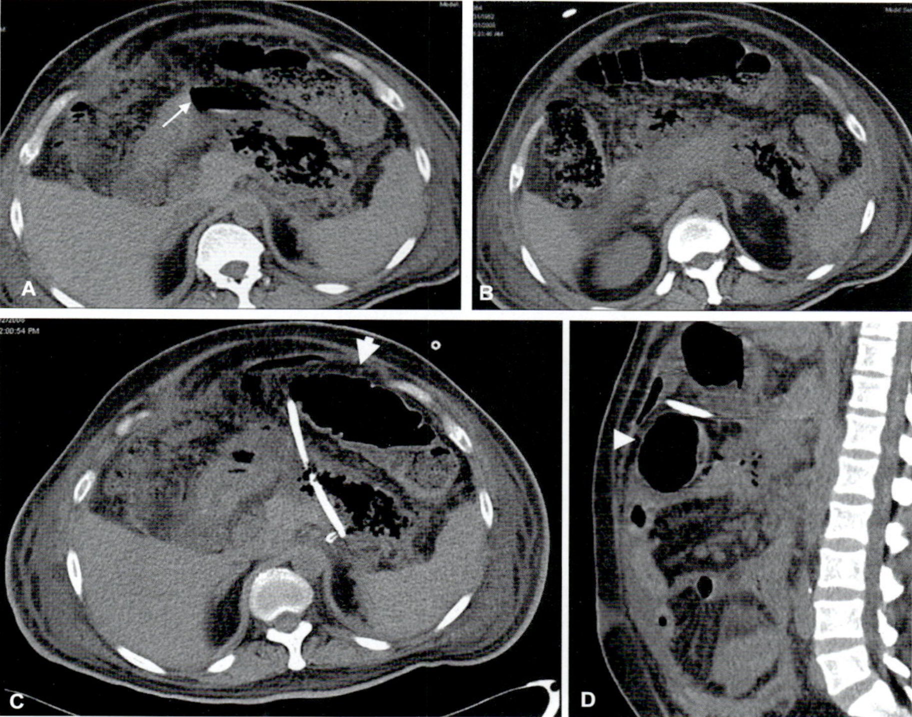

Figs 18.18A to D: NCCT(A and B) of a 48-years-old man showing extensive pancreatic necrosis with air-fluid level (arrow) and extensive air pockets within the pancreas with peripancreatic inflammation. Axial(C) and sagittal (D) NCCT showing a 8 F pigtail catheter placed under CT guidance (C&D). The catheter has been placed avoiding the transverse colon(arrowhead)

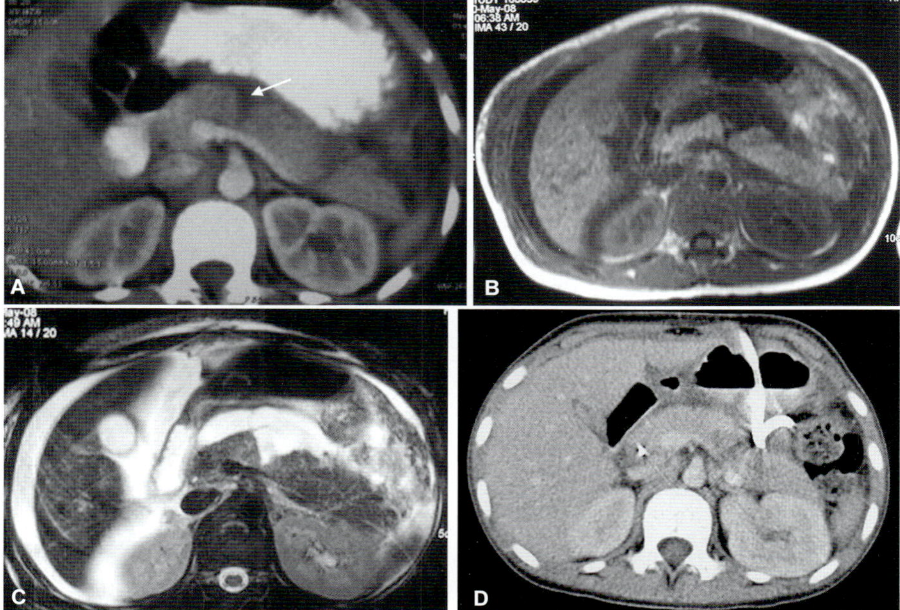

Figs 18.19A to D: Traumatic Pancreatitis with percutaneous drainage: CECT(A) of a 15-year-old boy obtained on the day of trauma showing lacerations in the pancreatic neck and distal body. A follow-up MRI after 3 days (B&C), when patient developed fever reveal progression of pancreatitis with accumulation of peripancreatic and mesenteric fluid. MRI in addition reveals fine septae with in the collection. A 8F pigtail catheter was placed under CT guidance using the transgastric route(D)

Once a drainage procedure has been performed, follow-up imaging is required in assessing procedural success. Persistent collections lasting for months may suggest pancreatic ductal communication.

CHRONIC PANCREATITIS

Chronic pancreatitis is a syndrome of destructive inflammatory condition arising from long-standing pancreatic injury.[52] According to the Marseilles classification it is defined as a continuing inflammatory disease of the pancreas characterized by irreversible morphological damage typically causing pain and/or permanent loss of function.[53]

Classically, the clinical presentation of chronic pancreatitis is abdominal pain which may be recurrent or persisting, malabsorption resulting from exocrine pancreatic insufficiency and in most severe cases diabetes mellitus may result due to endocrine insufficiency caused by progressive destruction of pancreatic parenchyma.

Etiology and Pathophysiology

A number of etiological factors have been implicated and long-standing alcohol abuse is a common cause of chronic pancreatitis. Other causes include chronic biliary tract disease, hereditary pancreatitis, cystic fibrosis, hyperlipidemia, hyperparathyroidism and pancreas divisum. Cases where no definite etiology can be identified are labelled as idiopathic chronic pancreatitis.

The pathogenesis of this condition is poorly understood and it is believed that regardless of the cause, the disease process leads to a final common pathway of irregular sclerosis or fibrosis, acinar and islet cell loss and inflammatory infiltrates. The manifestations are in the form of parenchymal loss or atrophy, ductal dilatation resulting from obstruction by protein plugs or calculi (calcified plugs), stricture or stenosis of ducts and cystic changes. These changes may be focal, segmental or diffuse. The clinical diagnosis of chronic pancreatitis is often difficult with clinically significant pancreatic insufficiency occurring only when about 85% of functioning tissue is lost.[54] Amylase and lipase levels are also usually normal unlike in acute pancreatitis.

The diagnosis is, therefore, based on a combination of clinical, functional and morphologic features. Endoscopic retrograde pancreatography (ERP) and pancreatic function tests although considered as gold standards for the diagnosis but are unfortunately insensitive or discordant in a number of cases.

Imaging in Chronic Pancreatitis

Various imaging modalities offer non-invasive means for making the diagnosis of chronic pancreatitis based on the changes in the pancreatic duct and parenchyma and the detection of ductal calculi. Unfortunately most imaging methods are insensitive and detect only advanced disease. Early opportunity of disease detection and therapeutic interventions is therefore missed. Plain radiographs, contrast studies and ultrasonography have a limited role here and the mainstay of imaging diagnosis is CT and ERP. Recent advances in imaging techniques including gadolinium enhanced MRI, MRCP and endoscopic ultrasound would prove helpful in early diagnosis of chronic pancreatitis.

Plain Films

Pancreatic calcification is the hallmark of chronic pancreatitis and can be seen in 27 to 65% of patients.[24] These calcific densities frequently represent calculi, intraductal in location and vary in size. They are common in alcoholic pancreatitis but occur quite late in the course of the disease. Calcification increases with disease progression. Calcification is less commonly seen with hereditary pancreatitis and cystic fibrosis (Figs 18.20 and 18.21).

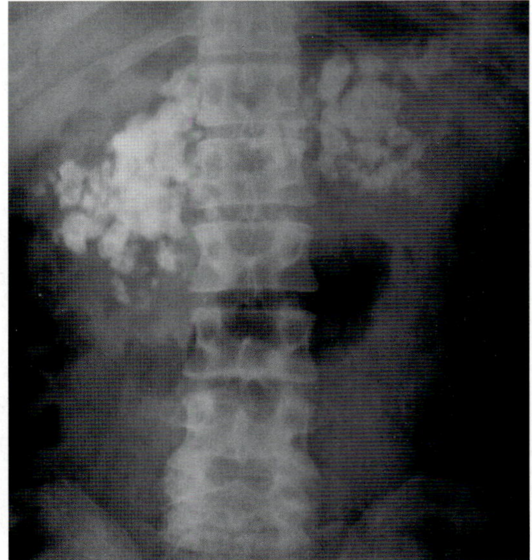

Fig. 18.20: Chronic calcific pancreatitis: Plain radiograph of abdomen reveals extensive calcification in distribution of the main pancreatic duct, its side branches and pancreatic parenchyma

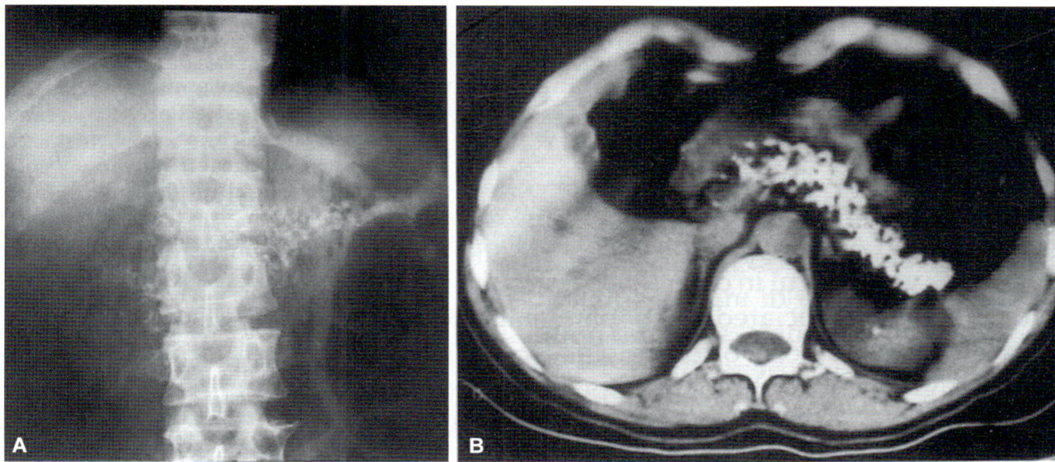

Figs 18.21A and B: Chronic Calcific Pancreatitis (A) Plain radiograph showing classical location of pancreatic calcification extending across the spine. (B) Non-enhanced CT of the same patient showing dense pancreatic calcification

Ultrasonography (US)

Transabdominal sonography (TAS) provides a low cost non-invasive method for screening of patients with suspected chronic pancreatic diseases. Using stomach as a window after intake of water or methyl cellulose aids the visualization of pancreas. The sonographic features of chronic pancreatitis include alteration in pancreatic size and echotexture, focal masses, calcification, ductal dilatation and pseudocyst formation.

Most commonly, the pancreas atrophies and demonstrates areas of heterogeneous echotexture. Increased echogenicity results from fibrosis and calcification whereas areas of diminished echogenicity represent focal inflammation. Ductal dilatation with intraductal calculi, seen as echogenic foci with posterior acoustic shadowing, may be focal or diffuse. This is the most specific feature on ultrasonography but is seen only in advanced stage of the disease.

A focal mass may be seen in up to 40% of patients with chronic pancreatitis which may be hypoechoic or hyperechoic. This may be a diagnostic problem and differentiating benign enlargement from malignant mass may be difficult (Fig. 18.22). Presence of calcification within the mass can help to exclude a neoplasm and presence of local adenopathy or hepatic metastasis favors the diagnosis of a neoplastic mass.[55]

Complications like bile duct dilatation, presence of fluid collections or pseudocyst and portal or splenic vein thrombosis may be picked up on TAS. Application of color Doppler can be very useful in detection of vascular complications associated with pancreatitis viz. venous thrombosis or pseudoaneurysm.

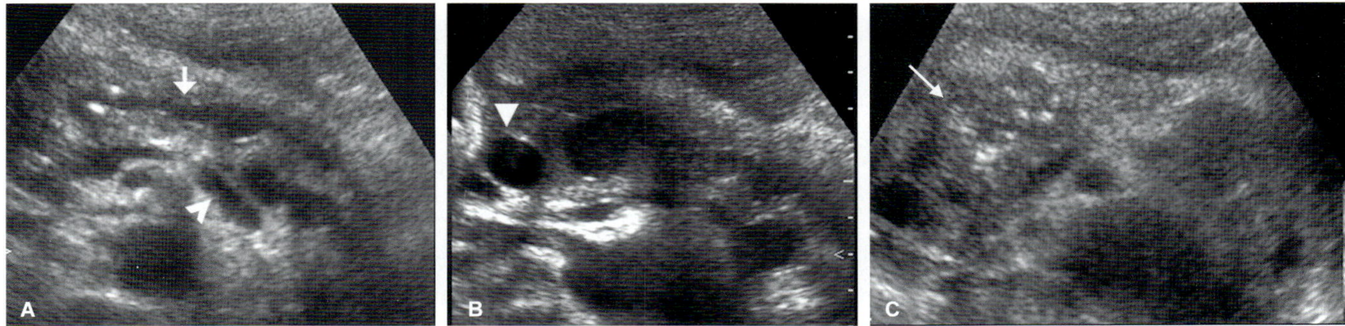

Figs 18.22A to C: (A-C Cranial to caudal): Chronic pancreatitis with focal mass: US of a 42 years old male showing dilated MPD (short white arrow), and CBD (large arrow-head) with hypoechoic mass in pancreatic head region (B) with calcific foci in the uncinate process (long white arrow). Small white arrow-head in Figure A shows the splenic vein

Although the morphological spectrum of chronic pancreatitis ranges from a normal study in early or mild disease to a grossly abnormal study in moderate or severe disease, overall sensitivity of TAS varies and is about 60 to 70%.[56]

Endoscopic Ultrasonography (EUS)

With the advent of endoscopic ultrasonography, this tool has increasingly been used for the diagnosis of chronic pancreatitis. High frequency US probes (7.5-12 MHz) attached to the tip of an endoscope enables good visualization of head and body of the pancreas. EUS offers the advantage over ERCP, of being able to visualize the parenchymal and ductal changes without cannulating the papilla or injection of contrast material. There are only few studies describing the sensitivity and specificity of EUS in chronic pancreatitis.[57] The technique is, however, operator dependent and is useful only for evaluation of head and body of pancreas, the tail region being technically not accessible.

The diagnosis of chronic pancreatitis is made by EUS when at least 3 or 4 of the following findings are present. These include both ductal and parenchymal changes. Ductal changes are dilatation (> 3 mm), tortuosity, intraductal echogenic foci, echogenic duct wall and side-branch ectasia. Parenchymal changes include inhomogeneous echo pattern, hypoechoic foci (1-3 mm), echogenic foci, prominent interlobular septae or echogenic strands, lobular gland margin and large echo poor cavities.[57]

Some authors have found that EUS is positive in a subgroup of patients with early chronic pancreatitis with normal ERP findings.[58] Also EUS may detect abnormality when CT is normal.[59] Therefore; EUS may play an adjunctive role to ERP and CT in the diagnosis of early chronic pancreatitis

The diagnosis of pancreatic malignancy complicating chronic pancreatitis is very difficult using techniques like US, CT and ERCP. The sensitivity of EUS for detection of pancreatic cancer has been reported to be quite high (over 90%) especially for small tumors (less than 2 cm). The image morphology of masses, i.e its shape, margin and echotexture have been used to qualify the nature of lesion with limited success only. Other EUS features suggesting malignancy are presence of calcification limited to the periphery of the mass and vascular involvement, but even these are not very sensitive and frequently EUS guided cytological evaluation is required.[60]

CT

CT confidently detects patients with severe or advanced chronic pancreatitis and is relatively insensitive in picking up early or mild chronic pancreatitis. The sensitivity of CT for diagnosis of chronic pancreatitis varies from 50 to 90% depending on the severity and specificity ranges from 55 to 85%.[61] The advent of helical CT and the advancement in detector technology now enables thinner collimation and allows acquisitions during different phases of contrast bolus and may improve the sensitivity of CT findings further.

The key CT findings of chronic pancreatitis are intraductal calcifications, parenchymal atrophy and MPD dilatation (Figs 18.21 and 18.23). Leutmer et al in their study on patients of chronic pancreatitis found dilatation of MPD in 68%, parenchymal atrophy in 54%,

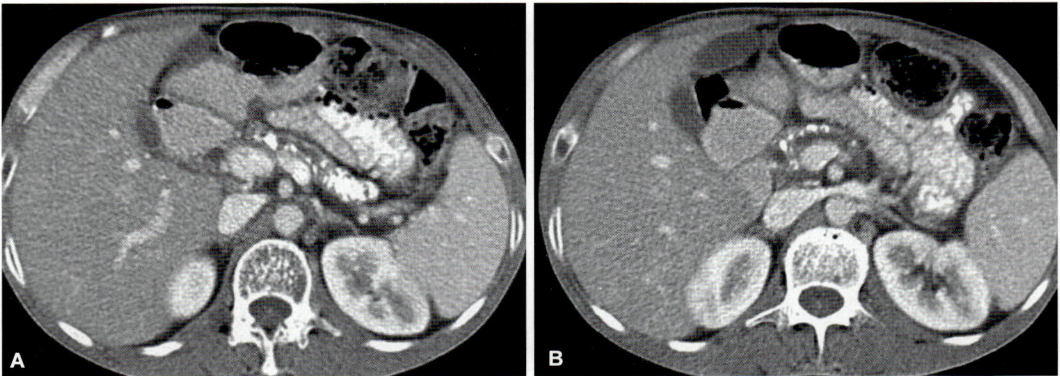

Figs 18.23A and B: Chronic calcific pancreatitis MDCT showing dilatation of the main pancreatic duct with intraductal calculi, and parenchymal atrophy

parenchymal calcification in 50%, focal pancreatic enlargement in 30%, biliary ductal dilatation in 29% and alteration in peripancreatic fat or fascia in 16% patients. Ductal dilatation and parenchymal atrophy were often found to coexist. Patients with exocrine insufficiency frequently revealed gland atrophy or ductal dilatation on CT but about 32% of such patients had no CT evidence of atrophy.[62]

Atrophy is common in advanced disease but is less important and less sensitive in the elderly patients in whom it may be a part of the normal aging process.

Pancreatic ductal dilatation (> 2 to 3 mm) is a frequent feature in chronic pancreatitis. Dilatation may be smooth or beaded and irregular. Calculi consisting of calcium carbonate, protein and polysaccharide are a common finding. CT is superior to US in detection of calculi. Non-calcified protein plugs may be seen as radiolucent filling defects on ERCP but are not well seen on CT. In hereditary pancreatitis, calculi occur early in the course of the disease, are usually large and tend to arrange themselves in a linear fashion within the main duct.

At times focal or diffuse enlargement of pancreas may be noted in chronic pancreatitis. Because of the increased risk of pancreatic cancer in chronic pancreatitis, focal enlargement becomes a diagnostic challenge and often percutaneous or endoscopic biopsy is necessary to distinguish pancreatitis from carcinoma.

CT detects most complications of chronic pancreatitis including pseudocysts, pseudoaneurysms of pancreatico-duodenal or splenic arteries, splenic vein thrombosis or biliary dilatation.

Pseudocysts are seen as well defined, rounded, fluid attenuation collections circumscribed by a detectable wall. They may be within the pancreas, in the retroperitoneum and even in distant locations (Fig. 18.24). Pseudocysts might contain necrotic debris, blood or septations which are more readily appreciated on US than on CT.

Pseudoaneurysms are most often seen near the pancreatic head or splenic hilum. They result from vessel wall destruction by inflammation and are seen as rounded areas iso attenuating to vascular structures. On unenhanced scans they may demonstrate attenuation like that of a hematoma. Splenic or portal vein thrombosis can be well visualised on a contrast enhanced CT. Chronic pancreatitis accounts for 65% of cases of splenic vein thrombosis.[63] This can lead to prehepatic portal hypertension and UGI bleeding.

Bile duct dilatation may result from chronic inflammation involving the pancreatic head. It may be relatively mild and may demonstrate a gradually tapering stenosis differentiating it from the malignant ductal dilatation which is more abrupt and irregular in appearance.

Endoscopic Retrograde Pancreatography (ERP)

ERP remains the most reliable method for visualization of the pancreatic duct by retrograde injection of contrast after cannulation of the ampulla of Vater. The main indications of ERP in chronic pancreatitis are to establish a diagnosis, to assess the pancreatic duct anatomy for pre-surgical evaluation and to perform endoscopic therapy such as stone removal, stent placement or stricture dilatation.

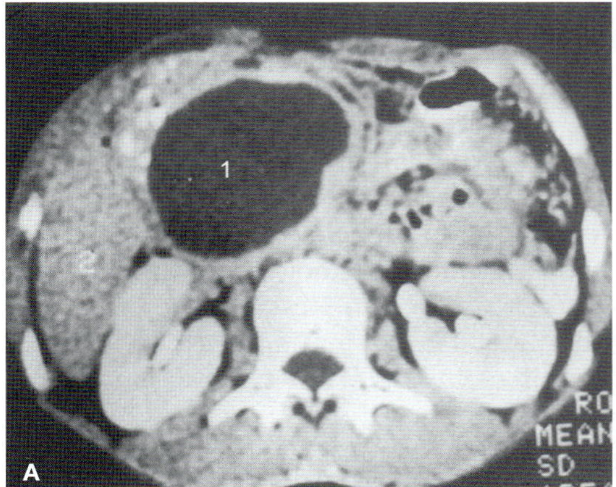

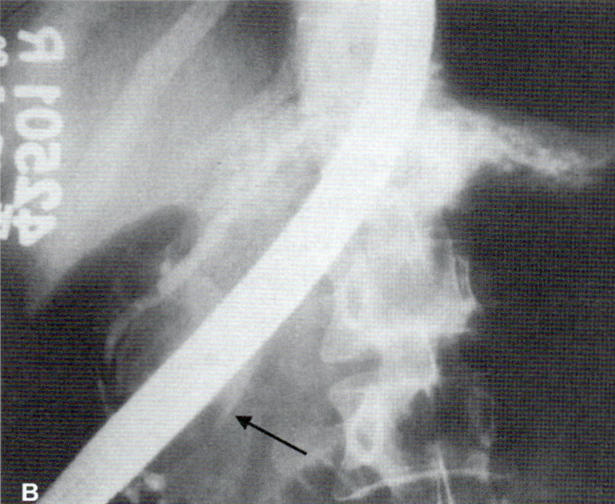

Figs 18.24A and B: Pseudocyst in chronic pancreatitis (A) CT showing a large well defined pseudocyst in the head and uncinate process of pancreas with adjacent pancreatic calcification. (B) ERCP of the same patient shows changes of chronic pancreatitis with involvement of MPD and displacement of the distal MPD by the pseudocyst. Opacification of pseudocyst with contrast suggests ductal communication (arrow)

The normal MPD measures 95-250 mm in length. Its diameter is greatest in the head (3-4 mm) gradually tapering towards the body (2-3 mm) and tail (1-2 mm). Progressive overall increase in the duct calibre is seen with aging. Normal physiologic narrowing occurs at the junction of major and minor ducts in the head and in midgland as the pancreas crosses the mesenteric vessels and spine. Side branches number 20 to 30 and join the main duct at right angles alternating from above and below. Even side branches taper away from the main duct and it is normal to see fewer branches in the body region than in the head and tail.

The Cambridge classification and its modifications are the most commonly used methods of classifying disease severity based on imaging findings. Morphologic changes that help in assessment of disease severity based on ERP, US and CT findings are described below (Table 18.3).

Chronic pancreatitis causes abnormalities on ERP that first affects the side branches and subsequently the MPD. The changes include dilatation, contour irregularity, clubbing, stenosis of side branches and opacification of small cavities. With progression of disease, MPD is involved with dilatation, mural irregularity, loss of normal tapering and areas of stenosis (Fig. 18.25). Multifocal stricture with intervening dilated segments of the main pancreatic duct results in a "chain of lakes" appearance. Strictures or smooth compression of the distal CBD may also be seen.[64] Solitary stricture of MPD may also be seen in a neoplasm or pseudocyst.

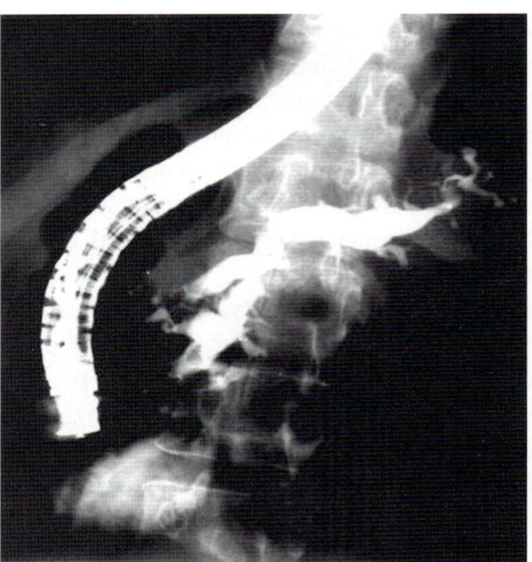

Fig. 18.25: Chronic Pancreatitis: ERCP image showing dilated MPD with dilatation and pruning of side branches. Few intraductal filling defects are seen in the side branches

Stenoses are shorter, smoother and more symmetric in pancreatitis than with neoplasm. Rarely MPD may be completely obstructed by calculus or fibrosis and differentiation from malignancy can be difficult.

ERP is more sensitive than CT for detecting the changes in the ductal system associated with chronic pancreatitis. In some situations however CT may provide additional information about the gland parenchyma and associated complications such as non-communicating cysts and vascular involvement. Hence, both serve as complementary modalities for a complete evaluation.[66]

Table 18.3 Cambridge classification of pancreatic morphology in chronic pancreatitis

Changes	*ERP*	*CT and US*
Normal	MPD normal, no abnormal lateral side branches (LSB)	MPD not more than 2 mm in diameter, normal gland size and shape, homogeneous parenchyma
Equivocal	MPD normal, < 3 abnormal LSB	Only one of the following signs : MPD 2-4 mm in diameter, gland enlarged (less than two times normal), heterogeneous parenchyma
Mild	MPD normal, > 3 abnormal LSB	Two or more signs: MPD 2-4 mm in diameter, slight gland enlargement, heterogeneous parenchyma, small cavities (less than 10 mm)
Moderate	MPD and LSB abnormal	MPD irregularity, focal acute pancreatitis, increased echogenicity of MPD walls, gland contour irregularity
Marked	Any of the above changes plus one or more of the following: cavity greater than 10 mm in diameter, intraductal filling defects, calculi, MPD obstruction or stricture, severe MPD irregularity, contiguous organ invasion	

(*Modified from Axon ATR et al, Gut 1984) [64,65]

Magnetic Resonance (MR) Imaging

MR is a sensitive modality for evaluating pancreatic disease. Although multiple sequences can be performed but pre- and post-gadolinium T1W sequences with fat suppression are the key sequences in the evaluation of pancreas. Gradient echo breath-hold sequences are extremely useful for the evaluation of chronic pancreatitis

Normal pancreas shows avid parenchymal enhancement early after contrast administration. In chronic pancreatitis the pancreas may show diminished signal intensity of the parenchyma and less intense, heterogeneous glandular enhancement than normal on T1W gradient echo breath-hold sequences. Loss of signal reflects the loss of acini secondary to fibrosis.[67] Morphologic findings in chronic pancreatitis on MR are same as those seen on CT and include enlargement or atrophy, ductal dilatation and signal voids corresponding to calcification and pseudocysts. Calcification is less conspicuous on MR than on CT.

Recent work using dynamic MR imaging in unenhanced and gadolinium enhanced arterial and early and late venous phase have shown promise in the detection of early chronic pancreatitis.[69] Contrast enhanced MR has been used to assess patients with focal abnormalities detected on other imaging studies especially differentiating between inflammatory or neoplastic mass. Features favoring chronic pancreatitis on T1-W fat suppressed images are diffuse diminished contrast enhancement on dynamic post contrast images, lack of definition of a solid mass with all sequences, frequent punctate signal void foci on the area of enlargement suggestive of calcification and a few low signal areas representing small pseudocyst.[67]

With all its advantages, MR serves as a problem solving technique; however CT remains the first line imaging modality in evaluation of pancreatic disease.

MR Cholangiopancreatography (MRCP)

MRCP offers a non-invasive method for ductal evaluation. ERP is invasive and is associated with a risk of complications (post ERP pancreatitis in upto 5% patients, sepsis and failure to cannulate the PD in 10-15% cases). MRCP takes advantage of the long T2 relaxation time of pancreatic secretions or bile to depict ductal structures. Current MRCP techniques utilize single shot RARE and half-Fourier acquisition single shot turbo-spin echo achieving image acquisition in a single breath-hold (< 20 seconds). Images may be acquired as contiguous thin slices (source images) which can later be used for maximal intensity projections or thick-slab projections. Negative oral contrast media can be administered in order to reduce contamination of MRCP signal from fluid in stomach and duodenum.[68]

Findings of chronic pancreatitis on MR pancreatography (MRP) examination are similar to those on ERP and include side branch abnormalities, dilatation and irregularity of the MPD, strictures and pseudocysts. Calcifications can be difficult to visualize due to signal void they cause but can be seen as filling defects surrounded by intraductal fluid (Fig. 18.26).

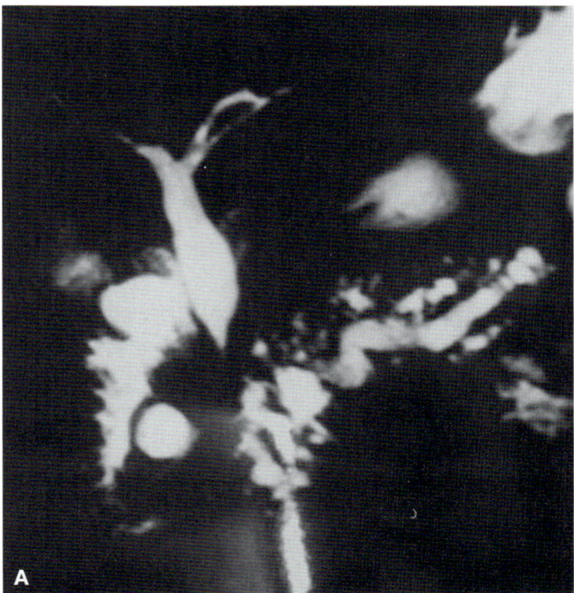

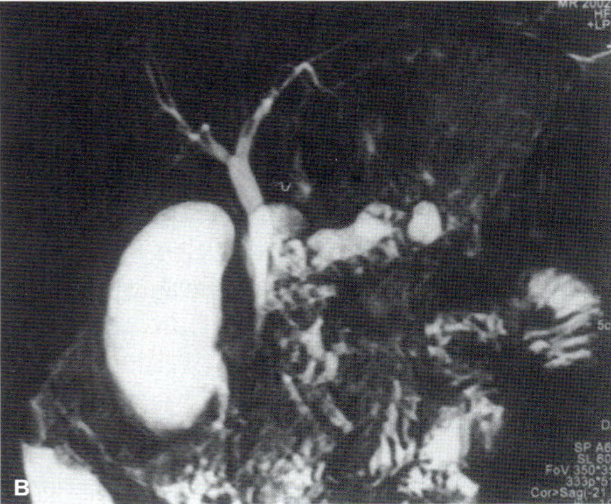

Figs 18.26A and B: MRCP images of two different patients showing dilatation and irregularity of MPD and side branches. In addition there is pruning of the side branches (A)

It has been observed that MRP tends to demonstrate a lesser degree of ductal dilatation in comparison with ERP and this is because of the pressure of contrast injection during ERP that distends the ducts thus improving visualization. Because of the limited ability to image side branches and detection of early pancreatitis the technique of MRP has been improved upon by use of intravenous secretin. Secretin simulates the secretion of fluid and bicarbonate by the exocrine pancreas. Images are obtained every 15-30 seconds till 10-15 minutes after injection. Over time, the pancreatic duct and fluid accumulation in the duodenum is assessed. This correlates well with the pancreatic exocrine function as well.

Also since the pancreatic duct distends in the first few minutes after secretin administration, its visualization is improved when compared with non-secretin stimulated MRP examination. Secretin also improves visualization of side branches, ductal narrowing and endoluminal filling defects in patients with severe chronic pancreatitis.

Advantages of MRP over ERP

- MRP is non-invasive and involves no ionizing radiation.
- MRP does not require any analgesia or premedication and has no risk of procedure induced acute pancreatitis.
- Resolution of MRP for main duct is comparable to that of ERP.
- MRP can be performed in patients in whom endoscopic access is unavailable or unsuccessful, i.e. previous gastric or pancreatic surgery or gastric outlet obstruction.
- MRCP can be combined with MRI of upper abdomen for a complete evaluation.
- MRP shows cysts or other fluid collections adjacent to the pancreas which do not communicate with the pancreatic duct and would not be opacified at ERP
- MRP demonstrates the upstream ductal anatomy in cases with total occlusion of the main pancreatic duct.[68,69]

Advantages of ERP over MRP

- Demonstration of ductal anatomy and resolution is superior to MRP, hence early changes are reliably detected.
- Opportunity for direct inspection of papilla and adjacent anatomy.
- Diagnostic samples of pancreatic juice or brushings for cytology can be obtained.
- Therapeutic maneuver like stent placement, papillotomy and calculi removal is possible.[68]

Positron-emission Tomography (PET)

PET appears promising in the evaluation of pancreatic masses or in differentiating focal enlargement due to pancreatitis from neoplastic process. However, the widespread use of this technology is limited by the need for a cyclotron and PET scanners. Fluorodeoxy-glucose (FDG) accumulation is regarded as a sign of malignancy and is quite sensitive in detection of pancreatic malignancy.[70] Compared with tracers like 201 Thallium used in SPECT imaging, PET was found to be significantly more sensitive (96% vs 64% for thallium) in the detection of pancreatic cancer.[71] Other tracers such as 11C-acetate may also be useful in pancreatic imaging and are currently being investigated.

Imaging in Special Situations and Variants

1. *Groove pancreatitis*: This is a form of segmental chronic pancreatitis localized within the groove between the head of the pancreas, duodenum and the CBD.[72] Patients present with pain, vomiting, jaundice and weight loss. The pancreatic duct system is normal and calcification or intraductal protein plugs are rare. Pancreatic duct stenosis and smooth tapering biliary stenosis may be seen. CT demonstrates a poorly enhancing lesion between the head of the pancreas and the duodenum. Cysts in the duodenal wall or the groove and duodenal stenosis due to wall thickening are commonly seen.

   In groove pancreatitis, the pancreatic head is variably involved and differentiation from pancreatic carcinoma is important. Usually the findings are confined to the groove and duodenum and pancreatic head enhance normally. On MR there is a sheet like lesion between the head of the pancreas and duodenum, which is hypo intense on T1W image, and Iso to slightly hyperintense on T2W images showing delayed enhancement after contrast administration.[73-75]
2. *Focal pancreatitis of head vs. carcinoma*: Often there is a problem in diagnosis of a focal mass in pancreas in an established case of chronic pancreatitis. It can be due to focal inflammatory mass or a malignancy superimposed on chronic pancreatitis (Fig. 18.27).

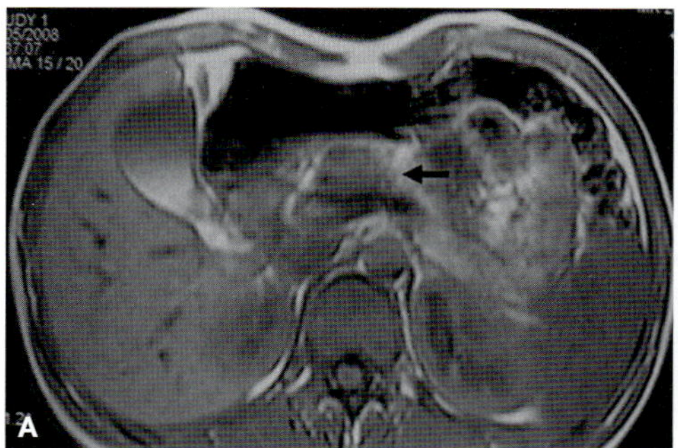
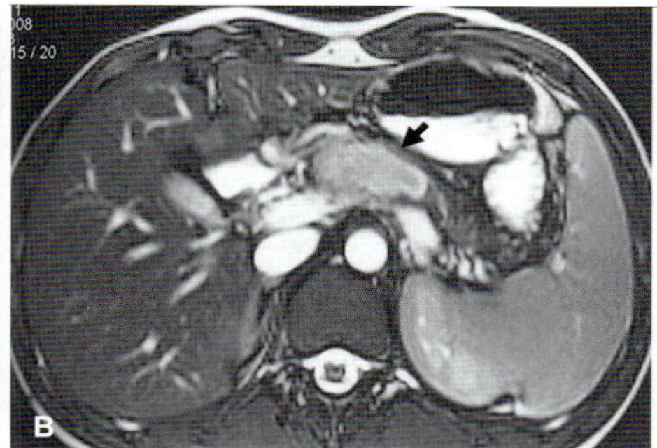
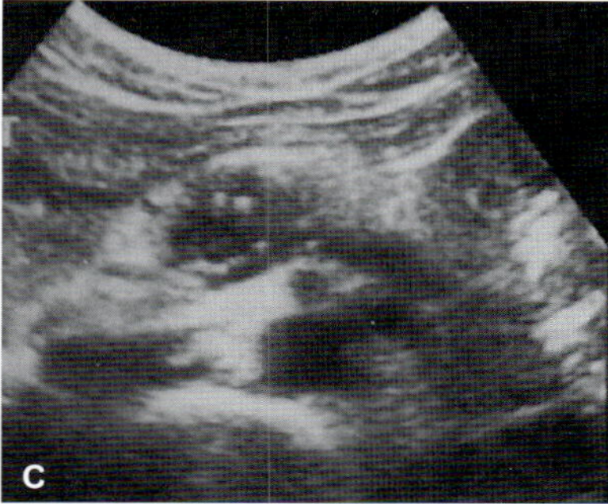

Figs 18.27A to C: Focal pancreatitis: T1W spoiled gradient echo(A) and TRU-FISP images (B) of a 19 years old boy showing focal lesion involving the body of pancreas, which appears hypointense on T1WI and hyperintense on TRU-FISP images. US(C) of the same patient reveal faint calcific specks within the focal lesion suggesting a diagnosis of focal pancreatiis

On CT, features like peripancreatic inflammatory changes, differential enhancement of the lesion and uninvolved gland, the character of ductal dilatation and vascular involvement have all been investigated but with limited success. Specific features of inflammatory mass like presence of calcification within the mass occur infrequently. An inflammatory mass may contain dilated intrapancreatic ductal branches with or without calculi, whereas ducts become obliterated when they are replaced by a neoplasm. Occasionally necrotic tumors may have a cavitary appearance but the thickness and irregularity of their walls should help to differentiate this from a pseudocyst related to chronic pancreatitis. Periarterial extension around the superior mesenteric artery occurs frequently in carcinoma but is rarely seen in chronic pancreatitis.

EUS shows a high sensitivity rate in detection of small tumors but even this modality is not without limitations.[60]

On MR the difference in signal on T1W and T2W images or pattern of enhancement on dynamic MR imaging also does not help to differentiate inflammatory from a neoplastic process. The appearance of pancreatic duct on MRCP may hold some promise here. If a nondilated MPD courses through a pancreatic mass then it is likely to be related to focal pancreatitis.[66]

FDG-PET is being investigated in its possible role in differentiating chronic pancreatitis and pancreatic cancer with variable success.[70-71] The only definite indicator of malignancy is presence of regional lymphadenopathy or hepatic metastasis. It is not always possible to differentiate the two by imaging alone and percutaneous or endoscopic biopsy/FNAC is often necessary.

SUMMARY

Pancreatitis can be a mild, self-limiting disease or can be severe with significant patient morbidity and mortality. The severity of the patient's condition is judged based on clinical, laboratory, and imaging criteria. Contrast enhanced MDCT is the imaging modality of choice for acute pancreatitis and is used to stage the severity of inflammation, detect pancreatic necrosis, and identify local complications. For chronic pancreatitis, combination of laboratory tests, radiological investigations and ERCP is necessary. Percutaneous CT-guided interventions provide therapeutic options in these patients. Other cross-sectional imaging modalities including MR imaging/ MRCP and ultrasound are used in specific clinical scenarios.

REFERENCES

1. DC. Whitcomb, Clinical practice. Acute pancreatitis, N Engl J Med 2006;354(20):2142-50.
2. Banks PA, Bradley III EL, Dreiling DA, et al. Classification of Pancreatitis: Cambridge and Marseille. Gastroenterology 1985;89:928-30.
3. NG Venneman E Buskens, MG Besselink et al. Small gallstones are associated with increased risk of acute pancreatitis: potential benefits of prophylactic cholecystectomy? Am J Gastroenterol 2005;100(11): 2540-50.
4. GH. Sakorafas and AG. Tsiotou, Etiology and pathogenesis of acute pancreatitis: current concepts, J Clin Gastroenterol 2000;30(4):343-56.
5. PA. Banks, Practice guidelines in acute pancreatitis. Am J Gastroenterol 1997;92(3):377-86.
6. PA. Banks, A new classification system for acute pancreatitis. Am J Gastroenterol 1994;89(2):151-52.
7. EJ. Balthazar, Acute pancreatitis: assessment of severity with clinical and CT evaluation. Radiology 2002;223(3): 603-13.

8. EL Bradley 3rd. A clinically based classification system for acute pancreatitis. Summary of the International Symposium on Acute Pancreatitis, Atlanta (GA), September 11 through 13, Arch Surg 1992;128(5):1993; 586-90.
9. C Dervenis, CD Johnson, C Bassi et al. Diagnosis, objective assessment of severity, and management of acute pancreatitis. Int J Pancreatol 1999;25(3):195-210.
10. CJ McKay, CW Imrie. The continuing challenge of early mortality in acute pancreatitis. Br J Surg 2004;91(10): 1243-44.
11. G Kloppel, R VonGerkan, T Dreyer. Pathomorphology of acute pancreatitis: analysis of 367 autopsy cases and through surgical specimens. In: KE Gyr, MV Singler, H Sarles, Editors, Pancreatitis: concepts and classifications, Elsevier Science Publishers, Amsterdam (The Netherlands) 1984;29-35.
12. JH Ranson, KM Rifkind, DF Roses et al. Objective early identification of severe acute pancreatitis, Am J Gastroenterol 1974;61(6):443-51.
13. SL Blamey, CW Imrie, J. O'Neill et al. Prognostic factors in acute pancreatitis, Gut 1984;25(12):1340-46.
14. Beger HG, Rau BM. Severe acute pancreatitis: Clinical course and management. World J Gastroenterol 2007;13(38):5043-51.
15. WA Knaus, EA Draper, DP Wagner et al. APACHE II: a severity of disease classification system, Crit Care Med 1985;13(10):818-29.
16. M Larvin, MJ McMahon. APACHE-II score for assessment and monitoring of acute pancreatitis, Lancet 1989;2 (8656):201-205.
17. C Wilson, DI Heath, CW Imrie. Prediction of outcome in acute pancreatitis: a comparative study of APACHE II, clinical assessment and multiple factor scoring systems. Br J Surg 1990;77(11):1260-64.
18. T Foitzik, DG Bassi, J Schmidt et al. Intravenous contrast medium accentuates the severity of acute necrotizing pancreatitis in the rat. Gastroenterology 1994;106(1):207-14.
19. T Foitzik, DG Bassi C. Fernandez-del Castillo et al. Intravenous contrast medium impairs oxygenation of the pancreas in acute necrotizing pancreatitis in the rat. Arch Surg 1994;129(7):706-11.
20. J Schmidt, HG Hotz, T Foitzik et al. Intravenous contrast medium aggravates the impairment of pancreatic microcirculation in necrotizing pancreatitis in the rat. Ann Surg 1995;221(3):257-64.
21. W Uhl, A Roggo, T Kirschstein et al. Influence of contrast-enhanced computed tomography on course and outcome in patients with acute pancreatitis. Pancreas 2002;24(2): 191-97.
22. TL Hwang, KY Chang, YP Ho. Contrast-enhanced dynamic computed tomography does not aggravate the clinical severity of patients with severe acute pancreatitis: reevaluation of the effect of intravenous contrast medium on the severity of acute pancreatitis. Arch Surg 2000;135(3):287-90.
23. PE Bize, A Platon, CD Becker et al. Perfusion measurement in acute pancreatitis using dynamic perfusion MDCT. AJR Am J Roentgenol 2006;186(1):114-18.
24. Bennett GL, Balthazar EJ. Imaging of acute and chronic pancreatitis. In Gazelle GS, Saini S, Mueller PR (Eds): Hepatobiliary and Pancreatic Radiology Imaging and Intervention. Thieme: New York 1998;746-82.
25. EJ Balthazar, JH Ranson, DP Naidich et al. Acute pancreatitis: prognostic value of CT. Radiology 1985; 156(3):767-72.
26. EL Bradley III, AC Gonzalez, JL Clements Jr. Acute pancreatic pseudocysts: incidence and implications. Ann Surg 1976;184(6):734-37.
27. M Yamamura, K Iki. Mediastinal extension of a pancreatic pseudocyst. Pancreatology 2004;4(2):90.
28. EK Paulson, KM Vitellas, MT Keogan et al. Acute pancreatitis complicated by gland necrosis: spectrum of findings on contrast-enhanced CT. AJR Am J Roentgenol 1999;172(3):609-613.
29. MW Buchler, B Gloor, CA Muller et al. Acute necrotizing pancreatitis: treatment strategy according to the status of infection. Ann Surg 2000;232(5):619-626.
30. P Buchler, HA Reber. Surgical approach in patients with acute pancreatitis. Is infected or sterile necrosis an indication–in whom should this be done, when, and why?, Gastroenterol Clin North Am 1999;28(3):661-71.
31. S Shankar E vanSonnenberg, SG Silverman et al. Imaging and percutaneous management of acute complicated pancreatitis, Cardiovasc Intervent Radiol 2004;27(6):567-80.
32. I Vujic. Vascular complications of pancreatitis. Radiol Clin North Am 1989;27(1):81-91.
33. JW Burke, SJ Erickson, CD Kellum et al. Pseudoaneurysms complicating pancreatitis: detection by CT, Radiology 1986;161(2):447-50.
34. A Gardner, G Gardner, E Feller. Severe colonic complications of pancreatic disease. J Clin Gastroenterol 2003;37(3):258-62.
35. EJ Balthazar, DL Robinson, AJ Megibow et al. Acute pancreatitis: value of CT in establishing prognosis. Radiology 1990;174(2):331-36.
36. J Ward, AG Chalmers, AJ Guthrie et al. T2-weighted and dynamic enhanced MRI in acute pancreatitis: comparison with contrast enhanced CT. Clin Radiol 1997;52(2):109-14.
37. A Saifuddin, J Ward, J Ridgway et al. Comparison of MR and CT scanning in severe acute pancreatitis: initial experiences, Clin Radiol 1993;48(2):111-16.
38. DE Morgan, TH Baron, JK Smith et al. Pancreatic fluid collections prior to intervention: evaluation with MR imaging compared with CT and US. Radiology 1997; 203(3):773-78.
39. GT Sica, J Braver, MJ Cooney et al. Comparison of endoscopic retrograde cholangiopancreatography with MR cholangiopancreatography in patients with pancreatitis. Radiology 1999;210(3):605-10.
40. AS Fulcher, MA Turner. MR pancreatography: a useful tool for evaluating pancreatic disorders, Radiographics 1999;19(1):5-24.

41. AS Fulcher, MA Turner, AM Zfass. Magnetic resonance cholangiopancreatography: a new technique for evaluating the biliary tract and pancreatic duct. Gastroenterologist 1998;6(1):82-87.
42. AS Fulcher, MA Turner, GW Capps et al. Half-Fourier RARE MR cholangiopancreatography: experience in 300 subjects, Radiology 1998;207(1): 21-32.
43. C Matos, O Cappeliez, C Winant et al. MR imaging of the pancreas: a pictorial tour, Radiographics 2002;22(1).
44. A Sodickson, KJ Mortele, MA Barish et al. Three-dimensional fast-recovery fast spin-echo MRCP: comparison with two-dimensional single-shot fast spin-echo techniques. Radiology 2006;238(2):549-559.
45. M Kanematsu, M Matsuo, Y Shiratori et al. Thick-section half-Fourier rapid acquisition with relaxation enhancement MR cholangiopancreatography: effects of iv administration of gadolinium chelate. AJR Am J Roentgenol 2002;178(3):755-61.
46. KJ Hellerhoff, H Helmberger 3rd and T. Rosch et al. Dynamic MR pancreatography after secretin administration: image quality and diagnostic accuracy. AJR Am J Roentgenol 2002;179(1):121-29.
47. Y Fukukura, F Fujiyoshi, M Sasaki et al. Pancreatic duct: morphologic evaluation with MR cholangiopancreatography after secretin stimulation, Radiology 2002; 222(3):674-80.
48. M Arvanitakis, M Delhaye, V De Maertelaere et al. Computed tomography and magnetic resonance imaging in the assessment of acute pancreatitis. Gastroenterology 2004;126(3):715-23.
49. A Chak, RH Hawes, GS Cooper et al. Prospective assessment of the utility of EUS in the evaluation of gallstone pancreatitis. Gastrointest Endosc 1999;49(5):599-604.
50. V de Ledinghen, R Lecesne, JM Raymond et al. Diagnosis of choledocholithiasis: EUS or magnetic resonance cholangiography? A prospective controlled study, Gastrointest Endosc 1999;49(1):26-31.
51. JH Kim, MJ Kim, SI Park et al. MR cholangiography in symptomatic gallstones: diagnostic accuracy according to clinical risk group. Radiology 2002;224(2):410-16.
52. Eternad B, Whitcomb DC. Chronic pancreatitis diagnosis classification and new genetic development. Gastroenterology 2001;120:682-707.
53. Sarner M, Cotton PB. Classification of Pancreatitis Gut 1984;25:756-59.
54. Singh SM, Reber HA. The pathology of chronic pancreatitis. World J Surg 1990;14:2-10.
55. Alpern MB, Sandler MA, Kellman GH, et al. Chronic pancreatitis. Ultrasonic features. Radiology 1985;155: 215-19.
56. Bolondi L. Sonography of chronic pancreatitis. Radiol Clin North Am 1989;27:815.
57. Catalano MF, Geenen JE. Diagnosis of chronic pancreatitis by endoscopic ultrasonography. Endoscopy 1998; 30(Suppl):A111–15.
58. Natterman C, Goldschmidt AJ, Dancygier H. Endosonography in chronic pancreatitis—A comparison between endoscopic retrograde pancreatography and endoscopic ultrasonography. Endoscopy 1993;25:565-70.
59. Muller A, Hatfieed ARW, Lees WR. Endoscopic ultrasonography of the pancreas and biliary tract. In Lees WR Lyons EA (Eds): Invasive Ultrasound Marlin Dunitz Ltd: London 1996;163-67.
60. Barthet M, Portal I, Boujaode J, et al. Endoscopic ultrasonographic diagnosis of pancreatic cancer complicating chronic pancreatitis. Endoscopy 1996;28:487-91.
61. Balthazar EJ. CT of pancreatitis. Categorical course on Gastrointestinal Radiology Am Coll Radiol 1991;109-14.
62. Luetmer PH, Stephens DH, Ward EM. Chronic Pancreatitis reassessment with current CT. Radiology 1989;171:353-57.
63. Gore RM, Marn CS, Baron RL. Vascular disorders of the liver and splanchnic circulation. In Levine MS, (Eds): Textbook of Gastrointestinal Radiology (2nd ed). WB Saunders Philadelphia 2000;2:1639-68.
64. Axon ATR, Classen M, Cotton PB, et al. Pancreatography in chronic pancreatitis: International Definitions Gut 1984;25:1107-12.
65. Jones SN, Lees WR, Frost RA. Diagnosis and grading of chronic pancreatitis by morphological criteria derived by ultrasound and pancreatography. Clin Radiol 1998;39: 43-48.
66. Remer EM, Baker ME. Imaging of chronic pancreatitis. Radiol Clin North Am 2002;40:1229-42.
67. Semelka RC, Shoenut JP, Kroeker MA, et al. Chronic Pancreatitis MR imaging features before and after administration of Gadopentate dimeglumine. J Magn Reson Imaging 1993;3:79-82.
68. Robinson PJA, Sheridan MB. Pancreatitis. computed tomography and magnetic resonance imaging. EurRadiol 2000;10:401-08.
69. Zhang XM, Shi H, Parker L, et al. Suspected early or mild chronic pancreatitis: Enhancement patterns on gadolinium chelate dynamic MRI. J Magn Reson Imaging 2003; 17(1):86-94.
70. Bares R, Klever P, Hanuptmann S, et al. F-18 Fluorodeoxyglucose PET in vivo evaluation of pancreatic glucose metabolism for detection of pancreatic cancer. Radiology 1994;192:79-86.
71. Inokuma T, Tamaki N, Torizuka T, et al. Value of fluorine 18-Fluorodeoxy-glucose and Thallium 201 in the detection of pancreatic cancer J Nucl Med 1995;36:229-35.
72. Stolte M, Weiss W, Velkholz H, et al. A special form of segmental pancreatitis "groove pancreatitis". Hepatogastroenterology 1982;29:198-208.
73. Yamaguchi K, Tanaka M. Groove Pancreatitis Masquerading as pancreatic carcinoma. Am J Surg 1992;163: 312-18.
74. Irie H, Honda H, Kuroiwa T, et al. MRI of groove pancreatitis. J Comput Assist Tomogr 1998;22:651-55.
75. Blasbalg R et al. MRI Features of Groove Pancreatitis. AJR 2007;189:73-80.

Chapter Nineteen

Tumors of Pancreas

Veena Chowdhury

The most common tumor of the pancreas comprising 75-90% of all non-endocrine pancreatic malignancies is ductal adenocarcinoma. Pancreatic tumors are the second most common malignancy of the gastrointestinal tract. Till date resection remains the only cure and the overall survival rate for 5 years is less than 5%. Cystic pancreatic tumors are a diverse group of lesions which are relatively rare as are the endocrine tumors of the pancreas.

Imaging of pancreatic tumors involves both diagnosis and staging. Computed tomography (CT) is the established technique for evaluation of pancreatic adenocarcinoma and the newer multidetector CT's (MDCT) allow accurate local and distant staging as well as assessment of resectability. Ultrasonography (US) endoscopic US, magnetic resonance imaging (MRI) provide complementary, additional and often characteristic information. A detailed understanding of the pancreatic topography, macro- and microanatomy and its physiology is mandatory for planning the strategies for evaluation of this relatively elusive organ and also to explain the hitherto insignificant impact on survival from malignancy of this organ, despite improved sensitivity and specificity of diagnostic modalities.

ANATOMY

Topography

The pancreas lies ventral to the first lumbar vertebra, deep in the epigastric region where it is located in the anterior pararenal space of the retroperitoneum. It is partially surrounded by duodenum and liver and lies behind the stomach. The gland is oriented slightly obliquely and cranially towards the left. It measures 15 cm in length, 7 cm craniocaudally and 2 to 3 cm in anteroposterior dimensions.

Head and uncinate process of pancreas lie within the duodenal C-loop, its anterior surface is limited by the transverse mesocolon and is crossed by the distal part of gastroduodenal artery while the posterior surface is fixed by the fascia of Treitz. The neck of pancreas is a focal area of narrowing caused by compression between Ist part of duodenum cranially and the mesenteric vessels caudally. It lies behind the antrum and pylorus of the stomach and its anterior surface is covered by transverse colon and mesocolon (Figs 19.1A and B). The posterior surface is bordered by the superior mesenteric vein and the retropancreatic segment of portal vein and inferior vena cava (IVC). The body of pancreas is covered anteriorly by parietal layer of lesser sac. Posteriorly it is in contact with superior mesenteric artery, splenic vein, left renal vein in the aortomesenteric space and the splenic artery. The upper part of the body is in close contact with the coeliac trunk. The tail of pancreas is completely covered by peritoneum and is, therefore, relatively mobile. Its caudal portion is oriented towards the splenic hilum, anterior surface lies close to the posterior part of the lesser sac while the posterior surface is in close contact with left kidney. The topography and relations of pancreas in the retroperitoneum are the major determinants of unresectability of its malignant lesions even when relatively small in size.[1]

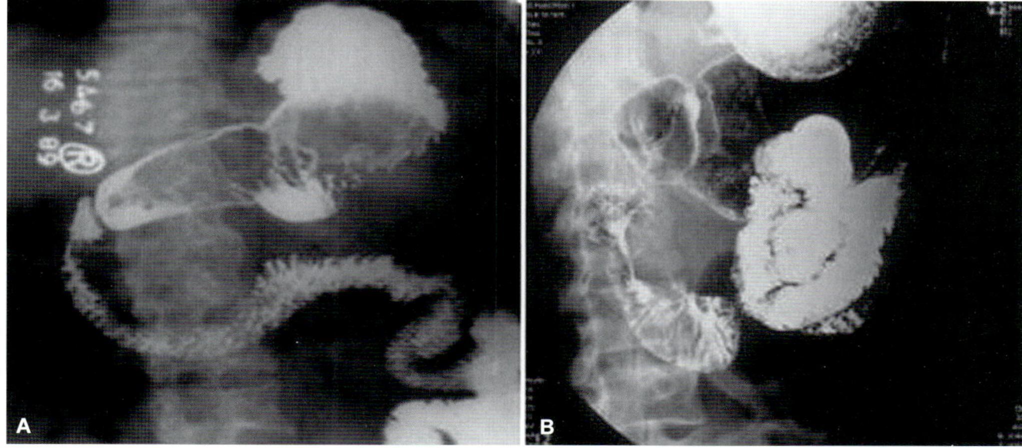

Figs 19.1A and B: Ba UGI showing widening of the C loop of duodenum with impression on the antrum and pylorus-antral pad sign: (A) Spiculated medial duodenal wall with traction and fixation, (B) Reverse 3 sign – pancreatic Ca

Histology

Pancreas is both an exocrine and endocrine gland. Acinar or exocrine unit constitutes the bulk of the organ (80%), ducts (4%), blood vessels and extracellular space (14%) while endocrine part or islet cells form about 2 % of its volume. The main islet cell types are glucagon secreting or A cells (15-20%), insulin secreting or B cells (70%) and somatostatin secreting or D cells. Polypeptide secreting PP or F cells and enterochromaffin secreting EC cells are the other cells described in these islets.[2]

Physiology

The exocrine pancreas plays an essential role in digestion and absorption through secretion of digestive enzymes and bicarbonates into the proximal duodenum. The endocrine pancreas releases hormones that regulate the metabolism and distribution of breakdown products of food.

MACROANATOMY

Ductal System

The excretory ducts are: the duct of Wirsung or main pancreatic duct and the duct of Santorini or accessory pancreatic duct. The duct of Wirsung is the main drainage duct of the embryologic ventral pancreas, which runs straight through the tail and body of gland, curves at the level of neck and then runs through the head into the duodenal wall where it is dorsal to the terminal common bile duct (CBD). The termination of the main pancreatic duct in the duodenum is situated at the major duodenal papilla. This termination is normally present as a common canal with distal CBD via the ampulla of Vater. This canal may be absent, and the two ducts then open separately. The accessory duct of Santorini drains embryologic dorsal pancreas and is rostral to the main duct in the superior part of head, extending from the curve of main duct to drain into the latter or separately at the minor duodenal papilla.

Vascular System

The pancreas derives its blood supply from the coeliac and superior mesenteric arteries. The head is supplied by gastroduodenal artery and direct branches of superior mesenteric artery (SMA). Gastroduodenal artery after giving its first branch, the postero superior pancreaticoduodenal artery, crosses the first part of duodenum and bifurcates into anterior inferior pancreaticoduodenal artery and the right gastroepiploic artery at the anterior surface of pancreas. The posterior inferior pancreaticoduodenal artery originates from the superior mesenteric artery, most frequently via a common trunk with the first jejunal artery. This artery visualises the uncinate process. The portal vein, splenic vein and superior mesenteric vein and its major trunks drain the pancreas.

At the microscopic level, the intralobular arteries contribute arterioles either to acini or to islets and the pancreatic parenchyma is supplied by an extensive capillary network. Several capillaries radiate from the islets to supply the periacinar capillary network. Thus an islet-acinar blood portal system exists in the pancreas (Fujita 1973)[1] and a large part of the blood first supplies the islets. Consequently, islet hormones may be distributed to the acinar tissue and they may interact with acinar cells. The parasympathetic nerve supply of the pancreas is derived from the vagus, and sympathetic fibers from the coeliac, superior mesenteric and the hepatic plexus. Nerve fibers are essentially distributed along the blood vessels around ducts, in the stromal, acinar and insular compartments.[1,2]

PATHOLOGY

Classification of tumors (Based on Predominant Cell Type and Radiological Appearances[1])

Epithelial Exocrine

A. *Duct Cell Origin*
- Solid neoplasms
  1. Adenocarcinoma
  2. Variant carcinomas
     - Pleomorphic giant cell carcinoma
     - Adenosquamous carcinoma
     - Colloid carcinoma
     - Anaplastic carcinoma
     - Small cell carcinoma
     - Ciliated cell adenocarcinoma
     - Oncocytic carcinoma
     - Clear cell carcinoma
- Cystic neoplasms
  1. Congenital cysts
  2. Pseudocysts
  3. Serous cystadenoma
  4. Mucinous cystic neoplasm
  5. Acinar cystadenocarcinoma
  6. Mucinous ductal ectasia
  7. Miscellaneous lesions presenting as cystic mass:
     - Ductal adenocarcinoma
     - Sarcoma
     - Lymphomas with necrosis and cystic de–generation
     - Cystic teratoma
     - Lymphangioma
     - Hemangioma
     - Paraganglioma
     - Papillary cystic tumor
     - Cystic islets cell tumor

B. *Acinar Cell Origin*
1. Acinar cell carcinoma
2. Acinar cell cystadenocarcinoma
3. Pancreaticoblastoma

C. *Indeterminate Origin*
1. Osteoclast-type giant cell carcinoma
2. Solid and papillary epithelial neoplasm
3. Mixed endocrine-exocrine neoplasm
4. Microadenocarcinoma.

Endocrine Islets Cell Tumors

1. Insulinoma
2. Gastrinoma
3. Glucagonoma
4. Vasointestinal peptidoma (VIPoma)
5. Somatostatinoma
6. Pancreatic polypeptidoma (Ppoma)
7. Carcinoids
8. Rare islet cell tumors
9. Multiple endocrine neoplasia syndromes.

Other Pancreatic Neoplasms

- Mesenchymal tumors
- Metastases
- Lymphomas

PANCREATIC ADENOCARCINOMA

The commonest tumor of the pancreas is an adenocarcinoma of ductal origin. It is usually seen in the middle aged and elderly and is among the five leading causes of death. It is twice as common in males as in females. The risk factors associated with pancreatic cancer include cigarette smoking, alcohol, high intake of animal fat in diet and hereditary pancreatitis. Ninety-nine percent of the tumors arise from the exocrine ductal epithelium and are histologically scirrhous infiltrative adenocarcinomas. One percent are seen in the acinar portion of the pancreatic gland while 0.1 % are malignant ampullary tumors. Jaundice is a common complaint in tumors of the pancreatic head while body and tail tumors may initially present with pain and weight loss.[3]

PATHOLOGICAL ANATOMY AND BIOLOGICAL BEHAVIOR

The strongest foundation for radiologic diagnosis and staging of pancreatic carcinoma is an understanding of the tumor's gross pathologic anatomy and its biological behavior.[4]

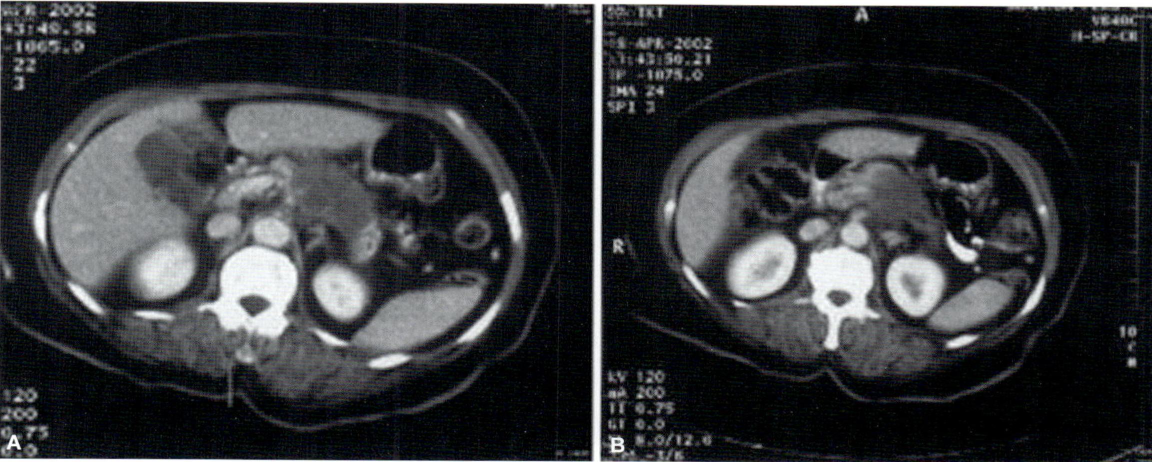

Figs 19.2A and B: Contrast enhanced CT scan showing a mass in the body and tail hypodense to the adjacent pancreatic tissue. The mass has definable margins though not encapsulated - pancreatic carcinoma

- The typical pancreatic cancer is a solid scirrhous tumor which has a decreased vascular perfusion as compared to the normal pancreatic tissue. The mass has definable margins although they are not encapsulated (Figs 19.2A and B).
- Some carcinomas are exceedingly infiltrative and may incite an inflammatory or desmoplastic reaction in adjacent parenchyma adding volume to the apparent mass. Most carcinomas have grown large enough to alter the contours of the gland by the time they are detected (Fig. 19.3).
- There is a strong tendency to constrict or obstruct the ducts that lie within their paths of growth and the main pancreatic duct is invariably involved. Dilatation occurs upstream from the occlusion and parenchyma surrounding the ducts is thinned. Side branches occasionally undergo cystic dilatation and increased pressure within obstructed ducts causes the system to rupture and allows fluid to escape into the substance of the pancreas or beyond its borders. Hence, tumors of pancreas are sometimes responsible for acute pancreatitis, extrapancreatic effusion or pseudocyst formation.
- Most pancreatic adenocarcinomas arise in the head and hence, obstruction of the CBD and concurrent neighboring pancreatic duct is frequently affected in this disease (Figs 19.4A and B). Metastatic lymphadenopathy adjacent to suprapancreatic part of the bile duct can also cause ductal obstruction.
- Direct extension into the neighboring structures, especially perivascular and perineural tissues is seen as encasement of one or more of the arteries that supply the gland. The precise nature of this form of extension is unexplained and it has been thought to represent tumors within perivascular lymphatic vessels (Figs 19.5A and B).
- The portal, splenic and superior mesenteric vein (SMV) lying adjacent to the pancreas are particularly susceptible to involvement. The confluence of the splenic and SMV to form portal vein at the posterior aspect of the pancreatic neck is a common location of venous involvement causing portal hypertension.
- Organs topographically adjacent to pancreas are likely

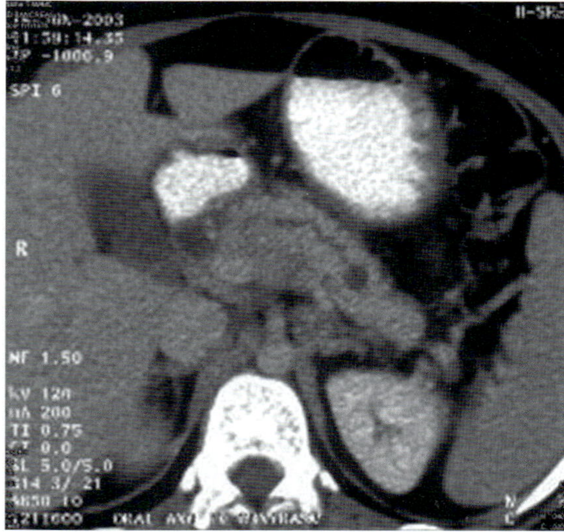

Fig. 19.3: CECT image showing an infiltrative hypodense mass in the pancreatic head which appears bulky. There is also upstream dilatation of the main pancreatic duct

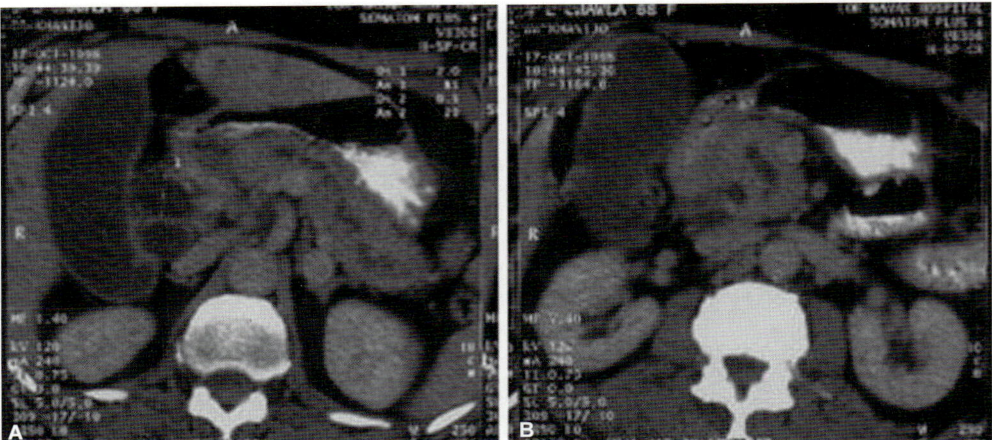

Figs 19.4 A and B: CECT images showing the "double duct sign", dilated CBD and MPD due to mass within the pancreatic head

to be invaded such as duodenum by head masses, stomach by body masses and hilus of spleen by tail masses.

- Metastatic dissemination of pancreatic carcinoma occurs to regional lymph nodes, i.e. coeliac, common hepatic, superior mesenteric and para-aortic; hepatic via portal venous drainage, omental and peritoneal via intraperitoneal shedding of tumor cells.
- The hallmark of pancreatic metastasis is the small size of individual lesions, so the regional lymph nodes with deposits may not be significantly enlarged and peritoneal seedlings are rarely more than a few millimeters in size.

Imaging: Imaging of pancreatic cancer involves both diagnosis and staging of the tumor. There have been advances in various imaging modalities used for the evaluation of pancreatic tumors. MDCT has the ability to obtain submillimeter imaging sections which have had a great impact in the diagnosis and staging. Multichannel coils, parallel imaging on MR allow more detailed and faster pancreatic imaging. The 3T imaging platform has further impoved the applications.[5,6]

Ultrasonography (US)

US evaluation of the pancreas, liver and biliary tract is useful for the diagnosis and evaluation of patients with suspected pancreatic disease. Using current–generation realtime scanners and meticulous techniques, highly detailed cross-sectional anatomy of the pancreas and surrounding organs can be depicted and the diagnosis of neoplastic and inflammatory pancreatic diseases made with a high degree of accuracy. The major limitation of

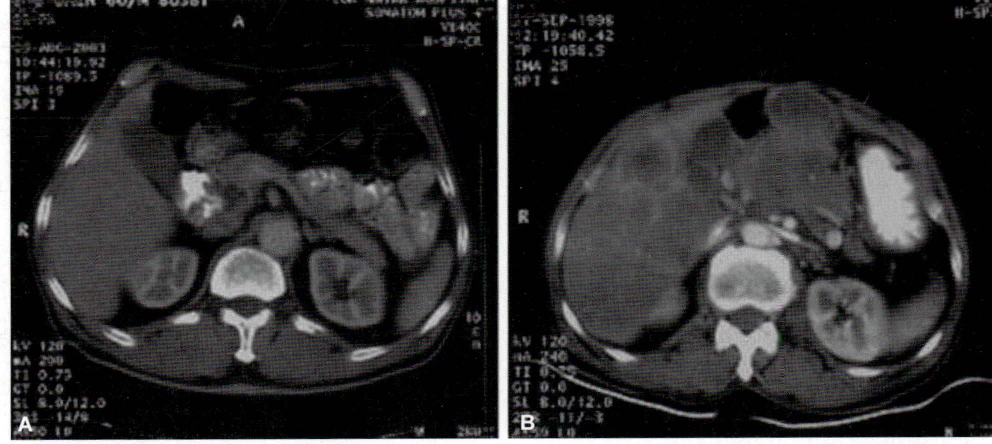

Figs 19.5A and B: (A) CECT image showing a mass at the pancreatic head with invasion of the duodenum suggesting direct extension into the adjacent organ (B) Another case showing encasement of the superior mesenteric artery and vein. Metastases in liver are also seen

pancreatic US is its inability to image the entire gland in about 15-20 % of cases.

Pancreatic carcinomas are usually hypoechoic as compared to normal parenchyma (Fig. 19.6). Necrotic tumors may show heterogenous echopattern, ductal obstruction and dilatation may also be visualized.

Vascular involvement is seen on US as thickening of periarterial tissues in which, normally echogenic fat immediately adjacent to the artery is replaced by tissue of lower echogenicity.

Color Doppler Flow Imaging (CDFI)

Color Doppler is now being extensively used for detection of vascular invasion of pancreatic tumors and relationship between tumor and neighboring vessels, namely the superior mesenteric, common hepatic, coeliac, splenic and gastroduodenal vessels (Figs 19.7A and B). The correspondence rates of CDFI with angiography for the presence of invasion, absence of invasion and overall evaluation are 78, 95 and 88 % respectively. A sensitivity of 60 %, specificity of 93 % and accuracy of 87 % have been obtained for detection of arterial invasion in comparing CDFI with surgical and histopathological findings. It may make angiography unnecessary, especially with advanced tumors if thorough evaluation for the large artery invasion is performed initially.[7]

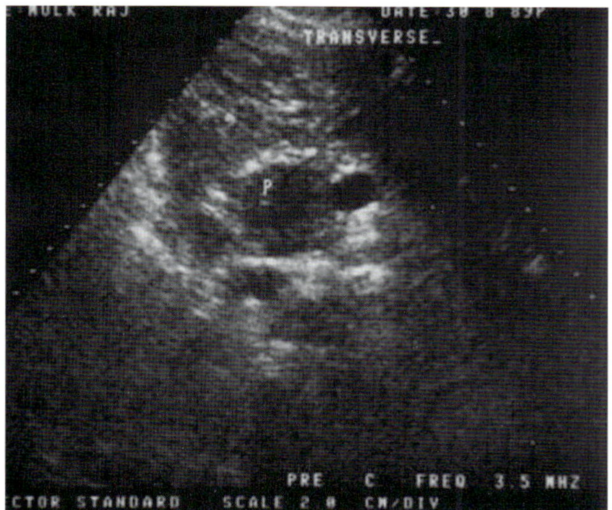

Fig. 19.6: Transverse sonogram showing an enlarged pancreatic head with a central hypoechoic area – Ca head of pancreas

Endoscopic US

EUS uses a 7-12 MHz 360o radial scanner, the tip of which is placed in the second part of duodenum for the pancreatic head, portal vein and papilla, in the duodenal bulb for the head, neck and distal CBD and through the stomach for imaging of body, tail and the pancreatic duct. EUS is especially sensitive for small (< 2 cm) solid tumors. Endosonographic criteria for nodal involvement are circularity, homogeneity, relative hypoechogenicity and proximity to the primary lesion. For vascular involvement, the endosonographic criteria are loss of the hypoechoic vessel wall/tumor interface, direct presence of tumor in the vascular lumen and non-visualization of a major portal vessel in the presence of collateral vessels.[8]

Roseh and colleagues compared EUS with US, CT and angiography in 60 patients with pancreatic and ampullary cancer. In the patients who were explored surgically, EUS was markedly superior to abdominal US and CT in determining tumor size, extent and LN status. Involvement of the portal vein was correctly predicted by EUS in 95 % of patients, with angiography in 85 % and CT in 75 % of cases. However, its assessment of arterial invasion

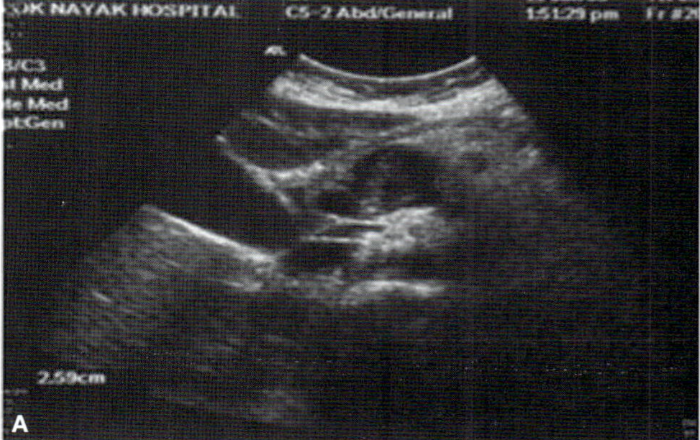

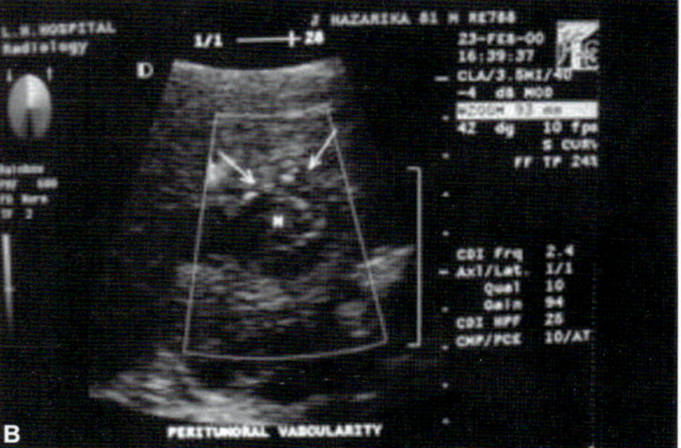

Figs 19.7A and B: Transverse sonogram showing a hypoechoic mass in the pancreatic head (A). On CDFI peritumoral vascularity and absence of internal vascularity seen. No vascular invasion was seen in this case *(For colour version see plate 3)*

is limited. Its main advantage is the assessment of small tumors < 3 cm that may be missed on CT scan, but EUS is an invasive procedure requiring sedation and monitoring and is highly operator dependent. Perhaps its real advantage lies in its ability to obtain accurate tissue for histological diagnosis. EUS FNAC is safe and reliable and improves the accuracy of noninvasive imaging techniques such as CT.[9]

Computed Tomography (CT)

CT is a widely used imaging technique for the evaluation of patients with suspected neoplastic pancreatic disease. Over the last decade, advancements in CT technology including the development of multidetector row CT (MDCT) scanners with 3-dimensional imaging software has significantly improved the ability of CT to evaluate a wide range of pancreatic pathology. CT is now considered to be the imaging modality of choice for the detection and presurgical staging of pancreatic cancer.[10]

Accurate imaging of the pancreas requires careful attention to technique. High resolution incremental dynamic CT is one of the most accurate procedure in the detection of pancreatic tumors. Although overall 5 years survival rate of pancreatic adenocarcinomas is as low as 5 %, studies have shown improved survival in patients with small tumors less than 2 cm.[11] Therefore, it is crucial to detect these small tumors and to identify patients eligible for surgical resection.[12] The overall accuracy of CT in the published literature for the detection of pancreatic tumors is approximately 80-91 %.[13,14] With the narrow collimation and faster scanning possible with new MDCT scanners, it is likely that the accuracy for detecting pancreatic tumors will improve further.[15]

When scanning a patient for suspected pancreatic cancer, maximum enhancement of the pancreatic parenchyma is essential to increase tumor conspicuity. The normal pancreas enhances to a greater extent than pancreatic adenocarcinoma, hence, tumors will be easier to detect when the normal pancreas is optimally enhanced (Figs 19.8A to C).

Routinely this is achieved by bolus infusion of 150 ml of 60 % iodinated contrast material at rates of 2-3 ml/sec. Slice thickness of 8 to 10 mm is usually satisfactory. Other protocols suggest 5 mm sections acquired in caudocranial direction beginning at the level of the transverse duodenum just below the pancreatic head and continuing superiorly through the liver to the dome of diaphragm.

Dual Phase Helical CT

The rationale behind the use of dual phase imaging is to obtain optimal pancreatic enhancement so that the tumor can be detected, and to obtain maximal vascular (arterial and venous) opacification to enable accurate assessment of vascular involvement. The optimal timing of the data acquisition, however, will depend on the scanner utilized, the rate of contrast administration and the patient's cardiac output.[16]

In this technique, spiral scans are obtained during the pancreatic arterial and portal venous phases. The arterial phase images are acquired 25 seconds after the start of injection of IV contrast material at 3 ml/sec. Venous phase images are obtained 70 seconds after the start of contrast infusion. This allows for optimal visualization of both the mesenteric arteries and veins and is essential for detecting vascular invasion.[17,18]

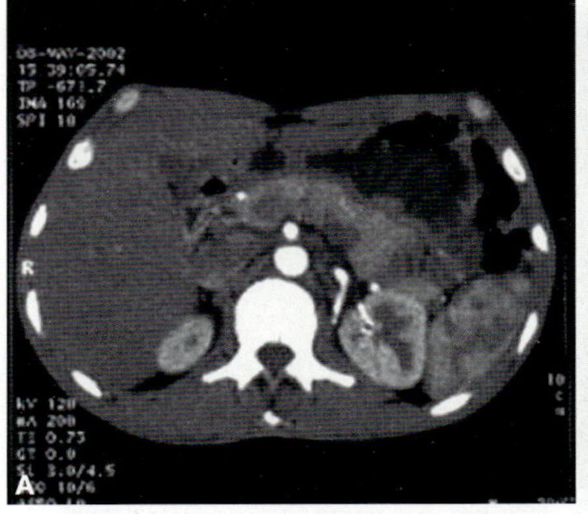

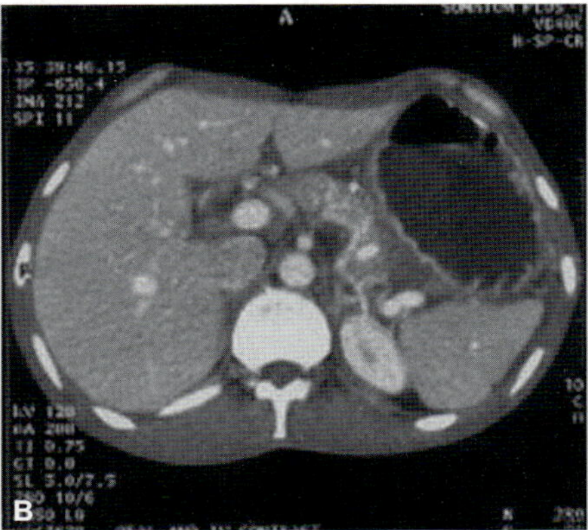

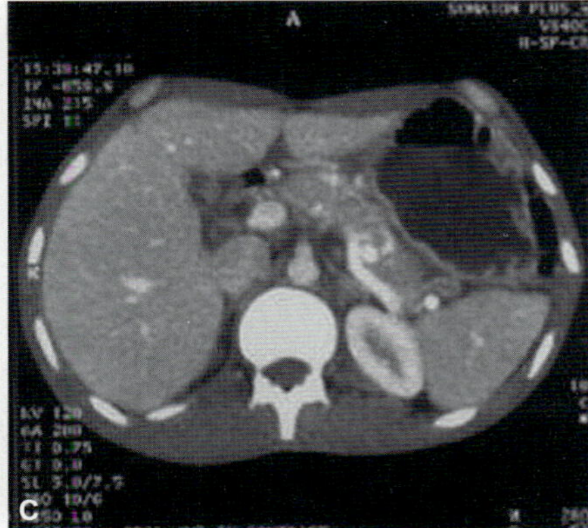

Figs 19.8A to C: Dynamic dual phase helical CT obtained in the arterial phase shows a small round mass within the pancreatic body. Optimal enhancement of the pancreatic parenchyma makes the lesion conspicuous. Venous phase images (B and C) show delayed enhancement of the lesion. No invasion of the mesenteric artery or the vein is seen in the arterial and the venous phases respectively

When performing CT evaluation of pancreatic tumors, high density oral contrast should be avoided and water should be used as oral contrast. Some centers perform a preliminary precontrast survey from the diaphragm to the kidneys using the following protocol: collimation 4 × 1 mm; slice thickness 25 mm; reconstruction interval 1 mm, table feed 10 mm/sec; 120 kVp; 160 mAs. Postcontrast scanning is then performed in the arterial and portal venous phases using the same parameters (Figs 19.8B and C). The 1 mm data sets are used for real-time interaction which include multiplanar reformats, multiplanar reconstructions and volume rendering for display and evaluation of arteries and veins.[20]

MDCT provides unparalleled capabilities for data acquisition with narrow collimation and consequently high resolution acquisition and near-isotropic voxels. The isotropy of the voxels allows a real-time interaction of the 3D data set with the possibility to reformat and visualize the images in any plane. With multidetector CT multiple discrete phases of vascular and parenchymal enhancement can easily be achieved. Scan timing can be determined by 3 methods either empirically, by a test bolus or bolus tracking. With 16-64 slice scanners bolus tracking is the technique of choice. The triple phase acquisition includes a nonenhanced phase, a late arterial phase, i.e. 10 second delay from the time of peak aortic enhancement and a portal venous phase with a 35 second delay (Fig. 19.9). Five millimeter axial images as well as coronal and sagittal reformatted images are obtained. The late arterial phase or pancreatic phase has the maximum conspicuity of the hypovascular tumor. The arterial and mesenteric venous enhancement is also seen which allows for detection of vascular invasion (Figs 19.10A and B). The portal venous phase is best for detection of liver metastasis and for visualization of venous structures.[15]

Multiplanar reconstructions and 3D images are extremely valuable for detection and staging of pancreatic tumors.[18]

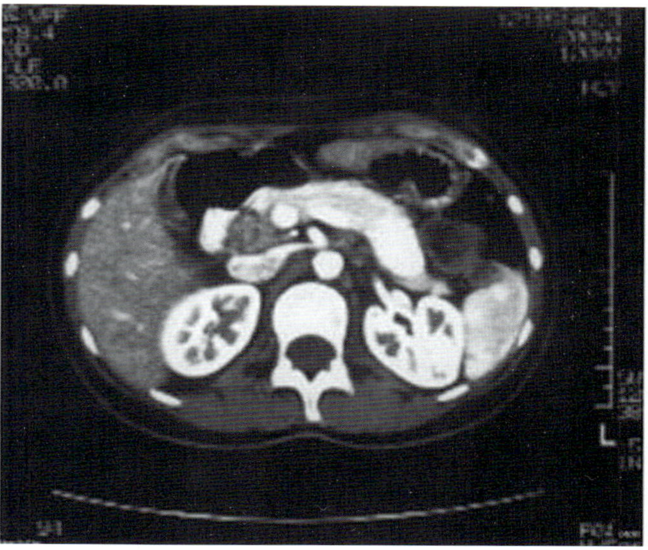

Fig. 19.9: Portal venous phase optimally detecting the venous structures. This phase is best for the detection of liver metastasis and for visualization of venous invasion

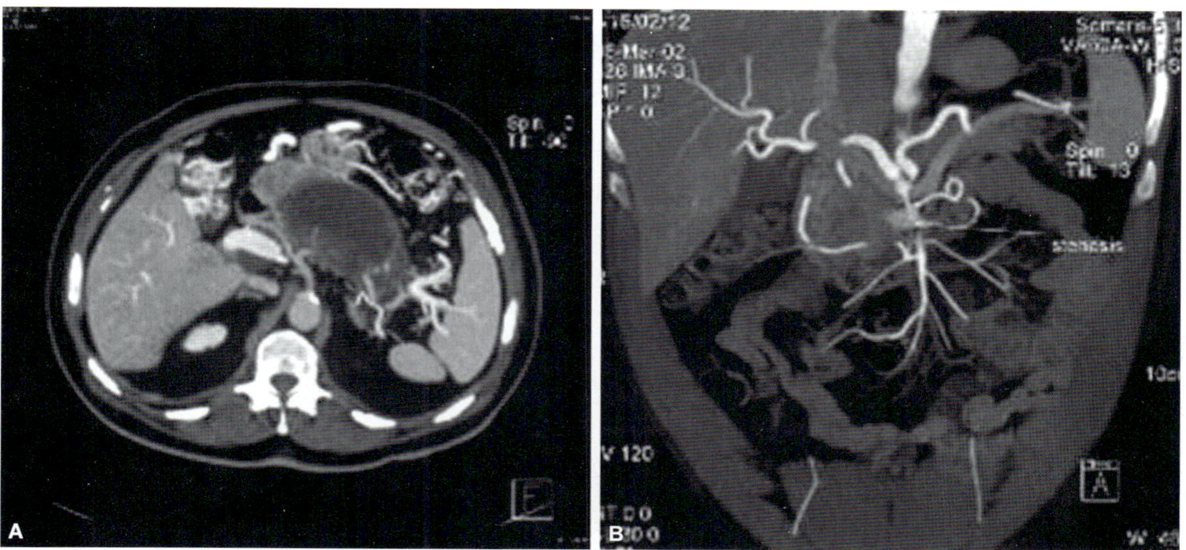

Figs 19.10A and B: MDCT images with coronal MPR showing a hypodense multilobulated mass arising from the pancreatic body and tail encasing the superior mesenteric and splenic vasculature

MAGNETIC RESONANCE IMAGING (MRI)

The pancreas is best imaged at field strength of 1.5 T or higher using high-speed gradient coils, phased array multicoils and parallel imaging. These advances allow for faster imaging, higher signal-to-noise and increased separation of water and fat frequencies. In addition, the use of breath-hold sequences, respiratory triggering, navigator technique and anti-peristaltic agents have resulted in images with less motion artifact. These tools have led to substantial advantages of MRI over other modalities, including high tissue contrast and the ability to assess vascular patency without the use of intravenously administered contrast material.[21]

No single pulse sequence is adequate to evaluate the pancreas. T1-weighted, T2-weighted, fat saturation with dynamic gadolinium-enhanced images, MRCP and MR angiography (MRA) are combined for the most successful protocol for MRI of the pancreas.[22]

Detection of cancer is best performed with T1-weighted fat-suppressed images and immediate post-gadolinium spoiled gradient echo images. Normal pancreatic tissue has increased signal on T1-weighted images compared with the liver, and intense enhancement during the arterial phase of a dynamic bolus of intravenous gadolinium (Gd) chelate (Figs 19.11A to C).[23] Pancreatic tumors being desmoplastic in nature are hypointense to normal parenchyma on T_1W fat saturated and non-fat saturated images. Contrast enhanced images 20-40 seconds after injection and 60 seconds after injection depict the lesion in the parenchymal and portal venous phase as hypo to isointense. The parenchyma upstream to the tumor obstruction may appear hypointense on T_1W images. The tumor may also obstruct the duct which appears beaded with smooth outlines.

MRI is especially suited for the detection of small, nonorgan deforming pancreatic ductal adenocarcinomas, detection of islet cell tumors and the differentiation of focal fatty infiltration of the pancreas from tumor. In addition, characterization of associated liver lesions is better performed with MRI. Ductal adenocarcinoma appears as an area of abnormally decreased signal on T1-weighted images and as a poorly enhancing hypovascular mass due to its desmoplastic fibrotic composition.

Differentiating adenocarcinoma from chronic pancreatitis on images is sometimes difficult. Typically, the chronically inflamed pancreas will demonstrate greater enhancement than that of pancreatic tumors on immediate post-Gd images, particularly, those tumors arising in the head. Chronic pancreatitis more frequently results in an irregularly dilated duct, often with intraductal calcification and the ratio of duct caliber to pancreatic gland width is higher (> 0.5) in patients with carcinoma.

On post-Gd fat-suppressed spoiled gradient echo images acquired in the delayed phase of a bolus injection, intermediate-signal intensity tumor tissue extending into the low-signal suppressed fat indicates local extension. MR was reported to be superior to helical CT for the determination of local tumor extension and nearby organ invasion. Liver metastases and peritoneal implants are better visualized on T1-weighted fat-suppressed post-Gd images than with CT[25] (Figs 19.12A to C).

MR angiography may also be done using 2D time of flight sequence or 3D gradient echo gadolinium enhanced technique. In patients with focal pancreatic lesions, Diehl *et al* have documented a significant increase in contrast to noise ratio with mangafodipir-enhanced MRI with and without fat saturation.[21]

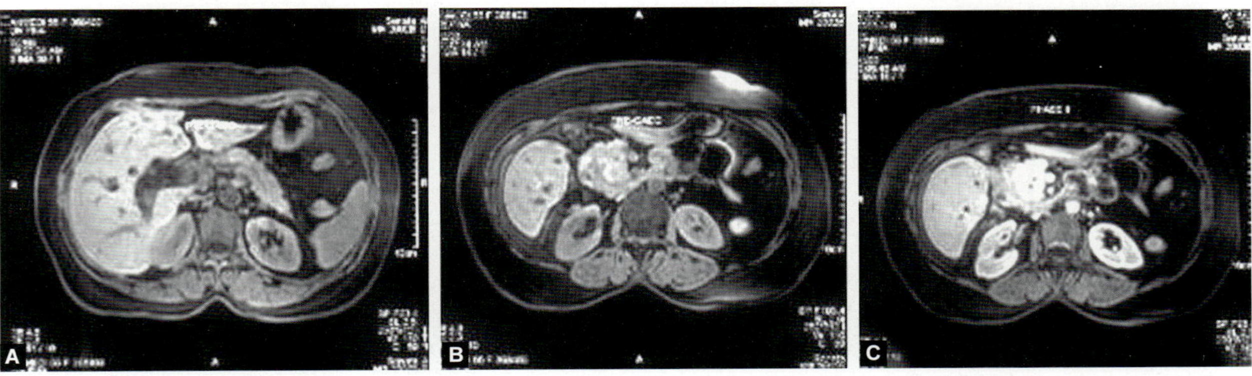

Figs 19.11A to C: T_1W fat suppressed images before (A and B) and after (C) contrast administration (dynamic scanning) reveal a poorly enhancing mass in the pancreatic head with duodenal infiltration

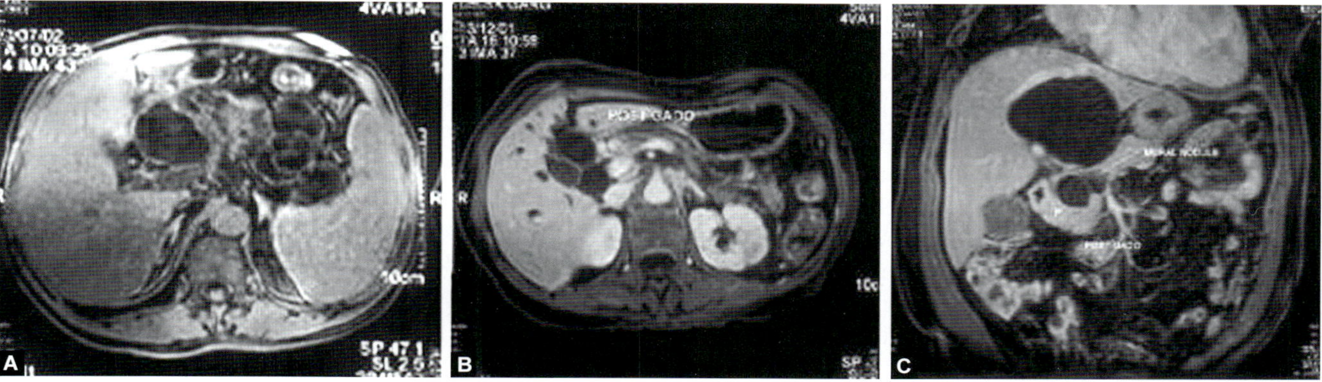

Figs 19.12A to C: T_1W fat suppressed spoiled gradient echo image before (A) and after (B/C) contrast administration reveal cystic lesion in the pancreatic head with an enhancing mural module within. A focal lesion with similar signal intensity as the primary tumor is seen in the liver S/o liver metastasis

MRCP

MRCP is a noninvasive technique for visualization of the biliary and pancreatic ductal system. MRCP is performed with heavily T2W sequences that depict the biliary and pancreatic ducts as high signal intensity structures. MRCP can be performed as a single shot or thick slab technique or using multislice thin slab technique. The thin slab images may be manipulated with maximum intensity projection algorithm and multiplanar reformatting techniques to generate 3D images of the ductal system[26-28] (Figs 19.13A and B).

MRCP offers a number of advantages compared with ERCP which is the standard of reference for imaging the biliary tract and pancreatic duct, because MRCP is a non-invasive examination which avoids the complications of ERCP that occur in up to 5 % of all ERCP attempts.[29] These include pancreatitis (1%) and rarely hemorrhage and GIT perforation. MRCP is performed rapidly and does not expose patients to ionizing radiation or contrast material.[30]

The major disadvantage of MRCP is that it is entirely diagnostic in comparison to ERCP which provides diagnostic information as well as access for therapeutic interventions.

MRCP has been shown to be accurate in identifying the presence and level of neoplastic obstruction of the pancreaticobiliary tract. In addition, MRCP performed in conjunction with a conventional abdominal MR and when necessary MRA, yields a comprehensive examination that permits not only diagnosis, but also staging of malignant neoplasms of the pancreaticobiliary tract.

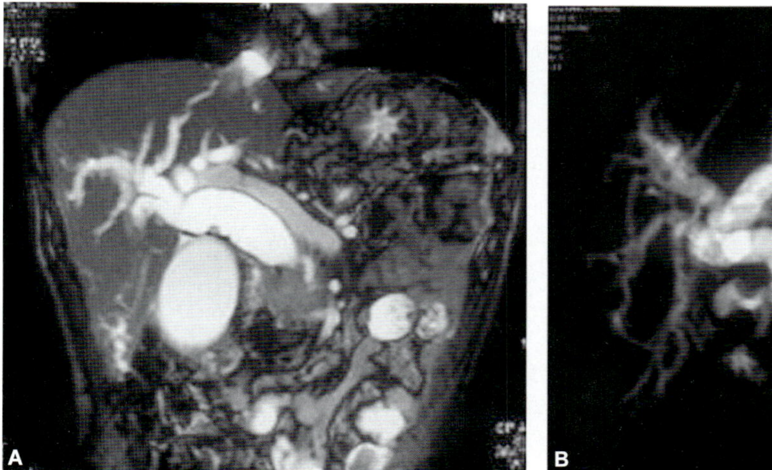

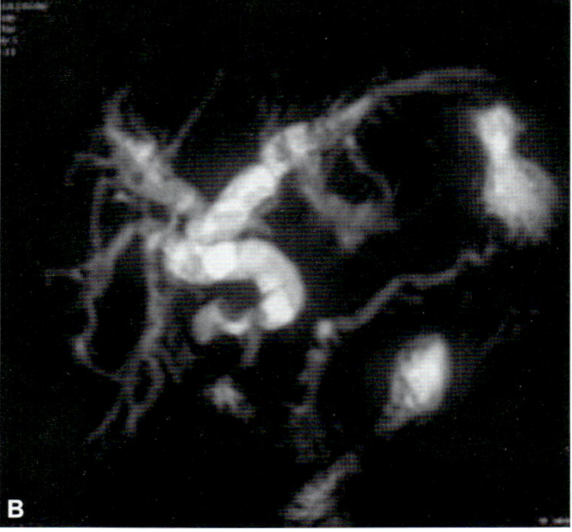

Figs 19.13A and B: MR-True FISP coronal image in a case of carcinoma pancreatic head showing an isointense mass causing obstructive biliopathy. MRCP image in the case showing dilatation of the common duct proximal to the lesion and the dilated main pancreatic duct (B)

MRCP identifies not only the dilated ducts located proximal to the obstruction, but also the ducts that are narrowed and encased by the tumor. The 'double duct' sign which represents dilatation of the biliary and pancreatic ducts is often observed when a mass is located in the pancreatic head (Figs 19.14A and B). The "duct-penetrating sign" was shown to be helpful in distinguishing an inflammatory pancreatic mass from pancreatic carcinoma (seen in 85% of chronic pancreatitis and only 4% of patients with cancer). This sign refers to a non-obstructed main pancreatic duct penetrating an inflammatory pancreatic mass, unlike its obstruction by pancreatic carcinoma[31] (Figs 19.14C and D).

When MR and MRA are performed in the same examination setting as MRCP, not only diagnosis of pancreatic carcinoma, but also an assessment for resectability can be made. In patients with unresectable disease, MRCP is useful in planning palliative, endoscopic and percutaneous procedures.

ERCP

There are several limitations in its use for diagnosis. Parenchymal abnormalities can only be detected by inference and a normal ERCP does not entirely exclude malignancy. Potentially silent areas on ERCP are the uncinate process, the accessory duct and the tail. The dilated pancreatic and biliary ductal system in pancreatic cancer is well demonstrated but it can be difficult to differentiate between chronic pancreatitis and pancreatic cancer on ERCP. Pancreatography may be frankly misleading in up to 13 % of patients and might be unable to make a diagnosis in 76 % of patients.

Diagnostic ERCP always carries the risk of pancreatitis and in an obstructed system, it might induce cholangitis by contaminating a nondraining biliary system. Therefore, ERCP should generally, only be undertaken with therapeutic intent after the tumor has been thoroughly assessed noninvasively.[29]

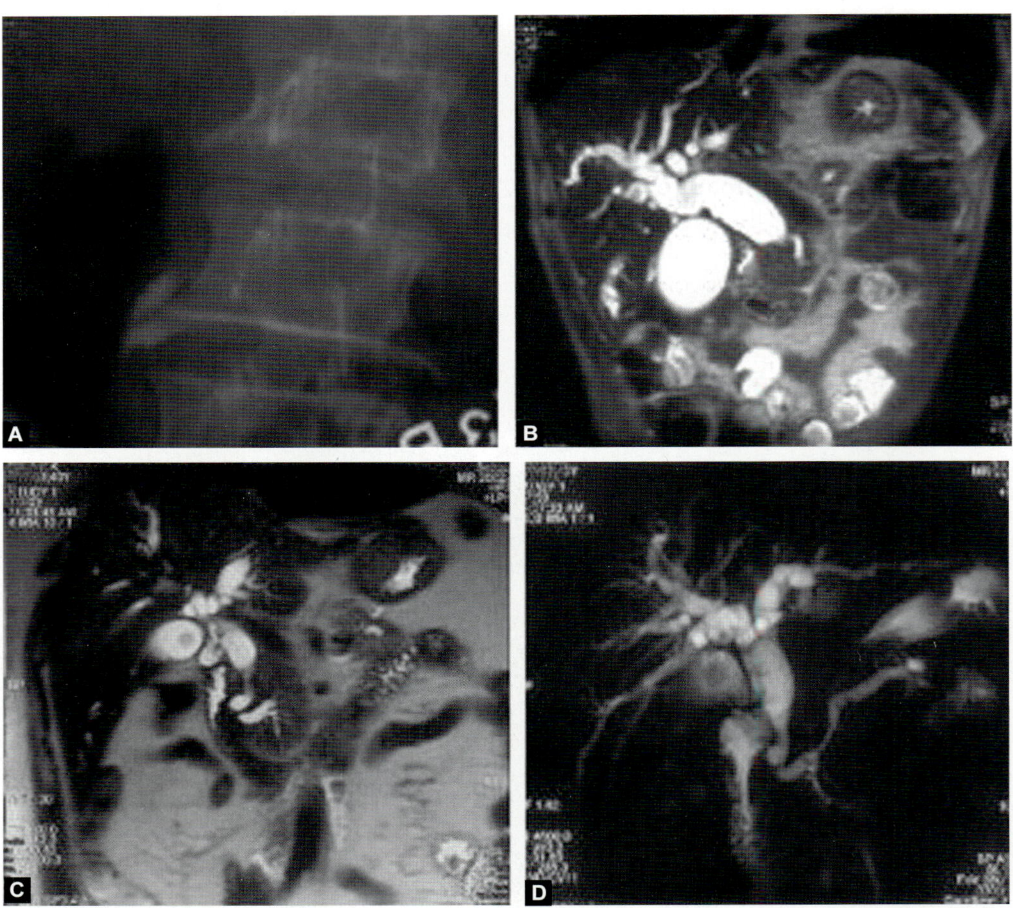

Figs 19.14A to D: (A) ERCP image showing the double duct sign. (B) TRUFISP MR coronal image revealing the same due to a pancreatic head mass (C and D) TRUFISP MR coronal image, revealing a non-obstructed pancreatic duct penetrating an inflammatory mass. MRCP image showing the 'duct penetrating' sign in the same

PET

PET provides an alternative in tumors < 2 cm in size. In lesions of this size, it is often difficult to distinguish focal pancreatitis from tumor. The development of PET with 2-[18F]– fluoro-2-deoxy-D-glucose (FDG-PET) has made it possible to demonstrate sites of increased glycosis from cancer. The glucose analogue, FDG enters the cell in the same manner as glucose, is trapped after phosphory-lation and cannot be further metabolized. Intracellular FDG concentration reflects intracellular glucose metabolism.

Hosten described a technique to superimpose images from CT and FDG-PET to help distinguish focal pancreatitis from tumor. In this, the images of CT and FDG-PET are superimposed allowing accurate localiza-tion of the tumor. This image overlay technique is experimental and requires sophisticated software.

In patients with pancreatic malignancy, PET helps in the evaluation of locoregional recurrence, distant metastases and in cases with equivocal diagnosis on CT and MRI. PET can localize recurrent disease, when abdominal CT is equivocal as a result of post-therapy anatomic alteration. Massey *et al* have reported that absence of FDG uptake at 1 month following chemotherapy for pancreatic cancer is an indicator of improved overall survival.[32]

DSA

Modern angiography equipment including DSA and magnification techniques are important for accurate evaluation of pancreatic tumors. Pancreatic angiography requires superselective cannulation of the branches of coeliac and SMA and familiarity with pharmacoangiography. Role of angiography is diminishing during the past decade with advent of dynamic CT, CDFI and MRA. Preoperative angiography is now recommended in special circumstances where operative difficulties are anticipated such as previous major abdominal surgery, doubtful resectability based on clinical grounds or CT appearances, major vascular structures anticipated to be resected, obese patient or preoperative radiotherapy.[33]

Tumor Markers in Pancreatic Carcinoma

No tumor marker has been shown to have sufficient sensitivity or specificity for screening purpose. CA 19.9 has been the most useful and important tumor marker in clinical setting with a sensitivity of 90 % and specificity of 75%. The specificity increases to 95 % in combination with other markers. Presence of progesterone receptor in the tumor tissue is seen in solid pseudopapillary tumor.[33]

Laparoscopy

Laparoscopy has its greatest utility in detection of hepatic and peritoneal metastases which are frequent sites of spread in pancreatic cancers. These implants may be seen in 27 % cases of carcinoma of head and 65 % cases of body and tail. Peritoneal cytology is positive in 20-30 % cases and suggests poor survival (median survival less than 6 months).

Fine Needle Aspiration (FNA)

Cytological confirmation of malignancy, when material is satisfactory, is not technically difficult, however, fine needle aspiration has a very high sampling error, hence a negative cytology does not exclude cancer. The utility of FNA is more for body and tail masses because resection is technically not possible when CT or angiographic evidences of unresectibility are seen. It obviates the need for a diagnostic laparotomy in a frail patient. FNA is, however, contraindicated in potentially resectable cancers to avoid sampling error which is misleading and may leave seedling along the tract in this highly vascular organ which is rich in lymphatics.

STAGING OF PANCREATIC TUMORS

The local spread of pancreatic carcinoma is determined by its site of origin. Anterior pancreatic head lesions grow towards the gastroduodenal and common hepatic arteries which are generally involved before the tumor invades the transverse mesocolon. Posterior lesions in the pancreatic head tend to involve the superior mesenteric and portal vein before the SMA is involved. Uncinate tumors spread along the inferior pancreaticoduodenal artery and extend into the jejunal mesentery.

Radiologists should use the TNM system for staging of pancreatic carcinoma.

The American Joint Committee on Cancer (AJCC) and Union Internationale Contre le Cancer (UICC) group the lymph nodes according to their anatomic location, whereas the Japanese Pancreatic Society System numbers the lymph nodes.[34]

T Staging: Imaging is highly sensitive for assessment of T stage. T1 and T2 are according to size less than 2 cm. or

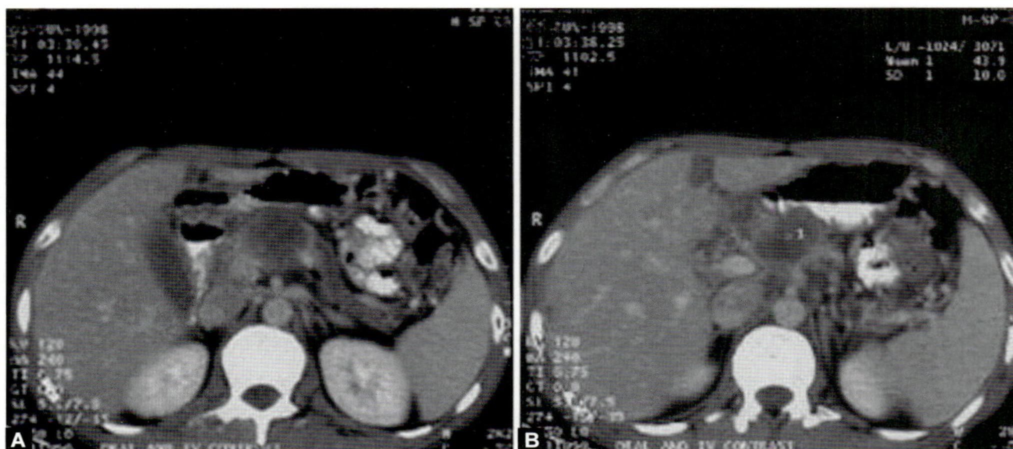

Figs 19.15A and B: CECT image showing a hypodense mass in the pancreatic head s/o carcinoma (A) with hepatic artery node which is a part of coeliac drainage located at the site of origin of the gastroduodenal artery (B)

more than 2 cm. confined to the pancreas. T_3 tumor extends beyond the pancreas with peripancreatic soft tissue involvement but celiac axis, SMA and stomach are not involved. T_4 tumor involves either the celiac axis or SMA.

N Staging: The lymph nodes are divided into 4 categories (AJCC and UICC) depending on whether they are:

i. Superior to the body and head of pancreas,
ii. Anterior including anterior pancreaticoduodenal, pyloric and proximal mesenteric,
iii. Inferior to the body and head of pancreas, and
iv. Posterior pancreaticoduodenal, common bile duct and proximal mesenteric.

The hepatic artery node which is a part of the celiac drainage is consistently located at the site of origin of the gastroduodenal artery. This node may be malignant without any increase in size (Figs 19.15A and B).

M Staging: Some patients may undergo laproscopy to rule out peritoneal implants and metastasis which may be missed on CT. However, MR detects liver lesions smaller than 1 cm as well as peritoneal and omental metastasis less than 1 cm. Improved visualization of these lesion is with the use of IV contrast or reticuloendothelial system specific contrast agents (ferumoxides) and hepatocyte selective contrast agents (mangafodipir trisodium). These hepatocyte or kupffer cell specific agents cause T1 and T2 shortening and metastasis appear hypointense (Figs 19.16A and B).

Vascular Resectability: The relationship of the tumor to critical arterial and venous structures is important as their involvement makes the tumor unresectable. Assessment of arterial involvement is done using axial and post processed images. Encasement of the hepatic artery, celiac trunk, proximal gastroduodenal artery and SMA makes

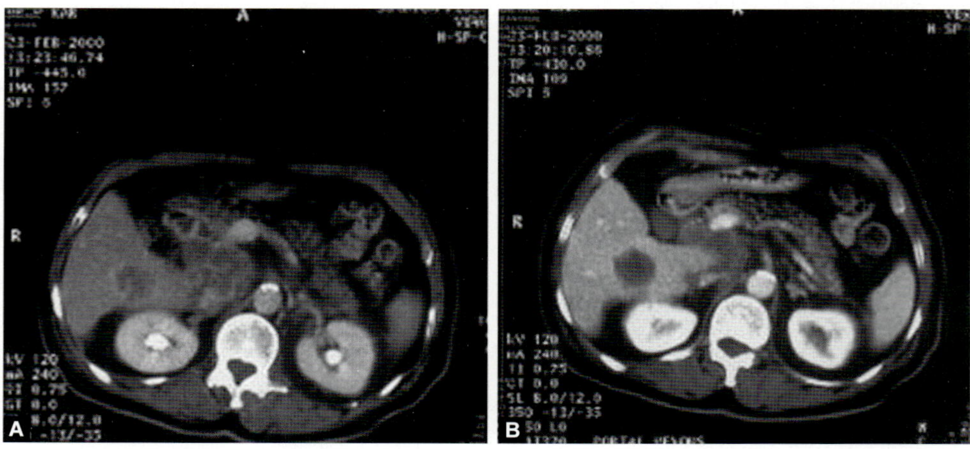

Figs 19.16A and B: CECT images showing a mass lesion in the uncinate process of pancreas with hepatic metastasis

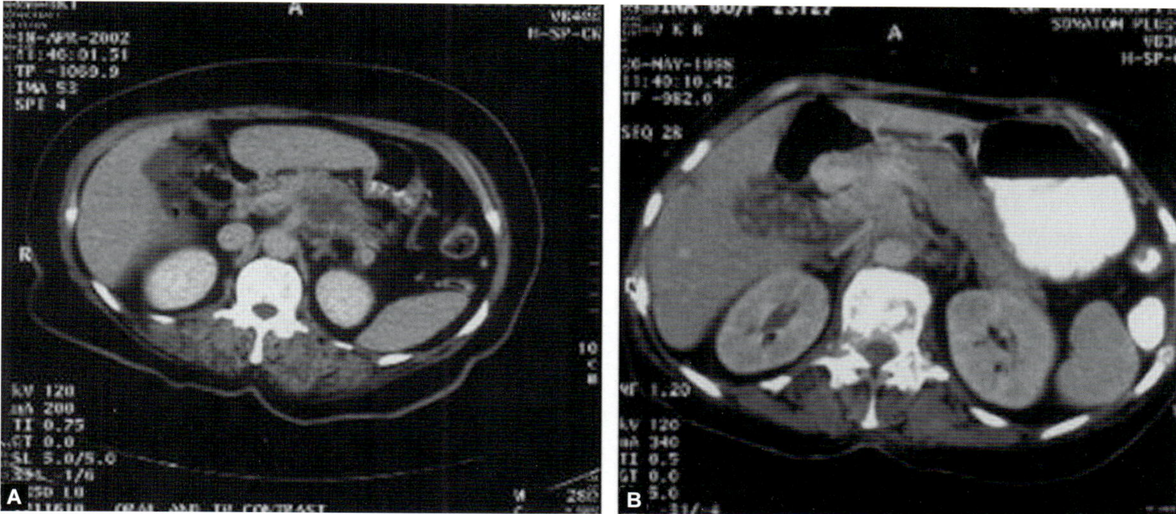

Figs 19.17A and B: CECT images in two cases of pancreatic carcinoma with soft tissue infiltration obscuring margins of vessel or perivascular fat suggesting vascular invasion. There is loss of planes between the mass and SMA in the Ist case. There is complete encasement of the superior mesenteric artery and vein in the 2nd case

the tumor unresectable. Post processed images allow better assessment of involvement than axial images. The venous phase shows waist like narrowing on axial images with extension to the left side of SMV implies SMA extension and circumferential narrowing or occlusion of SMV or portal vein implies unresectability (Fig. 19.17A). Increasing circumferential venous involvement leads to the "teardrop mesenteric vein sign" and this is a reliable sign to predict unresectability. The grading system proposed by Raptopoulos et al is used to assess axial images[17] (Table 19.1).

The scope of surgery has expanded in the recent years and SMV-PV en block resections are performed when this involvement is the only barrier to resection. The aim of preoperative staging is to ensure appropriate treatment with minimal risk, in the most cost effective manner. A rational sequence of testing for diagnosis and staging of pancreatic cancer always involves the use of non-invasive test as a first line of investigation. Ultrasonography is used first and if no metastases or major vascular invasion is observed it is followed by computed tomography to better delineate the pancreas and peripancreatic anatomy.

Patients with disseminated or locally advanced disease who are not candidates for resection or surgical palliation, ERCP with endoscopic stenting can be used for palliation of jaundice. Endoscopic or percutaneous

Table 19.1 **Grading of vascular involvement at ultrasonography and CTA**

Grade	*Involvement*	*Definition of resectability*	*Finding*
0	No vascular involvement	Resectable by CTA and ultrasonography	Normal, preserved fat plane around portal vein, superior mesenteric vein, their confluence superior mesenteric artery, and coeliac axis.
1	No vascular involvement	Resectable by CTA and ultrasonography	Loss fat plane, smooth displacement of the vessel
2	Vascular involvement	Resectable by CTA and ultrasonography	Flattening or irregularity on one side of vessel*
3	Vascular involvement	Unresectable by CTA and ultrasonography	Encased narrowed vessel with tumor >50% of the circumference
4	Vascular involvement	Unresectable by CTA and ultrasonography	Occluded vessel

Grading of vascular involvement according to the scale of Raptopoulos *et al.*[17]

*One side was defined as contiguous involvement of up to 180° of the circumference of the vessel.

biopsy under ultrasonic guidance can be used effectively to obtain a definite tissue diagnosis.[33]

CYSTIC TUMORS

The spectrum of cystic neoplasms of the pancreas encompasses a wide range of histologies from benign to malignant. The majority of cystic masses of the pancreas, excluding pseudocysts, will be either mucinous cystic neoplasms or microcystic adenomas. Cystic tumors are a diverse group of lesions which are relatively rare and constitute 10% of pancreatic cysts.

Within this group serious microcystic adenoma, mucinous cystic tumor (MCT); Intraductal papillary mucinous tumor (IPMT) and solid pseudopapillary tumor (SPT). Uncommon cystic tumors include the cystic endocrine tumors, cystic teratomas, metastasis and lymphangiomas. These may be categorized into two types: primarily cystic tumors and tumors with secondary cystic degeneration.

Mucinous Cystic Neoplasms (MCNs)

Mucinous cystic neoplasms are also known as macrocystic adenomas or mucinous cystadenomas/cystadenocarcinomas. These tumors are best referred to under the unifying term of mucinous cystic neoplasms, as the preoperative distinction between cystadenoma and cystadenocarcinoma is difficult in the absence of metastases.

MCNs are rare and comprise 2.5% of exocrine pancreatic tumors most often located in the body or tail of the pancreas (70-90%). They have a strong female predilection (> 95%). The mean age of occurrence is 50 years and they are referred to as "mother" lesion. Clinically, patients present with abdominal pain, a palpable mass, anorexia, or an incidentally found mass. MCNs have a spectrum from benign to malignant. These tumors have a much better prognosis than pancreatic ductal adenocarcinomas.[34]

Imaging: MCNs are typically large multilocular lesions at the time of diagnosis, (average–10 cm) or may be unilocular with well-defined borders, smooth external surfaces, and thick fibrous walls. Histologically, they are composed of tall, mucin–producing columnar cells.

Sonographically, MCNs usually appear as well circumscribed multilocular cysts that demonstrate the presence of anechoic cavities and posterior acoustic enhancement with occasional presence of echogenic debris, internal septations and papillary excrescences. These are often better appreciated on sonography than on CT (Fig. 19.18). Although uncommon at presentation, metastases may be seen in the liver, which may appear as cystic masses.

On CT, a round to slightly lobulated mass that is well encapsulated with smooth external margins and near water attenuation is seen, which shows capsular or septal calcifications in 10-25% cases. CECT demonstrates enhancement of the walls and the presence of thin, curvilinear septa in multilocular cysts (Figs 19.19 and 19.20). Although each cystic cavity can be of variable size, the entire lesion is usually composed of six or fewer cysts and the internal surface may demonstrate nodularity representing papillary projections. Disruption or distortion

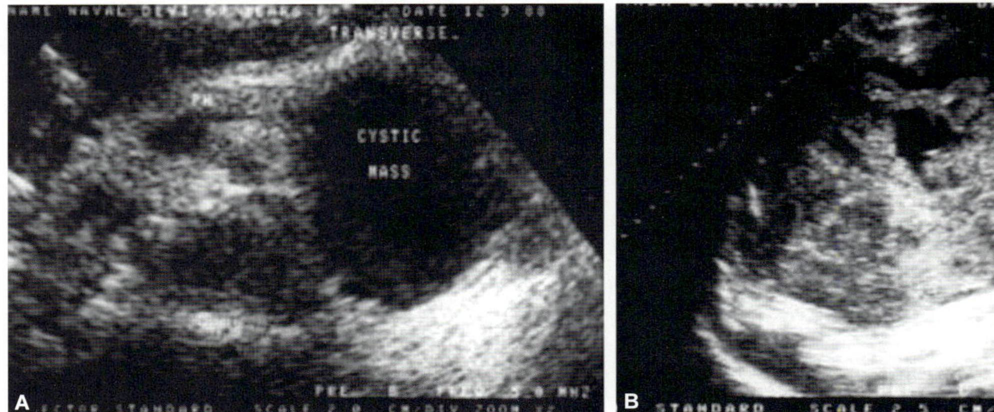

Figs 19.18A and B:US images showing an oval well marginated hypoechoic, predominantly cystic mass arising from the pancreatic tail (A) and another case revealing a well circumscribed mass with posterior acoustic enhancement and echogenic debris within (B) Mucinous cystic neoplasms

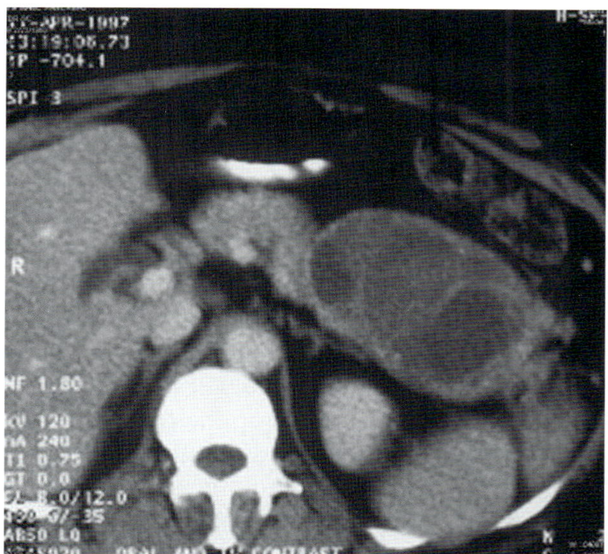

Fig. 19.19: CECT image in a case of mucinous cystic neoplasm (MCN) reveals a multiloculated cystic and solid mass arising from the pancreatic tail

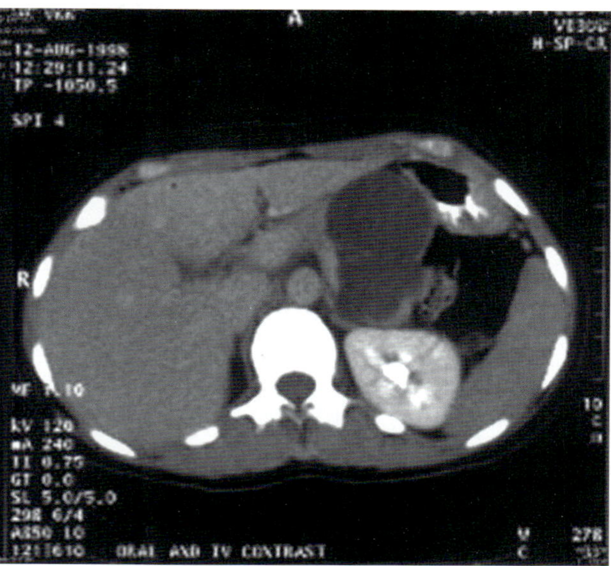

Fig. 19.20: CECT image showing a thin walled multiloculated hypodense mass arising from pancreatic body and tail – MCN

of adjacent organs with obliteration of adjacent fat planes suggests local invasion (Figs 19.21A and B).

MR signal characteristics can be variable depending on cyst fluid contents, with simple fluid showing decreased signal intensity on T1W images, and hemorrhagic or proteinaceous fluid showing increased T1 signal intensity. On T2W sequences, the fluid component is high signal intensity and internal septations are more conspicuous seen as low signal intensity curvilinear septa. Septa and mural nodules are typically seen as filling defects (Fig. 19.22).

The most important differential diagnosis is from pseudocysts in a unilocular lesion. In the proper clinical setting, the absence of radiographic signs of acute or chronic pancreatitis, presence of a solid component in the cystic mass, normal pancreatic tissue adjacent to the cyst, and lack of communication of the cyst with main pancreatic duct on ERCP favors the diagnosis of MCN.[35]

Peripheral calcification and the internal architexture of the cystic mass can be used to differentiate them from serious cystadenomas which have a central calcification.

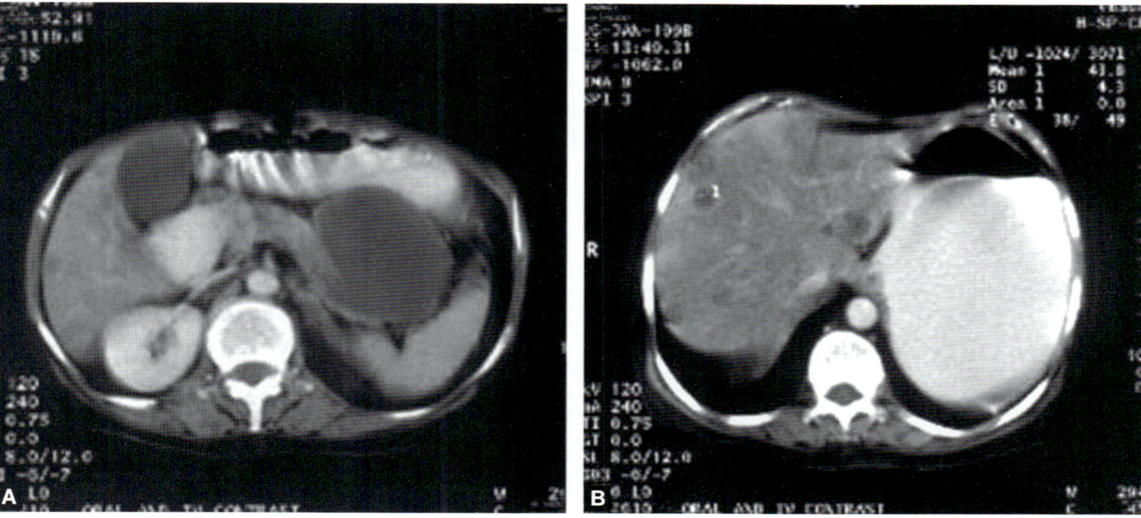

Figs 19.21A and B: (A) CECT image showing a well-encapsulated round to slightly lobulated mass with near water attenuation and enhancement of the wall (B) Liver shows multiple hypodense lesions with enhancing rim S/o metastases – MCN with liver mets

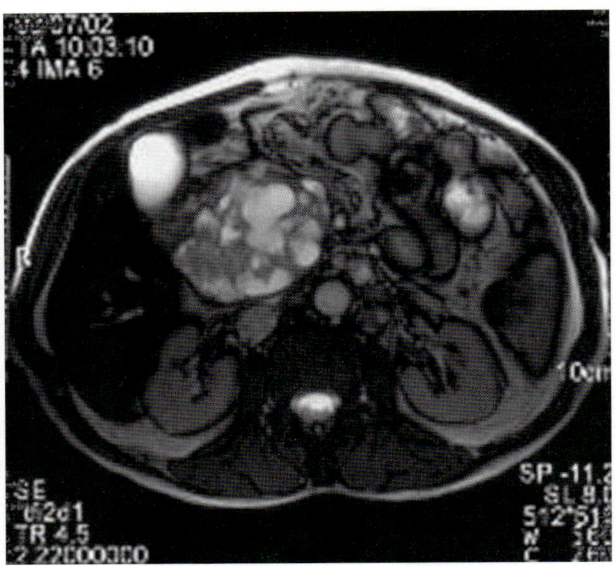

Fig. 19.22: Axial TRUFISP MR image revealing a multilocular cyst in the pancreatic head. The fluid component shows high signal and mural nodules show isointense signal – MCN

Small unilocular cyst should be differentiated from pseudocyst and IPMT (Figs 19.23 and 19.24).

Microcystic Adenoma (Serous Cystadenoma)

This is an uncommon cystic neoplasm constituting 1-2% of exocrine pancreatic tumors occurring most commonly in women over the age of 60 years as a benign incidental finding on imaging studies. This is termed as "grandmother lesion."

Clinically, when symptomatic, these patients present with abdominal pain, weight loss, a palpable abdominal mass, and rarely jaundice. An association with Von Hippel – Lindau disease has been reported.

Serous cystadenomas have a slight predilection for the pancreatic head and are typically large tumors (10.8 cm average size) with at least six or more cysts, each measuring 0.2-2.0 cm in size. The multiple cysts are separated by fibrous septa that radiate from the center forming a central stellate scar, that can calcify, which is a characteristic finding when present.

Grossly, these tumors are well circumscribed with lobulated margins, with a honeycomb or sponge like appearance on cut section. Histologically, the cysts are lined by glycogen rich cuboidal epithelial cells.

Duck et al stated that the difficulty in diagnosing microcystic adenomas lies not in differentiating them from other cystic neoplasms, but in appreciating that they are in fact cystic lesions because of the solid appearance of tumors with a high stromal content and multiple tiny cysts more than 6 measuring less than 2 cm in size separated by thin septa lined by epithelial cells. Grossly the tumor is described as having a "cluster of grapes" appearance. Accurate radiologic diagnosis and differentiation from mucinous cystic tumors are crucial to avoid aggressive surgical intervention in case of an asymptomatic serous cystadenoma which has low malignant potential.[34]

Imaging: Sonographically, the lesions may appear as solid echogenic masses secondary to the myriad of interfaces produced by the numerous microscopic cysts, or may appear as a multilocular cyst or a mixed solid and cystic lesion. Itai et al demonstrated posterior acoustic enhancement in the majority of microcystic adenomas, due to their fluid content.

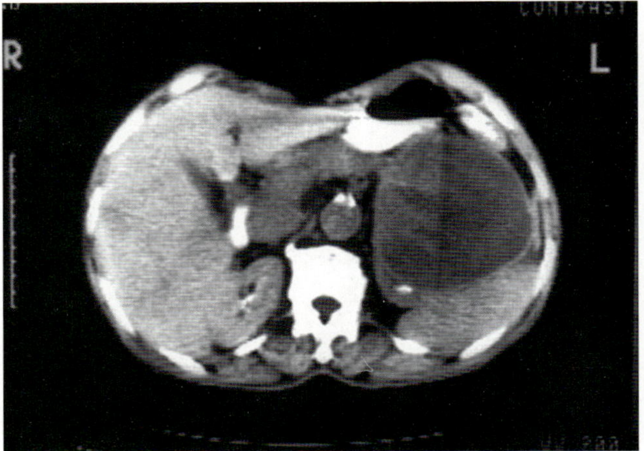

Fig. 19.23: CECT image showing a unilocular thin walled cystic mass in the pancreatic tail with small peripheral calcification in the inferior part of the cyst – MCN

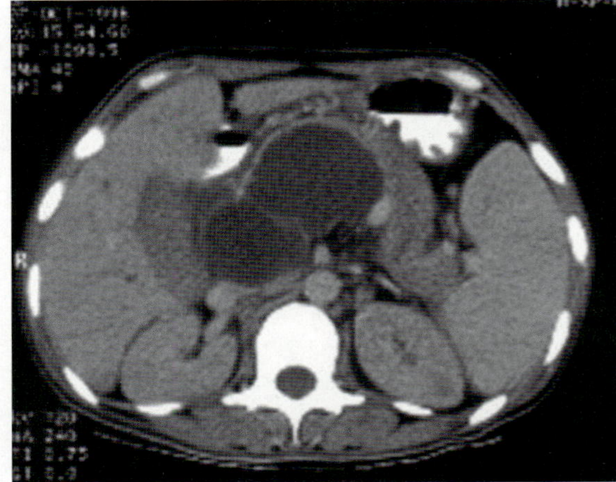

Fig. 19.24: CECT image in a case of MCN showing a thin walled cystic lesion with water attenuation and presence of thin enhancing septa within

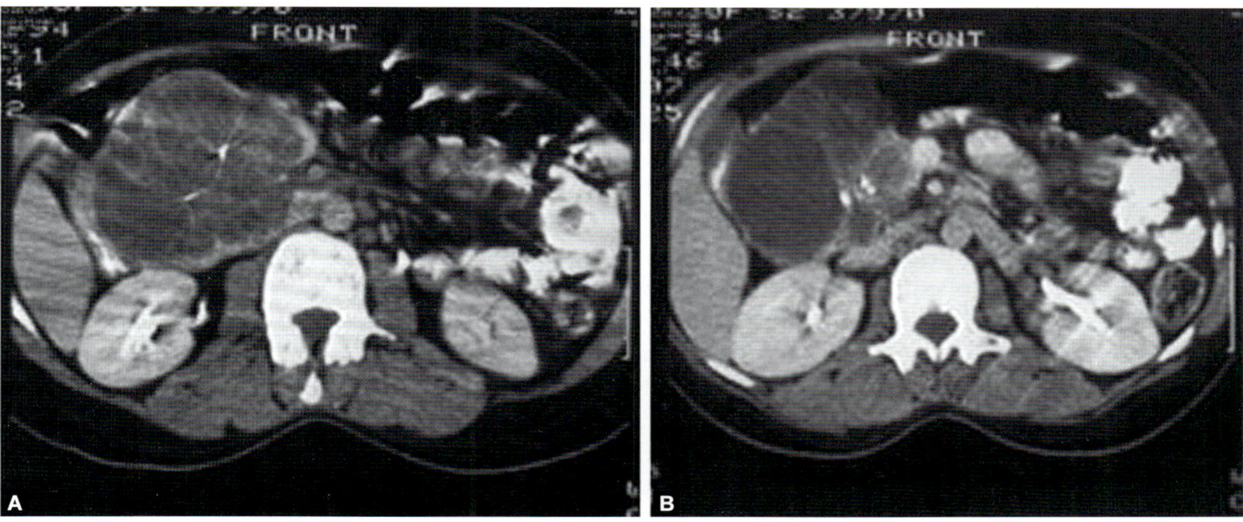

Figs 19.25A and B: CECT images showing a bulky, multiloculated hypodense predominantly cystic mass of the pancreatic head with a central calcified stellate scar – serous cystadenoma

On unenhanced CT, serous cystadenomas appear as hypodense, near water attenuation masses that frequently show central calcification. A central stellate scar that may calcify is seen in upto 20% lesions and is a characteristic feature of serous cystadenoma (Figs 19.25A and B). The tumor is hypervascular and contrast enhancement of the septations results in a typical "swiss cheese" or honeycombing appearance due to the presence of tiny cysts. The arrangement of cysts around a central fibrous scar in a sunburst pattern with coarse calcification is characteristic. CT can also be useful to exclude invasion of adjacent structures and the absence of metastases, to help confirm the benign nature of these lesions[35](Fig. 19.26).

On MRI, these tumors appear as a well-defined lesion showing predominantly low signal intensity on T1W images and high signal intensity on T2W images with a "cluster of grapes" appearance, best depicted on breathing-independent single-shot, echotrain spin echo sequence. The tumor is hypervascular secondary to its rich subepithelial capillary network and has a tendency to hemorrhage (Fig. 19.27). Tumor septa are seen as dark thin strands on T2-weighted images, which enhance minimally with delayed enhancement of the central scar observed occasionally. Calcifications are not well demonstrated on MR compared with CT.

On ERCP, the common bile duct or pancreatic duct may be displaced, encased, or obstructed by the tumor

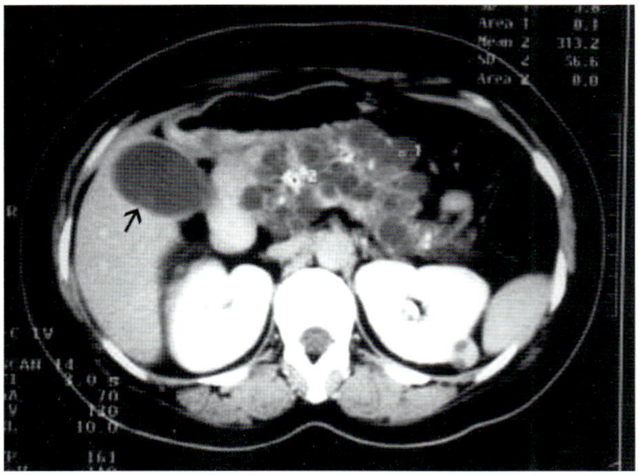

Fig. 19.26: Contrast enhanced CT showing a predominantly cystic lesion with contrast enhancement of the septations giving rise to the characteristic "swiss cheese" or honeycombing appearance. Few calcific foci are seen within the lesion - Serous cystadenoma

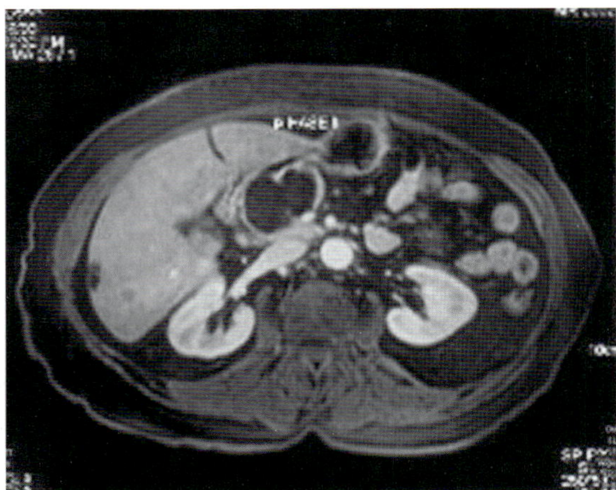

Fig. 19.27: Postgadolinium T_1W MR image showing a low signal intensity lesion in the pancreatic head with enhancing wall and minimal enhancement of the septa – serous cystadenoma

with no communication of lesion with the main pancreatic duct.

Differential diagnostic features that help in distinguishing serous from mucinous cystic tumors include older age group, and presence of multiple (> 6) cysts measuring less than 1 cm in diameter. The presence and location of tumor calcification is important. A central stellate scar is seen in serous tumors while 25% of mucinous tumors show peripheral calcification. Fishman et al reported that CT and sonography can correctly distinguish mucinous from serous cyst adenomas in approximately 90% of cases. Lesion enhancement particularly in septa is characteristic of microcystic (serous) cystadenoma, whereas enhancement of tumor nodules is typical of MCN's. The presence of cystic contents with high signal intensity on T1W images may favour MCNs because of old hemorrhage. Moreover, apparent diffusion coefficient (ADC) value calculated from echo planar imaging may differentiate viscous mucoid content of IPMT from fluid content of other cystic lesions and the main pancreatic duct.[34,35]

Tumors with similar histological characteristics as serous cystadenocarcinoma but with different gross appearances have been observed. These macrocystic serous cystadenomas can be mistaken for mucinous cystic tumors as they have large cyst without a central scar. Authors have found specific differentiating features and combination of three of the following four findings on CECT can differentiate the two. These macrocystic serious tumors are commonly located in the head with a wall thickness less than 2 mm, lobulated contour and absence of wall enhancement.[34]

Intraductal Papillary Mucinous Tumors/ Neoplasms (IPMT)/(IPMN)

IPMT is a distinct entity that is recognized as dilatation of the main pancreatic duct or branch ducts with the proliferation of pancreatic ductal epithelium and mucin overproduction.

IPMTs were classified by WHO in 1996 as an intraductal papillary mucus producing neoplasm arising from the main pancreatic duct or its major branches. The main duct type have further been subdivided into segmental or diffuse and the branch duct type into macrocystic or microcystic types by Procacci et al. IPMTs can also present as a combination of the branch and main duct types and they account for 1% of all exocrine pancreatic tumors.[36]

Males are more commonly affected between the ages of 60 and 80 years. Reported signs and symptoms include abdominal mass, diarrhea, diabetes and weight loss, but small early stage tumors can be asymptomatic and found incidentally. Histologically, IPMTs represent a spectrum of dysplasias ranging from simple hyperplasia to carcinoma with proliferation of dysplastic mucin-producing columnar epithelial cells lining the ducts and forming papillary projections.

Imaging: Sonography may reveal a cystic pancreatic mass, duct dilatation or the presence of echogenic intraductal contents due to mucin (Fig. 19.28). The branch duct type lesion demonstrates a hypoechoic mass with lobulated borders in the uncinate process or pancreatic head.

Imaging features that suggest malignancy include thick wall, solid mural nodules, diffuse main duct

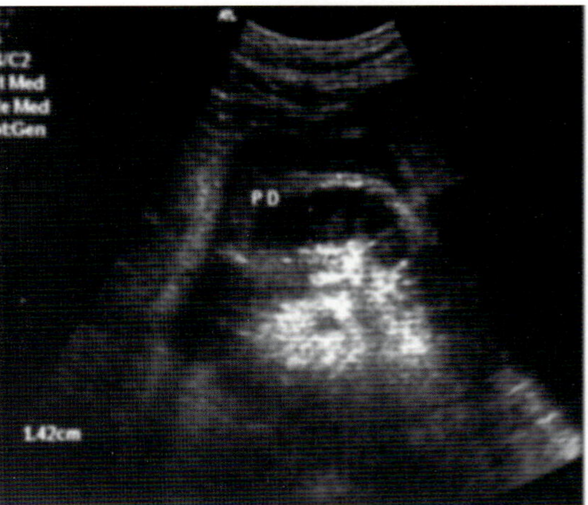

Fig. 19.28: Transverse gray scale sonogram showing a markedly dilated MPD with intraluminal papillary projections – IPMT

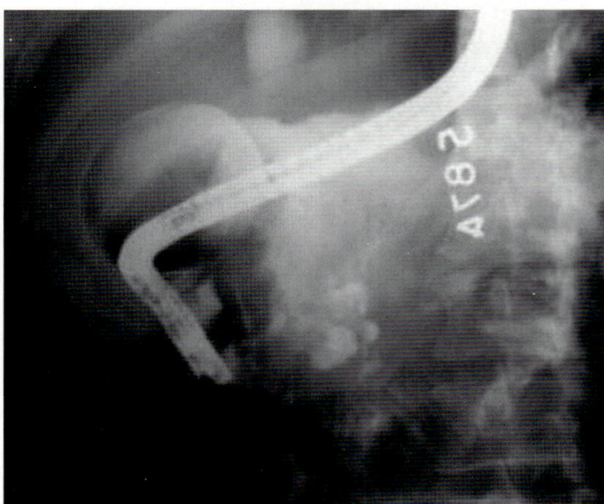

Fig. 19.29: ERCP shows filling of multiple cystic spaces within the pancreatic head in a case of IPMT

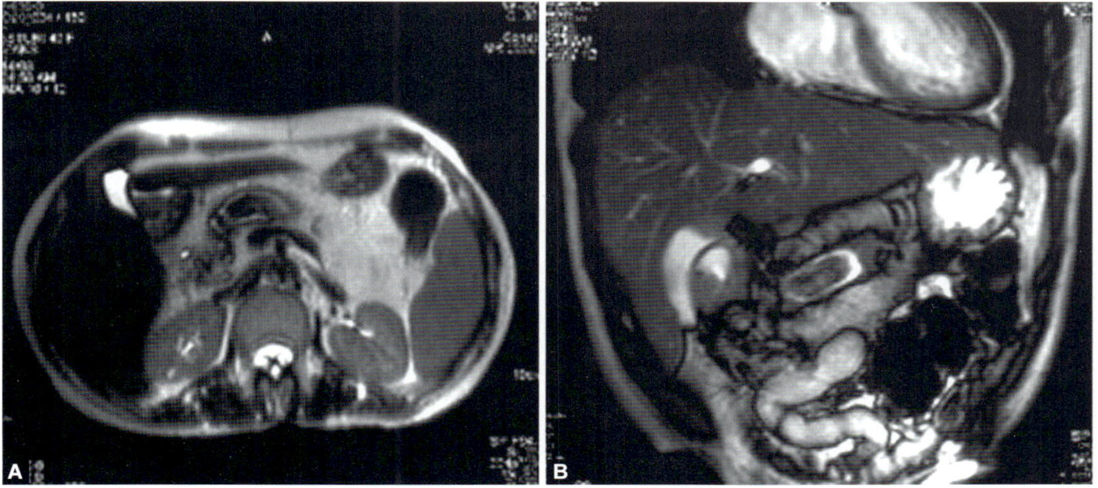

Figs 19.30A and B: Axial MR image (A) and coronal TRUFISP MR image (B) showing grossly dilated pancreatic duct with intraluminal filling defects and a non dilated biliary system

dilatation > 15 mm, intraductal filling defects, size > 6 mm and a bulging duodenal papilla.

The main differential dilemmas for IPMTs are distinguishing the main duct variant from chronic pancreatitis and the branch duct type from cystic neoplasms of the pancreas. The combination of clinical history and imaging findings, including the demonstration of intraductal filling defects, communication with the main duct, and a patulous papillary orifice with herniation into the duodenal lumen on ERCP should raise suspicion of an IPMT (Fig. 19.29).

MR cholangiography is an excellent imaging technique for characterization of IPMT. Assessment of the extent of ductal involvement and communication of the cyst with the duct are well visualized on MRCP (Figs 19.30 and 19.31). MDCT combined with 2D and 3D curved reformations are also very accurate. Malignancy is suspected when the MPD diameter is greater than 10 mm with mural nodules, papillary projections or a solid mass with the dilated duct or within a cystic lesion. Presence of vascular encasement, peripancreatic lymphadenopathy and metastases confirm malignancy. Side branch lesions > 30 mm diameter were considered malignant. Total resection is the treatment of choice for the main duct type. Local resection is often sufficient for main duct type with segmental involvement and in the case of branch duct type, total resection should be performed when the main pancreatic duct is dilated (Figs 19.32A to C). Small cystic lesion less than 2.5 cm in diameter with a normal pancreatic duct should be closely monitored.

Several authors have reported that endoscopic US is a useful modality for differentiating between benign and

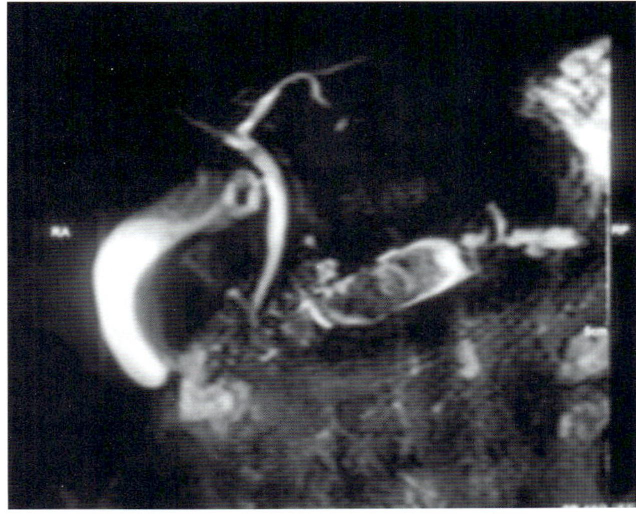

Fig. 19.31: MRCP image showing the extent of ductal involvement in the same

malignant IPMT. Main duct type tumors with ≥ 10 mm dilated MPD, branch duct type tumors (> 40 mm) with irregular septa, and large mural nodules (> 10 mm) strongly suggest malignancy on EUS.[37,38]

Solid and Papillary Epithelial Tumors/SPT's Neoplasms (SPEN)

SPENs are rare pancreatic tumors and are considered low grade malignancies which are thought to be hormone-dependent. Progesterone receptors are seen in > 90 % of tumors. These tumors are rare (1-2% of exocrine tumors) seen in the pancreatic tail in young females in the 2nd

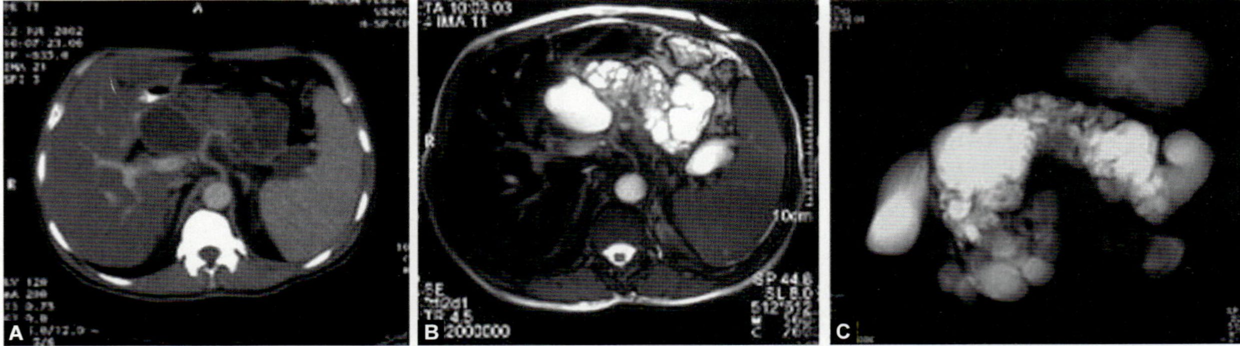

Figs 19.32A to C: CECT images showing multiple cysts replacing the entire pancreas (A). Axial TRUFISP MR image (B) revealing the entire pancreas to be replaced by multiple cysts. MRCP image (C) depicting the communication of the cysts with the main pancreatic duct – IPMT

and 3rd decades of life hence termed as "daughter" lesion. There is a predilection for Asians and Afro-Americans. They mostly exhibit a benign behavior but malignant degeneration does occur.

The patients with SPT are often asymptomatic or complain of discomfort or enlarging abdominal mass and the diagnosis is often made an imaging.

The mass is most frequently seen in the head or tail. It is well encapsulated and contains varying amounts of necrosis, hemorrhage and cystic changes. Both a capsule and intratumoral hemorrhage are important features which differentiate it from other pancreatic tumors. Complete resection is usually curative.[39]

Imaging: On USG, they are large well-marginated masses and may show solid, mixed solid and cystic or mainly cystic components. Hemorrhage within the mass is seen as echogenic areas. On CT, they show variable attenuation with thick enhancing capsules (Figs 19.33 and 19.34). Peripheral calcification is seen in up to one-third of the tumors. Detection of hemorrhage is important in differentiating SPENS from other cystic lesions of the pancreas. MR is more reliable than CT in demonstrating intratumoral hemorrhage and in showing the fibrous capsule which is hypointense on both T_1 and T_2 weighted images.[35]

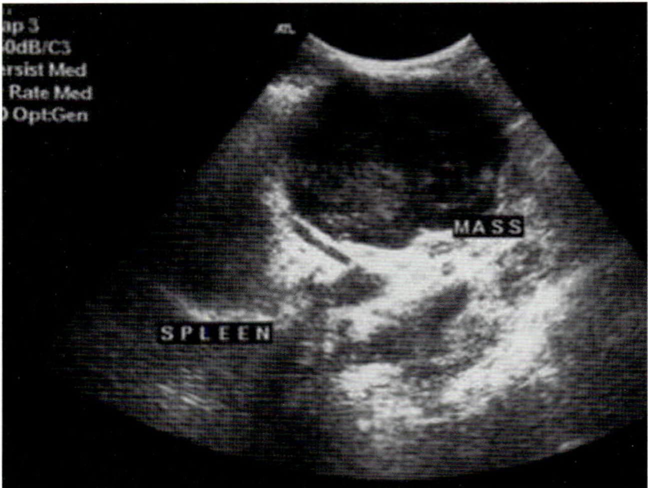

Fig. 19.33: Transverse sonogram image showing a mixed solid cystic mass in the pancreatic tail – SPEN.

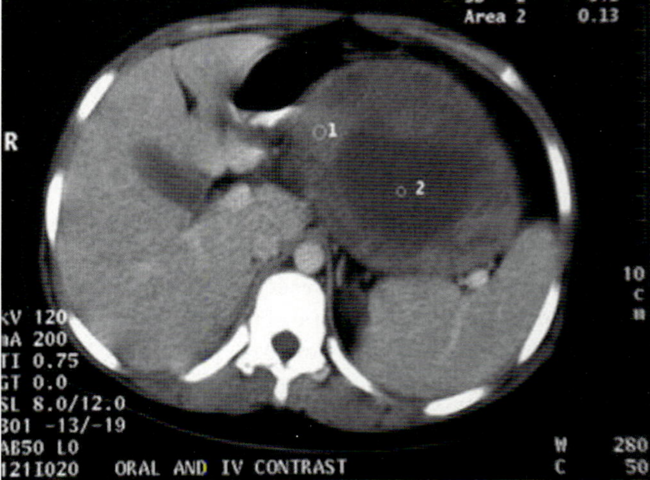

Fig. 19.34: CECT image showing a large solid mass with a necrotic area within arising from the pancreatic tail – SPEN

UNCOMMON CYSTIC PANCREATIC TUMORS

Cystic Endocrine Tumors

Islet cell tumors are usually solid but may develop a cystic appearance secondary to degeneration and necrosis and hence have to be considered in the differential diagnosis of cystic pancreatic neoplasms. There is equal distribution between genders and very few have been considered hormonally functional although immunohistochemically all of the tumor stains for one or the other pancreatic peptides. This contrasts with the reported 85 % incidence of clinical hormonal activity from islet cell tumors.

Cystic Metastatic: Disease occurs in cases of aggressive tumors such as sarcoma, melanomas or ovarian carcinomas. The imaging findings which can help differentiate primary from metastasis is the appearance of the shaggy peripheral wall and presence of lesions in other organs. With the exception of renal cell carcinoma where solitary metastatic disease to the pancreas is known majority have multiple foci of disease.[39,40]

Cystic Teratoma is a rare tumor of the pancreas which comprises tissue from any of the three germinal layers. Cystic lesions may be echogenic or hypoechogenic on ultrasound due to the variable amount of fat and sebum. On CT the lesions are cystic, multilocular, low attenuating with fat and peripheral calcification. On MRI the lesions have heterogenous signal on T1 are hyper intense on T2 with loss of signal intensity on fat saturated images. There may be a predominantly soft tissue mass with no involvement or dilatation of the biliary or pancreatic ducts.[34,39]

Lymphangioma: Less than 1% occur intra-abdominally twice as often in females than males at any age. They arise most commonly in the body and tail of pancreas and grow to large sizes up to 20 cm or more. They are typically multicystic with microcystic and macrocystic portions. US shows them as hypoechoic, anechoic cystic lesions in the pancreas. On CT multiple circumscribed cystic masses in, abutting or attached to the pancreas with this septations with variable enhancement. The cysts may be of fluid density or higher if there is hemorrhage[39](Fig. 19.35).

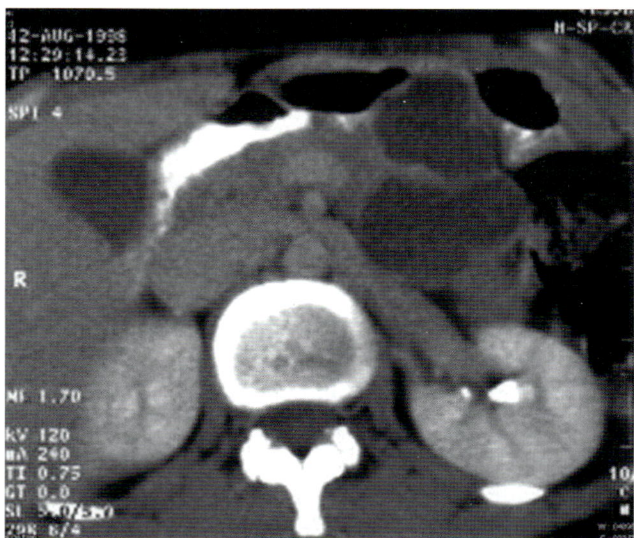

Fig. 19.35: CECT image showing multiple circumscribed fluid density cystic masses abutting the pancreatic tail with thin septations and variable enhancement – Lymphangioma

MRI displays a well-circumscribed predominantly cystic lesions hypointense on T1W1 and hyperintense on T2 W. In case of hemorrhage or infection there would be increased signal on T1 and decreased on T2 . The capsule is then with postgadolinium infusion.

Lipoma: Lipomas appear as well-defined masses of fat attenuation within the pancreatic parenchyma.

Imaging: MRI can be helpful in distinguishing true lipoma from focal fatty replacement of the pancreas. The T1 and T2 weighted images is homogenously hyperintense and isointense to abdominal fat. The signal typically is suppressed on fat-saturated images.[41]

Islet cell tumors (ICT): They are neoplasms of the neuroendocrine cells of the pancreas. ICTs are classified as functioning or nonfunctioning. Approximately, half of ICTs are functioning and half are malignant. Functioning islet cell tumors are named after the hormone they produce.

Hormonally active neoplasms are usually seen in the body and tail reflecting the distribution of islet cells. They are frequently multicentric and malignant islet cell tumors are classified based on the type of hormone synthesized.

Insulinomas are the most common ICTs and are usually benign. The clinical presentation is with hypoglycemic attacks and with atypical seizures associated with laboratory findings of low fasting plasma glucose and hyperinsulinemia. Gastrinomas are the second most common functioning ICTs and are malignant in 60 % of cases. They present with the Zollinger-Ellison syndrome with symptoms of peptic ulcers, malabsorption and diarrhea and are associated with elevated serum gastrin levels and gastric hypersecretions. Glucagonomas are uncommon tumors and show necrolytic migratory erythema and hyperglycemia. Vipomas are rare tumors with symptoms of watery diarrhea and flushing and may have elevated plasma peptide, hypokalemia and achlorhydria. Other functional islet cell tumors are somatostatinomas and corticotropinomas.[39,42]

Insulinoma

Insulinomas are small tumors most often less than 2 cm; large size or calcification suggest malignancy. Whipple's triad comprising symptoms of hypoglycemia, low blood glucose levels < 50 mg/dl and relief by glucose administration may be seen. They may be associated with MEN type I in adolescents and are more likely to be multiple and malignant in this syndrome. Only 5-10% of insulinomas are malignant and they can be found anywhere in the pancreas but more often in the body and tail (Fig. 19.36).

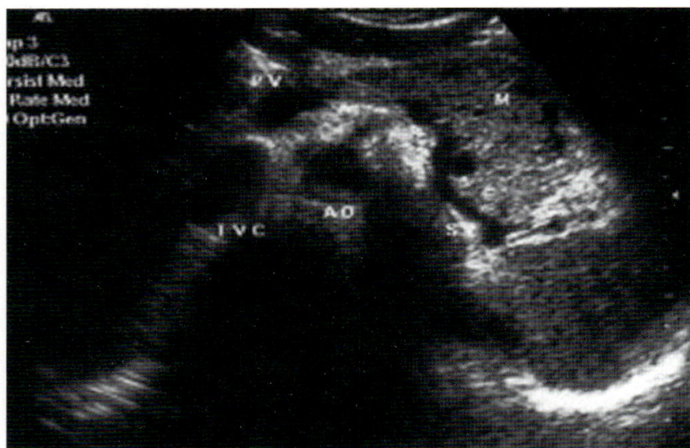

Fig.19.36: US showing an oval isoechoic mass in the pancreatic body – Islet cell tumor

Gastrinoma

Gastrinoma is the second most common islet cell tumor comprising 20% of all endocrine tumors. Seventy to ninety percent of gastrinomas lie in the gastrinoma triangle, which is an area bounded by the junction of cystic duct and CBD superiorly, SMA medially and junction of second and third part of duodenum inferiorly. These tumors are small in contrast to insulinomas, gastrinomas are frequently multiple and 30 % lie outside the pancreas. Gastrinomas frequently present with the Zollinger-Ellison syndrome. Gastrinomas is linked with MEN type I (Figs 19.37A to C).

Glucagonoma

These are more common in women and present with a mean age of 55 years and represent up to 3% of ICTs. They present with dermatitis, diabetes mellitus, weight loss and anemia. Blood glucagon levels are very high with elevated insulin levels. The most characteristic feature of the syndrome is necrolytic migratory erythema which occurs in 70 % of cases. Tumors are most commonly located in the body and tail and are large in size (mean 6.5 cm).

Vipoma

Represent 2% of islet cell tumors. This tumor is responsible for pancreatic cholera, also called Werner-Morrison syndrome. Seventy-five percent of vipomas are localized in the body or tail region and 10-20% arise in extra-pancreatic locations, e.g. adrenal medulla and sympathetic chain. The patient presents with watery diarrhea, achlorhydria, hypokalemia and acidosis.

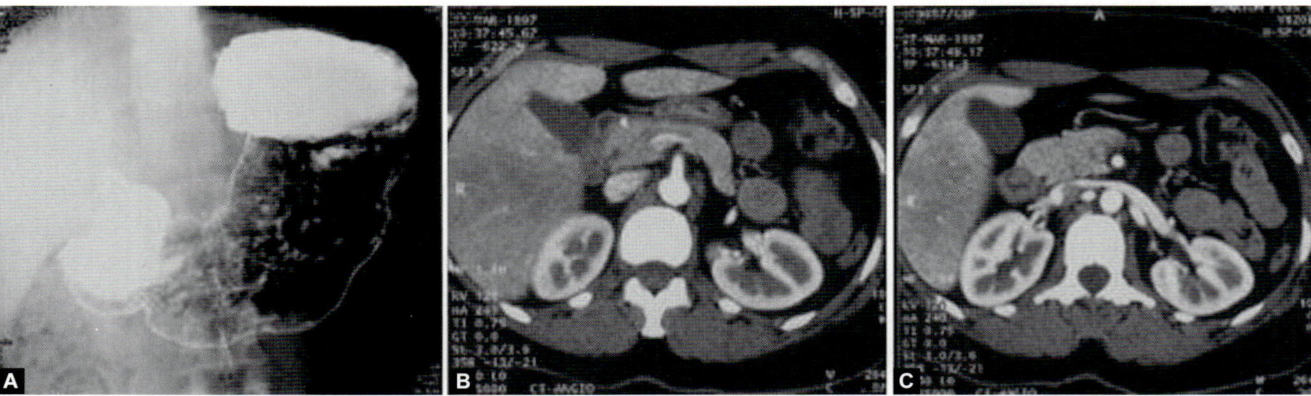

Figs 19.37A to C: Double contrast Ba UGI showing multiple small gastric erosions (A). Dual phase helical CT revealing a small enhancing lesion in the pancreatic body on the portal venous phase – GASTRINOMA

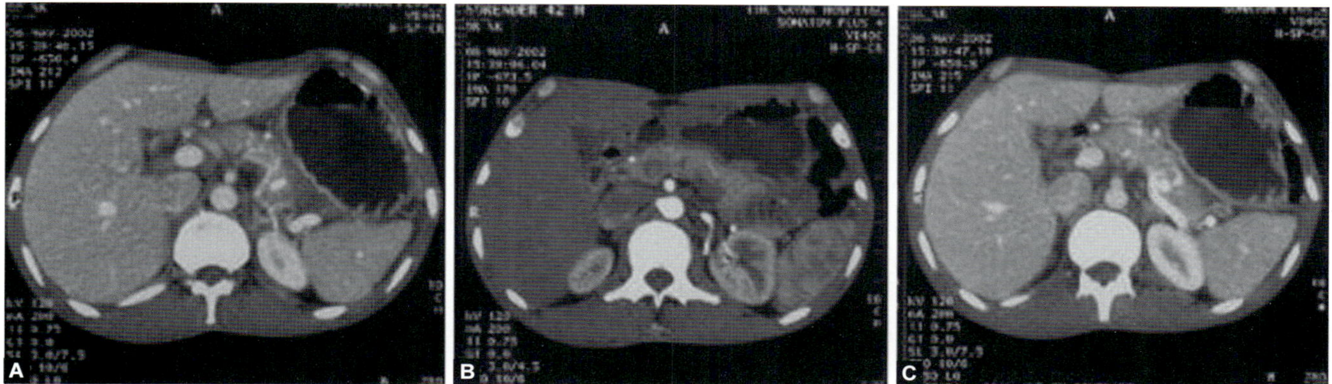

Figs 19.38A to C: Dynamic CT after intravenous contrast shows a small intensely enhancing round mass within pancreatic body causing slight contour abnormality – Islet cell tumor.

Somatostatinoma

Most tumors arise in the head and tend to be more than 3 cm. at the time of diagnosis. Somatostatin suppresses the release of insulin, growth hormone, glucagon, tsh, pepsin, secretin and gastric acid. Most patients have clinical features of diabetes mellitus, steatorrhea and gallbladder disease.[42]

Nonfunctioning ICTS

Asymptomatic ICTs usually reach a large size before diagnosis. Nonspecific signs and symptoms of abdominal pain, weight loss, jaundice or metastatic disease may be seen. Increased incidence of ICTs is seen in MEN type I and Von Hippel-Lindau (VHL) disease.

Imaging: The imaging appearance of islet cell tumors reflects their size and pathologic nature. Dual phase spiral CT scanning is indispensable for the detection of islet cell tumors and their hepatic metastases. On contrast enhanced CT, ICTs are hyper-attenuating in comparison with the normal pancreatic parenchyma because of their hypervascularity. This is particularly prominent in the arterial phase of dual phase scanning. ICTs are hyper-attenuating, even in the portal venous phase and this phase is particularly important because few lesions may exhibit delayed enhancement and are not easily diagnosed in the arterial phase (Fig. 19.38A to C). Nonfunctioning ICTs are easily detected by the mass effect they produce because of their large size at clinical presentation. Like the primary tumor, liver metastases are hypervascular and are best detected in the arterial phase. In addition to the liver, metastasis to the regional nodes are common, as is local extension and involvement of neighboring vascular structures (Fig. 19.39A and B). Nodular calcification is often associated with malignancy.

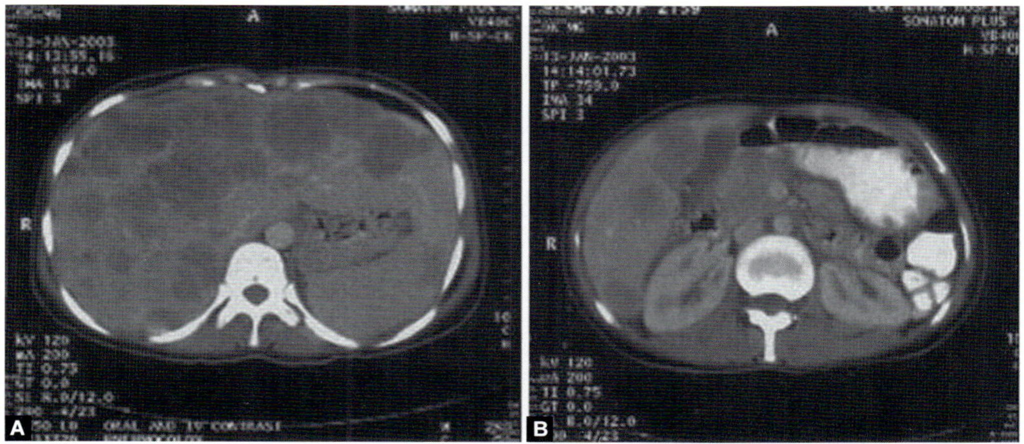

Figs 19.39A and B: CECT images in a case of ICT showing extensive liver metastasis involving both lobes

Three-dimensional CT angiography is useful for assessing arterial and venous involvement. The reported sensitivity of CT in localizing functioning ICTs varies from 71 to 82 %.[39]

On MRI, the lesions are hyperintense on both T2W and post-contrast T_1W images and are better seen on fat suppressed images.[40]

Arteriography and Venous Sampling

Large nonfunctioning ICTs and smaller functioning ICTs show increased vascularity with intense staining of the lesion which persists in late arterial and capillary phases for portal venous sampling. Transhepatic catheterization of the portal vein is done and the extrahepatic portal system is selectively catheterized. The hormone concentration in each sample is plotted on a diagram of the portal venous system. The sample that demonstrates the highest concentration of hormone comes from the vein draining the area of the tumor and the tumor can thus be localized.

Arterial Stimulation and Venous Sampling

The procedure is performed in the same sitting as that of angiography. A secretagogue is injected into each of the arteries that supply the pancreas one at a time. The secretagogue (calcium in the case of insulinomas) stimulates hormone production if it feeds the tumor area. Venous samples are taken from right and left hepatic veins and a two-fold increase in hormone production is taken as a reliable indicator.

Endoscopic US

Islet cell tumors are hypoechoic with well-defined smooth or slightly irregular margins. Small ICTs exhibit central echogenic areas resulting from necrosis, hyalinosis, calcification or microcysts. In larger tumors, irregularity of the margins is a reliable sign of malignancy.[38]

UNCOMMON SOLID PANCREATIC TUMORS

Pancreatoblastoma

This is a rare pancreatic tumor usually seen in young children in the first decade of life. It is a well-differentiated epithelial tumor of acinar origin seen in males of Asian origin. These tumors are difficult to differentiate from neuroblastma, Wilms tumor, hepatoblastoma or lymphoma. Cystic pancreatoblastomas tend to occur in newborn male with Beckwith-Wiedemann syndrome. Acinar cell carcinoma is pathologically similar but occurs in older patients

Imaging: On sonography these tumors have a well circumscribed heterogeneous appearance with solid and cystic components. On CT, the mass is well or partially circumscribed, with smooth lobulated margins. Uncommonly, infiltrative margin may be seen. The mass is heterogeneous with internal cystic areas due to necrosis. Small punctuate, clustered or curvilinear calcifications may be identified. tumors may appear multiloculated with enhancing septae. On MR, these tumors have a low to intermediate signal intensity on T_1 W images and hetergeneous high signal in T_2 weighted images. Invasions of adjacent organs and distant metastases may occur with pancreatoblastoma.[42,43]

Acinar Cell Carcinomas

Acinar cell carcinomas are found in old patients and are large, bulky masses with central necrosis. They may present with bone and skin lesions caused by metastatic fat necrosis due elevated lipase. These tumors are large mainly solid, but the appearance can be variable due to a large cystic component.[42]

Tumors of Neural Origin

Neural tumors are exceedingly rare in the pancreas and may be associated with neurofibromatosis in which pancreatic schwannomas and neurofibromas are seen.

Metastasis

Metastatic lesions are found in 3-12% of patients who have died of advanced malignancies. The common primary tumors which metastasize to the pancreas are from the lung, gastrointestinal tract, breast, kidney, osteosarcoma, melanoma and lymphoma. Majority of these lesions appear as large masses with well-defined margins. The enhancement pattern is variable and mimics the pattern of the primary tumor. The other imaging features which suggest the diagnosis include multiplicity of the lesions and hypervascularity. The most difficult to differentiate from a primary pancreatic tumor are metastasis from renal cell carcinoma and lymphomas (Fig. 19.40).

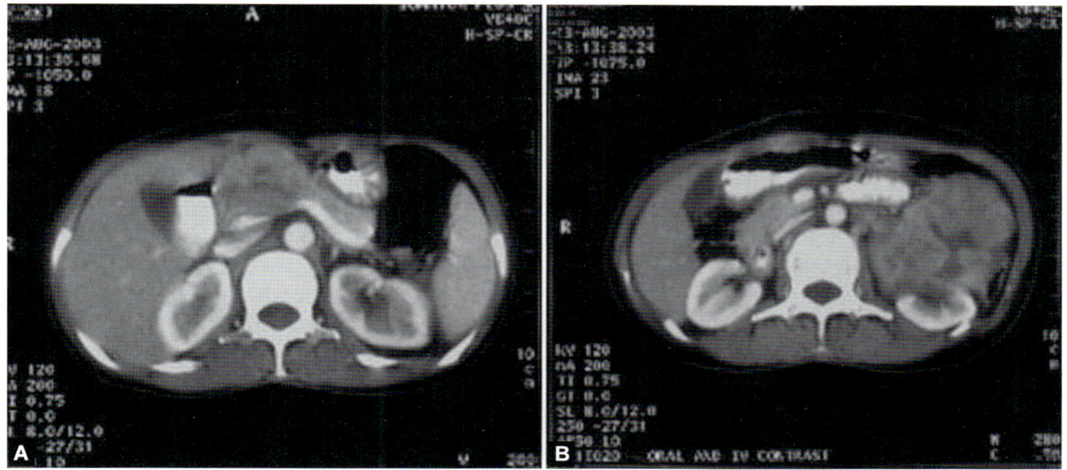

Figs19.40A and B: CECT images showing a bulky pancreatic head with multifocal hypodense lesions within (A) and a large solitary mass in the pancreatic tail (B)—Pancreatic mets

Lymphoma

The usual mode of involvement of the pancreas is by direct extension from peripancreatic B-cell type lymphadenopathy due to non-Hodgkin's lymphoma. Primary involvement of the pancreas is seen in immunocompromised hosts and in HIV positive patients.

Imaging: There are two distinct patterns of pancreatic involvement. Pancreatic lymphoma may present as focal mass or diffuse enlargement of the gland by an infiltrating tumor. The focal lesions enhance homogeneously to a lesser extent than the surrounding parenchyma. Diffuse enlargement in lymphoma is seen as homogeneous low attenuation on a non-contrast study (Figs 19.41A and B). Pancreatic lymphoma rarely causes ductal obstruction and is associated with lymphadenopathy below the level of the renal veins rarely seen in pancreatic adenocarcinoma.

On MR, the focal form demonstrates homogeneous hypointense signal on T_1W with low to intermediate signal higher than normal pancreatic parenchyma. In the diffuse form, the gland is enlarged with isointense $T_1$and T_2 signals, MRCP is helpful in assessing ductal dilatation.[44]

There is another subgroup of poorly differentiated pancreatic tumors called "small cell" tumor with similar histologic feature of pulmonary small cell tumor. These tumors are seen in men between 40 and 75 years and appear large (mean diameter 5.8 cm) with a appearance similar to malignant lymphoma, metastic small cell carcinoma and pancreatic adenocarcinoma. These tumors are treated with chemotherapy.

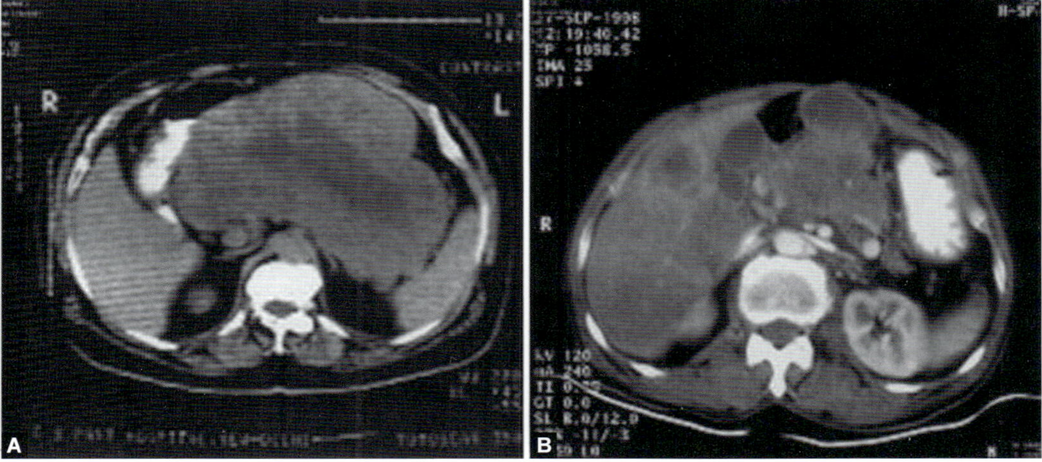

Figs 19.41A and B: CECT showing bulky lobulated centrally necrotic hypodense mass replacing entire pancreas except uncinate process (A) with extensive liver metastases (B)—Pancreatic lymphoma

REFERENCES

1. Baert AL, Delrome G. Radiology of the pancreas. Springer-Verlag, Berlin Heidelburg 1994;1-19.
2. Howard TJ, Stabile BE, Zinner MJ. Anatomic distribution of pancreatic endocrine tumors. Am J Surj 1990;159: 258-64.
3. Rosewicz S,Wiedenmann B. Pancreatic carcinoma. Lancet 1997;349:485-89.
4. Stephen DH: Pancreatic adenocarcinoma. Radiologic diagnosis and staging. Ailmentary tract radiology (5th edition). Margulis, Burhenne's (Eds) Mosby 1994; 1107-25.
5. Warshaw AL, Fernendez-del, Cassilo C. Pancreatic carcinoma — preoperative staging. New Engl J Med 1992;336-455.
6. Megibow AJ, Zhoui XH, Rotterdam H. Pancreatic adenocarcinoma: CT versus MR imaging in the evaluation of resectability — report of the radiologic diagnostic oncology group. Radiology 1995;195:327-32.
7. Tomiyama T, Ueno N, Tano S, et al. Assessment of arterial invasion in pancreatic cancers using colour Doppler US. Am J Gasteroenterology 1996;91(7):1410-16.
8. Palazzo L, Roseau G, Gayet B, et al. EUS in the diagnosis and staging of pancreatic adenocarcinoma: Results of a prospective study with comparison to US and CT scan. Endoscopy 1993;25:143-50.
9. Ahmad NA, Lewis JD, Seigelmann ES, et al. Role of EUS and MRI in the preoperative staging of pan-creatic adenocarcinoma. Am J Gasteroenterology 2000;95(8): 1926-31.
10. Boland GW, O' Malley ME, Saez M, et al. Pancreatic phase versus portal vein phase helical CT of the pancreas: Optimal temporal window for evaluation of pancreatic adenocarcinoma. AJR Am J Roentgenol 1999;172:605-08.
11. Tsuchiya R, Noda T, Harada N, et al. Collective review of small carcinomas of the pancreas. Annals Surgery 1986;203:77-81.
12. National cancer institute. Annual cancer statistics review: 1975-1988. Bethesda (MD). US Department of Health and Human Services; 1991.
13. Freeny PC, Marks WM, Ryan JA, et al. Pancreatic ductal adenocarcinoma: Diagnosis and staging with dynamic CT. Radiology 1998;166:125-33.
14. Diehl SJ, Lehmann KJ, Sadick M, et al. Pancreatic cancer: value of dual-phase helical CT in assessing respectability. Radiology 1998;206:373-78.
15. Darren DD, Brennan, Gulia A, Zamboni, Vassilios D, Raptopoulos, Jonathan B Kruskal. Comprehensive preoperative assessment of pancreatic adenocarcinoma with 64-section volumetric Ct. Radiographics 2007;27: 1653-66.
16. Tublin ME, Tessler FN, Chang SL, et al. Affect of injection rate of contrast medium on pancreatic and hepatic helical CT. Radiology 1992;210:97-101.
17. Raptopoulos V, Steer ML, Sheriman RG, et al. The use of helical CT and CT angiography to predict vascular involvement from pancreatic cancer: Correlation with findings at surgery. AJR Am J Roentgenol 1997;168: 971-77.
18. Fishman EK, Wyatt SH, Ney DR, et al. Spiral CT of the pancreas with multiplanar display. AJR 1992;159:1209-12.
19. Nino-Murcia M, Jeffrey Jr RB. Multidetector row CT and volumetric imaging of pancreatic neoplasms. Gastero-enterol Clin N Am 2002;31:881-96.
20. Horton KM, Fishman EK. Adenocarcinoma of the pancreas: CT imaging. Radiol Clin N Am 2002;40:1263-73.
21. Ly JN, Miller FH. MR imaging of the pancreas: a practical approach. Radiol Clin N Am 2002;40:1289-1306.
22. Tamm EP, Bhosale Priya, Lee H Jeffrey. Pancreatic ductal adenocarcinoma: Ultrasound, computed tomography and magnetic resonance imaging. Seminars in Ultra-sound, CT and MRI Vol. 2007;28.5:330-38.
23. Semelka RC, Kelekis NL, Ascher SM. Pancreas. IN: MRI of the Abdomen and Pelvis, New York, Wiley Liss 1997; 187-238.
24. Martin DR, Semelka RC. MR imaging of pancreatic masses. Magn Reson Im Clin N Am 2000;8:787-812.
25. Johnson PT, Outwater EK. Pancreatic carcinoma versus chronic pancreatitis: Dynamic MRI. Radiology 1999;212: 213-18.
26. Fulcher AS, Turner MA. MR Cholangio-pancreatography. Radiol Clin N Am 2002;40:1363-76.
27. Motochara T, Semelka RC, Bader TR. MRCP: Radiol Clin N Am 2003;41:89-96.
28. Fayad LM, Kowalski T, Mitchell DG. MRCP: Evaluation of common pancreatic diseases. Radiol Clin N Am 2003;41: 97-114.
29. Varghese JC, Farrell MA, Courtney G, et al. Role of MRCP in patients with failed or inadequate ERCP. AJR 1999;173: 1527-33.
30. Masci E, Toti G, Mariani A, et al. Complications of diagnostic and therapeutic ERCP: A prospective multicenter study. Am J Gasteroenterol 2001;96:417-23.
31. Ichikawa T, Sou H, Araki T, et al. Duct penetrating sign at MRCT: Usefulness for differentiating inflammatory pancreatic mass from pancreatic cancer. Radiology 2001;221:107-116.
32. Koyama K, Okamura T, Kawabe J, et al. Diagnostic usefulness of FDG-PET for pancreatic mass lesions. Annals Nucl Med 2001;15:217-24.
33. Rosch T, et al. Staging of pancreatic and ampullary carcinoma by EUS, CT and angiography. Gasteroen-terology 1992;102:188.
34. Christopher RS, Koenraad J Mortele. Cystic tumors of the pancreas: Ultrasound, computed tomography and magnetic resonance imaging features. Seminars in ultrasound, CT and MRI Vol 2007;28.5:339-55.
35. Hammond MD, Miller TH, Sica GT, et al. Imaging of cystic diseases of the pancreas. Radiol Clin N Am 2002;40: 1243-62.

36. Procacci CP, Megibow AJ, Carbognin G, et al. IPMT of the pancreas: A pictorial essay. Radiographics 1999;19: 1447-63.
37. Satomi Kawamoto, Karen MH, Leo P Lawler, Ralph H Hruban, Elliot K Fishman. Intraductal papillary mucinous neoplasm of the pancreas : Can benign lesions be differentiated from malignant lesions with multidetector CT? Radiographics : 2005;25:1451-70.
38. Kubo N, Chijiiwa Y, Akahoshi K, et al. IPMTs of the pancreas: Differentiating between benign and malignant tumors by EUS. Am J Gasteroenterol 2001;96:429-34.
39. Sheth S, Fishman EK. Imaging of uncommon tumors of the pancreas. Radiol Clin N Am 2002;40:1273-87.
40. Merkle EM, Boaz T, Kolkythas O, et al. Metastases to the pancreas. Br J Radiol 1998;71:1208-14.
41. Katz DS, Nardi PM, Hines J, et al. Lipomas of the pancreas. AJR 1998;170:1485-87.
42. Sejal Shah, Koenraad Mortele. Uncommon solid pancreatic neoplasms: Ultrasound, computed tomography and magnetic resonance imaging features. Seminars in ultrasound CT and MRI. Vol 2007;28.5:357-369.
43. Roebuck DJ, Yuen MK, Wong YC, et al. Imaging features of pancreaticoblastoma. Pediatr Radiol 2001;31:501-06.
44. Ferrozi F, Zuccoli G, Bora D, et al. Mesenchymal tumors of the pancreas: CT findings. J Comput Assist Tomogr 2000;24:622-27.

Chapter Twenty

Imaging in Portal Hypertension

Veena Chowdhury, Rashmi Dixit

Portal hypertension (PHT) is defined as an increase in portal pressure above the normal range of 6-10 mm Hg or a gradient of more than 5 mm Hg between hepatic veins and portal vein or portal vein pressure of more than 30 cm of saline measured at surgery.[1,2]

ANATOMY AND COLLATERAL CIRCULATION

The portal system consists of all the veins which carry blood from the abdominal part of the alimentary tract except lower rectum and anal canal. It also receives drainage from the pancreas spleen and gallbladder.[3] Figure 20.1 shows the normal portal venous system and its tributaries. The main portal vein is 6 to 8 cm long formed by the union of splenic vein and superior mesenteric vein dorsal to the neck of pancreas at the level of L_1-L_2 vertebrae. It ascends at an angle of 40°-90° with respect to the spine to reach the porta. Within the liver the portal venous branches have an intrasegmental course.

The normal liver receives blood from the hepatic artery and portal vein in a ratio of 1:3. The terminal branches of the portal vein and hepatic artery open into the hepatic sinusoids at different levels. The presence of these two different routes for blood inflow increases the complexity of liver hemodynamics. The sinusoids normally represent the only connection between hepatic artery and portal vein on one hand and the hepatic veins on the other, which carry blood away from the liver and drain into the IVC. Understanding basic aspects of liver hemodynamics is necessary to analyze diagnostic images.

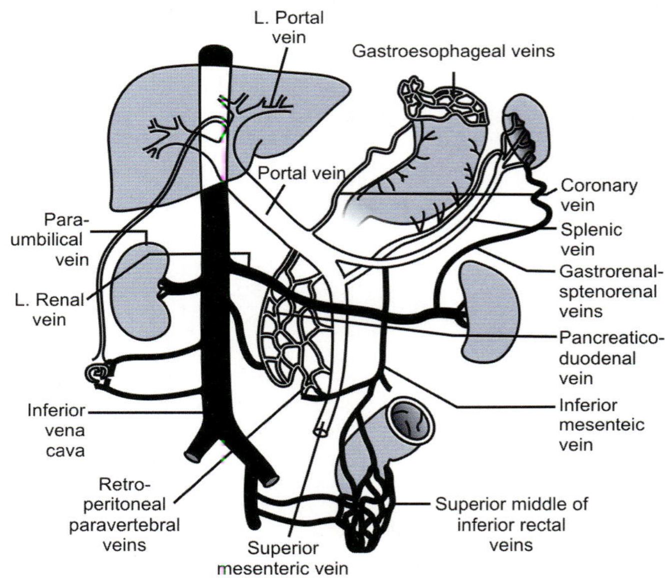

Fig. 20.1: Tributaries of the portal venous system with major sites of portosystemic collaterals

The portal system is unique in certain aspects as blood is not pumped into the portal system but is driven by a pressure gradient between the portal and systemic venous systems. Portal vein and its tributaries are devoid of valves. This plays an important role in the development of collaterals. Three types of collaterals may develop:[5]

Tributary Collaterals (Hepatofugal)

These are the normal tributaries of the portal venous system in which flow reversal occurs due to portal hypertension. These are:

a. The left gastric (coronary) vein (LGV) and short gastric veins. In PHT flow reversal occurs commonly to the submucosal venous plexus of the oesophagus, stomach and sometimes to the duodenum and subsequently via the azygos and hemiazygos system to the SVC.
b. Inferior mesenteric vein to superior/middle/inferior rectal venous communication and then to IVC.
c. Superior mesenteric vein (SMV) to retroperitoneal veins to IVC.

Developed Collaterals (Hepatofugal)

Developed collaterals are pre-existing channels (formed in the fetus) which are not used in normal individuals but re-open partially or fully in portal hypertension.

a. Left portal vein via recanalised paraumbilical vein to superior and inferior epigastric veins and then to SVC and IVC respectively.
b. Splenorenal collaterals
c. Gastrorenal collaterals
d. Splenoretroperitoneal collaterals.

Bridging Collaterals (Hepatopedal)

In extrahepatic obstruction of the portal venous system bridging collaterals help restore hepatopedal flow.

a. Splenic vein occlusion—Portal flow is diverted via the short gastric veins to portal vein via LGVor via gastroepiploic veins to SMV to portal vein.
b. Portal vein thrombosis—Blood flow is directed to the liver via parabiliary venous plexus (cavernoma).

Etiology of Portal Hypertension

Since pressure is a product of flow and resistance, portal hypertension may occur when portal flow or resistance within the portal system is increased. Table 20.1 shows the etiology of portal HT.

Common causes of portal hypertension in India include extrahepatic portal obstruction (45- 50% in North India),[7,8.] non-cirrhotic portal fibrosis or NCPF (15-30%)[9] and cirrhosis (25% approx.). Cirrhosis, in our country is most often the result of infective hepatitis while in the west it is most often due to alcoholic liver disease .

Table 20.1 Etiology and classification of portal hypertension[6]

i. **Hyperkinetic**
   A. Arterioportal fistula or malformation
ii. **Increased portal venous resistance**
   A. *Intrahepatic*
      1. Presinusoidal: Non-cirrhotic portal fibrosis, hepatic schistosomiasis, congenital hepatic fibrosis, sarcoidosis, and lymphoma
      2. Postsinusoidal hepatic cirrhosis (alcoholic, post-necrotic) and veno-occlusive disease
   B. *Extrahepatic*
      1. Prehepatic: Cavernous transformation (of portal vein) and splenic or superior mesenteric vein obstruction(segmental PHT).
      2. Posthepatic: Hepatic vein obstruction, suprahepatic inferior vena caval obstruction, congestive heart failure, and constrictive pericarditis

Nearly 15-30% of all patients with portal hypertension in India who undergo surgery or sclerotherapy have NCPF.[10,11] The mean age of patients varies from 25-30 years. A female dominance, male dominance or no sex prediliction has been reported by various investigators. It is characterized by well-tolerated episodes of gastro-oesophageal variceal hemorrhage in a young patient with prominent splenomegaly. Ascites, encephalopathy, jaundice and other signs of liver failure are not common. The main lesion is an obliterative portovenopathy of the liver with patchy segmental, subendothelial thickening of intrahepatic portal venous radicles with variable obliteration or recanalization and scarring and fibrosis resulting in presinusoidal abnormal blood flow. Fibrosis and nodule formation when present affect the subcapsular areas but not the deeper part unlike cirrhosis. Increased portal flow has been found in NCPF patients although it is uncertain whether it is a primary event or secondary change.[9,11]

A similar disease occurring predominantly in older females, in Japan has been called idiopathic portal hypertension (IPH) or hepatoportal sclerosis. Patients commonly present with a self-palpable mass (the enlarged spleen) rather than variceal bleed.

Noninvasive Radiological Evaluation

Radiological evaluation of patients with known or suspected portal hypertension may be used to establish the diagnosis, define the portal vascular anatomy for the surgical or angiographic creation of shunts or other therapeutic manoeuvres and evaluate the patency of these shunts.

Investigations include

i. Plain X-rays
ii. Barium contrast examinations
iii. Sonography and CDFI
iv. CT and CT portography
v. MR and MR portography.

Plain X-rays are of limited value. Chest X-ray may show a dilated azygos system while X-ray abdomen may show non-specific findings of hepatosplenomegaly and haze due to ascites.

Barium contrast examinations Barium swallow in the left anterior oblique position after administration of anticholinergic agents with Valsalva maneuver is optimally suited for demonstration of oesophageal varices which are seen as thickened serpiginous folds.

Gastric duodenal and rectal varices can also be detected using barium contrast studies however their role has become limited with the widespread use of endoscopy.

Sonography and CDFI

Sonography and CDFI have revolutionized the evaluation of portal hypertension and it is the most widely used investigation for non-invasive evaluation of portal hemodynamics. The cause of portal hypertension, vascular patency, presence of collaterals, and portal flow can be assessed non invasively. The examination is performed during quiet respiration with the patient supine. Ideally the patient should be fasting for about 12 hours before the examination.[12] Some investigators recommend repeat examination post prandially as well to document hemodynamic changes after a meal. Meticulous attention to the Doppler technique with use of correct pulse repetition frequency (PRF), color gain and adequately low Doppler angle i.e. less than 60° is essential for determination of portal flow and velocity. Doppler evaluation may be limited by obesity, ascites and interference by bowel gas. Doppler also does not provide 3-D depiction of vascular anatomy which is essential before any surgery and is operator dependent.

Computed Tomographic Imaging

CT can demonstrate the portal venous system and portosystemic collaterals in any part of the body with minimum interference from gas, bone or fat unlike sonography. Dynamic contrast enhanced scans are mandatory for detection of varices. Multislice scanners are ideally suited for this purpose.

The scan protocol consists of an initial non-contrast study to identify the liver location and volume of interest. Subsequently 100-120 ml of contrast medium is administered via a pressure injector at the rate of 3-3.5 ml/sec. Arterial phase images are initiated 25-30 sec after initiation of contrast material. Portal venous phase images are acquired after a delay of 60 sec after initiation of contrast and an additional acquisition may be made at 180 sec for hepatic venous phase images. Scanning can be done with 1.25-2.5 mm collimation. Patient may be given 750 ml of water orally before the scan as it allows visualization of even small varices in the gastric wall.[13]

Axial images acquired in the portal venous phase are sufficient for the diagnosis of portal hypertension, however three dimensional (3D) CT angiography especially multidetector CT angiography provides precise delineation of the distribution and extent of portosystemic collaterals with an accuracy comparable to conventional angiographic portography.[14-16]

MR Imaging

Like CT, MR imaging is not hindered by presence of ascites, bowel gas or obesity. In addition the absence of nephrotoxic contrast media and lack of ionizing radiation make it an attractive imaging modality.

On routine SE images the portal vein and variceal collaterals are visualized as signal free structures owing to flow void.[17] However if flow is very slow a paradoxic enhancement with increased signal may occur. On gradient echo pulse sequences flowing blood is bright while thrombus is hypointense.

MR Portography

In the past MR angiography was seldom used for the evaluation of mesenteric vasculature. Both TOF and PC techniques required an acquisition time upto several minutes. This made it impossible to acquire data in a single breathhold therefore MRA of the upper abdomen was limited by blurring from extensive motion artefacts. Furthermore it was impossible to obtain pure arterial phase or venous phase images.[18,19]

Gadolinium enhanced breathhold MR portography can now be achieved using fast imaging techniques within

20-30 s. There are some technical issues to consider when it is essential to obtain high quality images of the portal venous system. By the time the contrast agent reaches the portal vein it is considerably diluted, hence a higher dose of contrast (0.2 ml/kg) is required for dedicated imaging of the portal vein as compared to arterial studies. The acquisition volume should include the entire portal and mesenteric venous system. If the anterior abdominal wall is not included in the acquisition volume the paraumbilical collateral may be missed.

CEMR portography is superior to Doppler in management of patients with portal hypertension by identifying portosystemic collaterals more adequately and clearly demonstrates portal venous vessels that cannot be visualized at Doppler.[20] In a recent study MR portography was superior to Doppler in detecting almost all types of portosystemic collaterals such as short gastric, para-oesophageal veins and retroperitoreal veins. Doppler was superior to MR portography with regard to detection of umbilical vein only. Other advantages of MR portography include that it is an operator independent technique which allows better anatomic orientation preoperatively. Moreover images can be stored or transmitted for subsequent analysis.[20,21]

Pitfalls[22]

a. Insufficient enhancement of portal vein due to dilution of contrast.
b. Blurring: Breathholding twice in a row to capture both the arterial and venous phase is difficult for many patients. It is therefore important to keep scan times short.
c. Surgical clips are commonly present around the hepatic hilum due to their widespread use in cholecystectomy, stents used in TIPS also obscure visualization of the portal vein and IVC containing the stent.

INTRAHEPATIC PORTAL HYPERTENSION

Organ Parameters

Sonography can differentiate intrahepatic from extrahepatic portal hypertension in 98% cases with over all sensitivity of 92% and can also detect the presence of splenomegaly and ascites. Evaluation of the liver by ultrasound may reveal changes of cirrhosis such as coarsened echo texture with or without altered echogenicity, nodularity of liver surface (Figs 20.2A and B), presence of regenerating nodules and reduction in the number of visible portal or hepatic veins. Reduction of liver size with a combination of segmental hypertrophy and atrophy is seen. A caudate to right lobe ratio > 0.65 and reduction of the transverse diameter of segment IV, i.e left wall of gallbladder to ascending portion of left portal vein to less than 30 mm has been reported.[3]

On *CT* similar morphological changes such as lobular contour of the liver surface, a combination of segmental

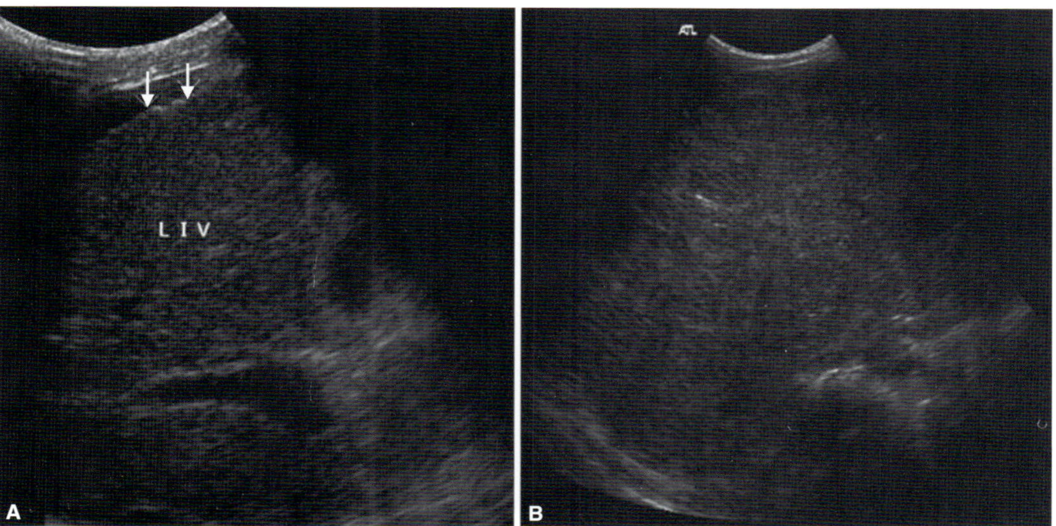

Figs 20.2A and B: (A) Sonogram showing a nodular hepatic surface (arrows) with coarsened hepatic echotexture in a patient of cirrhosis, (B)Heterogenous hepatic parenchyma with attenuation of hepatic veins seen on ultrasound of a patient with cirrhosis

hypertrophy(seg I-III)and atrophy(seg IV-VII) along with inhomogeneous attenuation of hepatic parenchyma on unenhanced CT, or occasionally regenerating nodules may be visualized in hepatic cirrhosis. *MR imaging* may reveal morphological changes of cirrhosis with regenerating nodules being better visualized on MRI than any other modality.[23]

Only limited literature is available regarding ultrasound findings in *NCPF*. The liver surface is smooth and subcapsular atrophy is seen at times. There is marked dilatation of the portal vein (≥ 19 mm) with selective dilatation of the left branch.[9,24,25] Thickening of the portal vein wall (> 3 mm) and sudden narrowing of intrahepatic second degree portal vein branches has been observed with increased periportal echogenicity (Fig. 20.3).

Conspicuously heterogeneous and decreased portal perfusion at the periphery of the liver with heterogeneously increased arterial perfusion has been described on CT arterioportography. This was not found in cirrhotics and may be an important feature of idiopathic portal hypertension.[26] Proximity of medium sized intrahepatic vessels to each other and to the liver surface, small vessels running parallel to second order branches of intrahepatic portal vein and periportal abnormal high signal intensity of T_2-weighted images have been reported in IPH.[27]

Splenomegaly

The size of the spleen is not well correlated with PHT. However, if splenomegaly is absent, PHT is unlikely though not ruled out. Siderotic Gamna Gandy nodules which represent small foci of perifollicular and trabecular hemorrhage may be seen as multiple faint hyperechoic spots on ultrasound or multiple faint calcifications on CT. They are seen as multiple low signal foci 3-8 mm in size on gradient echo MR images.

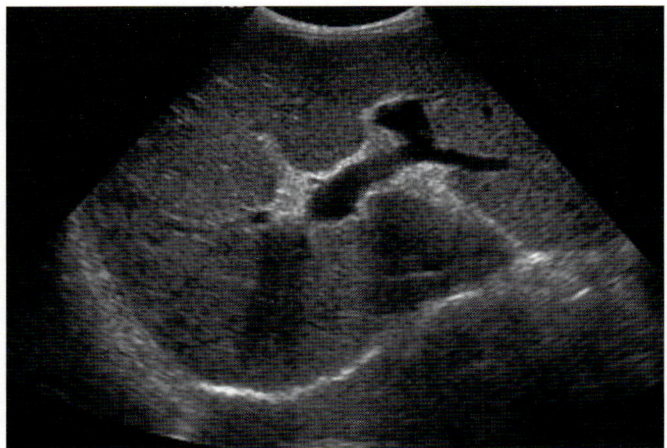

Fig. 20.3: Grey scale ultrasound showing an increase in periportal echogenicity with normal parenchymal echotexture in a case of NCPF

Ascites

Ascites in patients with portal hypertension secondary to cirrhosis usually occur secondary to underlying liver cell failure and increase in sinusoidal pressure leading to an increase in fluid in the space of Disse and to ascites formation. In prehepatic PHT, liver function remains normal and ascites is minimal.

Increased density of the mesentry (misty mesentry) and omentum may be seen. In addition, patients with PHT especially those with hypersplenism have an increased incidence of splenic artery aneurysms which may be visualized incidentally during imaging.[28]

Vascular Evaluation

Color and spectral Doppler ultrasound. The following vascular criteria have been found to be valuable for diagnosis of intrahepatic portal hypertension:

1. Portal vein diameter and response of portal, splenic or superior mesenteric veins to respiration.
2. Portal flow direction
3. Portal velocity and waveforms
4. Presence of portosystemic collaterals
5. Hepatic vein evaluation
6. Hepatic and superior mesenteric artery changes.

Portal Vein, Superior Mesenteric Vein and Splenic Vein Diameter

The normal portal vein diameter is 9-12 mm in quiet respiration. A portal vein diameter of more than 13 mm indicates portal hypertension with a high degree of specificity but low sensitivity and a caliber over 17 mm is 100% predictive for large varices.[12] Normal portal vein dimensions, however, do not exclude portal hypertension.

The upper limit of normal splenic and superior mesenteric veins ranges from 10 to 12 mm with these vessels becoming prominent in PHT (Fig. 20.4). In normal individuals, the diameter of these veins increases by 20 to 100% from quiet to deep inspiration. An increase of less than 20% indicates portal hypertension with 81% sensitivity and 100% specificity.[12]

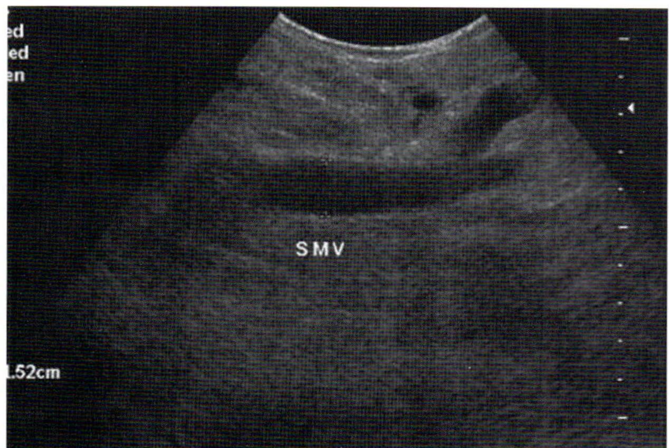

Fig. 20.4: Longitudianal grey scale ultrasound showing a dilated superior mesenteric vein measuring 15.2 mm with mesenteric thickening and collaterals in a patient with portal hypertension

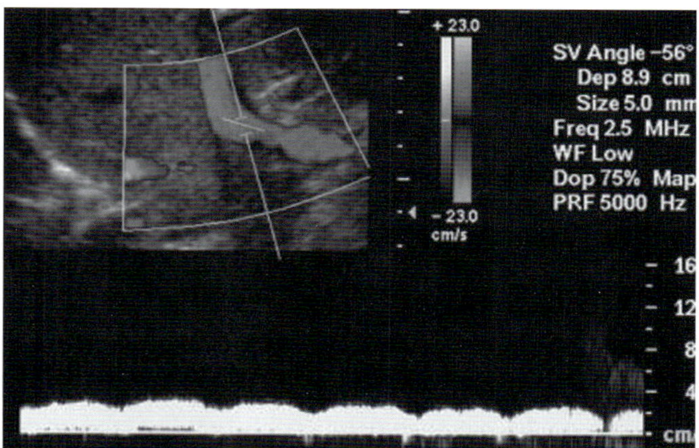

Fig. 20.5: CDFI of the main portal vein showing hepatopedal flow with a normal spectral trace *(For color version see plate 4)*

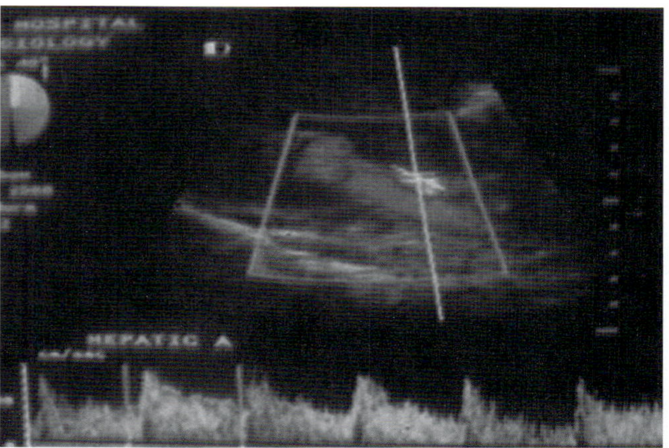

Fig. 20.6: CDFI in a patient of cirrhosis showing hepatofungal flow in the main portal vein. Note portal vein and hepatic artery show flow in opposite directions. Spectral trace from the hepatic artery is shown *(For color version see plate 4)*

Portal flow direction, velocity and wave form CDFI can easily establish the presence and direction of flow in the portal vein. The normal portal flow is always directed towards the liver (hepatopedal) and has a fairly uniform flow velocity with slight phasicity in the spectral tracing secondary to respiration and to a lesser extent cardiac activity (Fig. 20.5). Helical flow is present in some normal individuals and can simulate reverse or bidirectional flow. The fasting mean flow velocity is approximately 12-18 cm/sec (range 12-23 cm/sec) and has respiratory cycle variation decreasing on inspiration and increasing on onset of expiration. In normal subjects, the average portal flow is 500-900 ml/min.[6] Errors in measuring cross sectional area affect calculation of flow volume but repeated measurement of diameter can reduce errors. Portal vein diameter is done at the center of the portal vein at a known angle of insonation less than 60°. This is usually done 1 cm proximal to its bifurcation. Mean velocity should be calculated over tracing 4-6 sec long in order to avoid fluctuation in flow velocity. As portal hypertension develops, the flow velocity in the portal vein decreases and the flow in the portal vein loses its undulatory pattern and becomes monophasic. As severity of PHT increases, flow becomes biphasic and finally hepatofugal (Fig. 20.6). Flow reversal should be assessed throughout the portal venous system as reversal may be segmental.

As there is a wide variation of reported values for portal vein flow velocity, it is recommended that the threshold for defining a reduction of portal flow velocity is established in each ultrasound unit. Although a velocity below 12 cm/sec is highly suggestive.[28] Both the volume flow and velocity are affected by the type of collaterals that develop and may actually increase when there is a large paraumbilical collateral, but effective liver perfusion is lower as calculated from flow volume in portal trunk minus portal flow volume in the umbilical vein.[29]

Pitfalls of Portal Flow Assessment

The direction of flow in the portal vein may be ambiguous or may spuriously appear and the reversed due to technical reasons and the portal vein may appear occluded when the flow is very low. Portal vein dilatation and flow reversal may also be caused by CHF. However, in this case, the portal flow is markedly pulsatile and the IVC is dilated unlike in portal hypertension.[12]

Portosystemic Venous Collaterals[12]

Portosystemic venous collaterals are a clear indication of portal hypertension. Ultrasonography is reported to visualize 65% to 90% of portosystemic collaterals. The important collaterals are:

1. Left gastric (coronary vein)—Diameter of the normal coronary vein is less than 4 mm, while a diameter more than 7 mm is evidence of portosystemic pressure gradient exceeding 10 mm Hg. Normal flow is towards the portal vein, hepatofugal flow is also indicative of abnormal portosystemic pressure gradient (Fig. 20.7).
2. Short gastric veins may be visible between the upper pole of spleen and gastric wall. They are seen as anechoic tubes with venous flow towards the oesophagus. Gastroepiploic collaterals can also be visualized around the stomach (Fig. 20.8).

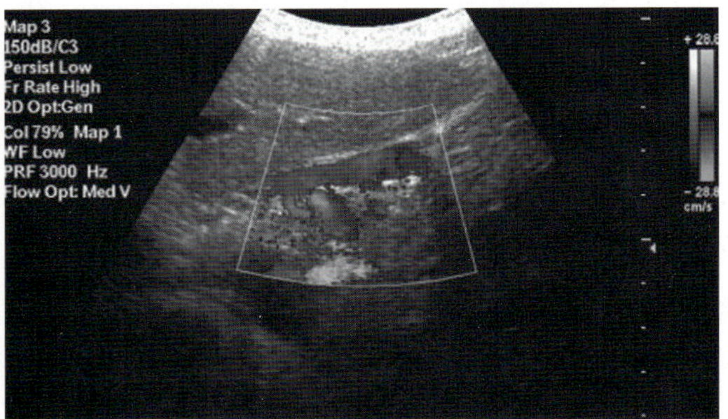

Fig. 20.7: Colour Doppler study showing a tortuous coronary collateral with prominent varices at the gastroesophageal junction *(For color version see plate 4)*

The coronary and short gastric collaterals result in esophageal and gastric varices and increase the risk of variceal bleed. When large, esophageal varices may be visualized as small anechoic tubular or rounded structures filling with color on CDFI. However, direct visualization of esophageal varices is often difficult though their presence may be inferred by demonstrating thickening of esophageal wall, irregularity of lumen and variation of esophageal wall thickness with respiration.

3. Paraumbilical vein—This runs in the ligamentum teres in the left lobe of liver and when recanalized is easily visible as a channel greater than 3 mm in diameter (Fig. 20.9). Recanalization of umbilical vein is a highly specific sign of portal hypertension. Hepatofugal flow on color Doppler is virtually pathognomic of portal hypertension. It may be followed distally along the abdominal wall towards the umbilicus.
4. Splenorenal shunts are tortuous, inferiorly directed vessels located between the spleen and upper pole of left kidney, accompanied by left renal vein enlargement (Fig. 20.10).

Paraumbilical and splenorenal collaterals decrease the risk of GI bleed. However, the risk of hepatic encephalopathy is increased.

5. Occasionally, collaterals may be seen within the gallbladder wall, and these are usually prominent in extrahepatic portal obstruction. Other collaterals that have been described include splenoretroperitoneal, splenocaval, omphaloiliocaval and splenoportal.

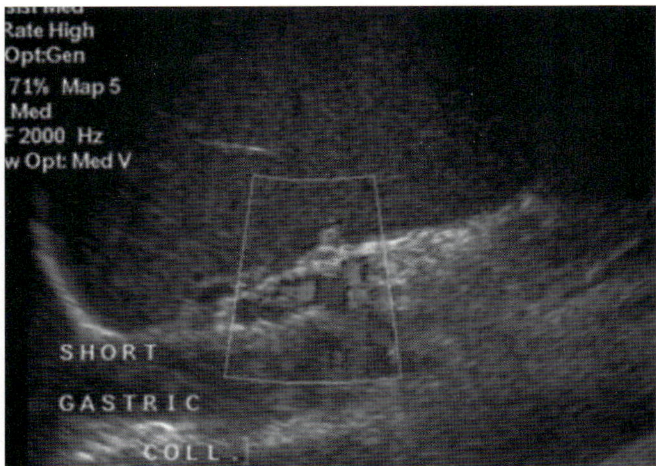

Fig. 20.8: Collateral vessels between upper pole of spleen and stomach consistent with short gastric collaterals *(For color version see plate 4)*

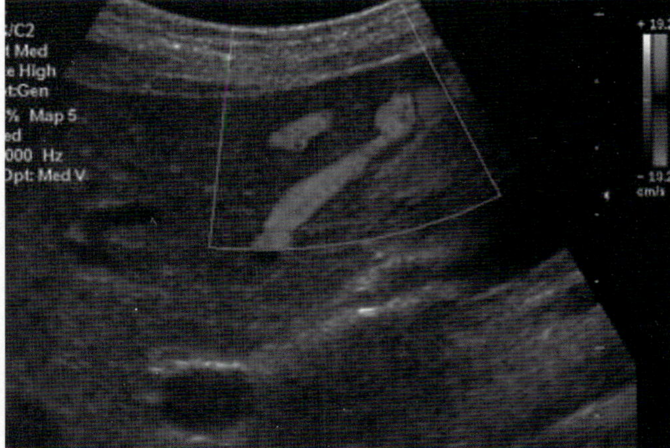

Fig. 20.9: Color Doppler study showing a paraumbilical collateral running in the ligamentum teres to the hepatic surface with hepatofugal flow *(For color version see plate 4)*

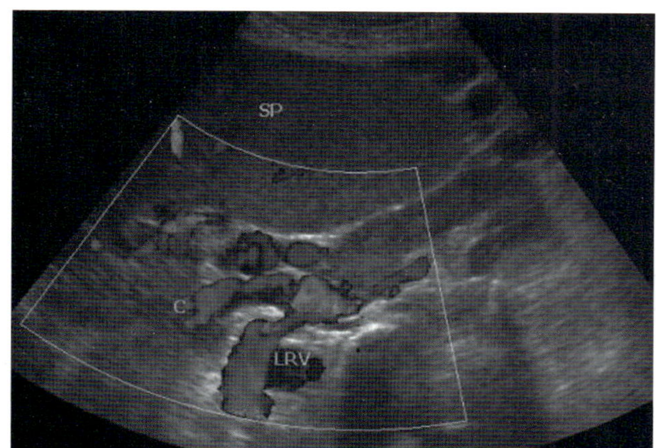

Fig. 20.10: CDFI showing a large lienorenal collateral draining into an enlarged renal vein *(For color version see plate 4)*

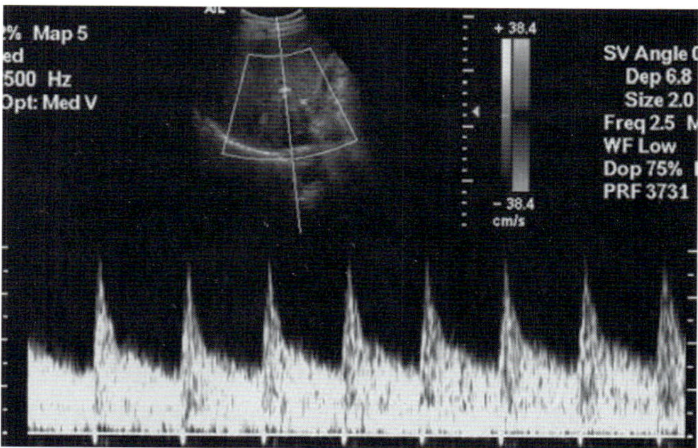

Fig. 20.12: Spectral Doppler trace from a normal hepatic artery *(For color version see plate 5)*

Assessment of Hepatic Veins

The hepatic veins (usually three in number) are thin-walled structures enclosed by hepatic parenchyma. They drain into the inferior vena cava immediately inferior to the diaphragm. Doppler spectral traces from normal hepatic veins have a triphasic appearance (Figs 20.11A and B) consisting of two large antegrade waves that represent atrial and ventricular diastole and a small retrograde wave that occurs in atrial systole.[30] Antegrade flow direction is defined as towards the heart and retrograde as away from the heart. Flow patterns in the hepatic veins depend on both cardiac physiology and liver histology. Altered hepatic vein waveforms are seen in at least 50% of patients with cirrhosis with flattening of the phasic oscillations. Similar changes are also found in Budd-Chiari syndrome.[30]

Arterial Evaluation

The normal hepatic artery (HA) supplies only about 25 to 30% of blood to the liver. It lies anterior to the portal vein and measures about 4.6 mm. In a fasting patient, HA has a systolic velocity of approximately 30 to 40 cm/sec and diastolic velocity of 10-15 cm/sec (Fig. 20.12). Hepatic artery diastolic velocity normally is less than the peak portal vein velocity of about 18 cm/sec. If the Doppler study shows hepatic arterial diastolic velocities greater than the portal vein, one should suspect parenchymal disease in the liver. Measurements of the right hepatic artery are taken where it crosses the portal vein near the porta hepatis. The resistive index of the hepatic artery in a fasting subject varies from 0.55 to 0.81 (mean 0.62-0.74) RI increases in normal subjects after a meal.[31,32] The pulsatility index (PI) of the hepatic artery varies from 1.16 to 1.24 in normal subjects.

The RI and PI of the hepatic artery are increased in chronic liver disease due to an increase in intrahepatic vascular resistance. The most commonly used measurement is the hepatic artery RI which is an indirect estimation of the impedence of arterial flow into the liver. In patients with advanced hepatic cirrhosis and chronic hepatitis the normal increase in RI after a meal is also absent. The

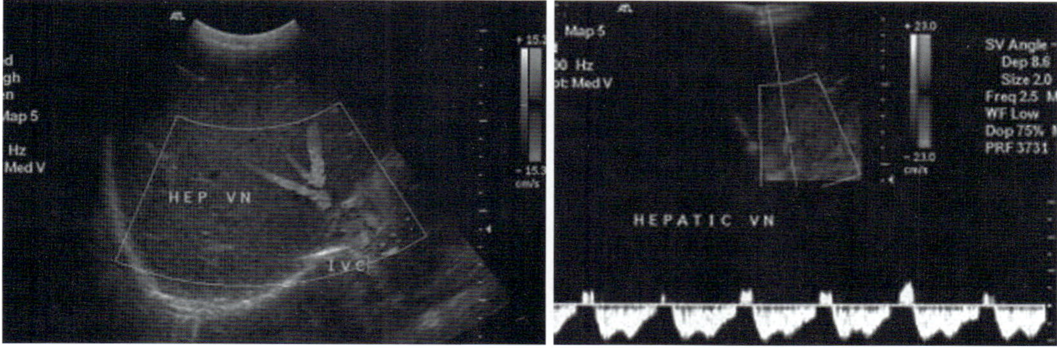

Fig. 20.11: CDFI study showing the normal hepatic veins with the triphasic flow pattern *(For color version see plate 5)*

hepatic artery RI falls steadily following acute portal vein thrombosis.[30]

Impedance changes in the superior mesenteric artery (SMA) and splenic artery have also been studied. SMA is measured 2 cm distal to its origin. The PI of the SMA is significantly reduced in cirrhosis and acute hepatitis but not in portal vein thrombosis, also the normal postprandial decrease in SMA resistive index is generally absent in cirrhosis.[30] Doppler impedance indices measured in the intraparenchymal branches of splenic artery were found to be increased in patients with cirrhosis.

Although ultrasound cannot directly measure portal pressure an 'indirect' assessment can be made using the '*congestive index*' which correlates with portal pressure or more strictly with portal resistance. The congestion index is the ratio between the cross-sectional area and the mean flow velocity of the portal trunk. It takes into account the fact that in portal hypertension, the portal vein tends to dilate and blood velocity to decrease, so that higher values are found in patients with more severe portal resistance, pressure and larger varices. Congestive index above 0.13 cm/sec has 67% sensitivity in predicting portal hypertension.[12]

The *Liver Vascular Index (LVI = PVVel/ Hepatic Artery PI)* aids in the diagnosis of cirrhosis and portal hypertension. A liver vascular index less than 12 cm/sec identified cirrhosis and portal hypertension with a specificity of 97% and a sensitivity of 93%.[30] Other indices described include *hepatic buffer index (HBI)* and *portal hypertension index*. However, according to some authors, hemodynamics of the PV is unrelated to degree of endoscopic abnormalities in patients with liver cirrhosis. Endoscopic findings followed by left gastric vein hemodynamics appear to be superior to those of the PV in predicting variceal bleed. The diameter and blood flow velocity of the LGV being significantly higher in the group with esophageal varies.[33]

On CT, the splenoportal axis is best visualized on portal phase images. Measurement of the diameter and length of the main portal vein can be performed on 2D multiplanar reconstructions and axial images.[23] Variceal collaterals are demonstrated as hyperdense structures that are easily distinguished from other nonvascular structures. Most varices are convoluted and their detailed course may be better visualized on CT than CDFI. Retroperitoneal and mesenteric collaterals may also be better visualized on CT than CDFI due to lack of interference by bowel gas or ascites. In a recent study, no statistically significant difference between CT-MIP and conventional angiography was apparent in the detection rates of gastric varices and their inflowing and outflowing vessels. 3D CT portography can depict portosystemic collaterals larger than approximately 3 mm in diameter. 3D vascular reconstructions both MIP and VRT can also augment the surgeon's perception of potentially problematic varices by detecting the course of these tortuous vessels (Fig. 20.13). However, direction of flow, flow velocity and volume flow cannot be ascertained.[13,14,34]

Both SE and gradient echo *MR images* can show collaterals well—as a signal void or flow-related enhancement respectively. Direct sagittal images are useful in the assessment of paraumbilical veins and coronal images are useful for mesenteric and splenorenal varices. Administration of gadolinium enhances detection of varices[35] (Fig. 20.14).

Portosystemic collaterals and their complex course is well-depicted on 3D MIP images generated by *CE-MR portography*. CE MRA can be combined with PC techniques to determine direction and volume of portal flow. A single 5 to 10 mm thick 2D phase contrast image is acquired in an oblique plane perpendicular to the portal vein. On the 2D phase contrast images, background tissues are grey while flow perpendicular to the image plane is bright in one direction and black in the other. Dynamic flow evaluation can also be done using the direct bolus imaging (DBI) method. This allows immediate visualization of fluid movement thereby enabling calculation of flow velocity from fluid movement. This method involves a bolus

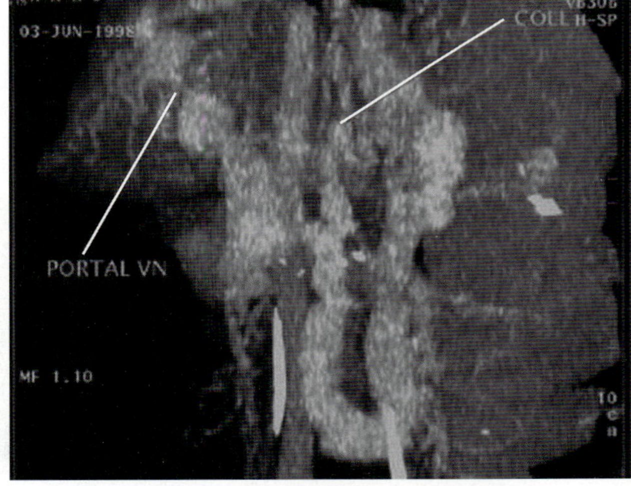

Fig. 20.13: CT portography MIP image showing attenuation of the MPV due to partial thrombosis with multiple collaterals, a tortuous splenic vein and massive splenomegaly

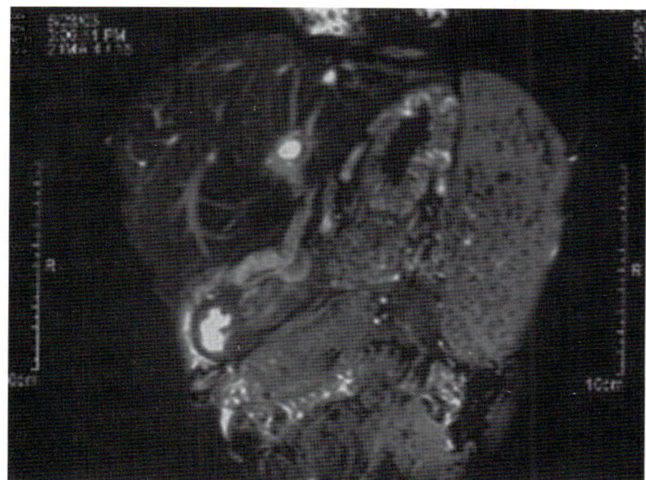

Fig. 20.14: Coronal GRE MR image showing a prominent coronary collateral with varices within the gastric wall seen as flow-related enhancement

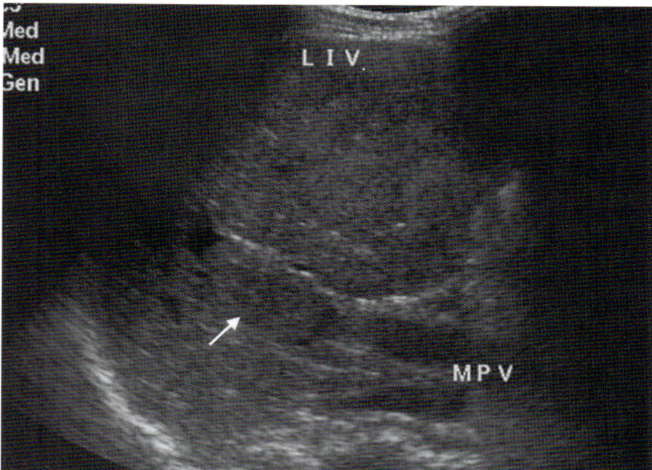

Fig. 20.15: Grey scale ultrasound showing a moderately echogenic thrombus occluding the right branch of PV (arrow)

tagging phase and a read out phase.[36] The values correlate well with duplex sonography. However, flow evaluation by MRI is more time consuming and rarely needed.

Extrahepatic Portal Hypertension: Prehepatic

Portal Vein Occlusion

Portal vein occlusion may be caused by thrombosis, tumor invasion or compression. There are several patterns of portal vein occlusion including main stem embolization, branch embolization, cast-like embolization, and partial obstruction. Thrombosis may be precipitated by stagnant portal flow in patients with cirrhosis. Other causes include infections such as neonatal/umbilical sepsis, intraperitoneal inflammatory processes such as pancreatitis and appendicitis hypercoagulable states and surgery.[12]

Tumour invasion of the portal vein occurs most commonly with hepatocellular carcinoma and pancreatic carcinoma. Malignancy may also result in portal vein thrombosis due to a hypercoagulable state or post-radiotherapy.

In children, extrahepatic portal vein occlusion (EHPO) is the most common cause of portal hypertension. The most common etiologic factor for portal vein thrombosis in children was found to be infection (approx. 50%).[37,38] Often, EHPO may be idiopathic.[39] Portal vein occlusion is usually permanent but recanalization may occur in some cases of thrombosis. Portal flow may be re-established via cavernous transformation of the portal vein.

Sonographic manifestations of acute portal vein occlusion include failure to visualize the portal vein and detection of echogenic intraluminal material (Fig. 20.15).

The normal portal vein is seen in 97% of upper abdominal sonograms. Therefore, when a normal appearing portal vein is not readily seen, one should consider portal vein occlusion. Occluding thrombus or tumour is generally low or moderate in echogenicity, however, recently formed thrombus may be almost anechoic and may be overlooked on grey scale examination alone (Fig. 20.16). On color Doppler examination, color fill may be absent in an occluded segment or a trickle of flow may be seen around the thrombus. The occluding thrombus frequently dilates the main portal vein and its branches noticeably.[12]

If portal vein thrombosis persists without substantial lysis, the portal vein undergoes fibrosis and may be

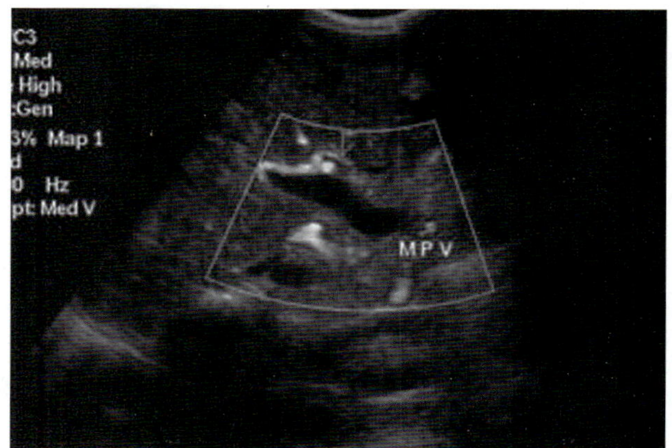

Fig. 20.16: Power Doppler study showing absence of color fill in the main portal vein due to anechoic thrombus *(For color version see plate 5)*

invisible sonographically. *Cavernous transformation* is the principle manifestation of chronic portal vein thrombosis producing a tangle of tortuous vessels in the porta hepatis. This appears 6 to 20 days after acute occlusion.[12] These channels demonstrate venous flow on CDFI (Fig. 20.17). Occassionally, a prominent collateral channel may mimic the main portal vein. Because the normal portal vein lies immediately posterior to the HA, when a venous structure thought to be the main PV lies anterior to the HA one should conclude that a variceal channel is present and the PV is occluded.[28]

A secondary sign of chronic portal vein occlusion is the development of portosystemic collaterals. These are mostly similar to those developing in intrahepatic portal hypertension. In addition, intrahepatic collaterals may develop connecting one portal segment with another (Fig. 20.18). Collaterals in the gallbladder wall are also more prominent in EHPO (Fig. 20.19). Partial trans-splenic shunting of venous blood due to flow reversal within intrasplenic tributaries of splenic vein draining to perisplenic surface collaterals has been reported in patients with portal cavernoma and also in cirrhosis.[12,38-41]

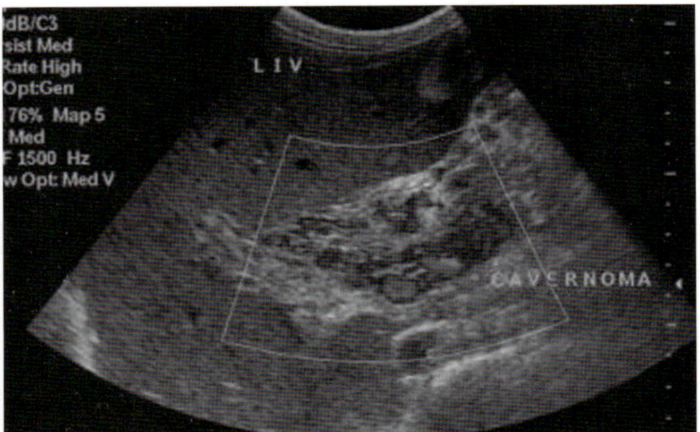

Fig. 20.17: Colour Doppler showing absence of MPV with a tangle of vessels at the porta hepatis suggestive of cavernous transformation *(For color version see plate 5)*

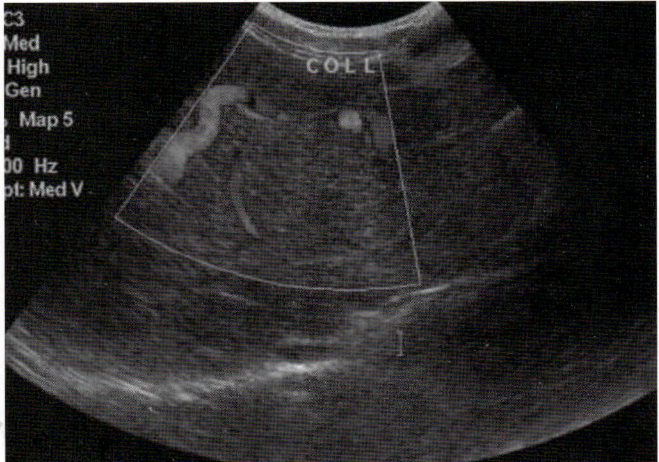

Fig. 20.18: Tortuous intrahepatic collateral coursing from the right to the left lobe in a patient of EHPO *(For color version see plate 5)*

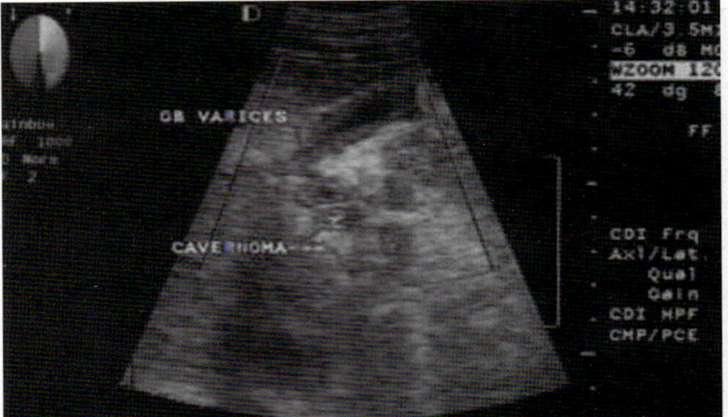

Fig. 20.19: Gallbladder varices in a case of EHPO seen as multiple rounded/tubular structures filling with color on CDFI *(For color version see plate 6)*

The ultrasonographic diagnosis of portal vein occlusion is highly accurate (sensitivity 89-100% and specificity 96-100%). However, certain pitfalls are noteworthy. Firstly, recently formed thrombus is anechoic and may remain undetected. Also, patients with portal hypertension may have low velocity flow or to and fro portal flow which may not be detected by Doppler unless appropriate settings for low flow/power Doppler is used. Thirdly, an inadequate Doppler angle may also preclude detection of portal flow.[12] While a complete thrombosis of the PV is easily diagnosed by color Doppler, a partial non-occluding thrombus especially in a branch vessel may be more apparent on CT or MR.

On helical CT or multislice scanner, a thrombus is best seen during portal phase appearing as a low attenuation defect or lack of enhancement of the portal vein (Fig. 20.20). Image-based evidence as to when the changes in hemodynamics begin to develop in portal vein occlusion are seen on CT arterioportography and CT hepatic arteriography. Liver parenchyma shows dense staining at the blocked site. Other features are a transient attenuation difference, segmental staining and retrograde portal branch filling, due to a relative increase in hepatic arterial flow which compensates for the decrease in portal blood flow. With chronic thrombosis, cavernous transformation of the portal vein occurs with multiple tortuous venous channels enhancing during the portal phase (Fig. 20.21). These are seen at the porta and in the region of portal confluence where they may be mistaken for

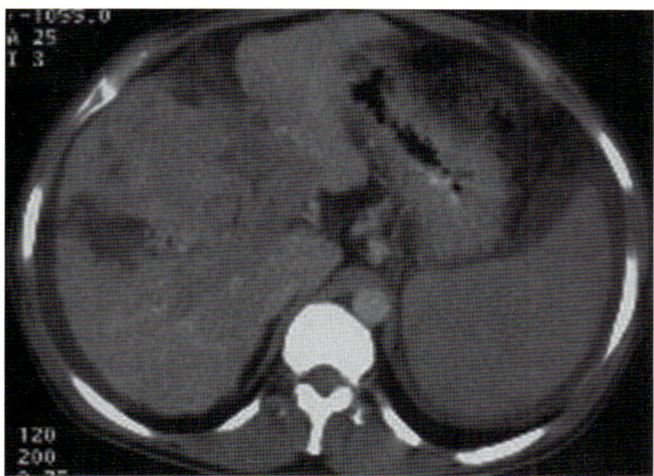

Fig. 20.20: Portal phase CECT of a patient with hepatocellular carcinoma showing enlargement and lack of enhancement of the portal vein branches due to tumor thrombus

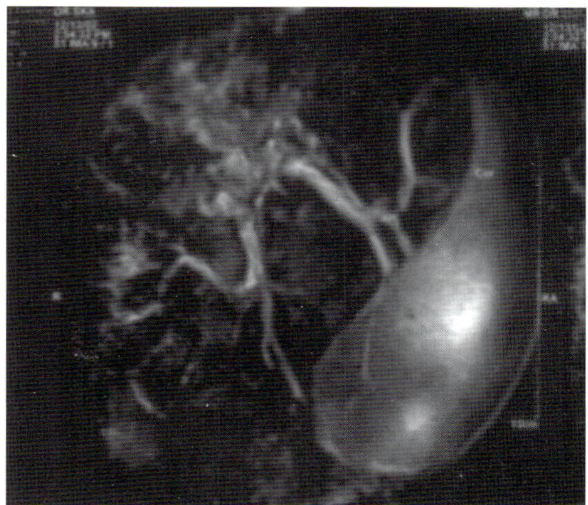

Fig. 20.22: MR portography showing replacement of the entire main portal vein by a tangle of tortuous vessel due to cavernoma formation. The splenic and superior mesenteric veins are normal

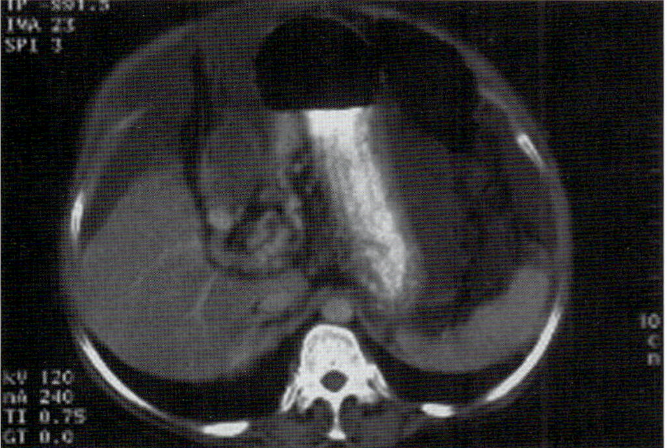

Fig. 20.21: Helical CT showing multiple tortuous channels replacing the main portal vein. Ascites is also noted in this patient

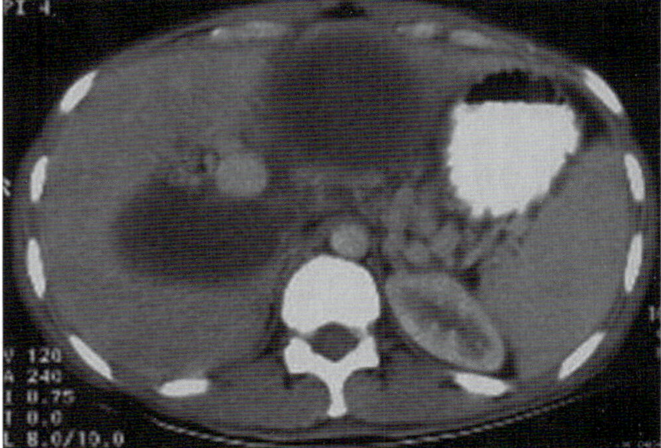

Fig. 20.23: Contrast enhanced axial CT in a follow-up case of acute pancreatitis showing multiple pseudocysts. Note that the splenic vein is replaced by multiple collaterals channels consequent to splenic vein thrombosis

a pancreatic mass on unenhanced or nondynamic scans.[20.23]

Thrombus can also be detected on routine *MR images* as a hypointense filling defect on gradient echo and as a hyperintensity on SE images. Portal vein thrombosis and cavernous transformation are easily recognized on portal phase images of MRA (Fig. 20.22).[17,23] In a recent study, MR portography was found to be slightly superior to CDFI in detecting parial thrombosis and occlusion in the main portal vein. [20]

Spleinic Vein Occlusion

Occlusion of one of the tributaries of the main portal vein like the splenic superior mesenteric or inferior mesenteric vein produces hypertension in the region of proximal venous drainage, sometimes referred to as regional portal hypertension (Fig. 20.23). The most common causes of splenic vein occlusion are pancreatitis and pancreatic carcinoma. Other less common causes include idiopathic thrombosis, retroperitoneal hematoma or tumor and hematological disorders.

The predominant collateral venous pathways that develop, i.e. short gastric and gastroepiploic veins return blood to the patient PV. Because short gastric collaterals feed the fundus and blood can be drained from the fundus by LGV to PV gastric varices are far more pronounced than esophageal varices. Blood flow in the LGV and PV remain hepatopedal.[42]

SMV Occlusion

Regional portal hypertension from SMV occlusion results in gastroepiploic and peripancreatic venous collaterals which return blood to the portal or splenic vein. Blood flow in the portal vein remains hepatopedal.[42]

Extrahepatic Portal Hypertension: Posthepatic

Posthepatic causes of portal hypertension include hepatic, vein or inferior vena caval obstruction or elevated caval and hepatic venous pressure caused by congestive heart failure or constrictive pericarditis. This is discussed in detail in chapter 22.

Hyperkinetic Portal Hypertension[6]

Hyperkinetic portal hypertension is usually caused by an intrahepatic or extrahepatic arterioportal fistula. The cause of the fistula may be traumatic, congenital, atherosclerotic or idiopathic. While CDFI may show the fistula in some cases with arterialization of portal vein flow, arterioportal fistulas are best evaluated by selective arteriography.

MEDICAL TREATMENT FOLLOW-UP

Doppler flowmetry is an excellent non-invasive technique to evaluate the effect of medical treatment such as beta blockers and vasopressin. Following treatment a reduction in portal flow and azygos vein flow has been reported.[29]

Evaluation of Surgical Portosystemic Shunts and Tips

A variety of surgical portosystemic shunts have been described in literature including portocaval, mesoatrial, proximal and distal splenorenal (the Warren shunt) and meso-caval shunt. Stenosis and thrombosis can occur at the level of shunt anastomosis. Assessment of shunt patency can be made by ultrasonography in about 75% cases and CDFI should be considered the primary modality for evaluating shunt patency. However, it can sometimes be difficult to visualize a shunt because of deep location or interference by abdominal gas.[29]

Provided preoperative baseline studies have been performed, it is possible within certain limits to assess flow through the shunt and to gauge changes in portal perfusion. A turbulent high speed flow towards the systemic circulation can be detected within the shunt itself. In some cases, this may show a phasic profile in response to variations in caval pressure.[29,30]

Indirect signs of shunt patency may be used when the shunt itself is not displayed. In portocaval shunts, a decrease in caliber of portal vein compared to preoperative value, widening of the IVC above the level of anastomosis, presence of hepatofugal flow in the intrahepatic portal branches is a reliable indicator of shunt patency. However, this may not be apparent in the immediate postoperative period. In patent, end-to-side portocaval anastomosis flow may be absent in intrahepatic portal vein branches. With distal splenorenal (Warren) shunts, a dilated left renal vein and phasic flow in the splenic vein synchronous with caval pulsatility is consistent with patent shunt. These shunts decompress the gastroesophageal varices while maintaining hepatopedal flow in the mesoportal venous bed in order to reduce incidence of hepatic encephalopathy.

Demonstration of flow reversal in the splenic and sometimes portal vein is proof of patency of conventional splenorenal shunts. Reversed flow in the superior mesenteric vein indicates patent mesocaval shunt.

All the above parameters are only valid if adequate preoperative measurements have been obtained for comparison.[29]

Transjugular Intrahepatic Portosystemic Shunt (TIPS)

Today TIPS is the treatment of choice in patients with portal hypertension when conventional endoscopic techniques fail to control gastrointestinal bleeding from portosystemic collaterals. TIPS is usually placed between right hepatic vein and right portal vein.

Blood flow in TIPS is easily confirmed with color Doppler. Spectral Doppler should be used to verify that the direction of flow in the shunt is from the portal vein to the hepatic vein. The first evaluation is usually done within 24 hours after shunt placement to establish baseline velocities within the portal vein, hepatic vein and shunt. Follow up studies are usually performed at 3-month intervals. Flow velocities in the shunt can vary widely ranging from 50 to 270 cm/s in the midportion. The mean velocity has been reported as 95 cm/sec near the portal vein and 120 cm/sec in the midportion. Flow in the main portal vein is hepatopedal with a velocity of 20-50 cm/sec. Stenosis of TIPS can be suspected when the peak shunt velocity is below 50 cm/sec, if there is an increase or decrease in shunt velocity greater than 50 cm/sec compared with initial post-procedure values, when portal vein velocity is lower than post-procedure levels and falls below 30 cm/sec, and when there is hepatofugal flow in the main portal vein.[30]

3D CT angiography is also promising as a screening modality for detecting TIPS stenosis or occlusion.[43] It is also extremely useful for evaluating surgical portosystemic shunts, especially where CDFI is equivocal due to interference by bowel gas, ascites or obesity by providing excellent 3D depiction of the entire portal venous system and the surgical shunt.

Surgically created portosystemic shunts can also be well-evaluated by *MR* portography. In a recent study, MR portography was able to demonstrate the patency of all surgical splenorenal and mesocaval shunts.[20] However, TIPS is difficult to assess as most often stainless steel Wall stents are used to bridge the portal and systemic venous system. Even with TE < 0.1 ms, the lumen of this metal stent cannot be evaluated by MRA.[22]

Evaluation of portal hypertension is complex and complete evaluation may require more than a single diagnostic investigation and an in-depth knowledge of hepatic hemodynamics. CDFI remains the most widely available and comprehensive diagnostic modality. However, CT and MR portography are being increasingly used and have an important role to play in problematic cases and in the preoperative workup of patients. Importantly, the role of the radiologist has now expanded beyond diagnosis to interventions in portal hypertension.

REFERENCES

1. La Mont JT, Koff RS, Isselbacher KJ. Cirrhosis. In Petersdorf, Adams, Braunwald, Isselbacher Martin, Wilson (Eds) Harrisons Principles of Medicine 10th ed. Tata McGraw Hill, 1983.
2. Boyer Thomas D. Portal hypertension and its complication. In Zakim and Boyer (Eds). WB Saunders Company. 1982;466.
3. Dick R, Watkinson A, Olliff JFC. Liver and spleen: In David Sutton (Ed). Textbook of Radiology and Imaging 7th ed. Churchill Livingstone.
4. Sherlock S, Dooley J. The portal venous system and portal hypertension. In Sheila Sherlock and James Dooley (Eds). 11th ed. 2002.
5. Mc Indoe AH. Vascular lesions of portal cirrhosis. Arch Path 1928;5:23.
6. Freeny PC, Itai Y. Portal venous system. In Margulis and Burhenne's (Eds): Alimentary Tract Radiology 5th ed, 1994.
7. Koshy A, Bhasin DK, Kapoor KK. Bleeding in extrahepatic portal vein obstruction. Ind J Gastro enterol 1983;3.
8. Nandy S. Background. In Nandy S, Tandon BN (Eds). Portal Hypertension in India, New Delhi: Raigarh Clinical Liver Research Unit 1978;18.
9. Dhiman RK, Chawla Y, Vashishta RK et al. Non-cirrhotic portal fibrosis (idiopathic portal hypertension). Experience with 151 patients and a review of the literature. Journal of Gastroenterology and Hepatology, 2002; 17:6-16.
10. Sama SK, Bhargava S, Gopi Nath N, et al. Non-cirrhotic portal fibrosis. Am J Med 1971;51:160-69.
11. Sarin SK, Sachdev G, Nanda R. Follow-up of patients with cirrhosis, non-cirrhotic portal fibrosis and extrahepatic obstruction. Ann Surg 1986;204:76-82.
12. Zwiebel WJ. Vascular disorders of the liver. In Zwiebel (Ed): Introduction to Vascular Ultrasonography 4th ed. WB Saunders Company, 2000.
13. Sheth S, Horton KM, Fishman EK. Vascular sequelae of cirrhosis: Evaluation with dual phase helical CT. Abdom Imaging 2002;27:720-27.
14. Henseler KP, Pozniack MA, Lee FT, et al. Three-dimensional CT angiography of spontaneous porto-systemic shunts. Radiographics 2001;21:691-704.
15. Ishikawa T, Ushiki T, Mizuno K, et al. CT maximum intensity projection is a clinically useful modality for the detection of gastric varices. World J Gastroenterol 2005;21;11(47):7515-19.
16. M Jain and Agarwal A. Multidetector CT portal venography in evaluation of portosystemic collateral vessels. Journal of Medical Imaging and Radiation Oncology 2008;52,4-9.
17. Bradley WG Jr., Waluch V. Blood flow. Magnetic resonance imaging. Radiology 1985:154:443.
18. Nghiem HV, Freeny PC, Winter TC III, et al. Phase contrast MR angiography of the portal venous system preoperative finding in liver transplant recipients. AJR 1994;163:445-50.
19. Waser MN, Geelkerken RH, Kouwenhoven M, et al. A systolically gated 3D phase contrast MRA of mesenteric arteries in suspected mesenteric ischemia. J Comput Assist Tomogr 1996;20:262-68.
20. Cakmak O, Elmas N, Tamsel S, et al. Role of contrast – enhanced 3D magnetic resonance portography in evaluation portal venous system compared with color Doppler Ultrasonography. Abdominal Imaging 2008; 33,65-71.
21. Liu H, Cao H and Wu ZY. Magnetic resonance angiography in the management of patients with portal hypertension. Hepatobiliary Pancreat Dis Int Vol 4 No. 2 2005;239-43.
22. Prince MR, Grist TM, Debatin JF. 3D contrast MR Angiography. Portal Vein 1999;123-34.
23. Merkle EM, Fleiter TR, Daniel TB. Hans Juergen Brambs: Liver: Normal anatomy imaging techniques and diffuse diseases. In Haaga JR, Kanzieri CF, Gilkeson RC (eds): CT and MR Imaging of the Whole Body 4th ed. Mosby, 2003.
24. Sarin SK. Progress report non-cirrhotic portal fibrosis. Gut 1989;30:406-15.

25. Sinha R. Grayscale and pulsed Doppler characteristics of non-cirrhotic portal fibrosis a preliminary report. Clin Radiol 1999;4(3):156-59.
26. Waguri N, Suda T, Kamura T, et al. Heterogeneous hepatic enhancement on CT angiography in idio-pathic portal hypertension. Liver 2002;22:276-80.
27. Arai K, Masui O, Kadoya M, et al. MR imaging in idiopathic portal hypertension. Journal of Computer Assisted Tomography 1991;15(3).
28. Baker EL, Kerlan RK Jr. In Gazelle Saini Mueller (Eds) Hepatobiliary and pancreatic radiology imaging and intervention. Imaging of Portal Hypertension, 1998.
29. Bolondi L, Gaiani S, Piscaglia F, et al. The portal venous system. In Meire H, Cosgrove D, Dewbury K, Farrant P (Eds): Abdominal and General Ultrasound 2nd ed. Churchill Livingstone, 2001.
30. Noguera AM, Montserrat E, Torrubia S, et al. Doppler in hepatic cirrhosis and chronic hepatitis. Seminars in Ultrasound CT and MRI 2002;23(1):19-36.
31. Iwao T, Toyanaga A, Oho K, et al. Value of Doppler ultrasound parameters of portal vein and hepatic artery in the diagnosis of cirrhosis and portal hypertension.
32. Paulson EK, Klicwer MA, Frederich MG, et al. Hepatic artery: Variability in measurement of resistive index and systolic acceleration time in healthy volunteers. Radiology 1996;200:725-29.
33. LI FH, HaO J, Xia JG et al. Hemodynamic analysis of esophageal varices in patients with liver cirrhosis using color Doppler ultrasound. World Journal of Gastroenterology: 2005;11(29):4560-65.
34. Matsumoto A, Kitamoto M, Imamura M, et al. Three-dimensional portography using multislice helical CT is clinically useful for management of gastric fundic varices. AJR 2001;176:899-905.
35. Danet IM, Sernellea RC, et al. MR imaging of diffuse liver disease. 2003;41(1):67-88.
36. Edelman RR, Zhao Bin, Liu C, et al. MR angiography and dynamic flow evaluation of portal venous system. AJR 1989;153:755-80.
37. Webb LJ, Sherlock S. The aetiology presentation and natural history of extrahepatic portal venous obstruction. QJ Med 1979;192:497-99.
38. Thompson EN, Sherlock S. The aetiology of portal vein thrombosis with particular reference to the role of infection and exchange transfusion. QJ Med 1964:132: 465-79.
39. Dilwari JB, Chawla YK. Extrahepatic portal venous obstruction—correspondence. Gut 1988;29:554-55.
40. Barakat M. Doppler sonographic findings in children with idiopathic portal vein cavernous deformity and variceal haemorrhage. Journal of Ultrasound in Medicine 2002;21(8):825-30.
41. Gaetano AN, Lafortune M, Patriquin H, et al. Cavernous transformation of the portal vein patterns of intrahepatic and splanchnic collateral circulation detected with Doppler sonography. AJR 1995;165:1151-55.
42. Kamee IR, Lawler LP, Cor L FM, Fishman EV. Patterns of collateral pathways in extrahepatic portal hypertension as demonstrated by multidetector row computed tomography and advanced image processing. J Comput Assist Tomogr 2004; 28, 469-77.
43. Chopra S, Dodd GD III, Chintapalli KN, et al. Transjugular intrahepatic portosystemic shunt accuracy of helical CT angiography in the detection of shunt abnormalities. Radiology 2000;215:115-22.

Chapter Twenty-one

Hepatic Venous Outflow Tract Obstruction

Naveen Kalra, Niranjan Khandelwal

INTRODUCTION

Hepatic venous outflow tract obstruction, Budd-Chiari syndrome (BCS), is a rare disorder of hepatic venous outflow obstruction which may involve the hepatic veins, inferior vena cava or both and is characterized by structural and functional abnormalities of the liver. The disease is more common in Northern India, South Africa and Japan as compared to the Western countries.

The clinical course of Budd-Chiari syndrome is determined by the degree of hepatic venous outflow obstruction and the rapidity with which it develops. Usually the clinical presentation of the syndrome is nonspecific. Large and sudden blockage of veins results in acute BCS, which is characterized by severe abdominal pain, ascites, jaundice, hepatomegaly and rapidly developing hepatic failure over a period of few days to few weeks. On the other hand, when there is insidious gradual venous outflow obstruction it leads to chronic BCS which is characterized by the development of portal hypertension, prominent abdominal veins, upper GI bleed, pedal edema, ascites and large nodular liver developing over a period of several months. Acute BCS is mostly reported from western countries, whereas cases of chronic BCS are reported mainly from Japan, China, South Africa and India. Differentiation of acute and chronic forms of the disease is important for determining the prognosis and planning the treatment. In patients with acute form, the prognosis is poor with high mortality if not treated, whereas chronic form is less ominous and 50% patients are alive after five years.[1]

The etiology of BCS also has geographical variation.[2] In Asian countries, the most common causes are web or membranous obstruction of the IVC (MOVC), pregnancy and infections, while in the West, primary myeloproliferative disorders, hypercoagulable states, steroidal contraceptives and tumors are responsible in majority of cases. Rarely, BCS may occur due to malignant thrombosis of the IVC or main hepatic veins secondary to hepatic, renal and adrenal neoplasms.[3] However, in 30-50% of patients etiology remains unidentified.[2] Hepatocellular carcinoma can produce an acute fulminant variant of BCS by causing obstruction of the main hepatic veins or inferior vena cava due to endoluminal invasion by the tumor.

DIAGNOSTIC TECHNIQUES

The recent advances in imaging techniques have enabled delineation of the exact vascular abnormalities and their treatment resulting in better and improved survival rates in patients of BCS. The available therapeutic options include medical treatment; radiological interventional methods like balloon angioplasty, stent placement, transjugular intrahepatic portosystemic shunt (TIPS) and surgical treatment which includes portosystemic shunts and liver transplantation. Imaging thus plays a crucial role in diagnosis and management. Till recently, IVC graphy, hepatic venography and liver biopsy alone or in combination were the definitive investigations available for anatomic and hemodynamic evaluation in patients of BCS, but these procedures are invasive and have risk of complications particularly in patients with coagulation abnormalities. Lately, several noninvasive imaging modalities-like ultrasound, CT and MRI are being increasingly used in the diagnosis of BCS as they can depict the hepatic vascular anatomy accurately without catheterization and thereby guide management decisions. The current chapter will discuss the role of these newer investigations in evaluating the hepatic veins, IVC and liver parenchyma in diagnosis of BCS and various interventional techniques used for treating this condition.

EVALUATION OF HEPATIC VEINS IN BCS

Real-time sonography is currently considered the investigation of choice for initial evaluation of BCS. The technique demonstrates the morphological hepatic changes as well as thrombosis or occlusion of hepatic veins or IVC. Simultaneously adjacent organs can also be assessed. The various findings depicted by routine ultrasound include hepatomegaly, heterogeneous liver and caudate lobe enlargement. In addition, findings that suggest hepatic vein thrombosis on US include non - visualization of confluence of hepatic veins with IVC, distorted or absent hepatic veins, stenosed hepatic veins with thick wall echoes (Fig. 21.1A), hyperechoic hepatic veins, portal vein thrombosis and ascites. Presence of comma shaped veno-venous intrahepatic collaterals is considered a very reliable sign of BCS (Fig. 21.1B).[4-9]

Liver is generally enlarged but may be normal in size or shrunken in advanced cases of chronic BCS. Right lobe may show atrophy with hypertrophy of the left lobe. Echotexture of liver is homogenously hypoechoic in acute BCS and heterogenous in chronic BCS. Surface of the liver may reveal fine nodularity due to cirrhotic changes. Caudate lobe enlargement is a common feature and a useful pointer towards the diagnosis, seen in 82-91% of the cases but is non-specific sign as it can be seen in cirrhosis due to other causes.[10]

Caudate lobe enlargement is explained by the fact that it has separate veins which are not affected by the thrombotic process and drain directly into the IVC just distal to the ostia of the main hepatic veins. Caudate lobe drainage thus serves as an outflow for intrahepatic venous collaterals. It has been reported that visualization of a caudate vein >3 mm in diameter strongly suggests the diagnosis of BCS is an appropriate clinical setting.[11] The overall accuracy of ultrasound for detecting hepatic venous thrombosis has been found to be 70-87% in the literature.[7,12]

The normal diameter of the right and middle hepatic veins is less than 10 mm while that of the left hepatic vein is less than 9 mm.[13] Though US has been extremely useful for evaluation of hepatic veins, it does not provide any information about blood flow in hepatic veins or IVC or portal vein. The technique has limitations in cases of

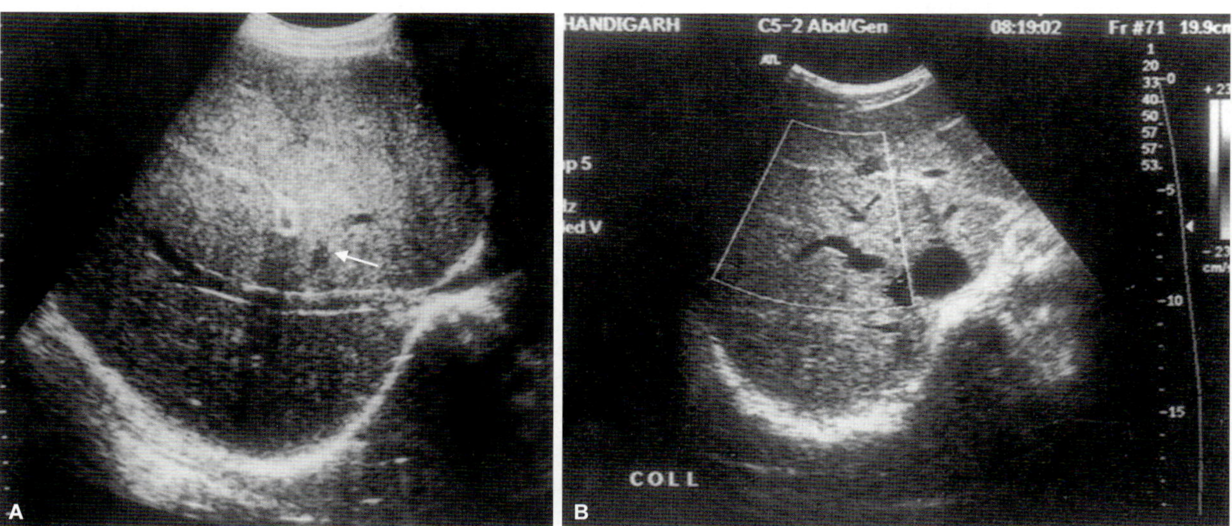

Figs 21.1A and B: Sagittal oblique ultrasound section shows echogenic walls of the RHV suggestive of thrombosed RHV. MHV and LHV are not visualized. A comma-shaped intrahepatic collateral is seen (arrow) (A), Transverse ultrasound section in another patient of BCS shows multiple comma-shaped intrahepatic collaterals, non-visualized hepatic veins and dilated IVC (B)

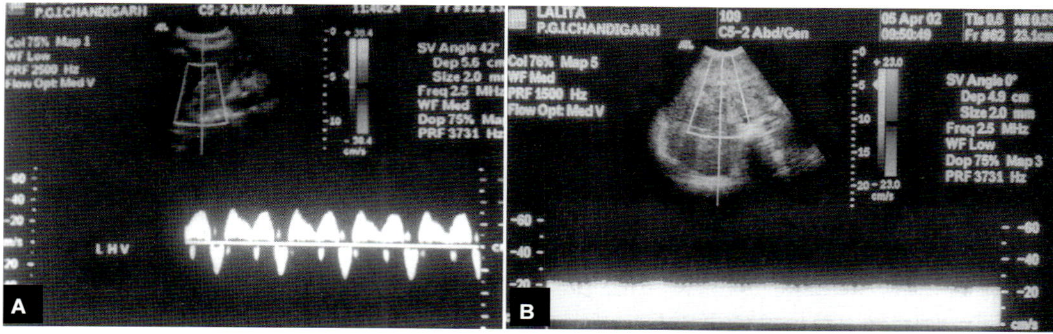

Figs 21.2A and B: Normal pulsed Doppler tracing in the left hepatic vein shows the triphasic waveform. The antegrade flow occurs during the ventricular systole and atrial diastole while retrograde flow occurs during the atrial systole (A), Color Doppler US with color box placed in the region of RHV and MHV in a patient of BCS shows no flow in RHV. MHV shows uniphasic flow (B)

swollen and nodular, or shrunken and scarred liver in which veins may be obscured within the hepatic parenchyma. Detection of intraluminal webs, thrombosis or membranes is also limited. Poor delineation of extrahepatic collaterals and possibility of an inadequate study due to bowel gas are other limiting factors.

Color flow duplex Doppler US combined with real-time imaging has increased the sensitivity and specificity of diagnosis of BCS as it allows better visualization of hepatic veins by automatically adding flow information. Doppler waveform of hepatic veins in healthy individuals is a triphasic waveform (two negative waves and one positive) (Fig. 21.2A).[14] Loss of the normal triphasic waveform is seen in BCS as well as in cirrhosis. Presence of flat waveform (uniphasic flow) without flutter or absent or reversed flow in hepatic veins are the most reliable signs of hepatic vein thrombosis (Fig. 21.2B). Veins that may be non-visualized on real-time ultrasound due to compression by hepatic nodules may reveal flow on color flow ultrasound and thus prove to be normal.[8] 3D ultrasound can also be used to show the entire morphology of the IVC and the hepatic veins.[13]

Recently MR has also been used for evaluation of hepatic veins.[15] MR has particular advantage of being able to show hepatic veins in three dimensions but its ability to determine the degree of flow is limited in the routine MR sequences. In our experience color flow Doppler US is superior to MR for evaluation of hepatic veins as the ostial narrowing can be better detected by US. The angiographic techniques used for delineation of the hepatic veins include IVC graphy with retrograde hepatic vein cannulation, percutaneous hepatography (injection of contrast in the hepatic parenchyma under fluoroscopy with serial filming to visualize the hepatic veins entering into IVC) (Fig. 21.3) and direct hepatic venography under US guidance. These techniques are the most definitive but are reserved for patients being considered for angioplasty or stent placement where exact delineation of the length of stenosed segment is mandatory for deciding the management. In BCS there is a collateral circulation between the tributaries of the hepatic veins which forms a 'spider web'. In the initial stage these collaterals are fine giving rise to a 'fine spider web'. With long standing BCS, these collaterals form a 'coarse spider web'.[16] Arteriography if performed in a patient with BCS would show larger diameter of the hepatic artery as compared to the splenic artery since the blood supply to the liver by the hepatic artery is increased.[17]

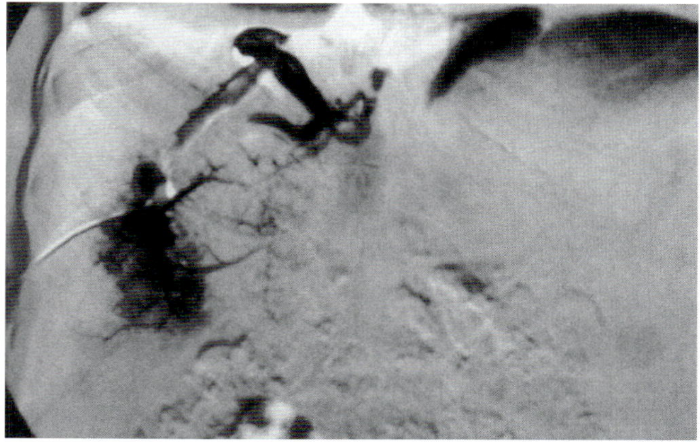

Fig. 21.3: Percutaneous hepatography shows non-opacification of the hepatic veins. There is filling up of multiple intrahepatic collaterals some of which have 'spider web' configuration

Scintigraphy and CT have also been used for diagnosis of BCS. Scintigraphy may reveal increased uptake by caudate lobe and left lobe, patchy uptake of radionuclide in the rest of the liver giving the appearance of hot spots. On CT, presence of enlarged caudate lobe with low attenuation areas elsewhere in the liver, atrophy of right lobe, non-visualization of hepatic veins and irregular surface of the liver may be seen. On CECT presence of patchy hepatogram, areas of linear, irregular or wedge-shaped hypoattenuation particularly in the peripheral portions of liver due to fibrosis and parenchymal destruction indicate hepatic venous thrombosis. Dynamic CT may demonstrate thrombus within the hepatic veins and comma shaped intrahepatic collaterals (Fig. 21. 4). Presence of areas of hypoattenuation surrounded by areas of increased enhancement can simulate presence of intrahepatic mass lesion. Although there is limited literature about the role of MDCT in BCS, the availability of volume imaging and 3D reconstructions will provide a useful adjunct to axial images in the near future.[17]

EVALUATION OF IVC IN BCS

Evaluation of IVC is an important and essential component of the imaging evaluation of a patient suspected to have BCS for two reasons. Firstly, IVC obstruction alone or in combination with hepatic vein obstruction may itself lead to BCS. Secondly, patency of IVC must be established before deciding upon the surgical procedure to be undertaken such as portocaval/ mesocaval shunt when IVC is patent and mesoatrial shunt when IVC is obstructed.

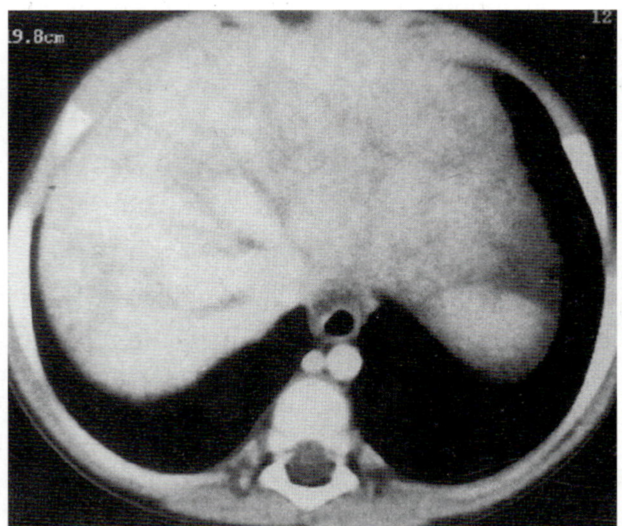

Fig. 21.4: CECT in a patient of BCS shows patchy hepatogram. The right hepatic vein and middle hepatic vein are thrombosed while the left hepatic vein is not visualized

Incidence of IVC obstruction in BCS varies from 33 - 56%.[18,19] IVC can be obstructed in its intrahepatic portion, suprahepatic portion or both. The causes of IVC obstruction are membranes, tumor thrombus and caudate lobe hypertrophy.[7,18,19] Suprahepatic obstruction is generally due to short segment stenosis or IVC webs. Intrahepatic IVC obstruction is most commonly due to compression from the enlarged caudate lobe. Chronic thrombosis of the IVC can evolve into calcification.[17]

Webs are visualized as dome shaped thin linear filling defects on contrast venography/MR angiography. On real-time imaging they appear as hyperreflective linear foci best seen in deep inspiration (Figs 21.5A to C). Whether these webs represent congenital lesions or they

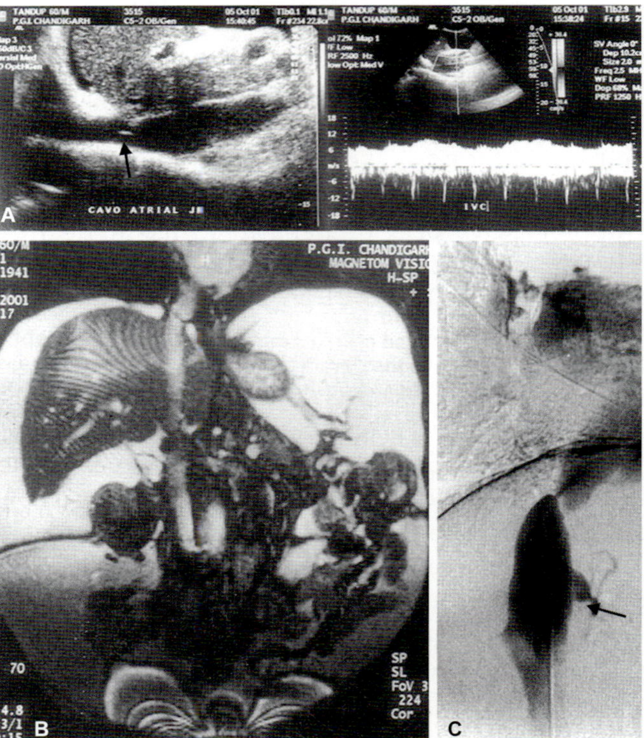

Figs 21.5A to C: A 60-year-old male presenting with abdominal distention. Sagittal US showing echogenic linear area in IVC proximal to cavo-atrial junction suggestive of a web in IVC (arrow). There is uniphasic flow with fluttering seen in the IVC (A), Coronal FLASH flow-sensitive MR image shows a hypodense linear signal in the IVC proximal to cavo-atrial junction suggestive of a web in the suprahepatic portion (B), IVC graphy lateral view shows dome shaped obstruction of suprahepatic IVC with a jet of blood flowing into right atrium confirming the presence of web. There is filling up of an intrahepatic collateral (arrow) (C)

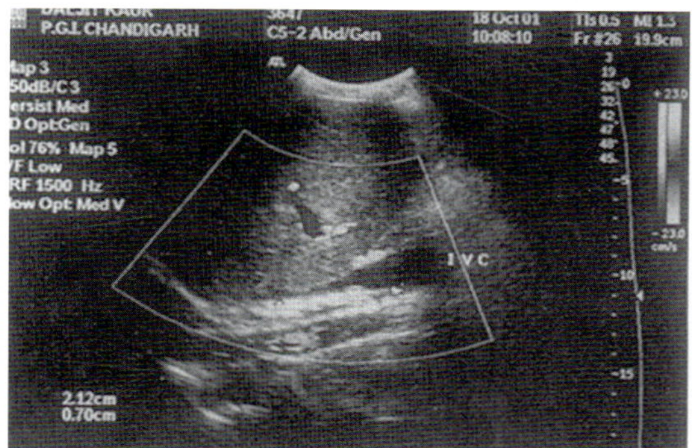
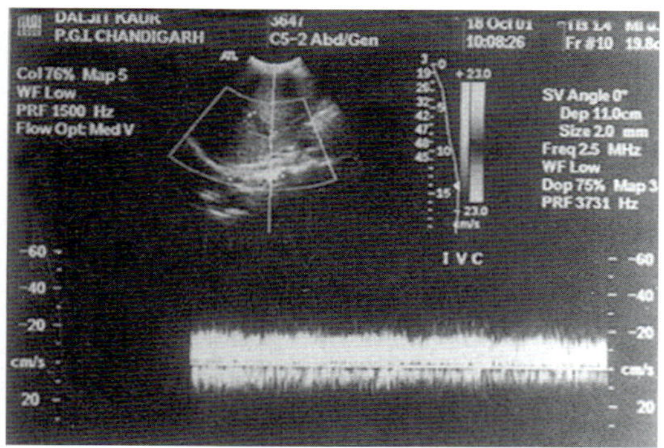

Fig. 21.6: Color Doppler shows a smooth long segment narrowing in the intrahepatic portion of IVC with loss of the normal phasic variation and a uniphasic flow pattern

are the result of thrombotic process is an issue which remains disputed.[20] It seems quite plausible to assume that both IVC web and segmental stenosis actually represent the spectrum of same pathological process, i.e. thrombosis.

On real-time ultrasound, short segment stenosis is seen as an area of narrowing and the caliber of IVC is dilated proximal to the obstruction with loss of phasic variation with respiration (Fig. 21.6). Long segment narrowing of the IVC due to caudate lobe enlargement is well depicted. When the IVC obstruction is due to tumor thrombi, extension of the tumor into the IVC is well demonstrated. However, ultrasound is unable to determine the length of stenosis, webs can be missed and the hemodynamic significance of IVC narrowing can not be assessed. Possibility of poor study due to bowel gas is also a limiting factor.

Color Doppler US combined with real-time imaging is superior to gray scale imaging as it provides better assessment of IVC impairment by adding flow information. The normal flow pattern of IVC is a triphasic waveform. The flow abnormality can be seen in the form of either absent (IVC occlusion), reversed or uniphasic flow (stenosis).[8,21] Turbulent flow may be seen at the site of short segment stenosis.[21,22]

IVC graphy has been considered the gold standard for evaluation of inferior vena cava. However, in patients of BCS, it has certain limitations particularly for evaluation of hepatic veins. Diagnosis of hepatic vein occlusion is inferred when there is failure to cannulate the hepatic veins selectively at the time of catheterization. Thus, overdiagnosis of hepatic vein thrombosis may result even when failure of cannulation is due to technical failure. The other limitations of IVC graphy include non-visualization of IVC distal to obstruction due to diversion of contrast into the collaterals. Thus, in case of suprahepatic obstruction due to web/membrane visualization of IVC above and below the lesion may require double catheter study. Lastly the intrahepatic collaterals which form important parameters for diagnosis of chronic BCS are not picked up with IVC graphy.

Recently MR venography has shown a great potential by overcoming many of the limitations of IVC graphy. MR venography accurately depicts the site and cause of IVC obstruction with clear delineation of IVC both above and below the obstruction (Fig. 21.7).[12,15]

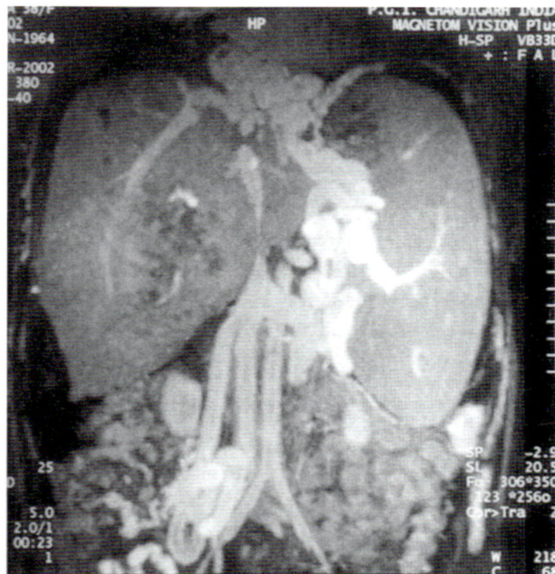

Fig. 21.7: Coronal contrast enhanced MR venography shows long segment narrowing of IVC in intrahepatic portion with filling defect proximal to cavoatrial junction. There are multiple collaterals in the retroperitoneum and at the splenic hilum

MR is excellent for detection of both intra- and extrahepatic collaterals, portal vein obstruction and detection of tumor thrombi within the IVC. Incidence of portal vein thrombosis in BCS is 5 - 20%. [21,22]

Five types of Collateral Pathways develop in Budd-Chiari syndrome[23]

i. Left renal- hemiazygous pathways
ii. Vertebrolumbar azygous pathways
iii. Intrahepatic collaterals
iv. Superificial abdominal wall collaterals
v. Inferior phrenic-pericardiophrenic collaterals. Intrahepatic collaterals have been noted in 80-93% cases of BCS [8,22,24] and are seen as comma shaped bridging veno-venous collaterals which reveal flat waveform on color Doppler ultrasound.

ASSESSMENT OF LIVER PARENCHYMA IN BCS

As a result of hepatic venous or IVC obstruction there is ischemic damage to the liver cells resulting in severe congestion, centrilobular necrosis followed by fibrosis and cirrhosis. In acute BCS, congestion predominates whereas patients of chronic BCS are more likely to develop cirrhosis and regenerative nodules.[19] Since the obstruction of the hepatic veins is usually asynchronous, liver biopsy may show areas of congestion and hyperplastic enlargement in the recently affected areas and fibrosis with atrophy in the older affected segments. As the distribution of the disease in the liver is inhomogeneous liver biopsy may even be normal.[25]

Development of regenerative nodules in BCS is known to occur in response to focal loss of portal perfusion and hyperarterialization in areas with preserved hepatic venous outflow.[17] Incidence of nodules greater than 5 mm have been seen on histology in 40-80% of patients.[22,26] Although the question of possible malignant transformation of the large regenerative nodule remains unsettled, it is generally believed that HCC is extremely rare in patients presenting with BCS due to hepatic venous obstruction alone. However, it may be co-existent in patients of BCS due to IVC obstruction particularly MOVC.[19] HCC in BCS accounts for 0.7% of all cases of hepatocelluar carcinoma.[27] Differentiation of HCC from regenerative nodules is important. US and conventional CT are both poor modalities for detection of these nodules. On the other hand MRI and biphasic CT have been reported to be more reliable. [3,28,29]

Benign regenerative nodules which are hyperintense on T1WI and iso- to hypointense on T2WI are likely to be benign (Figs 21.8 A and B) compared to HCC nodules which are hypointense on T1WI and hyperintense on T2WI (Figs 21.9 A and B). Multiple (>10) and small (< 4 cm) lesions are suggestive of benignity.[3] On biphasic CT large regenerative nodules are markedly and homogeneously hyperattenuating on arterial phase images and remain slightly hyperattenuating on portal venous phase images.[17,29] On histopathology these nodules have normal or hyperplastic hepatocytes, arteries extending radially from the center of the nodule and a central scar in the larger nodules.[26,30] The imaging characteristics of this scar may be similar to those of the

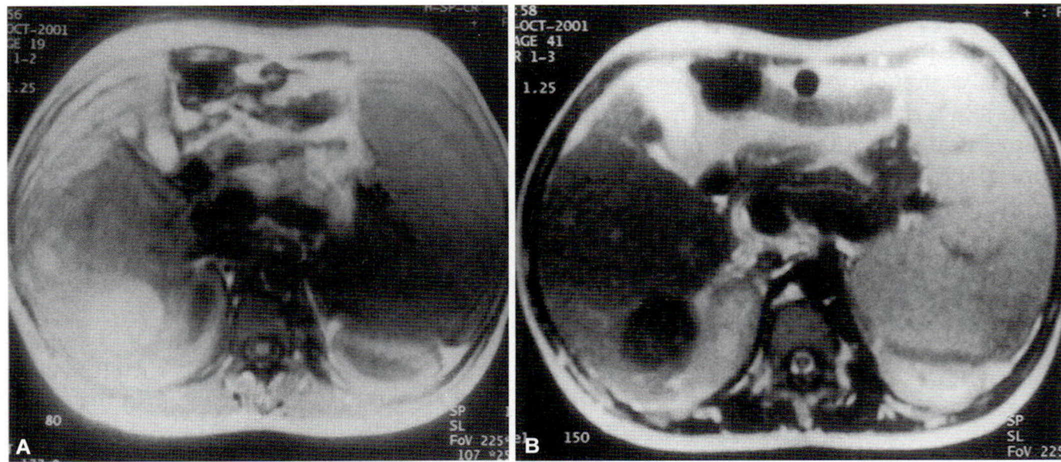

Figs 21.8A and B: Axial T1W flash image shows single large hyperintense nodule and multiple small hyperintense nodules of varying sizes in the liver. The hyperintensity of the nodules on T1WI is suggestive of their benign nature (A), Axial T2W HASTE image at the same level depicts the hypointense signal of the large nodule. Smaller lesions are not seen, probably due to being isointense to the liver parenchyma (B)

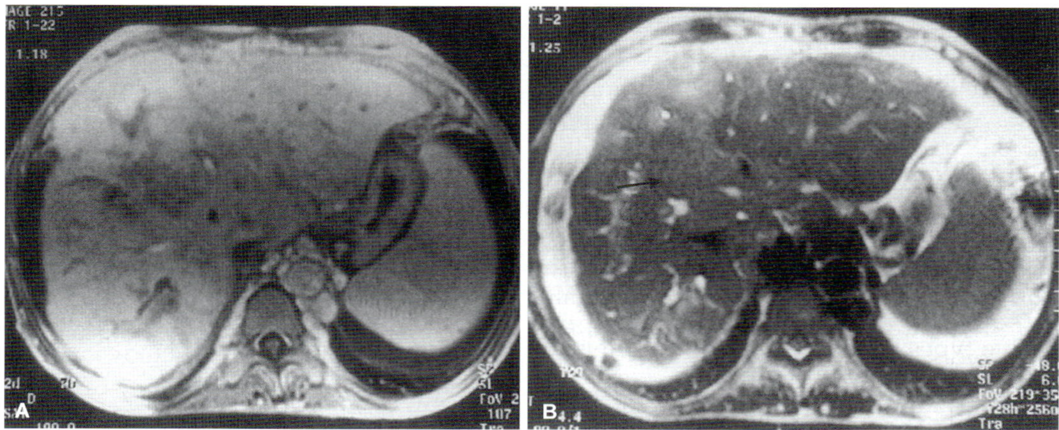

Figs 21.9A and B: Axial T1W FLASH MR image at the level of hepatic veins shows irregular outline of liver with multiple ill-defined hypointense focal lesions in the liver. Ascites is seen (A), Axial T2W HASTE image at the same level shows that the lesions are isointense to hyperintense in signal (arrow). FNAC proved these lesions to be HCC (B)

scar found in focal nodular hyperplasia on dynamic imaging.[26]

Liver biopsy has been used in the past to differentiate acute from subacute and chronic BCS. A liver biopsy is required only if radiological imaging is inconclusive.[31] Differentiation is important for deciding the plan of treatment. Acute BCS may be treated by infusion of thrombolytic substances at the site of block followed by stenting whereas, chronic BCS requires the creation of a shunt between the hepatic veins and portal vein by transjugular intrahepatic portosystemic shunt procedure. MRI and dynamic CT have shown potential to determine the chronicity of the hepatic changes.[12,32,33]

A study by Noone et al[12] has described the role of MRI in differentiation of acute, subacute and chronic BCS. In their experience in acute BCS there is decreased signal intensity on T1WI and heterogeneously increased signal intensity on T2WI peripherally with decreased enhancement of peripheral liver after gadolinium administration (Figs 21.10A to C). These changes were attributed to acutely increased tissue pressures and edema in the peripheral portions of the liver because of hepatic venous obstruction thus causing diminished inflow of blood. As the duration of disease increases there is reversal of flow in the portal vein and development of small collaterals permitting egress of blood. Thus in subacute BCS the signal characteristics on T1 and T2 - weighted images are similar to those observed in patients with acute disease, however, periphery shows marked heterogeneous enhancement unlike to that seen in acute

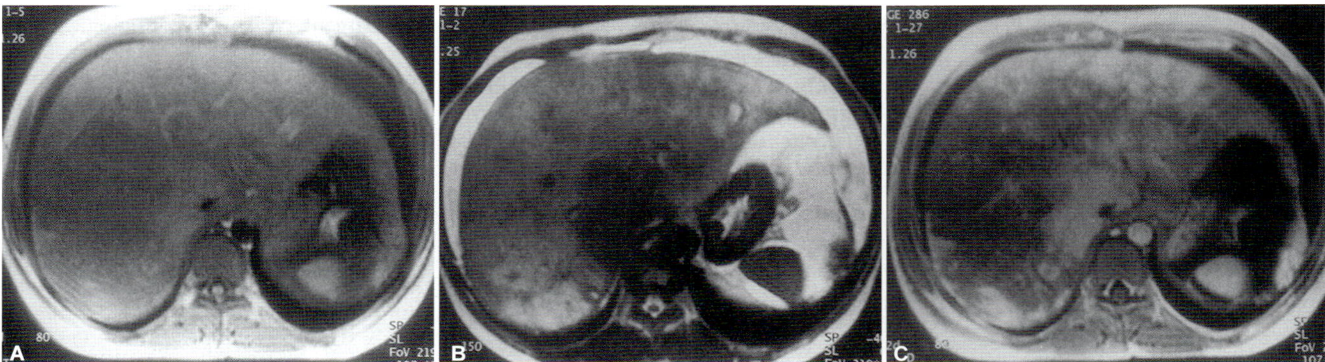

Figs 21.10A to C: Axial T1W FLASH sequence at a level caudal to the hepatic veins showing a differential signal intensity of the liver with hypointense signal in peripheral liver and hyperintense signal in central liver. Intrahepatic IVC shows narrowing (A), Axial T2W HASTE section at the same level shows hyperintense signal in the peripheral liver and hypointense signal in the central liver. Perihepatic fluid is also seen- findings suggestive of acute BCS (B), Axial post-contrast T1W image in the same patient shows diminished peripheral enhancement and marked patchy enhancement in the central liver. Biopsy confirmed acute BCS (C)

BCS. In chronic BCS there is no parenchymal edema and this stage is characterized by changes of fibrosis. Thus, there is no differential signal intensity and enhancement between peripheral and central liver. Using that criteria, in a study conducted at this institute 13/20 cases of chronic BCS were correctly diagnosed with MRI (Figs 21.11A and B).[34]

Abnormal patterns of parenchymal enhancement have also been reported on triphasic helical CT in different stages of BCS in a study by Camera et al.[33] They found abnormal enhancement of the caudate lobe in the arterial phase, the 'fan shaped pattern', in all cases of acute BCS. On the other hand 'patchy pattern' of enhancement was seen in patients of subacute and chronic BCS.

In conclusion, ultrasound with color flow Doppler imaging is the modality of choice for initial diagnosis of BCS. When combined with MR and MRA, need for diagnostic IVC graphy can be obviated which can be reserved for patients where surgical or radiological intervention is being contemplated. The role of dynamic helical CT in BCS appears promising and is presently under evaluation.

MANAGEMENT OF BCS

The treatment modality for BCS is determined by the status of hepatocyte necrosis and the stage of the disease.

Non-surgical management of BCS such as radiological intervention alone or in combination with medical management is indicated in patients, where biopsy shows no evidence of hepatocyte necrosis.

The medical management includes treatment for ascites by diuretics or paracentesis and control of gastrointestinal bleeding with balloon tamponade or sclerotherapy. Systemic thrombolytic therapy has been shown to have varying outcome. Treatment with heparin alone has been followed by recanalization of thrombosed hepatic veins and of thrombosed portal vein when associated with thrombosed hepatic veins.

Treatment of BCS by radiological intervention was first described in 1974 by Eguchi et al who reported the successful balloon membranotomy for obstruction of the inferior vena cava.[35] The aim of the radiological interventions is the restoration of hepatic blood outflow by means of repermeation of the obstructed hepatic veins or IVC or by portosystemic shunting. The methods include balloon angioplasty, stent insertion and TIPS (Transjugular Intrahepatic Portosystemic Shunt). Balloon angioplasty is used for short length stenosis of the hepatic veins. This results in immediate relief of the obstruction. However, the recurrence following this procedure is common. Griffith et al[36] in their study of 18 patients found that restenosis occurred in all patients treated with angioplasty when followed for longer than 10 months. The use of wall stents has resulted in better long-term patency rates of the order of 80-90% over a one year follow-up period (Figs 21.12A to F).[22,37,38] Baijjal et al[39] performed percutaneous angioplasty followed by primary stent placement in their study of 9 patients with IVC obstruction. There was residual stenosis of about 9-40% after the procedure. Revascularization was successful in all patients and the IVC remained patent during the follow-up period (3-31 months).

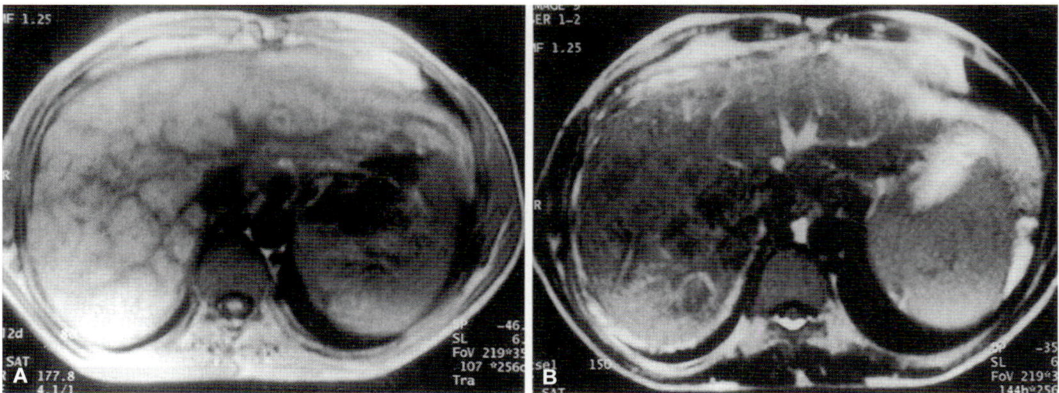

Figs 21.11A and B: Axial T1W FLASH and T2W HASTE MR images show uniformly heterogeneous signal intensity of the liver. There is no differential SI of the peripheral or central liver seen. Hepatic veins are not visualized — a case of chronic BCS due to hepatic vein thrombosis and IVC stenosis

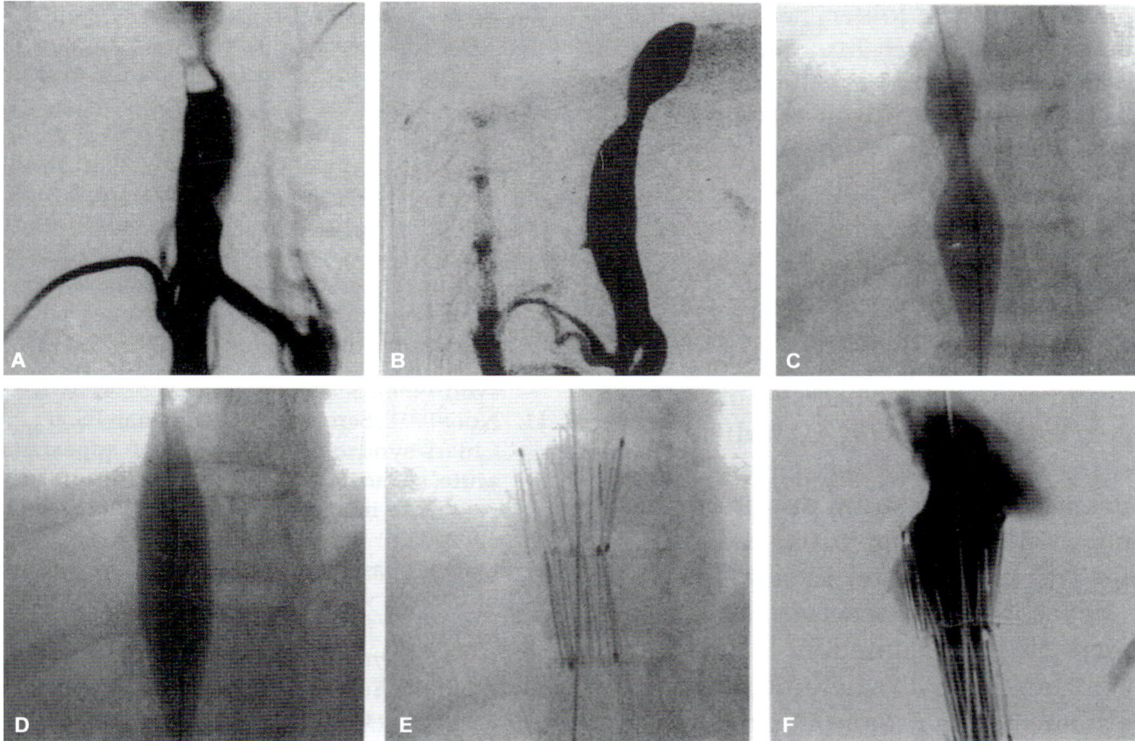

Figs 21.12A to F: Percutaneous stent placement in a patient with short segment stenosis of intrahepatic IVC. IVC graphy images in AP and lateral views (A,B), show the short segment narrowing of the intrahepatic IVC and filling up of multiple paravertebral collaterals. The stenosed segment was pre-dilated with a balloon (C,D). This was followed by stent placement across the stenosis (E,F). Check angiogram shows free flow of contrast across the IVC into the right atrium

Surgical management of BCS is indicated in patients with features of congestion, hepatocyte necrosis and fibrosis on liver biopsy. Decompressive surgical shunts like portocaval and mesocaval shunts relieve the sinusoidal congestion and thus halt the ongoing hepatocyte necrosis. The rationale for the side to side portocaval shunts is to transform the portal vein into an outflow tract for the hepatic circulation. A portocaval or mesocaval shunt is successful if the portal vein minus infrahepatic IVC pressure is >10 mm Hg. If this pressure gradient is <10 mm Hg, these infrahepatic surgical shunts should not be done.[16] These shunts are associated with a 25% mortality rate and shunt thrombosis which may occur in 10-25% of patients. Stenosis of the shunt is a late complication and is amenable for percutaneous balloon dilatation with or without stenting. In patients who have intrahepatic IVC abnormality these classical infrahepatic portocaval shunts do not work unless a stent is inserted in the IVC to correct the pressure gradient. Such patients require a suprahepatic shunt, i.e. mesoatrial shunt between the SMV and the right atrium. The criteria for the mesoatrial shunt are reduction of IVC diameter more than 75% or a caval atrial gradient exceeding 20 mmHg.[40] These shunts are, however, associated with poorer results and a higher incidence of shunt thrombosis.

Successful treatment of BCS with TIPS was described in 1993 by Peltzer et al and Ochs et al. [41,42] This involves the placement of an intrahepatic shunt connecting a hepatic vein stump through the liver to a branch of the portal vein. The shunt can also be created between the suprahepatic IVC and the portal vein when no hepatic vein stump is available. The transcaval approach is also technically more feasible in BCS. This is because the liver is enlarged and the intrahepatic IVC is surrounded by liver parenchyma providing stability for the transcaval puncture. In BCS the liver parenchyma is also relatively soft unlike that in other causes of cirrhosis.[43] The primary patency rate of these shunts has also increased with the use of polytetrafluoroethylene (PTFE) covered stents. The advantages of TIPS are its minimal invasiveness and the lower mortality rate as compared with surgical shunting.

In addition, intrahepatic caval stenosis can also be bypassed by using TIPS which is not possible with the surgical shunts. The most frequent complication of TIPS is hepatic encephalopathy which can occur in upto 30% of patients but can be treated medically. Other complications include stenosis or occlusion requiring revision in about 70% of cases by 6 months, intraperitoneal bleed, liver failure and subcapsular hematomas.

Liver transplantation is indicated for patients with fulminant hepatic failure, those who deteriorate after shunt procedure and in cirrhotics with end stage disease. In fact orthotopic liver transplantation is considered the only curative treatment for BCS.[43] Significant fibrosis and cirrhosis on liver biopsy with poor hepatocellular reserve can only be managed by transplantation. It is a useful option in patients with a hereditary thrombophilia state such as protein C, protein S, and antithrombin III deficiency which can be corrected with liver replacement. Ten-year survival rates upto 75% have been reported after liver transplantation.[22]

REFERENCES

1. Mulholland JP, Fong SM, Kafaghi FA, et al. Budd-Chiari syndrome: Diagnosis with ultrasound and nuclear medicine calcium colloid liver scan following non-diagnostic contrast CT scan. Australas Radiol 1997;41:53-56.
2. Mahmoud A, Elias E. Advances in hepatology—New approaches to the Budd- Chiari syndrome. J Gastroenterol Hepatol 1996;11:1121-23.
3. Vilgrain V, Lewin M, Vons C, et al. Hepatic nodules in Budd-Chiari syndrome: Imaging features. Radiology 1999;210:443-50.
4. Arora A, Sharma MP. Recent trends in the diagnosis and treatment of Budd- Chiari syndrome. J Assoc Physicians India 1992;40:533-36.
5. Floyd JL. The radiographic gamut of Budd-Chiari syndrome. Am J Gastroenterol 1981;76:381-87.
6. Menu Y, Alision D, Lorphelin JM, et al. Budd-Chiari syndrome: US evaluation. Radiology 1985;157:761-64.
7. Powell -Jackson PR, Karani J, Ede RJ, et al. Ultrasound scanning and ^{99m}Tc sulphur colloid scintigraphy in diagnosis of Budd-Chiari syndrome. Gut 1986;27: 1502-06.
8. Chawla Y, Kumar S, Dhiman RK, et al. Various imaging diagnostics in Budd- Chiari syndrome, liver cirrhosis and carcinoma-Duplex Doppler sonography in patients with Budd-Chiari syndrome. J Gastroenterol Hepatol 1999; 14:904-07.
9. Makuuchi M, Hasegewa H, Yamazaki S, et al. Primary Budd-Chiari syndrome: Ultrasonic demonstration. Radiology 1984;152:775-79.
10. Lupescu IG, Dobromir C, Popa GA, et al. Spiral Computed Tomography and Magnetic Resonance Angiography Evaluation in Budd-Chiari syndrome. J Gastrointestin Liver Dis 2008;17:223-26.
11. Bargallo X, Gilabert R, Nicolau C, et al. Sonography of the caudate vein: value in diagnosing Budd-Chiari syndrome. Am J Roentgenol 2003;181:1641-45.
12. Noone TC, Semelka RC, Siegelman ES, et al. Budd-Chiari syndrome: Spectrum of appearances of acute, subacute and chronic disease with magnetic resonance imaging. J Magn Reson Imaging 2000;11:44-50.
13. XU K, Ren K, Chen Y, et al. Application and evaluation of non-invasive examination for Budd-Chiari syndrome. Chinese Medical Journal 2007;120:91-94.
14. Ohta M, Hashizume M, Tomikawa M, et al. Analysis of hepatic vein waveform by Doppler ultrasonography in 100 patients with portal hypertension. Am J Gastero-enterol 1995;89:170-75.
15. Kane R, Eustace S. Diagnosis of Budd-Chiari syndrome: Comparison between sonography and MR angiography. Radiology 1995;195:117-21.
16. Kamath PS. Budd-Chiari syndrome: Radiologic Findings. Liver Transplantation 2006;12:S21-S22.
17. Brancatelli G, Vilgrain V, Federle MP, et al. Budd-Chiari syndrome: Spectrum of imaging findings. Am J Roentgenol 2007;188:W168-76.
18. Datta DV, Saha S, Singh SA, et al. Chronic Budd-Chiari syndrome due to obstruction of the intrahepatic portion of the inferior vena cava. Gut 1972;13:372-78.
19. Dilawari JB, Bambery P, Chawla Y, et al. Hepatic outflow obstruction (Budd-Chiari syndrome)- Experience with 177 patients and a review of the literature. Medicine (Baltimore) 1984;73:21-36.
20. Kage M, Arakawa M, Kojiro M, et al. Histopathology of membranous obstruction of the inferior vena cava in the Budd-Chiari syndrome. Gastroenterology 1992;102:2081-90.
21. Bolondi L, Gaiani S, Li Bassi S, et al. Diagnosis of Budd-Chiari syndrome by pulsed Doppler ultrasound. Gastroenterology 1991;100:1324-31.
22. Valla DC: Hepatic vein thrombosis (Budd-Chiari syndrome). Semin Liver Dis 2002;22:5-14.
23. Cho OK, Koo JH, Kim YS, et al. Collateral pathways in Budd-Chiari syndrome. CT and venographic correlation. Am J Roentgenol 1996;167:1163-67.
24. Clain D, Freston J, Kreel L, et al. Clinical diagnosis of Budd-Chiari syndrome. A report of six cases. Am J Med 1967;43:544-54.
25. Janssen HL, Garcia-Pagan JC, Elias E, et al. Budd-Chiari syndrome: review by an expert panel. J Hepatol 2003;38:364-71.
26. Maetani Y, Itoh K, Egawa H, et al. Benign hepatic nodules in Budd-Chiari syndrome. Radiologic-pathologic correlation with emphasis on the central scar. Am J Roentgenol 2002;178:869-75.
27. Tanju S, Erden A, Ceyhan K, et al. Contrast-enhanced MR angiography of benign regenerative nodules following TIPS shunt procedure in Budd-Chiari syndrome. Turk J Gastroenterol 2004;15:173-77.

28. Brancatelli G, Federle MP, Grazioli L, et al. Benign regenerative nodules in Budd-Chiari syndrome and other vascular disorders of the liver: radiologic-pathologic and clinical correlation. Radiographics 2002;22:847-62.
29. Brancatelli G, Federle MP, Grazioli L, et al. Large regenerative nodules in Budd- Chiari syndrome and other vascular disorders of the liver: CT and MR imaging findings with clinicopatholgic correlation. Am J Roentgenol 2002;178:77-883.
30. Cazals-Hatem D, Vilgrain V, Genin P, et al. Arterial and portal circulation and parenchymal changes in Budd-Chiari syndrome: a study in 17 explanted livers. Hepatology 2003;37:510-19.
31. Valla DC. Prognosis in Budd-Chiari syndrome after reestablishing hepatic venous drainage. Gut 2006;55: 761-63.
32. Artia T, Matsunaga N, Kobayashi H. Budd-Chiari syndrome: Peripheral abnormal intensity of the liver on magnetic resonance imaging. Clin Radiol 2000;55:640-42.
33. Camera L, Mainenti PP, Di Giacomo A, et al. Triphasic helical CT in Budd-Chiari syndrome: patterns of enhancement in acute, subacute and chronic disease. Clin Radiol 2006;61:331-37.
34. Anand A, Suri S, Chawla Y, et al. To evaluate the role of MRI and MR-angiography in the diagnosis of Budd-Chiari syndrome. PGIMER, (unpublished data) 2003.
35. Eguchi S, Takeuchi Y, Asano K. Successful balloon membranotomy for obstruction of the hepatic portion of the inferior vena cava. Surgery 1974;76:837-40.
36. Griffith JF, Mahmoud AEA, Cooper S, et al. Radiological intervention in Budd-Chiari syndrome: Techniques and outcome in 18 patients. Clin Radiol 1996;51:775-84.
37. Lopez RR, Benner KG, Hall L, et al: Expandable venous stents for the treatment of the Budd-Chiari syndrome. Gastroenterology 1991;100:1435-41.
38. Pisani-Ceretti A, Intra M, Prestipino F, et al. Surgical and radiologic treatment of primary Budd-Chiari syndrome. World J Surg 1998;22:48-53.
39. Baijjal SS, Roy S, Phadke RV, et al. Management of idiopathic Budd- Chiari syndrome with primary stent placement: Early results. J Vasc Interv Radiol 1996;7: 545-53.
40. Orloff MJ, Orloff MS, Daily PO. Long-term results of treatment of Budd-Chiari syndrome with portal decompression. Arch Surg 1992;127:1182-87.
41. Peltzer MY, Ring EJ, LaBerge JM. Treatment of Budd-Chiari syndrome with a transjugular intrahepatic portosystemic shunt. J Vasc Interv Radiol 1993;4:263-67.
42. Ochs A, Sellinger M, Haag K, et al. Transjugular intrahepatic portosystemic stent shunt (TIPS) in the treatment of Budd-Chiari syndrome. J Hepatol 1993;18:217-25.
43. Gandini R, Konda D, Simonetti G, et al. Transjugular intrahepatic portosystemic shunt patency and clinical outcome in patients with Budd-Chiari syndrome: Covered versus uncovered stents. Radiology 2006;241: 298-305.

Chapter Twenty-two

Gastrointestinal Hemorrhage

Deep Narayan Srivastava, Shivanand Gamanagatti

INTRODUCTION

Gastrointestinal hemorrhage, even if detected only by positive tests for occult blood, indicates a potentially serious disease and must be investigated further. Acute gastrointestinal bleeding is a major clinical problem that is responsible for 10-20% mortality in patients with massive gastrointestinal hemorrhage (GIH).

Endoscopy is the initial diagnostic procedure in suspected upper GI hemorrhage.[1] It determines the cause of bleeding with upto 90-95% accuracy.[2] Endoscopy is particularly useful in excluding lesions not, requiring angiography for diagnosis. It provides prognostic information as well as access for therapeutic interventions in gastroesophageal varices, nasopharyngeal abnormalities and anorectal lesions.

IMAGING MODALITIES

Angiography

Angiography plays a significant role in the diagnosis and management of patients with acute GIH by localizing the actual site of active bleeding and also helps in management by transcatheter embolization of the bleeding artery.[3] The role of angiography has diminished because of wider availability of endoscopy. However, it remains a valuable tool in patients with recurrent or continued GIH in whom source has eluded previous endoscopic, radionuclide and barium studies. Angiography is especially important in whom bleeding has continued after blind laparotomy.[4]

In acute gastrointestinal bleeding, angiography is diagnostic if bleeding exceeds 0.5 ml/min (blood loss exceeds four units within 24 hours).[2] If bleeding is intermittent and the patient is stable, other less invasive examinations can be used and emergency angiography may not be required.

Evaluation of recurrent hemorrhage may be time-consuming and expensive if bleeding is intermittent. Provocative pharmaco-angiography and intraoperative and capsule endoscopy may be useful in these situations.

Technical Considerations

Digital subtraction angiography (DSA) is sometimes not helpful in mesenteric studies because of the bowel gas and peristalsis. The motion artifacts may be misinterpreted as contrast extravasation and hence antispasmodic drugs are often used to reduce bowel peristalsis.

The renal function should be normal because angiography requires large amount of contrast medium. If renal function is deranged, use of alternative contrast media like carbon dioxide can also be used for angiography.

Usually a flush aortogram is done followed by selective and superselective arteriography. In flush aortogram, the tip of pigtail catheter tip is placed above the coeliac axis and a total of about 40 ml of contrast is injected using a pressure injector at the rate of 18-22 ml/sec. Depending on the initial findings on a flush aortogram, further selective and superselective studies are done using various visceral angiographic catheters. Flush aortograms are important, particularly in cases of suspected aortoenteric fistula. If a major splanchnic artery can not be catheterized or identified, a lateral aortography is used to accurately demonstrate and catheterize major aortic branches.

In mesenteric studies, the flow rate for contrast injection should be approximately 10 ml/sec for the coeliac, 8 ml/sec for the superior mesenteric artery and 3 ml/sec for the inferior mesenteric artery. The imaging must be rapid during the arterial phase (1-2 frames/sec) and reduced to (1 frame/2-5 second) for the capillary and venous phases. Imaging should be carried out up to at least 30 seconds, to identify slow extravasation, suspected venous occlusion and vascular malformations.

The suspected bleeding vessel should be injected first. The more selective the catheter is placed, the higher the probability that active bleeding will be recognized. The rate of blood loss must be at least 5-6 ml/min for it to be detected on the midstream flush aortogram. However, selective arteriography may reveal bleeding sources with rate of bleeding as low as 0.5-1 ml/min.

In approximately 70% of patients with gastric mucosal hemorrhage, bleeding occurs from left gastric artery (LGA). Hence, it is essential that LGA be well opacified during selective angiography. The celiac axis angiogram would not suffice if the tip of the catheter is distal to the origin of the LGA, or if the LGA originates from the aorta.

In bleeding duodenal ulcers, contrast extravasation is most commonly noted from the supraduodenal branch of gastroduodenal artery. In variceal bleeding, contrast extravasation is rarely demonstrated as contrast medium gets diluted by the time it reaches the bleeding veins. The purpose of angiography in variceal bleeding is very limited either to rule out any arterial source of bleeding or to define portal venous anatomy for urgent portosystemic shunt surgery.

Angiographic Findings in GIH

- Extravasation of contrast : It is seen as a puddling or staining that persists beyond the capiliary and venous phases.
- Delayed films may show opacified intestinal folds due to luminal extravasation of contrast medium.
- If the lumen of the gastrointestinal tract is filled with clotted blood, a 'pseudovein' appearance is often seen as the extravasated contrast flows through the clot to the most dependent part. However, unlike the venous phase, it persists for a much longer time.

Because bleeding may be intermittent, and spasm may preclude opacification of the target vessel, repeat injection or repeat angiography may be required to show the bleeding vessel (Figs 22.1A to C).

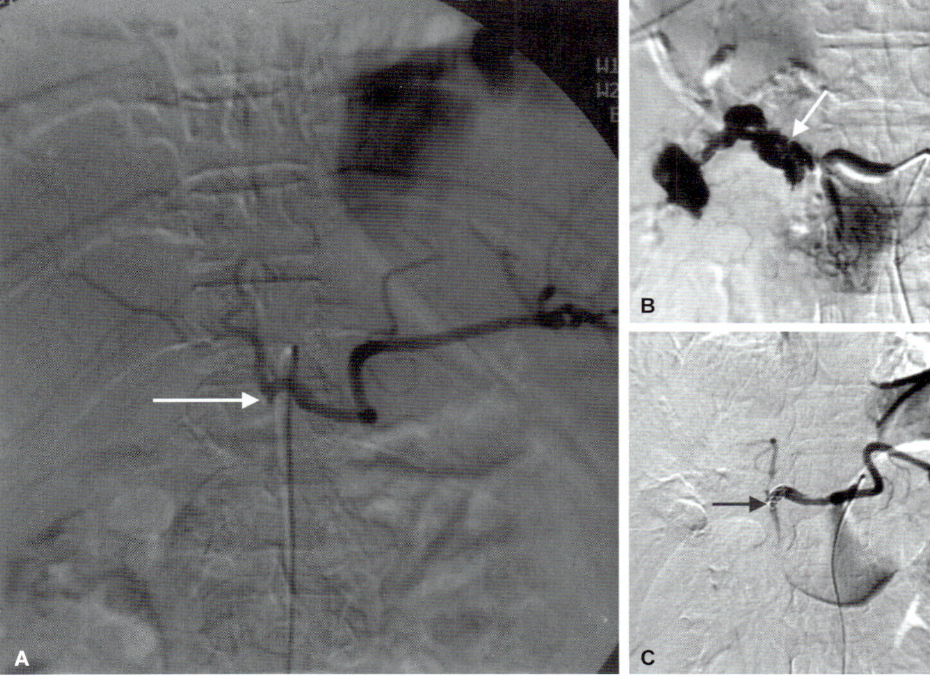

Figs 22.1A to C: Coeliac artery angiogram in a case of GIH is showing spasm of gastroduodenal artery (arrow), (B) Hepatic artery angiogram showing extravasation of contrast in subhepatic area (arrow), and (C) Coeliac artey angiogram after steel coil embolization not showing extravasation of contrast (arrow)

Radionuclide Studies

Radionuclide studies also play role in the evaluation of patients with GIH with minimal risk and invasiveness to the patient. The major indication is in cases where bleeding has stopped or is intermittent. It is not useful in patients with massive continuous bleeding. It has variable accuracy and sometimes proximal or distal movement of the radionuclide between imaging sessions impair precise localization of the actual bleeding site.

The common radionuclides employed in patients with GIH are as follows:

^{99m}Tc sulphur colloid: It is cleared from the blood pool by the reticuloendothelial system. The half-life of the tracer in the blood pool is approximately 2.5-3 min. If active bleeding is occurring during this short time, the tracer would extravasate in the bowel. Thus, like arteriography only active bleeding can be detected, but sulphur colloid scintigraphy can detect bleeding rates as low as 0.1 ml/min. In addition, isotope study can be repeated as often as required. The drawback is that bleeding into the hepatic or splenic flexures of the colon and upper gastrointestinal hemorrhage (UGIH) will be obscured because of the overlap by normal accumulation of the tracer in liver and spleen.

^{99m}Tc-labelled RBC: These labeled RBCs in circulation extravasate during bleeding and can be detected. The advantage is that images can be obtained upto 2 hours after the initial injection and hence is especially useful for evaluating intermittent GIH. The major limitation is that activity seen in the lower GIT, when it may have occurred from more proximal segments of small bowel and sources of bleeding may be missed if frequent views are not obtained.

^{99m}Tc-pertechnetate scanning : It is used in cases of bleeding of Meckel's diverticulum. This tracer accumulates in ectopic gastric mucosa.

Computed Tomography

Accurate localization of acute gastrointestinal and intraperiotoneal bleeding is also possible on arterial phase CT.[5] Many studies have suggested that good arterial phase abdominal CT can be used as the initial imaging technique in the diagnosis of active hemorrhage if the clinical condition of the patient allows.[6] Arterial phase CT can demonstrate extravasated contrast in the bowel lumen greater than 90 HU, focal dilatation of fluid filled bowel segment. Non contrast CT sometimes show acute hematoma.

In some cases CT,[7] MR[8] and Doppler sonography[9] may detect parenchymal abnormalities such as hepatic artery aneurysms, arterioportal fistulae, tumors, etc. and thus help in selection of patients for directed arterial treatment.

Barium Studies

The barium studies have no role in the management of patients with acute UGIH because: (i) the mucosal details are difficult to evaluate in the presence of blood and clots in the stomach, (ii) it is difficult to perform in acutely ill patients, (iii) it may render further radiological investigations like angiography inconclusive, and (iv) provide no clue about the detected lesion as a cause of bleed.[2]

Barium studies may be done in chronic GIH to detect other causes in cases where endoscopy is negative and active bleeding has stopped.

CONTROL OF GASTROINTESTINAL HEMORRHAGE

After the bleeding site has been localized, minimally invasive angiographic procedures should be used to control hemorrhage. This may avoid an emergency surgery in a patient with acute GIH. Endoscopic coagulation and mucosal injection of sclerosing agent can control bleeding in ulcer and variceal cases.

Angiography is beneficial in patients who fail to respond conservative or invasive endoscopic management. It is also valuable in patients who are unstable and are bleeding massively. Angiogrpahy in these situations can locate the bleeding vessel and provide access to transcatheter management either to obviate surgery or to stabilize the patient before surgery.[2]

The bleeding vessels can be treated with transcatheter embolization[3] and rarely by arterial infusion of vasopressin.

Transcatheter Embolization

Transcatheter embolization has been used for lesions of the stomach, colon and small bowel.[10] It is especially useful in the treatment of bleeding pancreatic or hepatic artery pseudoaneurysms.[11] The advantages are as follows:

- Control of bleeding is immediate
- Risk of visceral ischemia is minimal if embolization is superselective and collaterals are preserved.

Minimum amount of embolic material should be used to stop hemorrhage and should be injected as selectively as possible.

The most commonly used materials include gelatin sponge, a temporary occluding agent or steel coils for permanent embolization. Polyvinyl alcohol particles are also used and have shown good results.[11] The embolisation in conjunction with vasopressin infusion is not recommended. The major risks of bowel embolization are ischemia and stricture formation, but these risks must be weighed against the high mortality rate of emergency surgery.

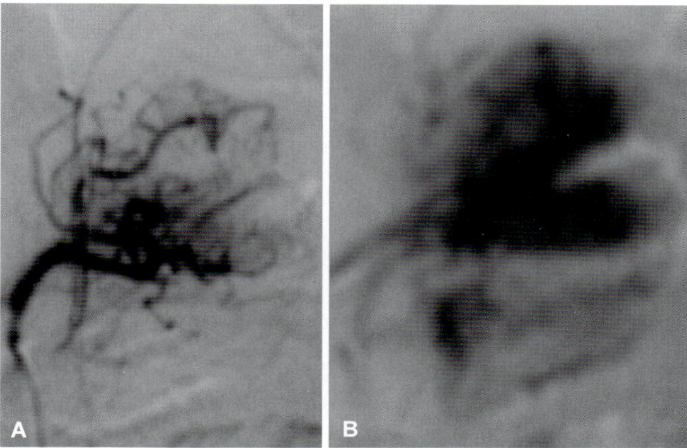

Figs 22.2A and B: Left gastric artery angiogram: (A) Early, (B) Delayed phase showing pooling of contrast in gastric arteriovenous malformation

SPECIFIC SITUATIONS IN GI HEMORRHAGES

Upper gastrointestinal hemorrhage (UGIH) can be differentiated from lower gastrointestinal hemorrhage (LGIH) by localizing the source of bleeding either proximal or distal to the ligament of Treitz. UGIH is ten times more common than LGHI. Before imaging, a distinction must be made between UGIH and LGIH based on clinical findings.

Upper Gastrointestinal Hemorrhage (UGIH)

Common causes of upper gastrointestinal hemorrhage are peptic ulceration, erosive gastritis, varices and esophagogastric mucosal tears. These entities account for up to 90% of all cases of UGIH in which a definite lesion can be found. Other less common causes of hemorrhage include neoplasms of esophagus, stomach and duodenum, aortoenteric fistula, pancreatitis, hemobilia, arterivenous malformations (Figs 22.2A and B), splanchnic arterial aneurysms and rarely mesenteric venous thrombosis and hepatobiliary and pancreatic tumors.[7,8,12] Acute UGIH due to penetration of a hepatic or left gastric artery aneurysm into the duodenal bulb[9] (Figs 22.3A to D) or stomach[13] (Figs 22.4A to D) is rare but has been reported. Rarely primary blood dyscrasias, vasculitis, connective tissue disorders, hamartoma, jejunoileitis and uremia may also produce significant bleeding.[14, 15]

Hemobilia

The causes are hepatic trauma, neoplasms, abscesses, hepatic artery aneurysm, laparoscopic and post-operative or interventional procedures of the liver (Figs 22.5A to 22.8F).

The presentation is characteristic, i.e. biliary colic, obstructive jaundice and UGIH.

The diagnosis is made either on endoscopy by the appearance of blood from the ampulla of Vater or by diagnostic hepatic arteriography. The rupture of hepatic arterial branches and hepatic arterial aneurysms can be treated by angioembolization or surgical ligation of hepatic artery.[3, 9]

Pancreatitis and UGIH

In pancreatitis a pseudocyst is frequently recognized on imaging, but a pseudoaneurysm is noted in less than 10% of cases. Intracystic hemorrhage has been reported in 6-10% of cases and this is due to extension of pancreatic inflammation to the nearby splenic artery. The pancreatic pseudocysts may present with the following five patterns of hemorrhage:[16]

- Hemorrhage within the pseudocyst presenting with intermittent severe abdominal pain due to elevated intracystic pressure.
- Gastrointestinal bleeding caused by fistula formation near the digestive tract.
- Rupture into the peritoneum.
- Hemorrhage caused by fistula formation with the bile duct.
- Hemorrhage into the duodenum via the pancreatic duct (hemosuccus pancreaticus).

Superior mesenteric angiography is the investigation of choice to diagnose and selective arterial embolization may control the hemorrhage (Figs 22.9 A to D).

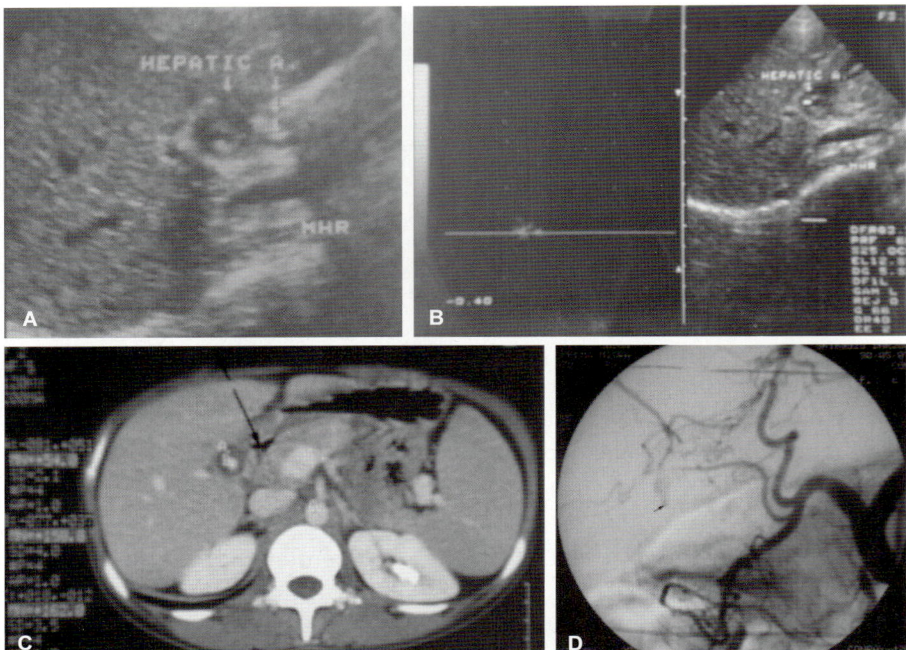

Figs 22.3A to D: (A) Abdominal sonography showing a round, cystic mass at the porta, (B) Doppler sonogrphy showing absence of signal in the echogenic area of the lesion, (C) Contrast-enhancing CT showing a low attenuating area with an enhanced center lateral to second part at the duodenum (arrow). Selective coeliac artery angiogram (D) is showing the aneurysm (arrow). At surgery the partially thrombosed aneurysm was communicating to duodenal bulb

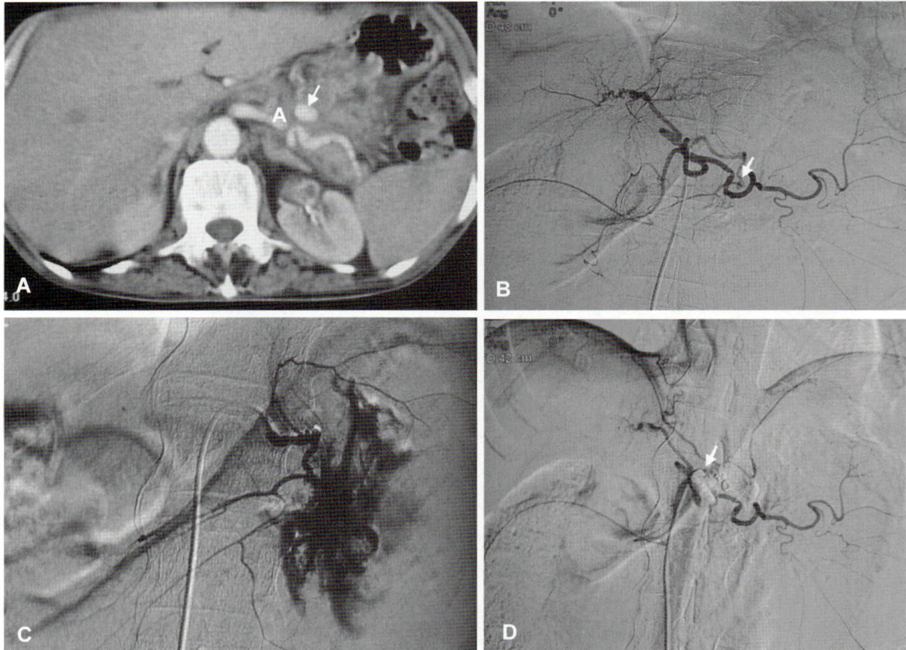

Figs 22.4A to D: Contrast enhanced arterial phase CT (A) and coeliac artery angiogram (B) of a case of massive gastrointestinal hemorrhage is showing an enhancing aneurysm posterior to stomach (arrows). Selective left gastric artery angiogram (C) is showing leakage of contrast into stomach due to aneurysmogastric fistula. The left gastric artery was embolized (arrow) with steel coils (D) and partial gastrectomy was done later

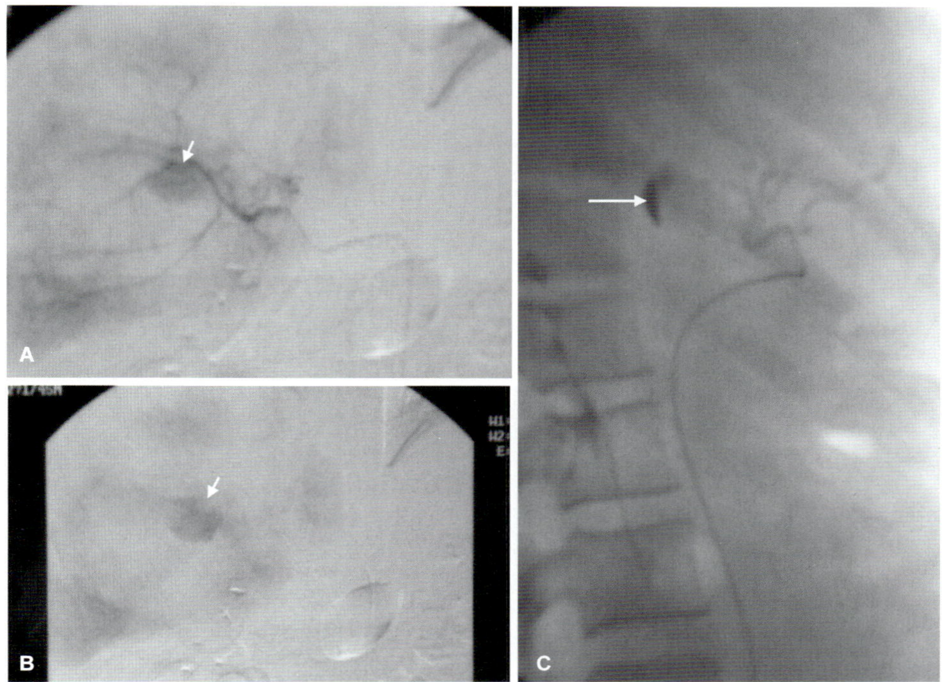

Figs 22.5A to C: (A-B) Hepatic artery angiogram in a postoperative patient of road traffic accident showing extravasation of the contrast in the right lobe of liver (arrows), and (C) Lateral film showing pooling of contrast in a cavity (arrow)

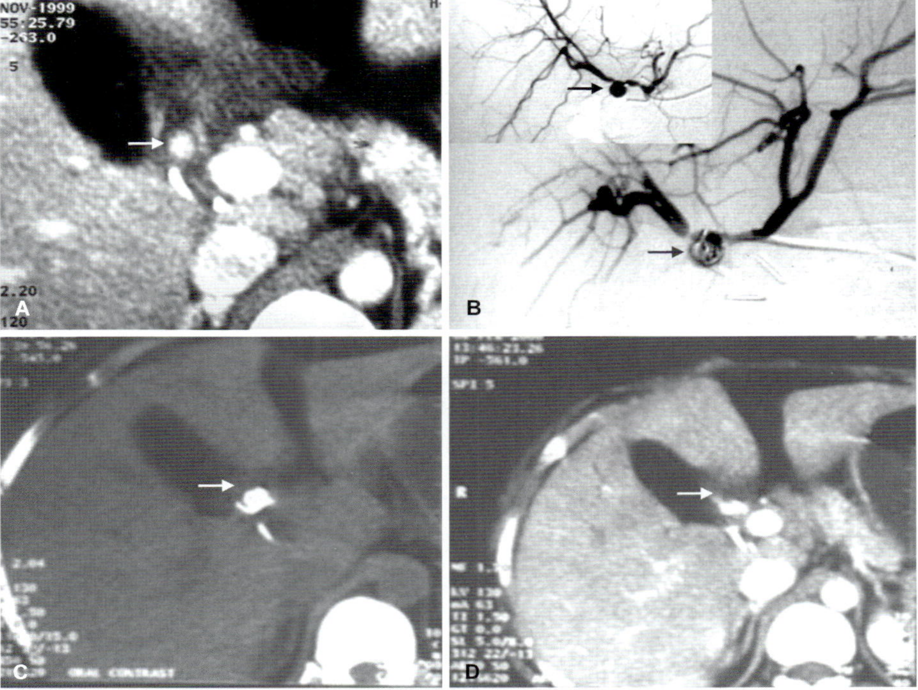

Figs 22.6 A to D: 42- year-old woman with hemobilia following open cholecystectomy done two months ago shows right hepatic artery aneurysm (arrow) on CT (A) and hepatic angiography (B, inset). It was embolized using steel coils (B, arrow). Four months following embolization the non-contrast enhanced CT (C) shows aneurysm packed with coils (arrow). There is no enhancement of aneurysm on contrast enhanced CT (D)

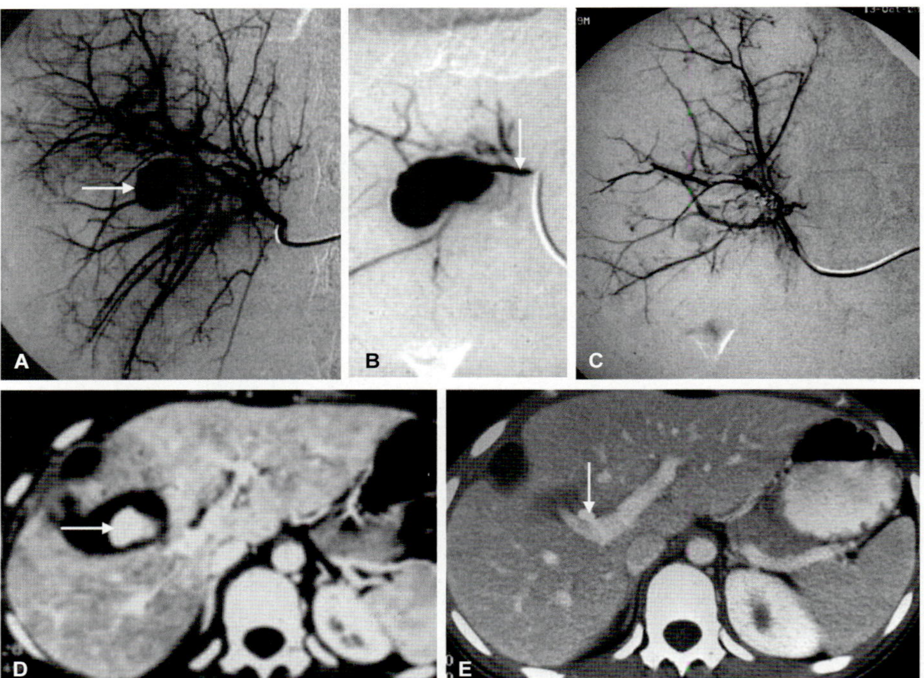

Figs 22.7A to E: (Upper row A-C) Hepatic angiogram of 28 years old male a road traffic accident victim with a large pseudoaneurysm (arrow) filling by middle hepatic artery (arrow head) was embolized with steel coil. (D-E) The aneurysm (arrow) and steel coil (arrow head) are seen on pre and postembolization three months CT

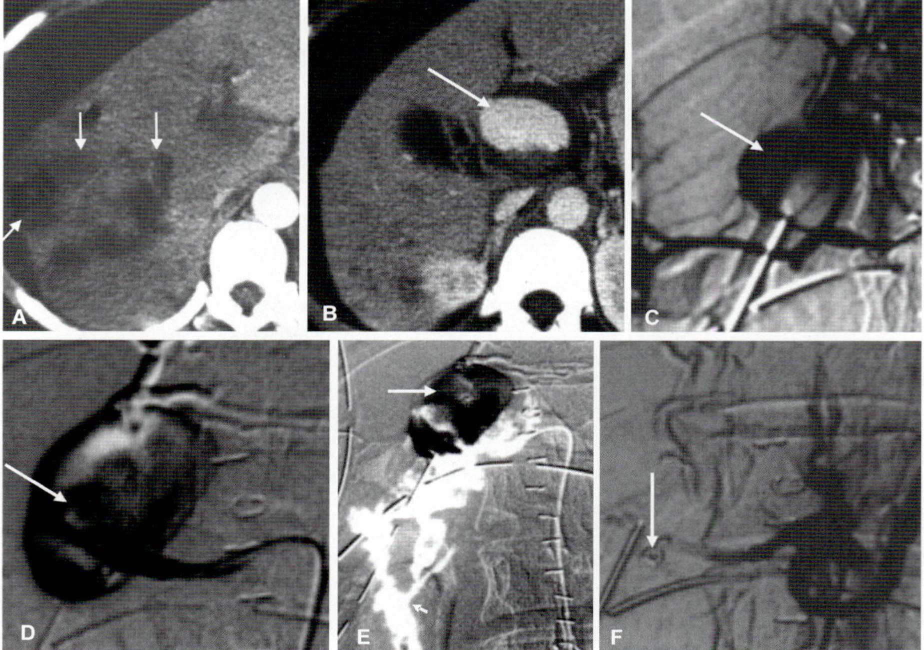

Figs 22.8A to F: (A to D) 35-year-old male with liver abscess (arrow head) on treatment developed a large hepatic artery aneurysm (arrow). (E) There is simultaneous opacification of duodenum (arrow heads) due to communication of aneurysm to duodenum. (F) The hepatic artery was embolized using steel coils (arrow)

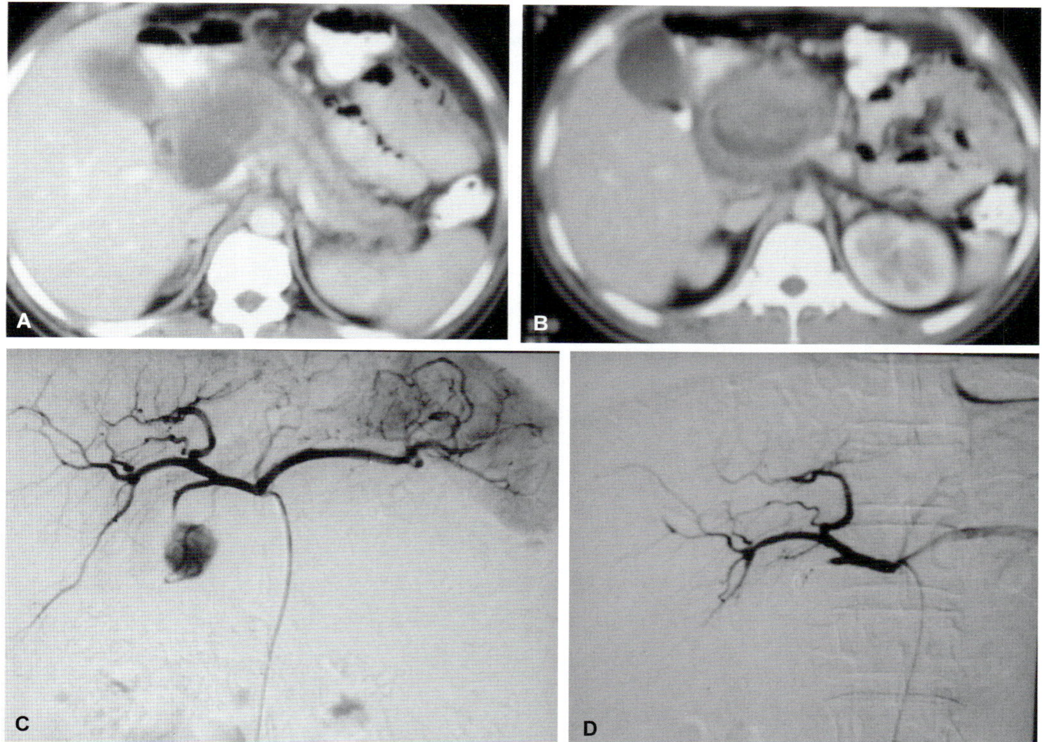

Figs 22.9A to D: Contrast enhanced CT (A-B) of a case of acute pancreatitis is showing a large pseudocyst with bleed and peripancreatic inflammation in head of pancreas. The pancreatic duct is dilated. Coeliac artery angiogram (C) is showing an aneurysm of gastroduodenal artery. The artery was embolized with steel coils (D). Superior mesenteric angiogram was normal

Lower Gastrointestinal Hemorrhage (LGIH)

Patients with lower gastrointestinal bleeding are usually older than those with gastric or duodenal lesions. Causes of LGIH in India are nonspecific ulcers (30%), enteric ulcers (15%), tuberculosis (6%), neoplasms (6%) and others (31%). In western literature the causes are diverticular (33%), colitis and ulcers (22%), neoplasms (20%), angiodysplasia and others (25%). Some of the causes of the LGIH are discussed below.

Colonic Diverticula

They are mostly in the left colon. Bleeding is typically abrupt in onset, massive and painless, and does not recur in 60% of patients. Active diverticular bleeding can be demonstrated either by direct endoscopic visualization or by filling of the bleeding diverticulum with contrast medium at the time of angiography.

Meckel's Diverticulum

It is a congenital anomaly of the distal ileum, present in about 2% of the population and is an important cause of acute hemorrhage in children and young adults. Although only about 15% of these diverticula contain gastric mucosa, half the lesions, which cause acute bleeding, contain gastric mucosa. The acid secretions from gastric mucosa result in peptic ulceration, most often in the ileal mucosa adjacent to the gastric mucosa and may lead to gastrointestinal bleeding. ^{99m}Tc-pertechnetate radionuclide scans can detect these bleeding diverticula. Angiography can show the vessel supplying the area of abnormally increased contrast medium accumulation in the distal ileum. Vitelline artery is a separate branch of the superior mesenteric artery, which is specific to Meckel's diverticulum, but in 80 per cent of diverticula this vessel is involuted and is replaced by a distal ileal branch[17] (Figs 22.10A to E).

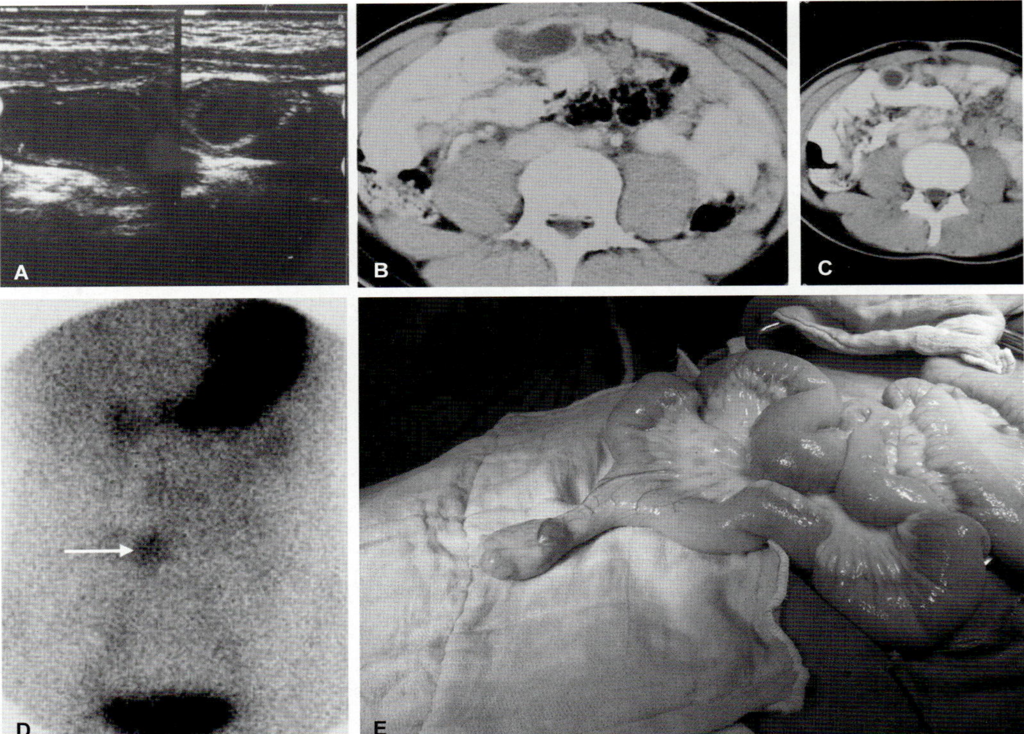

Figs 22.10A to E: USG (A) showing a tubular, non-compressible, thick walled blind ending structure in right paraumblical region. On CECT (B and C) it was fluid filled with enhancing wall and showed active uptake of tracer (arrow) on ^{99m}TC pertechnatate scan (D). The diagnosis of Meckel's diverticulum was confirmed at surgery (E)

Angiodysplasia

It is a mucosal telangiectasia, often multiple, usually involving the cecum or ascending colon. These lesions are often multiple and represent dilated pre-existing vascular structures (mucosal or submucosal venules). It is caused mainly by intermittent obstruction of venous outflow, but ischemia or toxic effects of bowel contents also have their role in its pathogenesis.

On angiography it is seen as a vascular tuft appearing in the arterial phase with an early opacification of a draining vein, and delayed emptying of a dilated and tortuous intramural vein. To diagnose bleeding from angiodysplasia, actual extravasation of contrast must be demonstrated. If extravasation is not detected, carcinoma or some other lesion should be considered, because about one-third of all elderly patients may have angiodysplasia without any history of bleeding. After angiographic diagnosis of the lesion, catheter may be left in place for arterial injection of methylene blue for intraoperative localization of the lesion. Treatment of incidentally found angioectasias is not indicated in patients with no history of LGIH.

Hemangioma and Arteriovenous Malformation

Gastrointestinal tract hemangioma and AVM are rare but can cause significant morbidity (Figs 22.11A and B). The clinical presentation may be acute, recurrent or chronic. MR imaging is sometimes useful in the evaluation of extent of the colonic lesion.[18]

Tumors

These can bleed spontaneously, but such blood loss is more likely to be chronic and intermittent rather than massive. On angiography some tumors like leiomyomas and leiomyosarcomas, adenoma and Kaposi's sarcoma are hypervascular and typically have an intense capillary stain (Figs 22.12A and B).

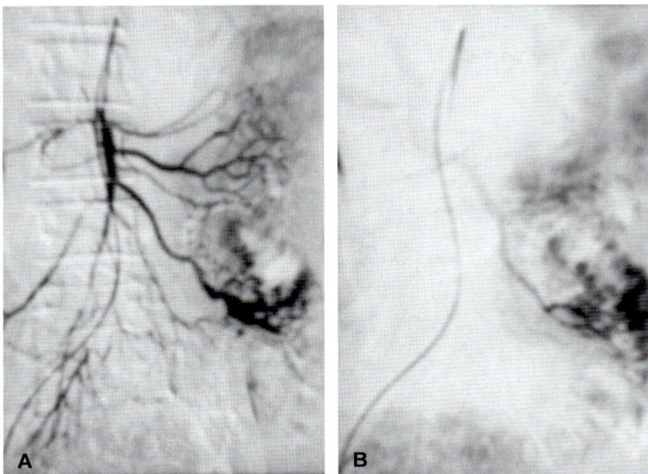

Figs 22.11A and B: Superior mesenteric artery angiogram: (A) Early, (B) Delayed phase showing pooling of contrast in jejunal arterivenous malformation

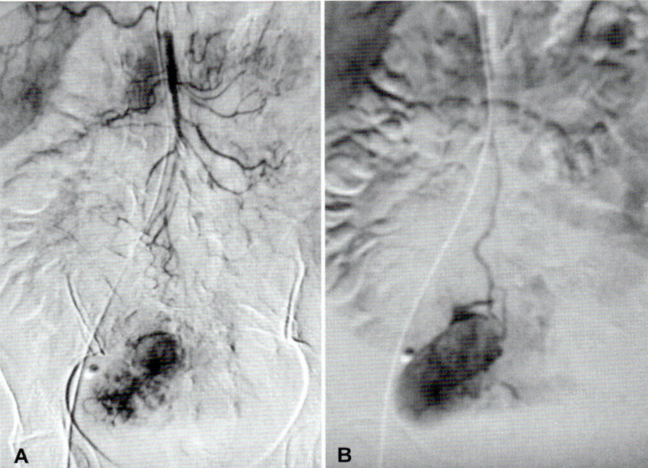

Figs 22.12A and B: Superior mesenteric artery angiogram: (A) Early, (B) Delayed phase showing tumor vascularity in a case of ileal adenoma

Inflammatory Bowel Diseases and Small Bowel or Colonic Ulcers

These produce nonspecific angiographic findings such as dilated arteries, mucosal outlining and sometimes pooling of contrast.

Others

Mesenteric varices are rare and bleeding from these sites is unusual. The common location of these is in the rectosigmoid area. The commonest cause of these varices is portal hypertension. Rarely these may be secondary to portal vein obstruction, congenital hepatic fibrosis (CHF), splenic vein thrombosis secondary to pancreatitis and splenorenal shunt block.[19] On angiography these can be demonstrated on delayed phase.

Ischemic colitis can be of occlusive or nonocclusive aetiology. The occlusive causes are iatrogenic interruption of inferior mesenteric artery during aortic surgery, embolizm, thrombosis, aneurysm of abdominal aorta, amyloidosis and vasculitis[20] (Figs 22.13A and B). Nonocclusive causes include low flow states due to cardiac dysfunction and hypovolemia. In the majority of patients, it is mild or transient. On barium enema, the hallmark of ischemic colitis is thumb-printing caused by submucosal hemorrhage and edema.

The rupture of arteriosclerotic aortic aneurysms into the small intestine (aortoenteric fistula) is almost always fatal. Rupture usually occurs after an arterial reconstructive surgery with fistula formation between synthetic graft and bowel lumen. A small bleed may precede a sudden massive hemorrhage from an aortoenteric fistula. It is often difficult to diagnose it angiographically and on CT angiography, but observation of a nipple-like projection or a pseudoaneurysm in the presence of a vascular graft is presumptive evidence of a fistula. Mycotic aneurysm of mesenteric vessels are rare and are usually managed by surgery (Figs 22.14A to C).

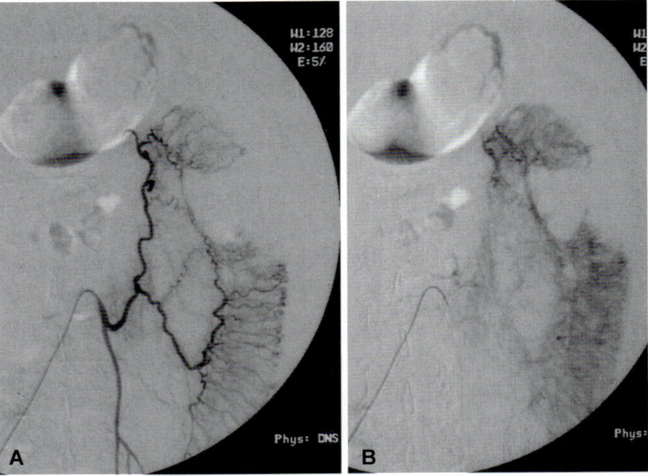

Figs 22.13A and B: Inferior mesenteric artery angiogram: (A) Early, and (B) Delayed phase, showing avascular segment of descending colon

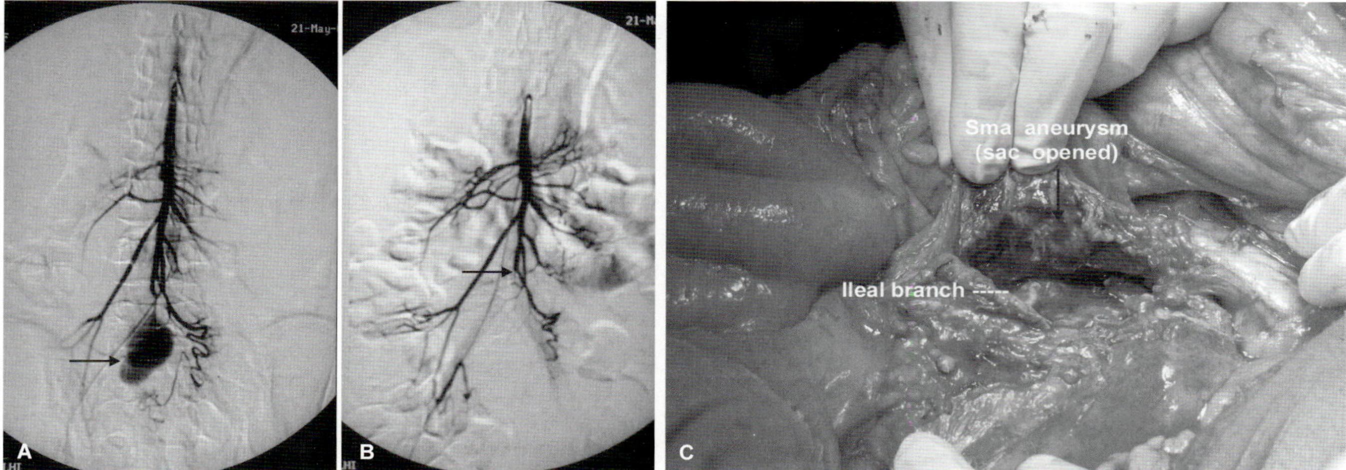

Figs 22.14A to C: Superior mesenteric artery angiogram (A) is showing a large aneurysm (arrow). The aneurysm was embolized (arrow) with steel coils (B) and later on surgically removed (C)

CONCLUSION

GIH is a common clinical problem and needs a unified systemic approach by the physician, surgeon and radiologist with special expertise in vascular interventions. In spite of many modern diagnostic techniques, quite often the cause of GIH remains undiagnosed.

REFERENCES

1. Perng CL, Lin HJ, Chan CJ, et al. Characteristics of patients with bleeding peptic ulcer requiring emergency endoscopy and aggressive treatment. Am J Gastroenterol 1994;89:1811-4.
2. Gore RM, Tutton SM, Rattner Z, et al. Gastrointestinal hemorrhage. In: Gore RM, Levine MS (ed) Gastointestinal Radiology. 2nd ed, WB Saunders, Philadelphia 2000; 2206-27.
3. Srivastava DN, Sharma S, Pal S, Thulkar S, Seith A, Bandhu S, Pande GK, Sahni P. Transcatheter arterial embolisation in the management of hemobilia. Abdominal Imaging 2006;31(4):439-48.
4. Lau WY, Ngan H, Chu KW, Yuen WK. Repeat selective visceral angiography in patients with gastrointestinal bleeding of obscure origin. Br J Surg 1989;78: 226-9.
5. Jaeckle T, Stuber G, Hoffmann MH, Jeltsch M, Schmitz BL and Aschoff AJ. Detection and localization of acute upper and lower gastrointestinal (GI) bleeding with arterial phase multidetector row helical CT. Eur Radiol 2008 Mar 20 (E pub).
6. Roy-Choudhary SH, Gallacher DJ, Pilmer J, Rankin S, Fowler G, Steers J, Dourado R, Woodburn P, Adam A. Relative threshold of detection of active arterial bleeding: in vitro comparison of MDCT and digital subtraction angiography. AJR 2007;189(5):W 238-46.
7. Srivastava DN, Gujral RB. Pancreatic carcinoma associated with situs inversus in a young adult. Am J Gastroenterol 1993;88:156-7.
8. Srivastava DN, Sharma S, Yadav S et al. Pedunculated hepatic hemangioma with arterioportal shunt treated with angioembolisation and surgery. Australas Radiol 1998;42:151–3.
9. Srivastava DN, Chakravarti AL, Gupta RK et al. Gastrointestinal bleeding from a false aneurysm of the hepatic artery after cholecystectomy. Am J Gastroenterol 1996;91:395-7.
10. Ibrahim AS, Allangawi MH, Al-Muzrakchi AM. Massive bleeding from an arteriovenous malformation in the gastric fundus following gastric biopsy treated by embolisation. Int J Clin Pract 2003;57: 354-5.
11. Guy GE, Shetty PC, Sharma RP, et al. Acute lower gastrointestinal hemorrhage–treatment by superselective embolisation with polyvinyl alcohol particles. Am J Roentgenol 1992;159:521-26.
12. Srivastava DN, Gandhi D, Julka PK and Tandon RK. Gastrointestinal hemorrhage in hepatocellular carcinoma: management with transhepatic arterioembolization. Abd Imaging 2000;25:380-84.
13. Falodia S, Garg PK, Bhatia V, Ramachandran V, Dash MR and Srivastava DN. EUS diagnosis of a left gastric artery pseudoaneurysm and aneurysmogastric fistula seen with a massive GI hemorrhage. Gastrointestinal Endoscopy 2008;26. (E pub).
14. Gandhi D, Srivastava DN, Choudhary VP, Pande GK and Datta Gupta S. Haemangio-lymphangiomatous hamartoma of jejunum : an unusual cause of massive gastrointestinal hemorrhage. Trop Gastroenterol 2001;22(2): 95-7.
15. Chandrasekharm W, Srivastava DN, Mathur M, Bhatnagar V. Angiographic and immunologic studies in acute necrotizing jejunoileitis. J Trop Pediatr 2002;48(2): 88-92.

16. Rao RCK, Kumar A, Berry M: Pseudoaneurysm of anomalous right hepatic artery as a cause of hemosuccus pancreaticus. Gastrointest Radiology 1987;12:313-4.
17. Bree RL, Reuter SR. Angiographic demonstration of a bleeding Meckel's diverticulum. Radiology 1973;108: 287-8.
18. Kandpal H, Sharma R, Srivastava DN, Sahni P, Vashisht S. Diffuse cavernous hemangioma of colon : magnetic resonance imaging features. Report of two cases. Australas Radiol 2007;51:147-51.
19. Srivastava DN, Yadav S et al. Emergency percutaneous occlusion of surgical portosystemic shunt using steel coils and balloon catheter. Am. J Roentgenol 1999;172:1453– 4.
20. Srivastava DN, Gulati MS, Tandon RK. Colonic infarction in acute pancreatitis : an unusual cause of gastrointestinal hemorrhage. Am J Gastroenterol. 1998;93(7);1186-7.

Chapter Twenty-three

Interventions in Obstructive Biliopathy

Mandeep Kang, Naveen Kalra

The past few decades have witnessed a revolution in minimally invasive surgeries and techniques with image guided interventions having emerged at the forefront of these developments. Percutaneous biliary interventions had their origin way back in 1921 when direct puncture of the gallbladder was first performed to opacify the biliary tree. This was followed by reports describing percutaneous direct puncture of the biliary tree. The technique of percutaneous biliary drainage for the relief of obstructive jaundice was introduced in the 1970s followed by percutaneous cholecystostomy in the 1980s. The development of biliary stents has further enlarged the scope of percutaneous applications in the management of biliary diseases.

In the present day, percutaneous biliary interventions include percutaneous transhepatic cholangiography (PTC) and biliary drainage (PTBD) for the diagnosis and management of biliary obstruction and percutaneous cholecystostomy. This route can also be used for percutaneous transhepatic cholangioscopy or biliary ultrasonography; biopsy of the biliary duct and as an access for the application of intraluminal brachytherapy.

INDICATIONS FOR BILIARY DRAINAGE

The presence of cholestasis, whether due to benign or malignant etiology, causes biliary infection. Secondly, protracted hyperbilirubinemia causes impairment of the renal function. The surgical morbidity and mortality rates are also high (40-60% and 15-25% respectively) in the setting of hyperbilirubinemia, therefore decompression should be done as early as possible in patients with obstructive biliopathy. This will not only avoid the above mentioned complications but also relieve symptoms such as pruritus and improve the nutritional status of the patient.

Common causes of benign biliary obstruction include choledocholithiasis, sclerosing cholangitis and inflammatory conditions such as pancreatitis, iatrogenic causes (post laparoscopic cholecystectomy, liver transplantation or anastomotic strictures) and infections such as HIV infection, oriental and parasitic cholangitis. The common causes of malignant biliary obstruction include gallbladder carcinoma, cholangiocarcinoma, carcinoma of the pancreas and metastatic disease.

Percutaneous Transhepatic Cholangiography (PTC)

Percutaneous transhepatic cholangiography is a diagnostic procedure which involves placement of a fine needle into a peripheral biliary radicle under image guidance followed by contrast injection to opacify the biliary tree. The procedure is used for:

1. To define the level of obstruction in patients with obstructive biliopathy.
2. To evaluate for presence of suspected choledocholithiasis.
3. To determine the etiology of cholangitis.
4. To evaluate suspected bile duct inflammatory disorders.
5. To demonstrate site of bile duct leak.

6. As the preliminary step for draining the biliary tree (most common indication).

Although PTC has been shown to be an effective technique which reliably demonstrates the level of obstruction, it is more invasive and painful than endoscopic retrograde cholangio pancreatography (ERCP). It also involves the risk of significant complications such as hemoperitoneum and bile peritonitis. Hence, PTC is nowadays reserved for patients in whom an ECRP is not possible due to anatomy altering surgeries or in unsuccessful cannulation.

Pre-procedure Evaluation and Preparation

The initial workup of a patient with obstructive biliopathy includes a clinical evaluation with history taking, physical examination and pertinent laboratory tests. Cross-sectional imaging such as ultrasonography, CT and MRI should be performed to provide information about the pattern of dilatation and level of obstruction of the biliary tree and determine the cause. Coagulation parameters including prothrombin time, prothrombin time index and activated partial thromboplastin time as well as platelet counts should be checked prior to the procedure and corrected with fresh frozen plasma or platelets if deranged.

Antibiotics are routinely administered in all patients as bacteremia and sepsis can develop during the procedure. Broad spectrum antibiotics covering both gram positive and gram negative organisms should be started prior to the procedure. A venous access should be secured.

Conscious sedation should be used for adequate pain control. Over-dosage of the sedative should be avoided as the patient needs to follow the instructions of the operator such as breath holding. General anesthesia may however be required in selected cases.

Technique

With the patient lying supine on the fluoroscopy table the upper abdomen is cleaned and draped. The skin puncture site is anesthetized with a local anesthetic (2% lidocaine) upto the liver capsule. If the peripheral biliary radicles are dilated they can be punctured under ultrasonographic guidance. If not dilated, the procedure is performed under fluoroscopic guidance. Most PTCs are performed from the right mid-axillary approach through an intercostal space which is caudal to the costophrenic sulcus. This can be identified on fluoroscopy on deep inspiration. A fine (22G) Chiba needle is advanced into the liver aiming for the right lateral aspect of the 12th thoracic vertebral body. After the stylet is removed the needle is slowly withdrawn while injecting a small amount of contrast. When contrast is seen to opacify the biliary tree, needle withdrawal is stopped and cholangiography performed to delineate the biliary anatomy. If the first puncture is unsuccessful, a second or third puncture can be made by changing the needle angulation once the needle tip is near the liver capsule.

The success rates for PTC are reported to be more than 90% in a dilated system and 67-80% in a non-dilated system. Major complications are seen in 2% of procedures and include sepsis, cholangitis, bile leak, hemorrhage or pneumothorax.

Percutaneous Transhepatic Biliary Drainage (PTBD)

PTBD is a therapeutic procedure that consists of sterile puncture of a peripheral biliary radicle under image guidance followed by placement of a catheter or stent for internal or external drainage of bile. Percutaneous therapy of bile duct lesions is often staged, requiring multiple sessions to achieve therapeutic goals. The indications include:

1. To decompress the biliary tree
2. To dilate biliary strictures
3. To remove bile duct stones
4. To divert bile from and stent bile duct defects

The patient preparation and pre-procedure work up are as for PTC. As with PTC, the endoscopic route is preferred for drainage, particularly in lesions involving the mid or distal CBD. However, with lesions involving the hilum, the percutaneous approach is associated with a higher success rate and is therefore preferred. In cases of failed ERCP or where ERCP is not possible due to anatomy altering surgeries, PTBD is the only approach available.

Technique

The first step of the procedure is performing a PTC. If the peripheral ducts are sufficiently dilated, sonographic guidance may be used to puncture the biliary radicle. In lesions distal to the confluence, either the left or the right system can be accessed. The left system is accessed from an anterior, sub-xiphoid approach while the right is accessed from the right mid-axillary approach. In cases of lesions involving the hilum with isolation of the right and left systems, the approach should be based on a careful assessment of the volume of the liver which will be drained by the catheter. At least 30% of the liver volume should be drained with a single catheter as placement of multiple catheters increases the morbidity and mortality in a patient. This assessment assumes even more significance in patients in whom the secondary confluence is involved or with multilevel isolation (e.g. due to metastases).

After anesthetizing the skin, a 18G puncture needle is used to enter the selected biliary radicle. In a dilated system, allowing a little amount of bile to drain after the puncture before injecting contrast is beneficial as it prevents over-distension of the biliary system which can result in bacteremia and sepsis. A little contrast is injected to opacify the biliary tree. A 0.035 inch hydrophilic guidewire is then passed through the needle and manipulated into the biliary tree. After safely anchoring the guidewire the needle is withdrawn and a 4F or 5F sheath or cannula introduced. The slippy guidewire can then be exchanged for a stiffer (Teflon coated) guidewire over which a 7F or 8F drainage catheter can be placed after dilatation of the tract with fascial dilators (Figs 23.1A and B). If the tip of the catheter is in the CBD, a catheter of the pigtail type is placed. If the tip of the catheter is in an intrahepatic duct a straight type catheter is selected.

Fluoroscopic Guidance

Fluoroscopic guidance can be used in patients with or without biliary dilatation for performing PTBD. There are two methods by which the procedure can be done.

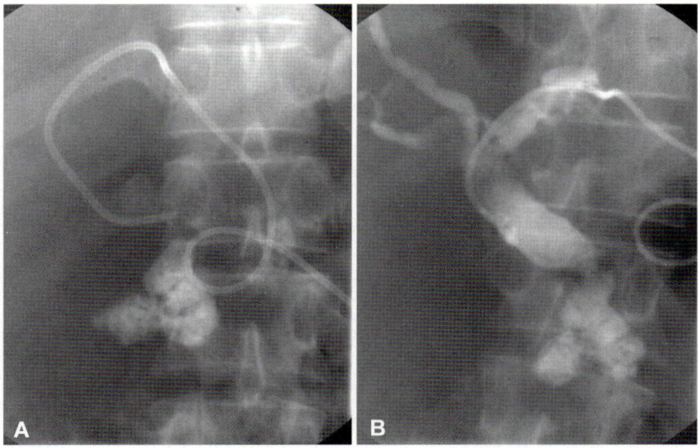

Figs 23.1A and B: External biliary drainage: (A) An 8F drainage catheter has been placed via the left hepatic duct into the CBD. (B) Cholangiogram shows complete block of the distal CBD due to chronic calcific pancreatitis

In the one step method, a 21G chiba needle is used for the puncture. A 0.018 inch guidewire is then passed through the needle and manipulated into the biliary tree. The needle is then removed and a 4F percutaneous access set manipulated over the guidewire. The sheath of the access set allows passage of a 0.035 inch stiff guidewire and the rest of the procedure is as described under US guidance.

In the two step method, a 22G chiba needle is used for puncture of the biliary radicle. After opacification of the biliary tree a second 18G puncture needle is used for re-puncture of a suitable biliary radicle.

Minimal contrast injection and minimal possible manipulation should be done on the initial day of procedure to place an indwelling catheter to avoid over-distension of the biliary tree and cholangio-venous reflux.

Two points should be kept in mind while doing the procedure. The site of puncture of the biliary radicle should be as far as possible from the obstructing lesion so as to allow safe anchorage of the external drainage catheter. Also, a longer passage makes subsequent internal drainage easier to perform. Secondary, the puncture should not be done in deep inspiration as the liver will move cephalad, thereby causing a difference in the level between the site of punctures of the skin surface and the liver. Therefore, the puncture should be performed in shallow inspiratory breath hold.

Internal and External Drainage

Internal drainage should ideally be attempted a few days after the PTBD. This allows decompression of the biliary system and the inflammatory changes to subside particularly the edema around the obstructing lesion. Injection of contrast through the drainage catheter at this stage will demonstrate the true picture. The drainage catheter is replaced with 4F or 5F catheter with a curved or angled tip over a stiff guidewire. The stenosis is crossed using a 0.035 inch hydrophilic guidewire which is rotated at the obstruction site. Once the guidewire successfully crosses the stenosis, it is manipulated into the duodenum along with the catheter. The slippy guidewire is then exchanged for a stiff guidewire over which a 8.3F ring biliary catheter or 10F pigtail catheter is placed with the loop in the duodenum (Fig. 23.2). Contrast injection to check that side holes are present both proximal and distal

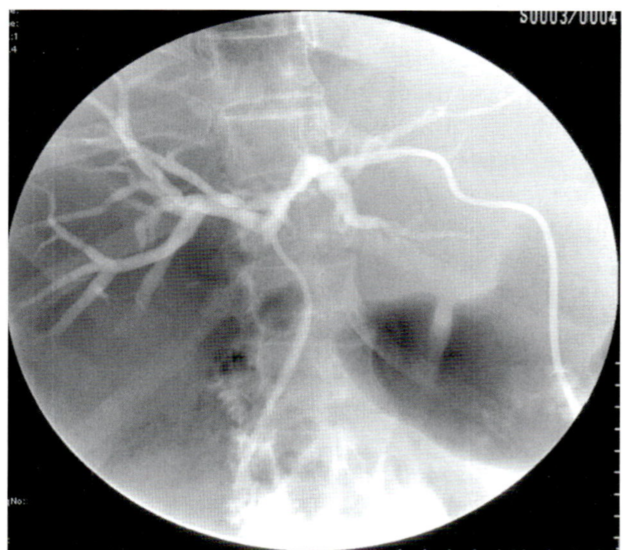

Fig. 23.2: External-internal drainage: Cholangiogram in a case of carcinoma gallbladder shows complete block of the common hepatic duct just distal to the confluence. An external-internal drainage has been instituted with the tip of the catheter in the duodenum

to the obstruction completes the procedure (Figs 23.3A and B). The catheter should initially be left to external biliary drainage. It can be capped to allow internal drainage once the bile is clear from blood or debris and the patient is afebrile. The reported technical success rate of internal drainage is above 90%.

Complications of Biliary Drainage

The complication rate for PTBD can be substantial and depends upon the pre-procedure patient status and diagnosis. The rate is higher in cases with malignant obstruction, cholangitis or coagulopathy. Major complications include hemorrhage, shock due to injection of contrast medium or sudden biliary decompression, sepsis and bile peritonitis due to slippage of catheter. Pancreatitis can occur after internal and external drainage and may be due to oedema of the CBD or obstruction of the MPD by the catheter. Pneumothorax or pleural effusion can result from inadvertent transpleural puncture. Cholangitis can develop if there is blockage of the catheter or if some intrahepatic ducts remain undrained. The reported rate of major complications is 2.5-10% while the reported mortality is 1.7%.

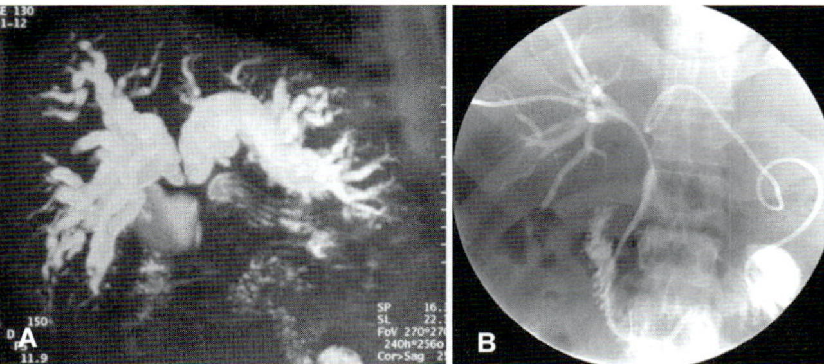

Figs 23.3A and B: A case of carcinoma gallbladder. (A) MRCP image shows a hilar "b" lock with isolation of the ductal systems. (B) An external-internal drainage catheter has been placed in the right ductal system with its tip in the second part of duodenum. An external drainage catheter is seen in the left ductal system with its tip just proximal to the confluence

Follow Up of Biliary Catheters

Patients who have undergone percutaneous biliary drainage procedure require close monitoring and regular follow-up to be able to detect catheter migration or obstruction at an early stage. Bile output, color and body temperature should be recorded every day and a watch kept on the serum bilirubin and amylase levels. The normal daily output of bile is 400-800 ml and it is clear and yellow in color. Any decrease in the output, change in color or increased turbidity are signs of cholangitis. Regular sonographic examination to look for any dilated intrahepatic radicles which denote undrained ducts or development of catheter obstruction should be performed. Some authors advocate daily gentle flushing of the catheter with 5-10 ml of normal saline or sterile water to prevent collection of debris which causes catheter blockage. If the patients are being discharged home with the catheter *in situ,* they should instructed in catheter care. In case of development of fever, the patients should be instructed to open the cap of the catheter to allow external drainage and to report back to the hospital. Catheters should be exchanged every 2-3 months to prevent blockage or breakage.

Biliary Stenting

Biliary endoprostheses may be either plastic or metallic and various kinds of both types are available. An external drainage tube can be uncomfortable or of psychological disadvantage to the patient particularly in cases of malignant obstruction. An internal stent also prevents the complications of peri-catheter biliary leakage or slippage. The disadvantage of stents is the need for performing a new procedure (PTBD or ERCP) in case of stent obstruction.

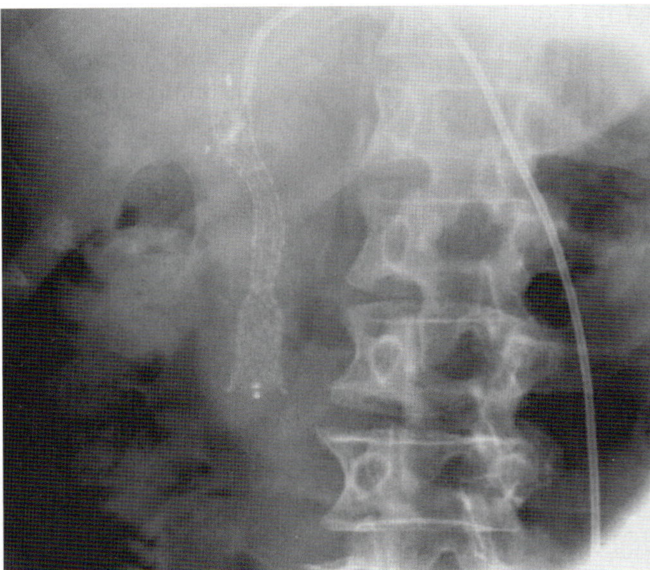

Fig. 23.4: A single metallic self-expanding stent placed in the distal CBD in a case of carcinoma head of the pancreas

Metallic stents are used almost exclusively for malignant obstruction, as they have poor long-term patency rates and are therefore not used for the treatment of benign disease. The major advantage of metallic stents is that they can be inserted in a contracted state through a small calibre tract and can achieve a large lumen (upto to 10mm) following expansion. They are available as self expanding or balloon mounted stents (Fig. 23.4). These stents are less prone to migration and show a better patency rate than plastic stents. The disadvantages include the high cost and difficulty in removal. Plastic stents are cheap but have many disadvantages including early occlusion due to the small luminal diameter (Figs 23.5A and B), frequent migration and a traumatic insertion procedure due to the large tract size required. Because of the large calibre, endoscopic insertion is done more frequently than the percutaneous route.

In cases of CBD obstruction, a single stent usually suffices. In cases of hilar obstruction two stents may be required which can be placed in a 'T' or 'Y' configuration (Figs 23.6A to D). Multiple stents may be placed in cases of involvement of the secondary confluences. The reported patency rate for palliative metallic stents in malignant obstruction is about 50% at 6 months. Causes of stent obstruction include tumor in-growth through the stent, tumor overgrowth either proximal or distal to the stent, and biliary sludge and debris. Recently the role of PTFE covered stents is being investigated in an attempt to prolong patency.

Intraluminal Brachytherapy with PTBD

In cases with unresectable tumors causing biliary obstruction, high dose rate intraluminal brachytherapy (ILBT) using Iridium-192 can be delivered selectively to the tumor whilst avoiding the side effects of external radiotherapy. This treatment can be offered in patients who have a single tumor with an overall stricture length

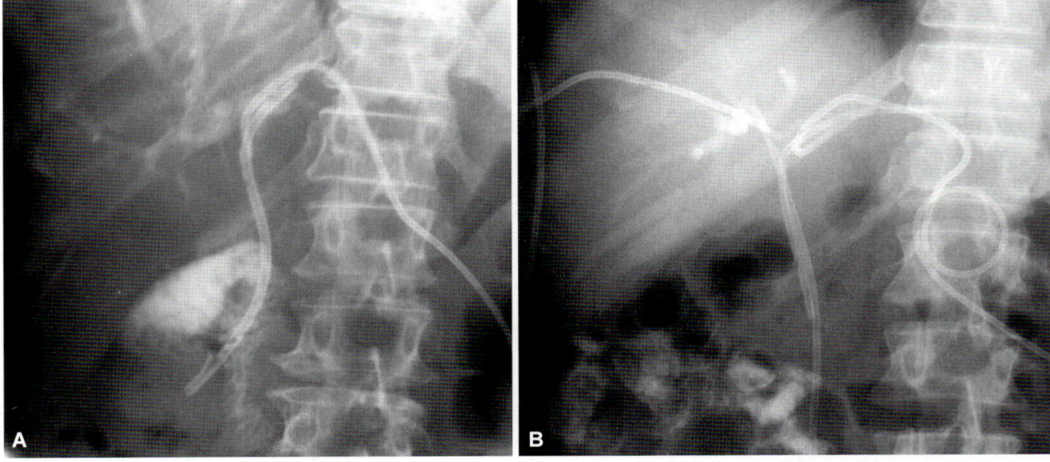

Figs 23.5A and B: Plastic biliary endoprostheses. (A) A single plastic endoprosthesis has been inserted via the left duct. The distal end is in the duodenum while the proximal end is in the left main duct. An external drainage catheter has also been placed as a safety measure in the immediate post-procedure period (B) Two plastic stents have been placed via both right and left ducts in a case of hilar obstruction. Safety external drainage catheters are also seen

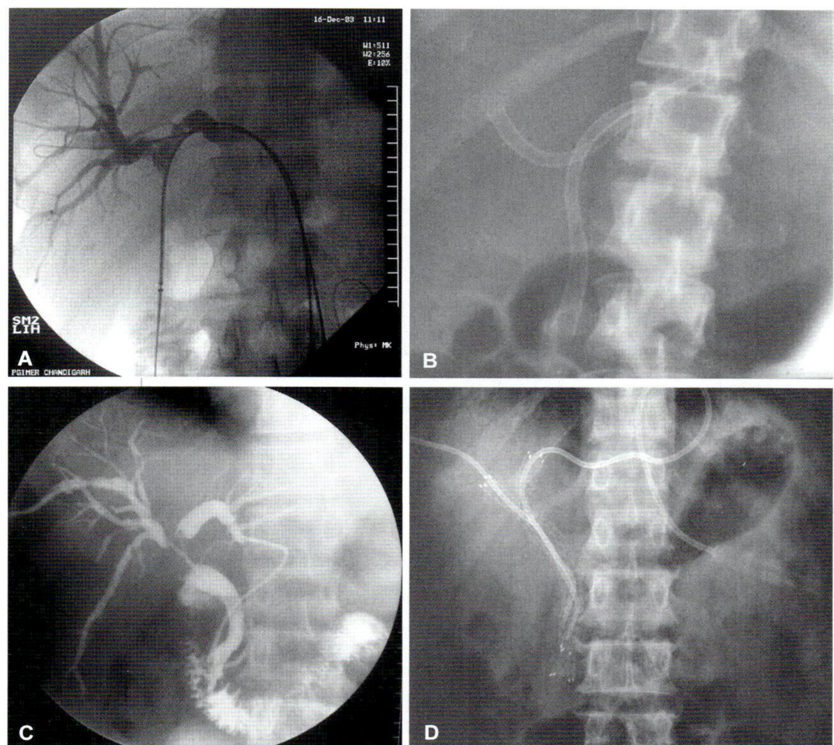

Figs 23.6A to D: Hilar obstruction. (A) T-stenting: An external-internal drainage is present on the left side along with a left to right drainage. A stiff guide-wire has been anchored in the right ductal system and a stent has been placed across the proximal CHD block. (B) Two metallic stents placed in a 'T' configuration. (C) Y-stenting: Cholangiogram shows an external-internal drainage catheter *in situ* in both ductal systems. (D) Two metallic self-expanding stents have been placed in a 'Y' configuration

of less than 6 cm and the absence of distant disease. After PTBD, an internal-external drainage is instituted. The brachytherapy catheter is passed through the drainage catheter and positioned with its tip 1 cm beyond the distal end of the stricture (Figs 23.7A and B). The unit is programmed to treat the stricture length and 1 cm beyond and proximal to the stricture. Studies have shown a significant improvement in the quality of life when ILBT is combined with PTBD though there is no significant improvement in survival or stent patency.

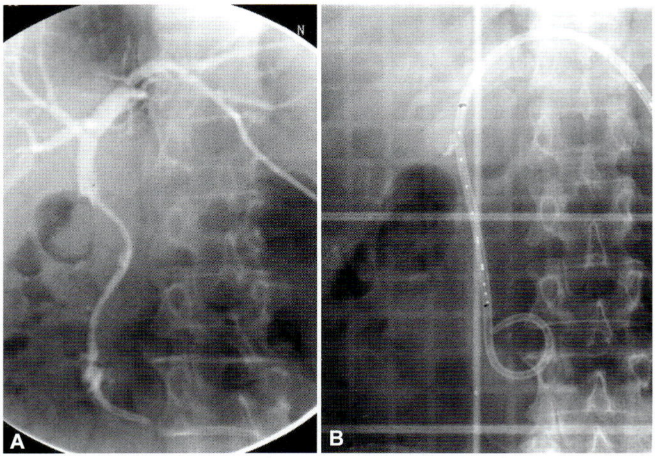

Figs 23.7A and B: Intraluminal brachytherapy. (A) Cholangiogram after external-internal drainage demonstrates a 4cm stricture in the mid CBD. (B) A 10F pigtail catheter has been placed with its tip in the duodenum. Simulator film shows placement of the brachytherapy catheter with its tip 1cm beyond the distal end of the stricture

Dilatation of Benign Biliary Structures

Most benign biliary strictures are treated surgically with creation of biliary enteric anastomoses. A considerable number suffer recurrence of the stricture after surgical treatment and these are even more difficult to treat surgically. Balloon dilatation of these strictures is a therapeutic option. The technique consists of crossing the stricture with a guidewire after performing a PTBD. The stricture is inflated with an 8-10 mm balloon and a large diameter catheter is placed across the stricture to induce non-stenosed fibrosis (Figs 23.8A and B). This can provide an easy access for re-intervention. The catheter is kept across the stricture for a few weeks and then retracted proximal to the stricture and capped. The patient is monitored for a few days to ensure that the bile is flowing internally. The external catheter is removed if the patient remains asymptomatic. Success rates of 70-93% have been reported in literature.

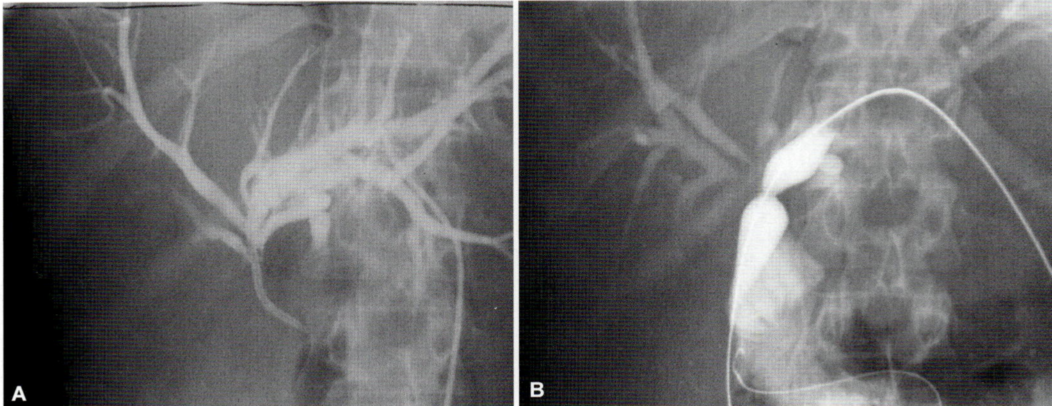

Figs 23.8A and B: Balloon dilatation of benign biliary stricture in a case of postoperative choledochojejunostomy stricture. (A) Drainage catheter has been placed across the stricture with its tip in the jejunal loop via the left hepatic duct. (B) Balloon dilatation of the stricture. Note the "waist" formation in the balloon at the stricture site

Percutaneous Cholecystostomy

Cholecystostomy may be used as a temporizing measure in patients of acute cholecystitis who are critically ill and therefore cannot undergo surgery. After the patient's condition is stabilized, cholecystectomy as the definitive treatment will still be required. However in acalculous cholecystitis, percutaneous drainage may be the only treatment required. Cholecystostomy can also provide a temporizing preoperative maneuver in patients with obstructive jaundice in whom the bile ducts are not dilated and the level of obstruction is distal to the insertion of the cystic duct.

Technique

The gallbladder is punctured under US guidance. There are two approach routes available for puncturing the gall bladder. The transhepatic route is usually preferred as the transperitoneal approach carries a greater risk of bile peritonitis. Using the transhepatic route the gallbladder is punctured where it is fixed to the liver, generally at the junction between the cephalic and middle third of the body. In the transperitoneal approach, the gall bladder is punctured at the point where it lies closest to the anterior abdominal wall. The trocar technique is generally used for direct puncture while the seldinger technique is preferred for the transhepatic route.

An 18G needle is used to puncture the gallbladder and sample collected for gram staining and culture. A small amount of contrast is then injected to opacify the gallbladder for the subsequent steps for which fluoroscopic guidance is used. A J-shaped soft tip guidewire is then inserted through the needle and coiled within the lumen. After dilating the tract, a 7F or 8F catheter having an anchor mechanism or of the pigtail type is placed within the gallbladder and sutured to the skin. The catheter is left to drain by gravity (Figs 23.9A to C).

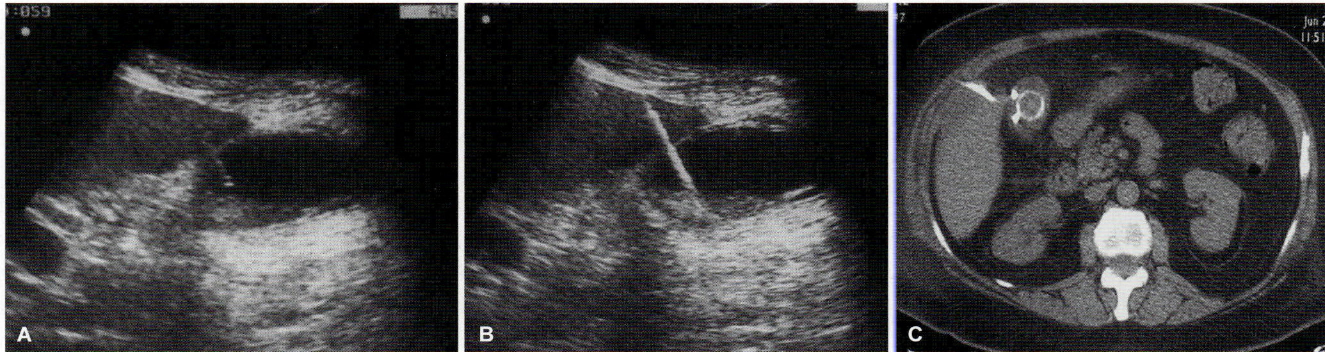

Figs 23.9A to C: Percutaneous cholecystostomy in a case of empyema of the gallbladder. (A) Sonogram demonstrates tip of the puncture needle in the lumen of the gallbladder placed via the transhepatic approach. (B) Guide-wire is seen *in situ*. (C) Follow-up CT image shows the loop of the drainage catheter in the lumen of the gallbladder

If surgery is not considered as in acalculus cholecystitis, the catheter can be removed once the patient's signs and symptoms resolve and a sufficient time has elapsed for the tract to mature. Removal of the catheter before tract maturation may result in leakage of bile and peritonitis.

Complications

The complications which can occur following percutaneous cholecystostomy include bile peritonitis, hemobilia and gall bladder perforation. Vaso-vagal reaction due to tube placement can be managed with atropine. Hemorrhage can at times be fatal. Minimal manipulations should be done at the time of initial drainage to avoid complications.

Gallbladder Biopsy

Percutaneous image guided fine needle aspiration biopsy of the gallbladder is a widely used and effective method for the diagnosis of gallbladder masses. The accuracy for diagnosing malignancy is more than 90%. It is particularly recommended in patients with inoperable disease for obtaining a histological diagnosis.

BIBLIOGRAPHY

1. Baijal SS, Dhiman RK, Gupta S, et al. Percutaneous transhepatic biliary drainage in the management of obstructive jaundice. Trop Gastroenterol 1997;18(4): 167-71.
2. Becker CD, Glattli A, Maibach R, Baer HU. Percutaneous palliation of malignant obstructive jaundice with the wallstent endoprosthesis: follow up and re-intervention in patients with hilar and non-hilar obstruction. J Vasc Interv Radiol 1993;4(5):597-604.
3. Bezzi M, Zolovkins A, Cantisani V, et al. New ePTFE/ FEP- covered stent in the palliative treatment of malignant biliary obstruction. J Vasc Interv Radiol 2002;13(6): 581-9.
4. Boggi U, DiCandio G, Campatelli A, et al. Percutaneous cholecystostomy for acute cholecystitis in critically ill patients. Hepatogastroenterology 1999;46(25):121-5.
5. Born P, Rösch T, Brûhl K, et al. Long term results of endoscopic and percutaneous transhepatic treatment of benign biliary strictures. Endoscopy 1999;31(a):725-31.
6. Burke DR, Lewis CA, Cardella JF, et al. Quality improvement guidelines for percutaneous transhepatic cholangiography and biliary drainage. J Vasc Interv Radiol 2003;14:243-6.
7. Coons H. Metallic stents for the treatment of biliary obstruction: a report of 100 cases. Cardiovasc Intervent Radiol 1992;15(6):367-74.
8. Davis CA, Landercasper J, Gundersen LH, Lambert PJ. Effective use of percutaneous cholecystostomy in high risk surgical patients: techniques, tube management and results. Arch Surg 1999;134(7):727-31.
9. Gabelmann A, Hamid H, Brambs HJ, Rieber A. Metallic stents in benign biliary strictures: long-term effectiveness and interventional management of stent occlusion. AJR Am J Roentgenol 2001;177(4):813-7.
10. Garber SJ, Matbieson JR, Cooperberg PL, et al. Percutaneous cholecystostomy: safety of the transperitoneal route. J Vasc Interv Radiol 1994;5:295-8.
11. Golfieri R, Giampalma E, Renzulli M, et al. Unresectable hilar cholangiocarcinoma: multimodality approach with percutaneous treatment associated with radiotherapy and chemotherapy. In Vivo 2006;20(6):757-60.
12. Harbin WP, Mueller PR, Ferrucci JT. Transhepatic cholangiography: complications and use patterns of the fine-needle technique: a multiinstitutional survey. Radiology 1980;135(1):15-22.
13. Inoue H. Diagnosis of cancer spread using percutaneous transhepatic biliary cholangioscopy-guided ultrasonography for malignant bile duct stenosis. Diagn Ther Endosc 2001;7(3-4):159-64.
14. Kiviniemi H, Makela JT, Autio R, et al. Percutaneous cholecystostomy in acute cholecystitis in high risk patients: an analysis of 69 patients. Int Surg 1998;83(4):299-302.
15. Kim ES, Lee B, Won JY, Choi JY, Lee D. Percutaneous transhepatic biliary drainage may serve as a successful rescue procedure in failed cases of endoscopic therapy for a post-living donor liver transplantation biliary stricture. Gastrointest Endosc 2008. [Epub ahead of print].
16. Kocher M, Cerná M, Havlik R, Král V, Gryga A, Duda M. Percutaneous treatment of benign bile duct strictures. Eur J Radiol 2007;62(2):170-74.
17. Lee BH, Choe DH, Lee JH, et al. Metallic stents in malignant biliary obstruction: prospective long-term clinical results. AJR Am J Roentgenol 1997;168(3):741-5.
18. Lee W, Kim GC, Kim JY, et al. Ultrasound and fluoroscopy guided percutaneous transhepatic biliary drainage in patients with nondilated bile ducts. Abdom Imaging 2008. [Epub ahead of print].
19. Lillemoe KD, Melton GB, Cameron JL, et al. Postoperative bile duct strictures: management and outcome in the 1990s. Ann Surg 2000; 232(3):430-41.
20. Moore AV Jr, Illescas FF, Mills SR, et al. Percutaneous dilatation of benign biliary strictures. Radiology 1987;163(3):625-8.
21. Mueller PR, Ferrucci JT Jr, Teplick SK, et al. Biliary stent endoprosthesis: analysis of complications in 113 patients. Radiology 1985;156(3):637-9.
22. Mueller PR, vanSonnenberg E, Ferrucci JT Jr. Percutaneous biliary drainage, technical and catheter-related problems in 200 procedures. AJR Am J Roentgenol 1982;138:17-23.

23. Mueller PR, vanSonnenberg E, Ferrucci JT Jr, et al. Biliary stricture dilatation: multicentre review of clinical management in 73 patients. Radiology 1986;160(1):17-22.
24. Saluja SS, Gulati M, Garg PK, et al. Endoscopic or percutaneous biliary drainage for gall bladder cancer: a randomized trial and quality of life assessment. Clin Gastroenterol Hepatol 2008. [Epub ahead of print].
25. Sawada S, Tanigawa N. Percutaneous transhepatic biliary drainage. In Interventional Radiology. Han MC, Park JH (Eds). Seoul, Korea: Ilchokak :1999.
26. Tsuyuguchi T, Takada T, Kawarada Y, et al. Techniques of biliary drainage for acute cholecystitis: Tokyo guidelines. Hepatobiliary Pancreat Surg 2007;14(1):46-51.
27. vanSonnenberg E, D'Agostino HB, Goodacre BW, et al. Percutaneous gall bladder puncture and cholecystostomy: results, complications and caveats for safety. Radiology 1992; 183:167-80.
28. Yee AC, Ho CS. Complications of percutaneous biliary drainage: benign vs malignant diseases. AJR Am J Roentgenol 1987; 148(6):1207-9.

Chapter Twenty-four

Interventional Treatment of Liver Tumors

Deep Narayan Srivastava, Shivanand Gamanagatti

INTRODUCTION

In the treatment of patients suffering from liver tumors various therapeutic interventional techniques have been developed employing angiographic and percutaneous routes. These are:

- chemical ablation with ethanol (PEI) or acetic acid (PAI)
- radiofrequency ablation (RFA)
- transcatheter arterial chemembolization (TACE)
- transcatheter arterial embolization (TAE)
- transcatheter arterial radionuclide therapy (TART)
- right portal-vein embolization
- hepatic vein stenting.

TREATMENT OF LIVER TUMORS

Hepatocellular Carcinoma (HCC)

Recent advances in diagnostic imaging have improved the detection rate of small HCC in high-risk populations;[1] as a result the number of patients undergoing surgery have increased. However, there are patients with extensive lesions or with concurrent cirrhosis or intrahepatic metastases who cannot undergo surgical resection of HCC. To improve the survival rate of such patients, various methods have been developed employing angiographic and percutaneous techniques of therapeutic intervention.[2] These are described below:

Chemical Ablation

This technique involves direct percutaneous injection of ethanol or acetic acid into a liver tumor under ultrasound or CT guidance. Percutaneous injection of ethanol (PEI) and percutaneous injection of acetic acid (PAI) result in coagulative necrosis and fibrosis of tumor by promoting denaturation of protiens and small vessel thrombosis. Ninety-five percent ethanol is the most commonly used agent and it is highly effective for the treatment of small liver tumors. HCC initially shows regional growth so local therapy is beneficial. The features of HCC that rationalize the ethanol therapy are its hypervascularity and the difference in consistency between neoplastic and cirrhotic tissue. Since HCC is softer than the surrounding cirrhotic tissue, ethanol diffuses within it easily and selectively and at the same time; hypervascularity ensures its uniform distribution within the rich network of neoplastic sinusoids.[3] PEI is indicated in majority of patients except in candidates for liver transplantation and surgical resection. This technique is particularly useful for small lesions (< 3 cm in diameter) but not of much help in larger lesions because alcohol diffusion is often incomplete and residual viable neoplastic tissue can persist along the periphery of the nodule or in portions isolated by septa. It is contraindicated in surface lesions, tumor with ascites or coagulopathy. PEI can be done alone or in combination with other angiographic (TACE or TAE) and percutaneous (RFA) therapeutic techniques.[4-7] Alcohol is injected in multiple sessions under radiological guidance using long needle (spinal/closed tip with few terminal side holes). Alcohol injection is started from deepest to superficial portion of the tumor avoiding direction injection into hepatic vein. The total amount of alcohol is calculated by using a formula:

$4/3\pi (r + 0.5)^3$ ml, where r = radius of lesion in cm and 0.5 is an added "safety factor". Multiple sessions of ethanol injections are frequently required for complete ablation. These may be performed once or twice a week depending upon liver function tests and patient's general condition.

In percutaneous acetic acid injection 50% concentration of acetic acid is normally used. The amount of acetic acid in milliliters required to achieve complete response is equal to three times the diameter of lesion in centimeters. Mechanism of action of acetic acid is essentially identical to that of ethanol.

The procedure can be done on an outdoor basis, however short admission for six hours after the procedure is preferred. The patient is instructed for overnight fasting, premedication is given and the procedure is done under aseptic conditions and local anesthesia. At a time one to eight milliliters at different sites is injected by one or more injections. The perfused area usually spreads within a radius of 2-3 cm and is seen as a patch of hyperechogenicity on ultrasound (Figs 24.1A to D). The injection should be stopped if there is leakage outside the lesion or when diffusion is not clearly visible. Direct injection into the hepatic vein may lead to cardiopulmonary collapse and should be avoided. The needle is slowly withdrawn after 10-30 seconds of the alcohol or acetic acid injection to avoid reflux into adjacent tissues.

Radiofrequency Ablation (RFA)

Radiofrequency ablation is a newly developed commonly used percutaneous image guided tumor ablation technique for small HCC as well as metastatic deposits. It induces necrosis of the tumor by deposition of thermal energy around the tip of the electrode inserted in the tumor. There are mainly two basic types of electrodes: cooled tip/noncooled tip and nonexpendable/expandable array electrodes. In cooled tip type electrodes there is continuous cooling of the needle tip by circulating saline allows tissue heating and necrosis far from the electrode without tissue charring. Bipolar and multipolar technology is the latest addition in radiofrequency ablation. This eliminates the need of a grounding pad and is also more effective with ablation of large area.[4,6]

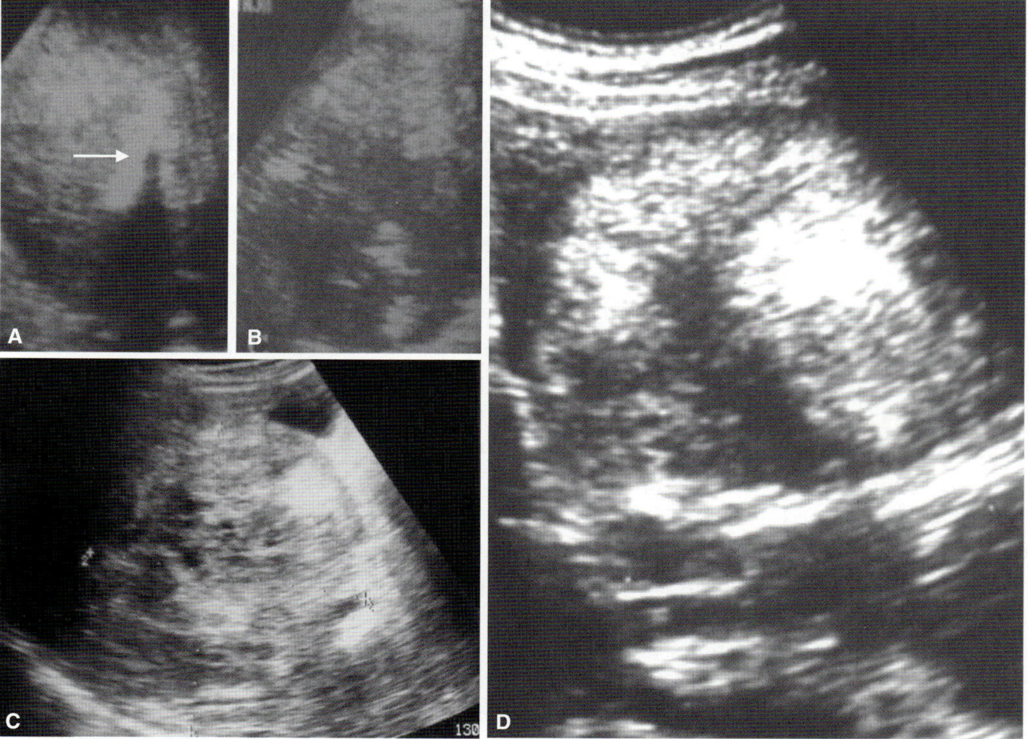

Figs 24.1A to D: Percutaneous alcohol injection under ultrasound guidance in HCC. Alcohol is injected in the deepest portion (A) followed by superficial portion (B) and (C) of the tumor with the help of a long needle (arrow). The perfused areas are seen as patches of hyperechogenicity (D)

RFA is ideally suited for smaller (< 3 cm) lesions. Although tumors up to 5 cm diameter can be ablated with RFA, chances of complete ablation diminish with increase in tumor diameter. The technique can also be used to treat multiple lesions and up to five lesions can be safely treated in single or multiple sittings. Lesions close to main branches of portal or hepatic veins are difficult to treat as continuous high blood flow in these vessels will have cooling effect because the thermal energy will be dissipated away. If the lesion is close to liver capsule or gall bladder, chances of peritonitis or cholecystitis respectively are high. For these reasons, lesions that do not have atleast 1 cm of normal liver parenchyma separating it from the liver capsule, gall bladder, porta hepatis or major vessels are considered unsuitable for RFA.

Technique

The radiofrequency probe is electrically insulated in its proximal part while the short distal part near the tip is uninsulated from which the electric current is passed into the tumor. It is inserted into the lesion under either ultrasound or CT guidance. The procedure is usually performed under adequate sedation. A grounding pad is applied to patient's thigh to complete the electric circuit in monopolar type of electrode. Alternating current is passed through the probe with energies ranging from 60 to 100 watts for a period of 6 to 12 minutes. Rapid change in the polarity of electric current results in fast oscillations of intracellular molecules, which in turn causes friction and heat generation. Local temperature of more than 60°C is maintained for more than 5 minutes.

High temperature in close proximity of probe tip may result in charring of tissue. This increases the impedance and decreases the deposition of heat. To avoid this, some probes have inbuilt mechanism to continuously circulate cooled water in the tip. These types of probes are called cooled tip electrodes. Other modifications in probe design include multiple prongs or branches of the electrodes, which flare out like umbrella inside the lesion. These help to deposit heat at multiple points and ensure uniform ablation over large volumes. Injection of saline in tumor has been shown to decrease its impedance and hence one design of a probe also has facility to inject saline in the tumor through side channels during the procedure. In multipolar technology, multiple electrodes can be placed inside the tumor and at a time any two electrodes can be selected. This technology is useful in the treatment of large lesions.

Complications of the procedure are rare and include severe pain after the procedure, local hemorrhage, peritonitis, cholecystitis, colitis, vascular injury or thrombosis. These can be avoided with careful selection of the lesions. The procedure is usually well tolerated. However, good pain management after the procedure is essential. The risk of tumor seedling during or after the procedure can be reduced by ablating the track.[8]

Follow-up

Follow-up imaging is required to assess the degree of necrosis and completeness of the ablation. Follow up CT shows low-density non-enhancing area, which corresponds to necrosis (Figs 24.2A to C). A peripheral thin hyperemic rim is usually seen which represent inflammatory reaction to the thermal injury. It may be difficult to differentiate it from residual tumor, however, it usually disappears within a month.

Tumor response rates for RFA appear to be inversely proportional to the tumor size. Tumors of less than 2 cm diameter show 85% response rate but it decreases to 35% for tumors of 3 cm diameter. Overall survival rates of 94% and 40% are reported for tumors of less than 3 cm diameter at the end of 1 and 5 years respectively.[8] Long-term results of multipolar technology are awaited.

Transcatheter Arterial Chemoembolization (TACE)

TACE has become the mainstay of therapy for unresectable HCC. It involves intra-arterial delivery of high concentrations of chemotherapeutic agent emulsified in lipiodol, combined with an embolic agent directly to the tumor. The principle is based on differential blood supply to the liver and to the tumors. Whereas the normal liver receives most of its blood supply from portal vein, hepatic arteries primarily feed the liver tumors. Commonly used chemotherapeutic agents are adriamycin, epirubicin, mitomycin-C and cisplatin, etc.[6] The role of preoperative chemoembolization is controversial.[6]

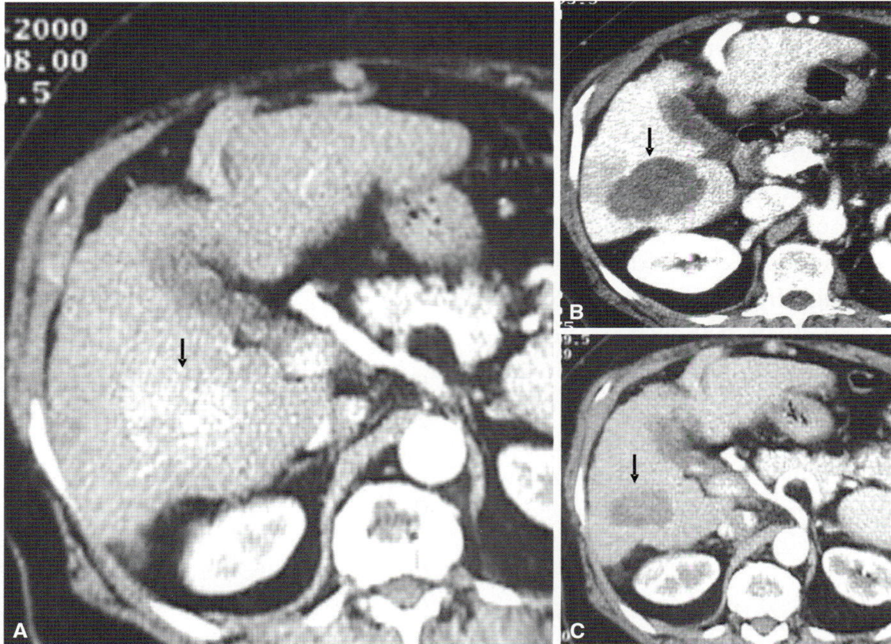

Figs 24.2A to C: Pre-ablation arterial phase CT liver showing vascular tumor (arrow) in segment VI, complete necrosis and reduction in size (arrow) one year (B) and 2 year (C) after radiofrequency ablation. The patient died after two and half year due to hepatic failure secondary to advanced cirrhosis

This treatment is contraindicated in few situations, viz. poor hepatic function, serum bilirubin > 2.0 mg/dl and thrombosed main portal vein.

Technique

Lipiodol is mixed with chemotherapeutic drug and is infused in hepatic artery followed by gel foam embolization under angiographic guidance (Fig. 24.3). The lipiodol is iodine containing lipid (475 mg/ml, 38% by weight) which is derived from poppy seed oil and is commercially available in 10 and 20 ml sterile ampoules.

TACE results in selective tumor necrosis due to ischemia and is associated with preservation of most of the normal liver. Lipiodol along with chemotherapeutic drug concentrates in malignant cells due to tumor vascularity and lack of lymphatics. However, it is cleared from non-malignant cells of the liver. This enables chemotherapeutic agent to remain in contact with tumor cells for prolonged period of time. Multiple sessions may be required depending on the follow-up imaging.

Large exophytic masses and surface lesions may get extrahepatic arterial supply. These feeding vessels are also used for TACE to prevent tumor recurrences.

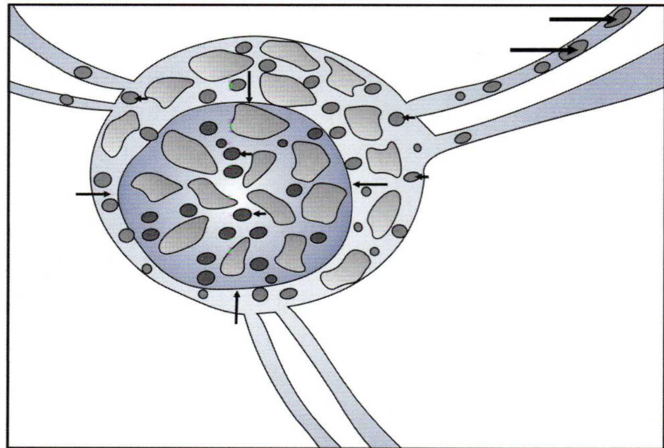

Fig. 24.3: Diagrammatic representation of transcatheter chemoembolization. Lipiodol is mixed with chemotherapeutic drug and is infused in hepatic artery (arrow heads) followed by gel foam embolization (long arrows) of the arterial branches. The dark area represents the tumor (small arrows)

Recently polyvinyl alcohol (PVA) microspheres are available in different sizes. These microspheres can be loaded with doxorubicin and can be infused into feeding tumor arteries. These doxorubicin beads (DC beads) allows accurate and controlled loading of doxorubicin thereby achieving better tumor response rates.[9]

Follow-up

Patients are followed with CT or MRI. Imaging features that need to be analyzed include reduction in size, amount of necrosis and lipiodol retention (Figs 24.4A to D). Clinical factors like symptomatic improvement, decrease in tumor markers, improved quality of life and patient survival are also assessed. TACE has shown better tumor response rate than systemic chemotherapy. TACE achieves substantial tumor necrosis while preserving normal liver, thereby delaying progression to liver failure. Although the true effect of TACE on patient survival remains unclear, TACE is an effective bridge to potentially curative treatments, including surgical resection and liver transplantation. These are still unanswered questions on how to improve its efficacy and ultimately prolong patient survival. A recent randomized controlled trial on unresectable HCC has shown that TACE has survival benefits of 57% and 26% at 1 and 3 years against 32% and 3% respectively in patients receiving other forms of supportive care.[10]

Transcatheter Arterial Embolization (TAE)

In this, tumor is embolized with intra-arterial temporary or permanent embolizing materials in single or multiple sessions. It has been proved to be a less effective palliative treatment especially for large and peripherally located HCC due to development of collateral circulation.

Transcatheter arterial embolization of the tumor may be done as an emergency procedure to reduce gastro-intestinal hemorrhage in selected patients. Gastro-intestinal hemorrhage from hepatocellular carcinoma (HCC) during the natural course of the tumor is unusual. The causes of massive intermittent gastrointestinal bleeding may be either due to varices or due to direct invasion of duodenum, transverse colon and stomach by the tumor. The variceal bleeding may be consequent to portal hypertension secondary to intra-tumoral arterioportal shunts (Figs 24.5A to D). These patients may respond well to TAE.[6] Some studies have shown that TAE is an effective method for palliative treatment in such patients.[6,7]

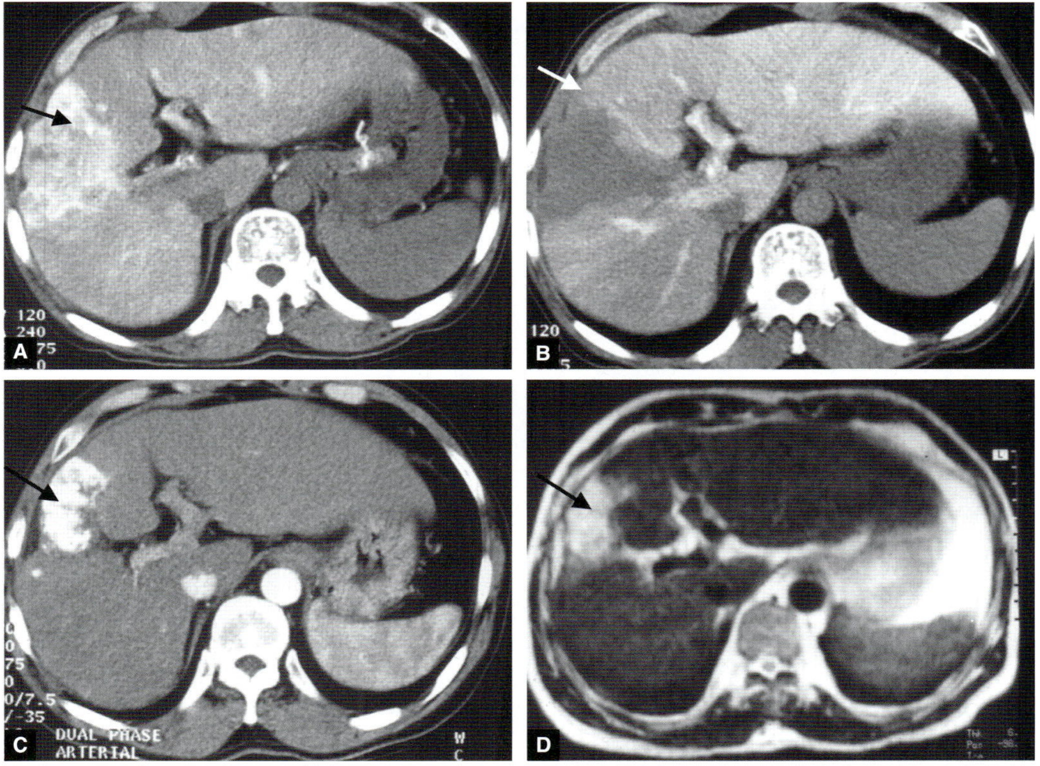

Figs 24.4A to D: Pre (A and B) and Post-treatment CT (C) and MR (D) of Liver showing vascular mass (arrows) in segments IV and V. The mass is reduced in size after TACE

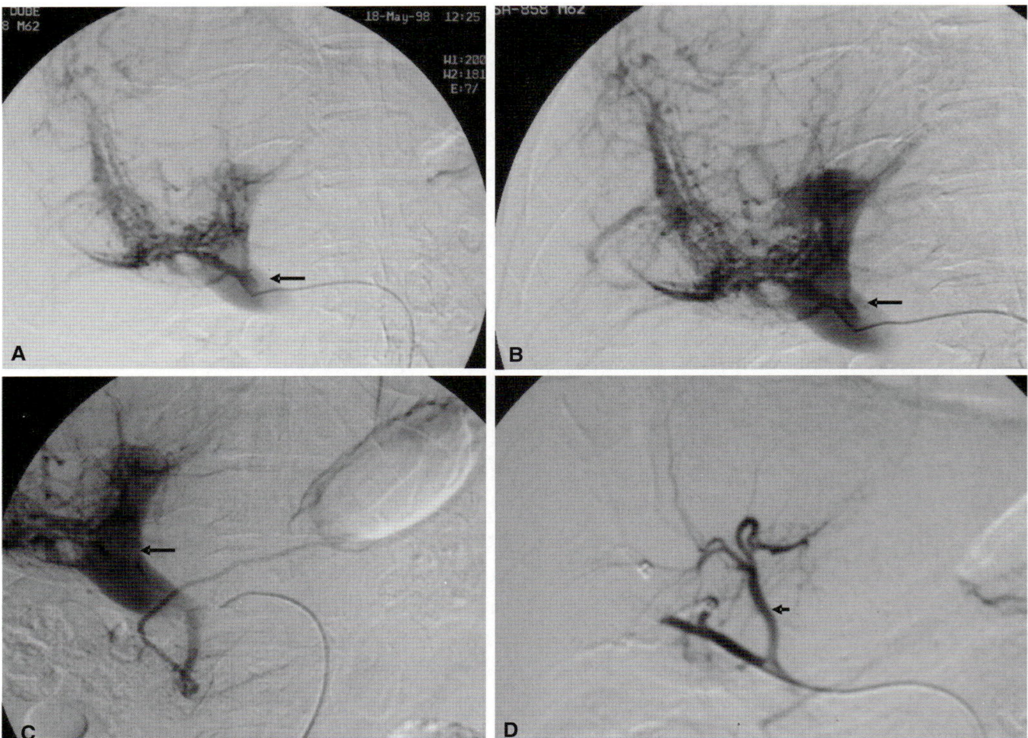

Figs 24.5A to D: A 62-year-male presented with massive upper gastrointestinal hemorrhage (GIH) due to variceal rupture secondary to intratumoral arterioportal shunts causing portal hypertension. The tumor (HCC) was embolized and GIH was stopped. Hepatic arteriograms (A-C) are showing tumor vascularity with simultaneous opacification of portal vein (arrows). The right hepatic artery branches were embolized with fibred steel coils. The postembolization angiogram is not showing opacification of portal vein (D). The left hepatic artery was not embolized (arrowhead)

Transarterial Radionuclide Therapy (TART)

External radiotherapy of whole or part of the liver with or without systemic chemotherapy or surgery has not shown good results.[11] Hemodynamic principles and techniques of TART are similar as TACE. Internal radiotherapy by injection of isotopes ([131]Iodine-lipiodol,[188] Re-lipiodol and[90] Yttrium) into the hepatic artery has shown improvement in survival. The technique is new and many multicenter prospective studies are being conducted. Results of these studies have shown that TART appears to be a safe, effective and promising therapeutic option in patients with inoperable HCC (Figs 24.6A to E).[11] TART can also be used in HCC with portal vein tumor thrombosis.

Right Portal Vein Embolization

Percutaneous right portal vein embolization has become an important preoperative treatment in patients who are to undergo extensive liver resection due to hepatic malignancy. It reduces post-operative hepatic failure in major right hepatectomy in patients with small left lobe. The aim is to occlude the branches of right lobe, which is to be resected and to preserve the branches of left lobe. This results in compensatory hypertrophy of the left lobe and hence subsequent increase in the functional reserve of the liver. The procedure is done percutaneously using both ultrasound and angiography guidance usually three weeks before surgery (Figs 24.7A to E).[6] This technique is mainly useful in noncirrhotic livers with malignant tumor confined to segments of right lobe.

Hepatic Vein Stenting

The association of Budd-Chiari syndrome and HCC is favored by two conditions. First, HCC can cause obstruction of the main hepatic veins or inferior vena cava due to endoluminal invasion by the tumor. This produces an acute or fulminant variant of Budd-Chiari syndrome, which has a poor prognosis. Second, HCC

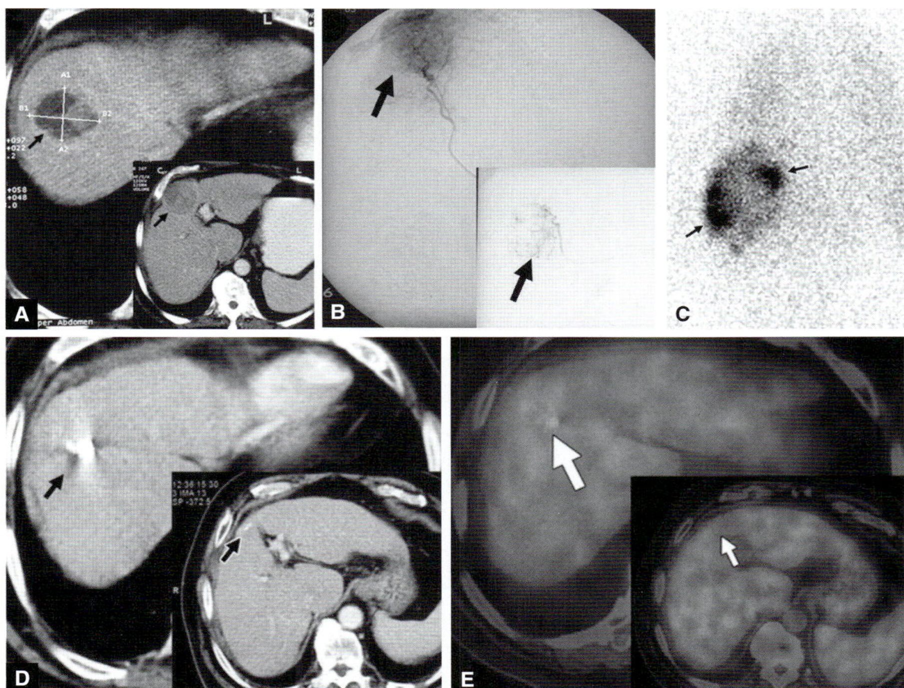

Figs 24.6A to E: A 69-year-old man with two HCC lesions involving both lobes of the liver. Both lesions were completely ablated after two doses of ^{188}Re HDD iodized oil at three-monthly intervals. At the time of this writing, the patient was alive and ambulatory with normal serum AFP levels and no evidence of mass at 3-year follow-up CT. (A) Pretherapy axial contrast enhanced CT shows two lesions (arrows) : One each in segments IV and VIII. (B) Angiogram shows increased vascularity in both lesions (arrows). (C) Posttreatment Re^{188} whole-body scan shows radiotracer accumulation in the tumors (arrows), with faint visualization of lungs and no radiotracer uptake in the thyroid, gastrointestinal tract, or anywhere else. (D) Repeat CT obtained 3 months after the second dose shows complete disappearance of both lesions (arrows). Small radiopaque area in segment IV lesion (appearing to be enhancing HCC mass in larger arterial phase image) is actually a small amount of iodized oil, which was seen in all CT scanning phases (non contrast, arterial, portal venous, and delayed). (E) Positron emission tomography / CT scan obtained 2 years after treatment also shows no evidence of residual or recurrent disease (arrows). Inset images show segment IV lesion

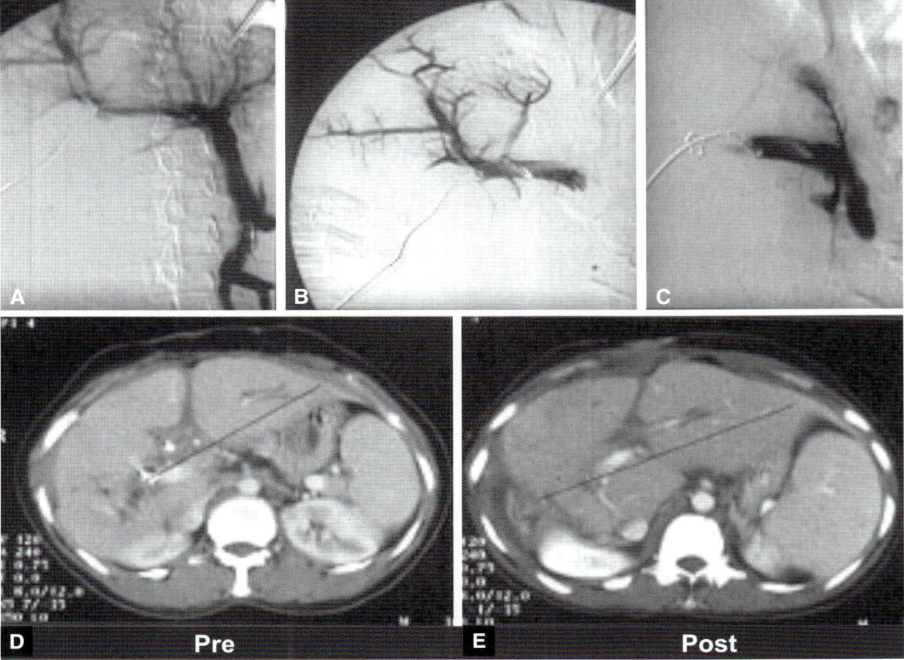

Figs 24.7A to E: Right portal vein was punctured and a portogram was taken (A). The catheter was withdrawn and right branch was embolized (B and C). Preprocedure (D) and first week post operative (E) CT showing significant left lobe hypertrophy

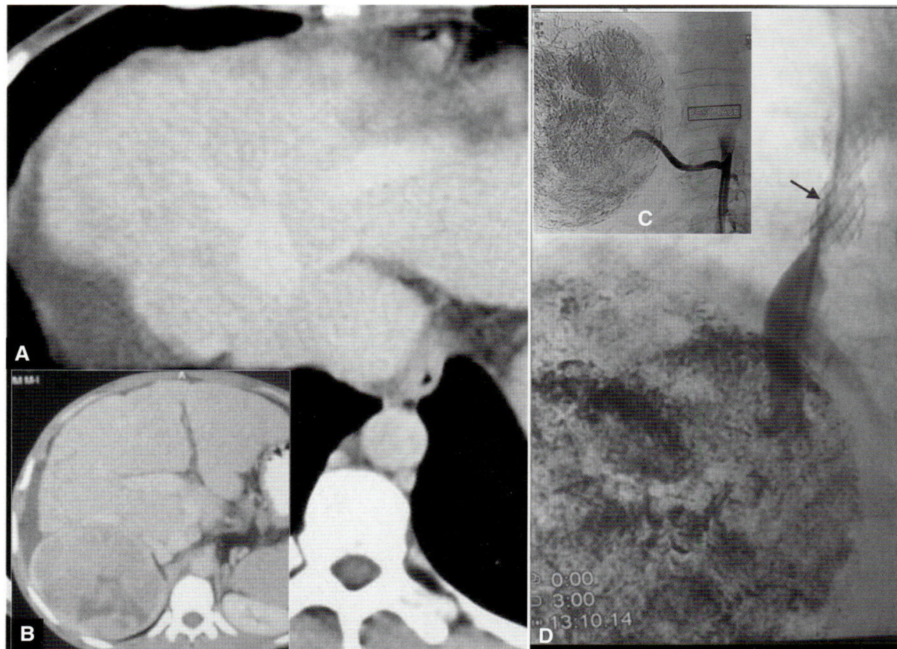

Figs 24.8A to D: A 32-year-male with HCC secondary to hepatic vein outflow tract obstruction (HVOTO) was treated with TACE and hepatic vein stenting. He developed lung metastases on one year follow-up CT and is presently on systemic chemotherapy. Contrast enhanced CT liver (A & B) showing right lobe HCC with HVOTO. The tumor was treated with chemoembolization (C) and HVOTO by right hepatic vein stenting (arrow) (D)

can develop in patients with chronic Budd-Chiari syndrome and accounts for 0.7% of all the cases of HCC. HCC is most common in patients with membranous obstruction of the vena cava. These patients can be managed effectively by combined interventional techniques; hepatic vein stenting or IVC dilatation to relieve the venous obstruction combined with trans-arterial chemoembolization for the hepatocellular carcinoma (Figs 24.8A to D).

METASTATIC TUMORS OF LIVER

Various angiographic and percutaneous interventional techniques used for HCC are also used for metastatic tumors of liver. In a study the results of radiofrequency ablation in the treatment of hepatic metastases were evaluated. Though complete necrosis, defined as an absence of detectable disease on computed tomography at 6 months follow-up was achieved in majority, treatment failure was also observed due to the development of new metastases on follow-up. It was concluded that radiofrequency ablation was safe and effective adjunct to systemic chemotherapy for the loco-regional treatment of liver metastases (Figs 24.9A to D).[12]

TACE using various chemotherapeutic agents has also shown good results in some vascular metastases from gastrointestinal tract, carcinoid and renal cell carcinoma (Figs 24.10A and B).

TART with Rhenium-188-HDD-lipiodol was also used in the management of multiple intrahepatic recurrences after radiofrequency ablation[13] and surgery[14] of hepatocellular carcinoma and was found to be a promising new therapeutic option[15] (Figs 24.11A to G).

BENIGN TUMORS OF LIVER

Cavernous Hemangiomas are usually asymptomatic but may become symptomatic with rapid tumor enlargement. These patients may present with abdominal pain, fever, anemia, obstructive jaundice, hemobilia, spontaneous rupture with subsequent life threatening hemorrhage, thrombocytopenia, hypofibrinogenemia and rarely portal or systemic hypertension due to intratumoral arterioportal or arteriovenous fistula. Hepatic artery embolization using both temporary and permanent occluding material may be indicated in the management of symptomatic hemangioma, hemangioma with high risk of bleeding and for preoperative embolization (Figs 24.12 and 24.13).

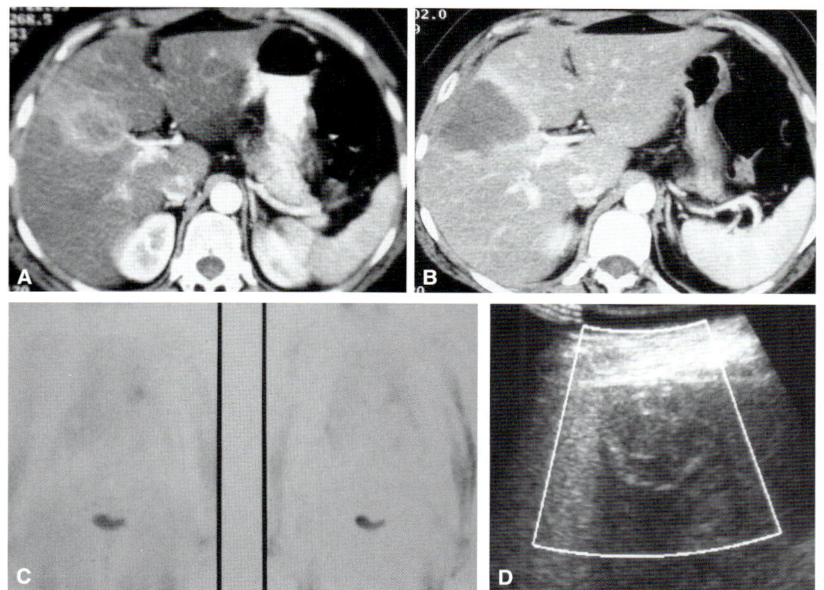

Figs 24.9A to D: A 46-year-female with single liver metastasis from carcinoma of breast (mastectomy done one yr. back) was treated with single session of RFA. Arterial phase CT (A) is showing single lesion (3.1 x 3 cm) in right lobe of liver (arrow). Post RFA 3 months arterial phase CT (B) is showing complete ablation of tumor (arrow). Seven year follow up PET (C) and color Doppler ultrasound (D) are normal

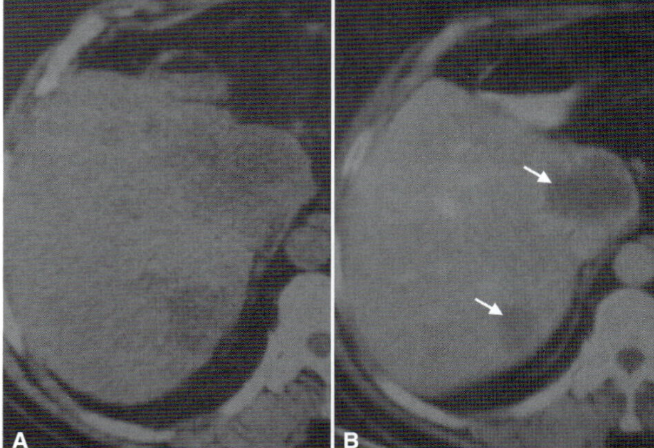

Figs 24.10A and B: A 52-year-male with liver metastases from leiomyosarcoma of intestine operated six months back was treated with TACE. CT liver four weeks post TACE shows multiple metastatic deposits with lipiodol (A). Repeat CT after six weeks (B) shows significant necrosis and reduction in the size of lesions (arrows)

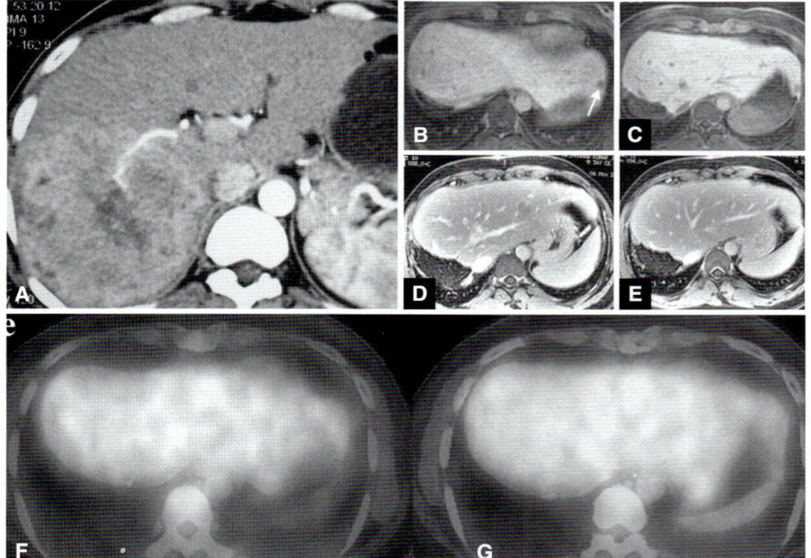

Figs 24.11A to G: Arterial phase CT liver (A) is showing HCC in right lobe of liver. One year post right hepatectomy MR (B and C) is showing two metastatic deposits (arrows) in left lobe of liver. The lesions disappeared on follow-up MR (D and E) and PET/CT (F and G) after Re HDD^{188} treatment

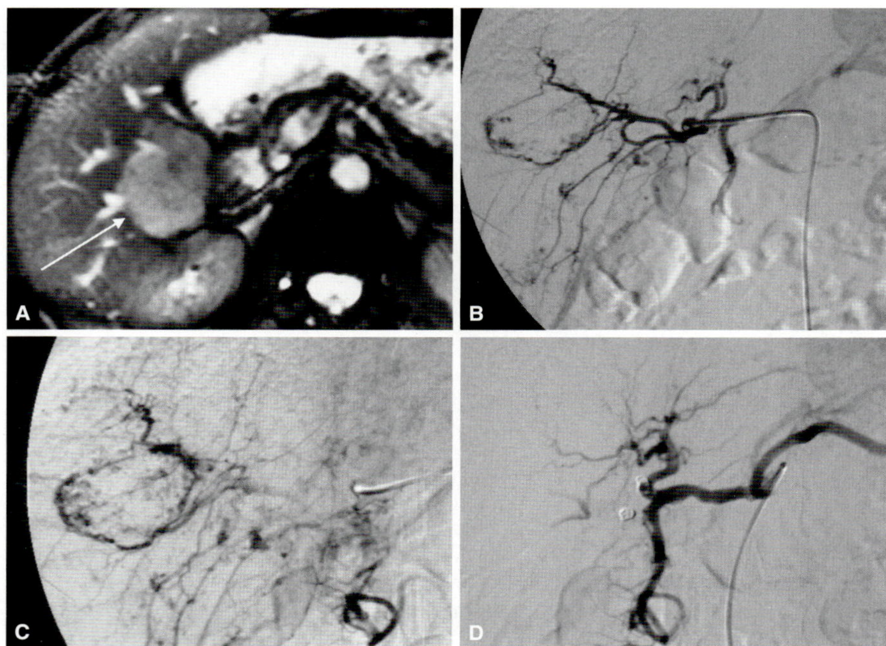

Figs 24.12A to D: Large cavernous hemangioma of right lobe of liver extending up to porta hepatis causing recurrent pain and cholangitis was embolized. (A) MR shows exophytic component of mass (arrow). (B&C) Hepatic artery angiograms show arterial supply from right hepatic artery. (D) Tumor was embolized with multiple steel coils and PVA particles. There was significant reduction in size of mass on follow-up imaging

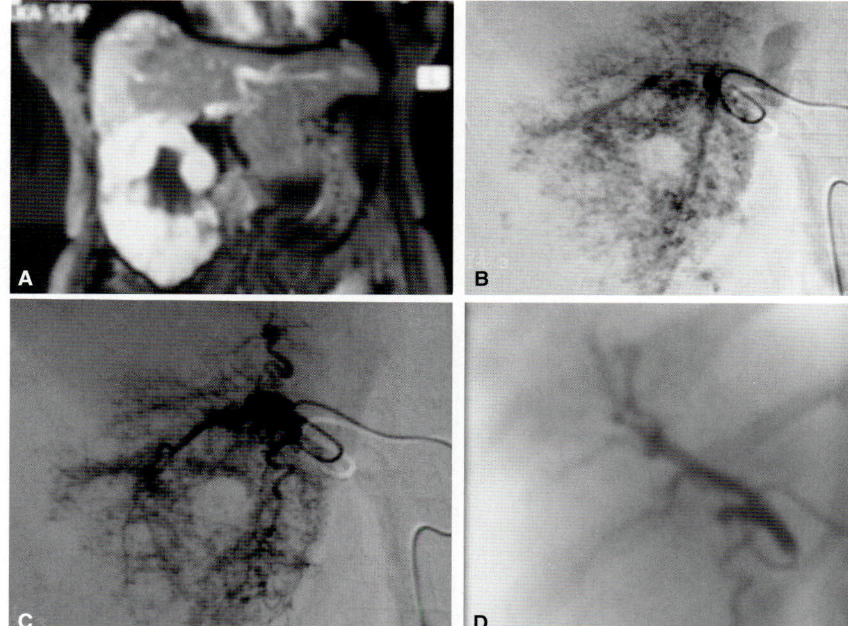

Figs 24.13A to D: Large symptomatic pedunculated hepatic hemangioma was embolized preoperatively and surgically removed later. (A) Contrast MR showing enhancing pedunculated mass in right lobe of liver with hypertrophied left lobe. (B and C) Right hepatic arteriogram showing large cavernous haemangioma with retrograde filling of portal vein, and (D) Complete preoperative embolization of the tumor. The tumor was surgically removed with less blood loss

Various studies have shown that TAE of hepatic cavernous hemangioma is a useful procedure in the therapy of symptomatic hemangiomas.[16, 17]

Pre-operative embolization of focal nodular hyperplasia, hepatic adenoma or other vascular tumors may help in surgical removal of the tumor (Fig. 24.14).[2]

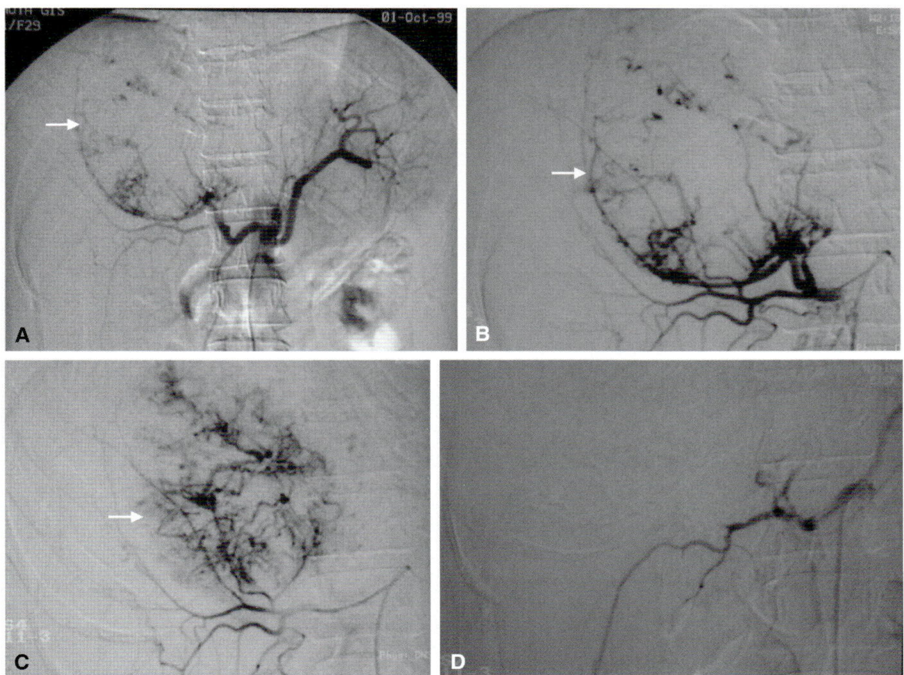

Figs 24.14A to D: A 32-year-female with Hepatic adenoma left lobe of liver. Hepatic angiograms shows (arrow) marked tumor vascularity (A-C). The tumor was embolized with gel foam and the post embolization angiogram (D) is not showing tumor vascularity. Complete surgical removal of the tumor was done with less blood loss

CONCLUSION

A variety of single and combination therapies are performed in the treatment of liver tumors. Selection of treatment options depends on clinical presentation, histology, site, size, number of lesions, surrounding liver, age, and performance status of patient. The treatment option should be selected on a case-by-case basis and must fulfill the needs of the individual patient.

REFERENCES

1. Srivastava DN, Mahajan A, Berry M, Sharma MP. Colour Doppler flow imaging of focal hepatic lesions. Australas Radiol 2000;44:285-89.
2. Srivastava DN. Imaging and therapeutic interventions in hepatic tumors. Tropical Gastroenterology 2000;21:103-13.
3. Shiina S, Niwa Y. Percutaneous ethanol injection therapy in the treatment of liver neoplasms. In Howard E (Ed): Current Techniques in Interventional Radiology. Cope C, Philadelphin 1994;3.1-3.14.
4. Seror O, N'kontchou G, Ibraheem M, Ajayon Y et al. Large (> = 5.0 – cm) HCCs: Multipolar RF Ablation with Three Internally Cooled Bipolar Electrodes – Initial experience in 26 patients. Radiology 2008 (E pubahead of print)
5. Srivastava DN, Julka PK, Berry M. Transcatheter arterial embolization with alcohol and steel coils followed by systemic chemotherapy in the treatment of Hepatocellular carcinoma (abstract). Radiology 1998;209:252.
6. Srivastava DN, Thulkar S, Sharma S, Pandey GK, Sahni P, Julka PK, Acharya SK. Therapeutic radiological interventional procedures in hepatocellular carcinoma. Indian J Gastroenterol 2002;21:96-98.
7. Srivastava DN, Gandhi D, Julka PK et al. Gastrointestinal hemorrhage in Hepatocellular carcinoma management with transhepatic arterioembolization. Abdominal Imaging 2000;25:1-6.
8. Ramsey DE, Geschwind JH. New interventions for liver tumors. Semin Roentgenoloy 2002;37:303-11.
9. Andrew L, Gonzalez V, Lloyd AW et al. DC Bead: In vitro characterization of a drug delivery device for transarterial chemoembolization. J Vasc Interv Radiol 2006;17:335-42.
10. Lo CM, Ngan H, Tso WK, et al. Randomized controlled trail of transarterial lipiodol chemoembolization for unresectable hepatocellular carcinoma. Hepatology 2002;35:1164-71.
11. Kumar A, Srivastava DN, Chau TTM, et al. Inoperable hepatocellular carcinoma: transarterial^{188}Re HDD-Labeled iodized oil for treatment—Prospective multi-center trial. Radiology 2007;243:509-19.
12. Gunabushanam G, Sharma S, Thulkar S, Srivastava DN, et al. Radiofrequency ablation of liver metastases from

breast cancer: results in 14 patients. J Vasc Interv Radiol 2007;18(1):67-72.
13. Kumar A, Bal C, Srivastava DN, Thulkar SP, Sharma S, Acharya SK, Duttagupta S. Management of multiple intrahepatic recurrences after radiofrequency ablation of hepatocellular carcinoma with rhenium-188-HDD-lipiodol. Eur J Gastroenterol Hepatol 2006;18(2):219-23.
14. Kumar A, Srivastava DN, Bal C. Management of postsurgical recurrence of hepatocellular carcinoma with rhenium 188-HDD labeled iodized oil. J Vasc Interv Radiol 2006;17(1):157-61.
15. Srivastava DN and Madhusudan KS. Oncologic Imaging. Ind. J of Medical and Paediatric Oncology 2008;29(1): 65-66.
16. Srivastava DN, Sharma S, Yadav S, et al. Pedunculated hepatic haemangioma with arteriportal shunt – treated with angioembolization and surgery. Australasian Radiology 1998;2:151-53.
17. Srivastava DN, Gandhi D, Seith A, Pande GK, Sahni P. Transcatheter arterial embolization in the treatment of symptomatic cavernous haemangioma of the liver: a prospective study. Abdominal Imaging 2001;26:510-14.

Chapter Twenty-five

Percutaneous Non-vascular GIT Interventions

Shivanand Gamanagatti, Deep Narayan Srivastava

In the treatment of patients suffering from gastro-intestinal tract diseases various therapeutic interventional techniques have been developed using percutaneous routes. There are:

1. Percutaneous gastrostomy
2. Percutaneous jejunostomy
3. Esophageal stent insertion
4. Duodenal stent insertion
5. Colorectal stent insertion
6. Percutaneous enterocutaneous fistula closure

Percutaneous Gastrostomy

Its procedure is used to provide nutritional support for patients with swallowing disorders. Enteral feeding is preferred in those with adequate small-bowel function to absorb sufficient water, electrolytes, and nutrients from a normal or elemental diet.[1-3]

Enteral feeding can be provided through nasogastric, nasojejunal, gastrostomy, or jejunostomy tubes. Nasogastric intubation is simple but poorly tolerated when used for long-term; it may potentiate gastroesophageal reflux and cause peptic esophagitis or aspiration of gastric contents.[4] The best method for long-term enteral feeding is directly through the stomach or jejunum by using gastrostomy or jejunostomy.

Three methods of gastrostomy are currently available. surgical, endoscopic, and fluoroscopic (using the Seldinger technique).

Surgical gastrostomy involves an abdominal incision usually performed under general anesthesia and is associated with significant morbidity; most patients are malnourished and the gastrostomy heals poorly, causing leakage and morbidity.[5,6]

Percutaneous endoscopic gastrostomy (PEG) was introduced in 1980 by Gauderer et al.[7] In PEG, the stomach is punctured percutaneously and, with the aid of a gastroscope, a string is brought up out of the patient through the mouth. The feeding tube is attached to the string and is pulled downward into the stomach and out through the anterior gastric and abdominal wall. PEG has fewer complications than surgery as it is performed under IV sedation instead of general anesthesia.

Percutaneous transgastric jejunostomy, another alternative to surgery, is a method that uses the Seldinger's technique. In this technique, under image guidance a feeding tube is placed in the stomach and sometime up to the jejunum.[8-10]

Indications

Nutritional support: For patients with swallowing disorders, like abnormal peristalsis associated with cerebrovascular accidents, anoxic brain damage, trauma, and neurosurgery. It can be used to provide enteral nutritional support for patients with anorexia nervosa, severe depression, and advanced malignancy.

Decompression of the stomach or small intestine Patients with chronic small-bowel obstruction may benefit from drainage with large-bore (24- to 28-French) gastrostomy tubes, which obviates long-term nasogastric suction. This indication is more common in patients with chronic intestinal obstruction secondary to carcinomatosis.

Other Indications

Innovative use of percutaneous gastrostomy has been reported in few unusual clinical settings, like retrograde dilatation of a gastroplasty stoma constructed for weight reduction in morbidly obese patients, to divert bile into the duodenum in patients with an external biliary drainage catheter where attempts to internalize the catheter are unsuccessful.

Contraindications

In cases of massive ascites and abnormal coagulation parameters.

Technique

Preprocedure preparation include overnight fasting. Procedure is performed under local anesthesia. Whenever possible, the esophagus should be intubated under fluoroscopic guidance using a 5 F multipurpose or cobra catheter. After administration of 40 mg butylscopolamine (Buscopan) the stomach is fully inflated with 500–1000 ml room air and then a puncture is made equidistant from the greater and lesser curvatures of the stomach at the junction of the upper two-thirds and lower one-third of the stomach with an 18 G needle. The correct needle position is checked by air aspiration and contrast injection. The T-fastener mounted in the needle is then pushed into the stomach (Cope gastrointestinal suture anchor set; Cook, Bloomington, MA) using the stiff guide wire that comes with suture anchor set. The needle is withdrawn and the T-fastener is retracted and sutured to the abdominal wall. The stiff guidewire is still inside the stomach and the stomach wall is retracted to the anterior abdominal wall with suture anchor. The tract is dilated over the guidewire serially using Seldinger technique. Preferably 12F -14F Malecot catheter or loop forming pigtail catheter is inserted as gastrostomy tube. Technical success is checked fluoroscopically at the end of the procedure and fluoroscopic contrast examination is done on the following day, before feeding is commenced. T-fasteners are usually cut after 7–12 days, under fluoroscopic gastrostomy control.[11,12]

Complications

Minor complications are abdominal pain with or without peritoneal tenderness, wound discharge, wound infection, fever, peristomal leakage, gastroparesis, simple dislocation, tract disruption without peritonitis, delayed catheter dislocation or catheter fracture.

Major complications are hemorrhage requiring blood transfusion or other intervention, peritonitis, aspiration pneumonitis, cardiac failure, anaphylaxis and collapse.

Percutaneous Jejunostomy

Percutaneous jejunostomy using fluoroscopic guidance was introduced by Gray et al. In 1987 and was modified by Coleman et al in 1990.[13,14] However, reports focusing on this technique are limited due to both the inherent technical difficulties, such as puncture of the mobile and compliant jejunum, and the difficulty of maintaining the position of the jejunum during the catheter insertion.

Indications

In cases where, percutaneous gastrostomy is not be possible due to unfavorable position of the stomach or because of previous partial or total gastrectomy.

Other indications included diversion of succus from a leaking anastomosis after esophagectomy and access to a limb of a Roux-en-Y anastomosis to facilitate biliary interventions.

Technical Difficulty

The normal, undistended jejunum is difficult to transfix because the bowel loops are so mobile and slippery that a puncturing needle will usually slide off.

Technique (Figs 25.1A to D)

General preparation should include overnight fasting and, whenever possible, insertion of a nasogastric tube. Interposition of colon or liver between the stomach and the anterior abdominal wall should routinely be excluded by both sonographic and fluoroscopic assessment of the upper abdomen. Procedure is performed under local anesthesia.

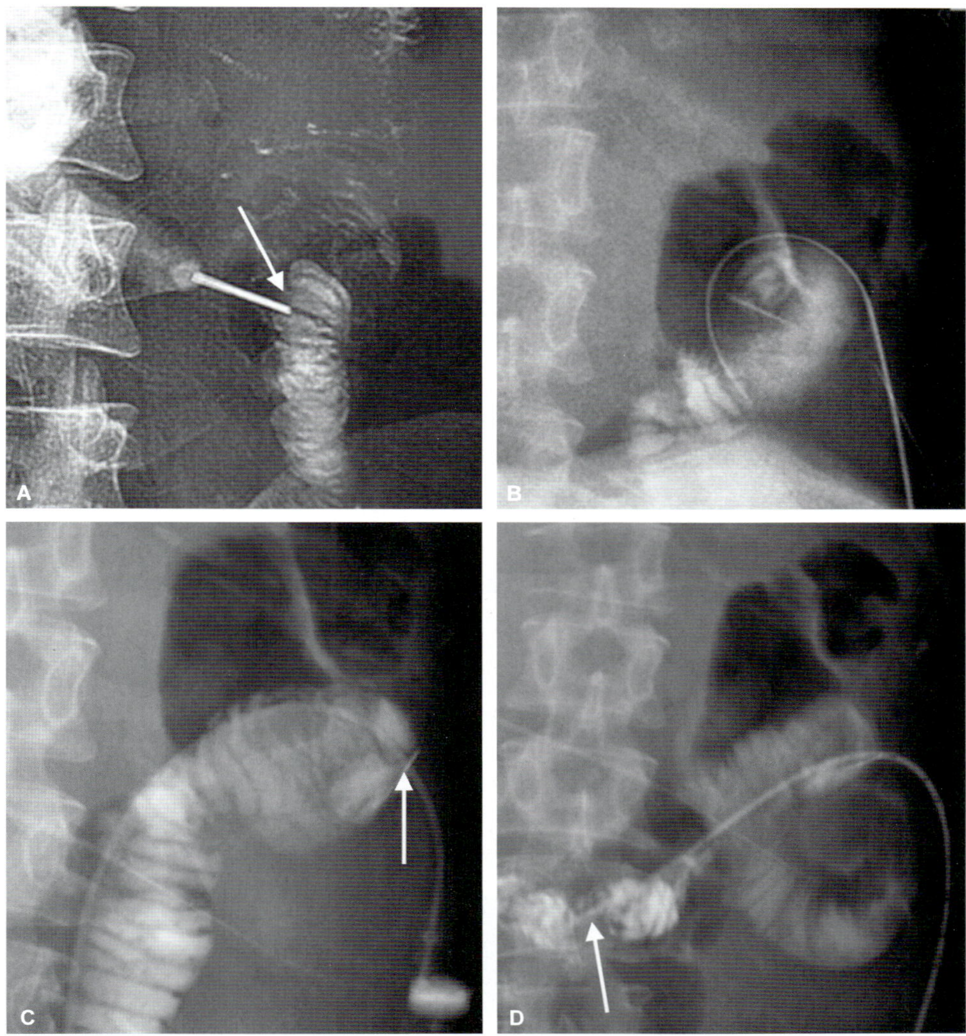

Figs 25.1A to D: Showing technique of percutaneous jejunostomy: Jejunal loop is punctured and the correct needle position is checked by contrast injection (A) (arrow). The T-fastener mounted in the needle is then pushed into the jejunum using the stiff guide wire that comes with suture anchor set (B). The needle is withdrawn and the T-fastener retracted and sutured to the abdominal wall (C) (arrow). The tract is dilated over the guidewire serially using Seldinger technique till the desired size of catheter to be inserted (D) (arrow)

A 120 cm long, jejunal tube is used to catheterize the duodenum or proximal jejunum through the nose. After administration of 40 mg butylscopolamine (Buscopan), the proximal jejunum was opacified with dilute, iodinated, aqueous contrast material and distended. Using the 18G needle preloaded with suture anchor set (Cope gastrointestinal suture anchor set; Cook, Bloomington, MA), one of the jejunal loop which is close to anterior abdominal wall is punctured under fluoroscopy and ultrasound. The correct needle position is checked by air aspiration and contrast injection (Fig. 25.1).

The T-fastener mounted on the needle is then pushed into the jejunum using the stiff guide wire that comes with suture anchor set. The needle is withdrawn and the T-fastener retracted and sutured to the abdominal wall. The stiff guidewire is still inside the jejunum and the jejunal wall is retracted to the anterior abdominal wall with suture anchor. The tract is dilated over the guidewire serially using Seldinger technique till the desired size of catheter to be inserted. Preferably 12F - 14F Malecot catheter or loop forming pigtail catheter is inserted as jejunostomy tube. Technical success is checked fluoroscopically at the end of the procedure. A fluoroscopic contrast examination is done on the following day, before feeding is commenced. T-fasteners are usually cut after 7–12 days, under fluoroscopic jejunostomy control.[1-3]

Complications

Are same as in case of percutaneous gastrostomy.

Esophageal Stenting

In 1959, Celestin[13] described the palliation of esophageal malignancy with a plastic endoprosthesis introduced at laparotomy. In the 1970s, Atkinson introduced an endoscopically inserted plastic prosthesis.[16] The first description of the endoscopic placement of an expanding metallic spiral stent was made by Frimberger in 1983.[17]

Indications

Stents are used primarily in patients with advanced or inoperable malignant esophageal obstruction and in those patients in whom surgery is contraindicated.

Other indications are:

1. Anastomotic tumor recurrence following surgery.
2. Primary or secondary tumors within the mediastinum causing extrinsic esophageal compression.
3. Esophageal perforation, which is usually iatrogenic, from direct endoscopic trauma or following stricture dilatation.
4. Treatment of symptomatic malignant gastro-esophageal anastomotic leaks.
5. Benign esophageal strictures: Esophageal stent placement is often a last resort if strictures are refractory to conventional treatment and surgery is contraindicated.

Stent Designs

Stents are available in an uncovered bare form or with a plastic coating on the inside and/or the outside of the stent. The advantage of uncovered stents is that they are less liable to migration, especially across the cardia. However, uncovered stents have a higher incidence of tumor in-growth and most stents now placed are of the covered type. Stents are usually inserted under fluoroscopic/endoscopic guidance, which allows for accurate positioning.

Commercially available stents are (Fig. 25.2):[18]

Gianturco-Z stent (Cook): This is made from stainless steel and a polyethylene covering with barbs on the outside or

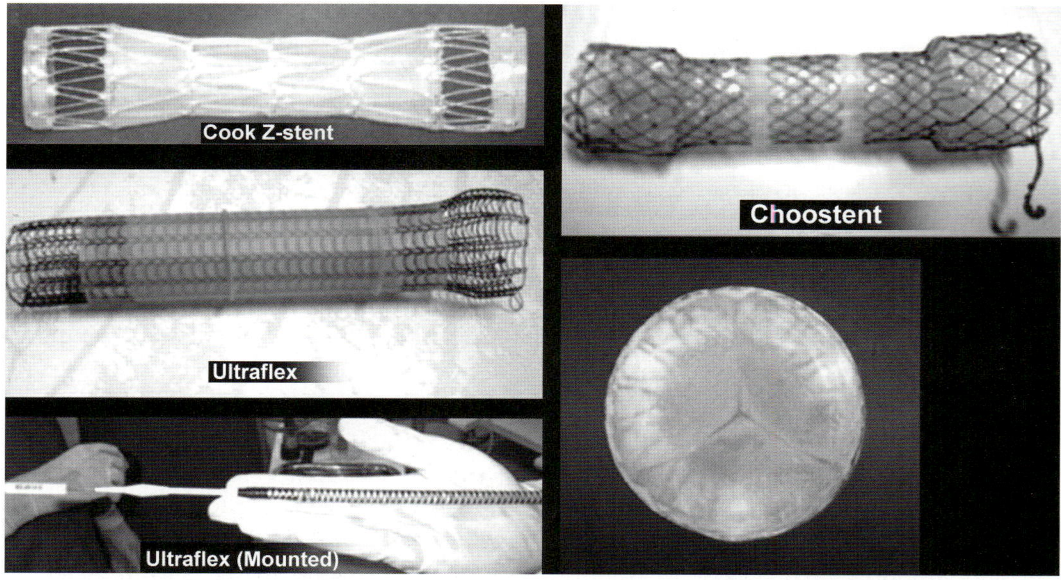

Fig. 25.2: Showing various designs of stents: Gianturco-Z stent (Cook). This is made from stainless steel and a polyethylene covering with barbs on the outside or uncoated flared ends to prevent migration. Ultraflex (Boston Scientific Ltd). This stent is made from a knitted Nitinol mesh and is available in both uncovered and covered. It has the weakest radial force but greater flexibility. These stents may be best for tortuous and upper third strictures.

Choo Stent (Diagmed) . This is a polyurethane-covered stent made from Nitinol and has a retrievable attached thread. These stents also come with an internal distal anti-reflux valve. *(For color version see plate 7)*

uncoated flared ends to prevent migration. This stent is also available with an anti-reflux distal long sleeve for positioning across the cardia.

Ultraflex (Boston Scientific Ltd). This stent is made from a knitted Nitinol mesh and is covered type. It has the weakest radial force but greater flexibility. These stents may be best for tortuous and upper third strictures.

Flamingo Wallstent (Boston Scientific). This is a tapered stent made from a braided stainless-steel alloy and is covered on the inside only. It is designed for use across the cardia only, as its conical shape prevents distal migration.

Wallstent (Boston Scientific). This stent has an internal silicon-based covering with flared ends and is made from a stainless-steel alloy woven into a tubular mesh.

Choo Stent (Diagmed) . This is a polyurethane-covered stent made from Nitinol and has a retrievable attached thread. These stents also come with an internal distal anti-reflux valve.

Memotherm (CR Bard). This is a flared Nitinol stent with an internal and external PTFE covering.
Song stent (Stentech), which is a modified Gianturco Z-stent made from stainless steel with a polyurethane covering. This stent has also been made in a retrievable form with a single thread attached to the tubular wire configuration.

Stent Selection

It is advisable to use an uncovered stent, e.g. a Flamingo or a Gianturco stent, at the cardia to reduce the risks of distal migration. Gastro-esophageal reflux occurs in most patients when the cardia has been crossed. This may lead to aspiration, and anti-reflux medication should be given prophylactically in all such cases. However, there are three new anti-reflux stents (Gianturco, FerX-Ella and Choo stents) that can be used as the stent of choice across the cardia.

Stents positioned in the upper third of the esophagus may result in a persistent foreign body sensation, especially if the cricopharyngeus is crossed. Endoscopy during stent placement is useful to identify the level of cricopharyngeus. These symptoms may be difficult to treat. The more flexible Ultraflex stent may be best for such high strictures.

The retrievable covered stents (Choo and Song stents) may become the stent of choice in the management of refractory benign strictures.

Technique (Figs 25.3 and 25.4)

Pharyngeal anesthesia is routinely provided with lidocaine aerosol spray (Xylocaine 10% spray; Astra, Linz, Austria) before the procedure. With fluoroscopic guidance, a 5-F angiographic catheter and a 145-cm-long, 0.035-inch-diameter hydrophilic guide wire are inserted and passed

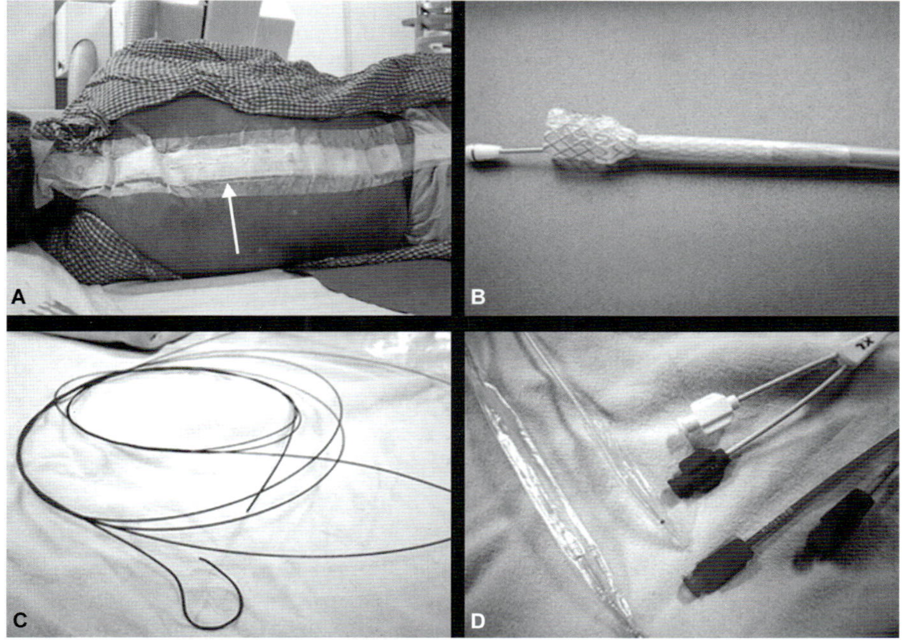

Figs 25.3A to D: Showing the preparation of esophageal stenting: Metallic marker pasted over the back of the patient (A) (arrow), Delivery system loaded with self expandable fully covered metallic stent (partially released) (B), Metallic and terumo guide wire (C) and Balloon catheter (D) *(For color version see plate 7)*

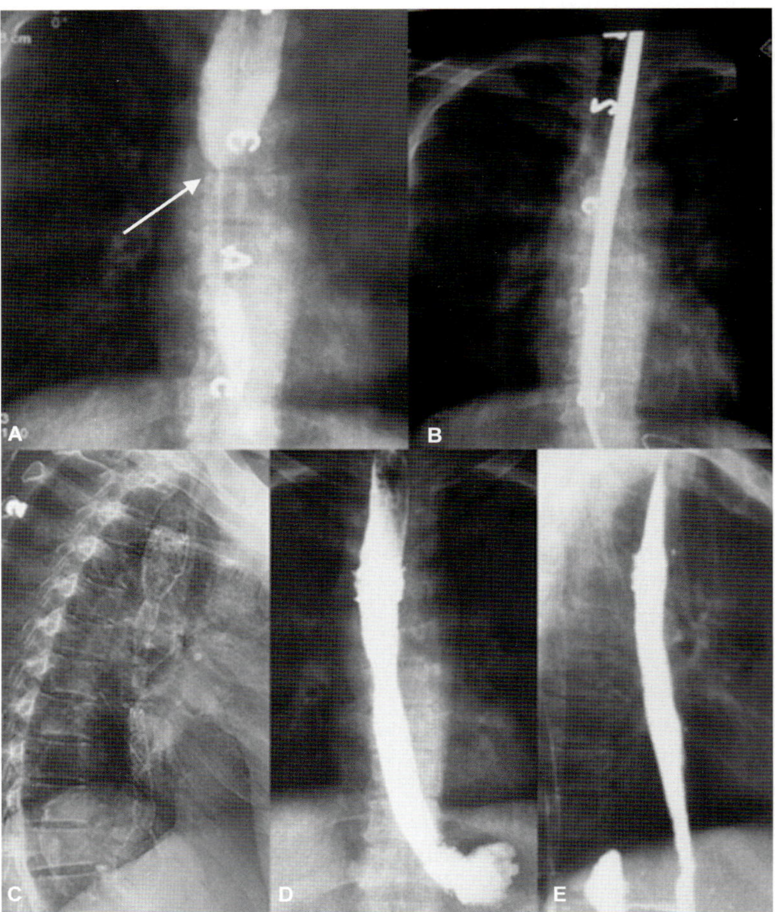

Figs 25.4A to E: Technique of esophageal stenting: Barium swallow shows irregular narrowing in mid third of thoracic esophagus with proximal hold up of barium column (A) (Arrow). Dilatation of the stricture with bougie (B). Completely deployed Choostent seen in situ. (Note: Lead markers placed on the patient's back for exact localization of stricture) (C). Esophagogram showing free flow of contrast across the stent (D, E).

through the stenotic segment. The guide wire is removed and a barium study is done with barium suspension to help correct localization of the lesion and measurement of the stenotic segment. Then, a 0.038-inch guide wire (Amplatz Superstiff) is introduced till the stomach and a flexible covered stent 4 cm longer than the stricture is usually selected, so that the proximal and distal parts of the stent is rested on the proximal and distal margins of the stricture (Fig. 25.3B). After being lubricated with jelly, the delivery system is advanced over the guide wire and properly positioned across the stricture with fluoroscopic guidance. The introducing tube is withdrawn while the pusher catheter is held in place. This maneuver releases the stent and allowed it to expand within the stricture. After the stent is deployed, the delivery system and guide wire are removed and a barium study is obtained in supine and erect positions to verify the position and patency of the stent.[19]

Postprocedure Care

Patients are allowed to take fluids immediately after the procedure and are kept on a soft diet for 2 days, then advanced to a solid diet. Progressive change in diet is recommended after stent placement. It is important to instruct patients to avoid leafy, uncooked vegetables and meat.

Patients are evaluated immediately after stent placement and every month thereafter. Patient's symptomatic improvement is assessed based on dysphagia score.

Complications

Early Complications

Early chest pain is the major-minor complication, that settles with analgesics. Major complications such as bleeding, perforation, aspiration, fever and fistula are uncommon.

Late Complications

Re-intervention following stent placement is common. This is predominantly due to tumor in-growth with uncovered stents and tumor over growth with covered stents. Other late complications include hemorrhage, esophageal ulceration, perforation or fistula, stent torsion, stent migration and stent fracture.

GASTRODUODENAL STENTING

Malignant obstruction of the stomach or duodenum causes nausea, vomiting, esophagitis, electrolyte imbalance, poor nutrition, and severe dehydration.[20] With the development of newer stent designs and delivery systems, metallic stent placement has now expanded into the palliative treatment for malignant gastroduodenal and colorectal obstructions.

Indications

1. Gastric, duodenal malignant obstructions caused by nonresectable tumors. Causes include primary tumors of the stomach and duodenum, malignant infiltration by neoplasms from adjacent organs (e.g. pancreas, gallbladder), and compression by malignant regional lymphadenopathy.
2. Patients with previous surgical anastomosis who later develop gastric outlet obstruction symptoms due to tumor recurrence.[21]
3. Patients with benign gastroduodenal obstructions who are at prohibitive surgical risk.

Contraindications

1. The only absolute contraindication for stent placement is evidence of gastrointestinal perforation.
2. Distal gastrointestinal obstruction is a partial contraindication; one of the main causes of clinical failure after stent placement.
3. Patients with peritoneal carcinomatosis or advanced metastatic disease are at high risk for multilevel small bowel obstruction.

Available Devices

The commonly used stent for enteral use is the enteral Wallstent (Microvasive/Boston Scientific) (Fig. 25.2). Advantages of this stent include its flexibility, ease of deployment, and small introducer system. This stent is an uncovered, braided metallic mesh. Available stents range from 18 to 22 mm in diameter and from 6 to 9 cm in length. The 20- and 22-mm-diameter stents are most commonly used. The delivery system is a 10-F Unistep set (Microvasive/Boston Scientific), which allows reconstraint of the stent before it has been completely deployed. Because of its braided design, the stent shortens approximately 40% after deployment. The delivery system is available in a 230-cm length designed for endoscopic placement and a 160-cm length for peroral fluoroscopic placement.

Endoscopic versus Fluoroscopic Placement

The technical success rates are similar whether fluoroscopy alone or a combination of endoscopy and fluoroscopy is used. Endoscopy is routinely used when the procedure is performed by gastroenterologists.[22] After the level of obstruction is identified, the endoscope is usually passed distal to the lesion (Fig. 25.2); balloon dilation is required to cross the stricture with the endoscope in 30% of cases (2). Submucosal injection of contrast material is then performed under fluoroscopic guidance to identify the stricture. The stent is usually deployed through the large (4.2 mm) working channel of the endoscope, which facilitates advancement of the stent through the tortuous anatomy and a distended stomach. However, the high friction between the working channel of the often angulated endoscope and the 230 cm delivery system increases the difficulty of stent deployment. Actual stent deployment is usually performed under fluoroscopic guidance. Technical failure rates are low (3%) and are usually related to failure to cannulate the stricture with the guide wire.

Accurate gastroduodenal stent placement depends mainly on fluoroscopic guidance. Many authors have reported a high technical success rate with peroral stent placement under fluoroscopic guidance without the use of endoscopy. [23,24] Interventional radiology is well suited for gastroduodenal stent placement because of the catheter techniques, skills, and materials are adequate for successful stent placement in the majority of patients. The reported technical success rate with fluoroscopy is the same as that with endoscopy. In some cases, fluoroscopic insertion is successful after failed endoscopic procedures, or vice versa.

Technique (Figs 25.5A to D)

An upper gastrointestinal study performed before the procedure is very useful for identifying the length and location of the stricture. Because of the prolonged obstruction, atony of the stomach is very common. Most patients have markedly distended and elongated stomachs, which significantly increases the difficulty of the procedure due to buckling of the delivery system in the greater curvature of the stomach.

Nasogastric tube placement with continuous suction is essential, not only to facilitate stent placement, but more importantly, to prevent aspiration. The procedure is performed with the patient under conscious sedation and with continuous monitoring of the vital signs and oxygen saturation.

An angiographic catheter with a guide wire is advanced perorally into the antrum after the pharynx has been numbed with topical anesthesia. A limited amount of diluted contrast material is injected to identify the location and length of the stricture, which is then traversed with a curved, 100 cm long angiographic catheter. We commonly use either a Multipurpose or Head Hunter catheter and a stiff Glidewire (Terumo, Piscataway, NJ; distributed by Boston Scientific). The catheter is advanced distal to the stricture, ideally into the first portions of the jejunum. An exchange-length

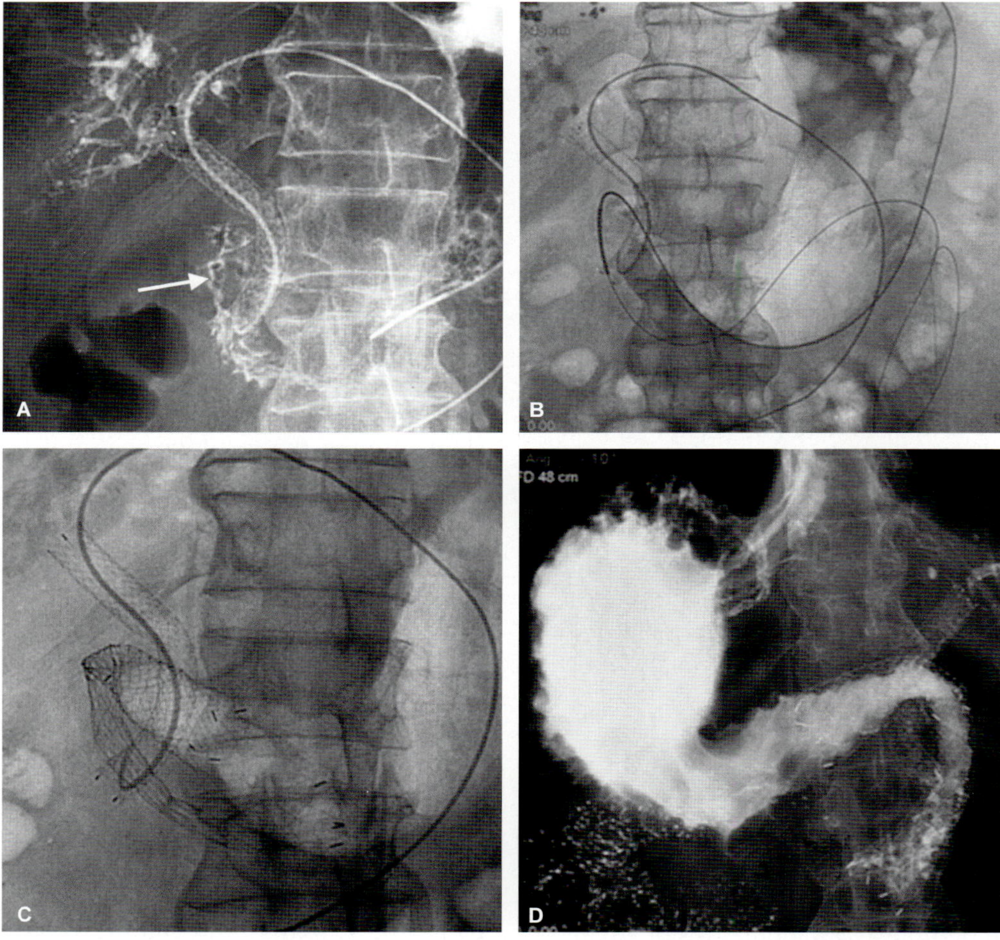

Figs 25.5A to D: Technique of duodenal stenting: Contrast study showing narrowing of D2 segment , proximal to ampulla (A) (arrow), Guide wire negotiated across the stricture (B), Completely deployed Wall stent seen in situ (C) and barium study showing free flow of contrast across the stent (D)

(260 cm) Amplatz superstiff or a Lunderquist extra-stiff guide wire is then advanced. In markedly distended stomachs, the introducer system will tend to buckle in the greater curvature, making the exchange-length guide wire too short for the procedure. In these cases, the use of a 500-cm-long Amplatz superstiff wire may solve the problem. The use of a 10-F (80 cm) introducer sheath is recommended to decrease the discomfort of the patient and to prevent buckling of the stent delivery system in the greater curvature of the stomach. If there is difficulty in negotiating the delivery system across the tight stricture, turn the patient to right lateral decubitus, that helps in unfolding the duodenal curvature and thereby delivery system can be pushed easily without much difficulty.

The mid section of the stent is centered in the stricture, and the stent is deployed under continuous fluoroscopic monitoring. It is important to "overstent" the lesion by placing the stent at least 2 cm distal and 2 cm proximal to the stricture to prevent recurrent obstruction due to tumor overgrowth. It is not necessary to dilate the stent after deployment because it will slowly expand over the next 24–48 hours.[25]

Postprocedure Care

A follow-up upper gastrointestinal study is usually performed the next day. The patient may resume oral intake almost immediately, advancing from liquids to semisolids. Dietary counseling is important because a semisolid or pured diet is usually recommended. Although many patients resume a normal diet, it is important to instruct patients to avoid leafy, uncooked vegetables and meat.

Rates of technical success, defined as the correct placement of the stent in the intended location with patency confirmed at fluoroscopy, vary from 94-100%.

Clinical success in relieving gastrointestinal obstruction, defined as the improvement of the patient's ability to resume oral intake and experience objective weight gain, has been reported in 80-100% of cases. A clinical failure rate of about 10% is expected despite adequate technical success. The most common causes of clinical failure are related to distal gastrointestinal obstruction, gastric paresis due to chronic distention of the stomach, and functional gastric outlet obstruction due to neural involvement of the celiac axis.[26,27]

Complications

Reported complications are rare, and no procedure-related deaths have been reported to date. Possible complications include perforation, migration, bleeding, ulceration, food impaction, and obstruction. Unlike with esophageal stents, most patients do not experience significant pain after placement of duodenal stents. Migration is rare with uncovered stents.

COLORECTAL STENTING

Indications

The primary indications for endoluminal metallic stent placement in the colon and rectum are:[26]

- For temporary colonic decompression in patients with an acute potentially resectable malignant colonic obstruction to allow laxative preparation and a single-stage surgical resection.
- For long-term colonic decompression in patients with unresectable malignant obstruction of the colon or rectum.

Contraindications

- Clinical or radiologic evidence of perforation
- Tumors that are too long or kinked or that are too proximal within the colon.

Technical Considerations

A variety of stents have been used effectively in the colon, including the enteral Wallstent, Ultraflex stent, and Memotherm stent.[28-31] Stent placement in distal colonic and rectal lesions can be guided with fluoroscopy or endoscopy alone. Because of the difficulty in accessing more proximal portions of the colon because of sigmoid colon tortuosity, these lesions are best handled with combined endoscopic-fluoroscopic guidance.

A radiologic water-soluble enema (one part 76% contrast material with two parts water) examination is performed to localize and characterize the length and caliber of the obstructive lesion. The enema is also useful for determining the best position in which to place the patient to display the lesion such that the stricture is perpendicular to the beam. This position facilitates visualization of the stricture during stent placement. On the basis of the length of the stricture and its distance from the anus, the appropriate device and delivery system can be selected.

Fluoroscopic guidance: With the patient placed in a good position to visualize the obstructive lesion, an angiographic catheter or guiding catheter is placed into the colon. High-torque, 70–100 cm-long catheters are often needed. The colonic segments are negotiated with the catheter–guide wire combination. Conventional or hydrophilic 0.035- or 0.038-inch wires are used.

Following successful catheterization past the obstructive lesion, contrast material is injected through the diagnostic angiographic catheter to better define the lesion (length, location, optimal position) and to rule out a perforation. The location of the lesion is marked and noted. An exchange length stiff guide wire is advanced well beyond the lesion. A stent with an adequate length and diameter (20–24 mm) is advanced under fluoroscopic guidance and deployed such that the middle of the stent covers the lesion with 1–2 cm of the stent extending beyond both the proximal and distal margins of the lesion. Long lesions may require two stents.[26]

Postprocedure Follow-up

A water-soluble enema examination is performed immediately after the procedure or the following day to check for patency and leakage. Patients who are candidates for resection are treated medically, and a bowel-cleaning preparation is instituted for subsequent surgery. Patients with unresectable disease who receive stents only for palliation are placed on a low-residue diet and receive mineral oil to lessen the likelihood of stent obstruction. Follow-up radiographs are obtained in symptomatic patients if needed to check for stent migration, perforation, or colonic obstruction.[26]

Complications

Minor complications, including mild abdominal pain and transient rectal bleeding, generally require no treatment. Perforation, stent migration, and restenosis are the major complications encountered with colonic stent placement.

Percutaneous Enterocutaneous Fistula Closure with N-butyl-2-Cyanoacrylate

Enterocutaneous fistulae usually occur as complications of complex alimentary tract surgery but may also arise spontaneously in patients with inflammatory bowel disease or after trauma or radiation therapy.[32,33] Gastrointestinal fistula are classified into high out put and low output fistulas, based on amount of output from fistula per day. Most fistulae that originate in the duodenum, jejunum, and ileum are classed as high-output and may drain as much as 4,000 ml of intestinal contents per day.

The problems posed by such fistula include massive losses of fluid, electrolytes, and nutrients are formidable and, frequently, management is complicated by the presence of one or more intraabdominal abscesses. Currently, most authors recommend a trial of conservative management before surgical therapy is attempted; accurate fluid and electrolyte replacement and prevention of malnutrition are combined with attempts to reduce the drainage of intestinal contents by nasogastric intestinal intubation.[33-36] Although this approach is occasionally successful, both the quantity and quality of bowel effluent and the presence of ongoing infection usually prevent the development of a mature, fibrous, external tract and spontaneous closure.

Radiologic involvement in the care of patients with enterocutaneous fistulae has largely been limited to opacification of the fistulous tract and identification of the morbid anatomy.[37] However, recent technical advances in interventional radiology techniques have made the treatment of low output fistula closure more practically feasible. The Cyanoacrylates have been shown to be successful in the closure of pancreatic fistulas, biliary fistulas and gastrointestinal fistulas.[38,39]

Mechanism of Action of the Glue (N-butyl-2-cyanoacrylate)

Intravascular injection of N-butyl-2-cyanoacrylate produces an immediate cast of the vessel. Total occlusion of the vessel occurs within hours. Mild eosinophilic inflammation is observed at 24 hours. By day 7, tissue reaction is minimal. After 1 to 2 weeks, the cyanoacrylate casts extrudes into the lumen, leaving behind a patent variceal lumen generally without re-bleeding.[40]

Prerequisites

1. Fistula should be low output
2. The fistulous tract should be short in length (longer the tract lesser the chances of success)

3. Tract should be linear, non-branching
4. No associated abscess cavity
5. Non-epithelialized tract (if the tract is epithelialized, it is traumatized the tract to make the surface raw).

Technical Consideration

Percutaneous closure of fistulous tract is performed as an out patient procedure and no anesthesia is required.

Preparation

The potency (i.e. "stickiness") of cyanoacrylates necessitates dilution before application. Most endoscopists mix cyanoacrylates with the lipid soluble lipiodol to retard polymerization and enhance imaging. Various mixtures of Histoacryl and lipiodol (range: 1:1 to 1:1.6) have been recommended. Whereas a mixture that is too concentrated risks premature polymerization, a mixture too dilute increases the risk of embolization. 50% dextrose solution is used to flush the catheter and to prevent the risk of polymerization inside the catheter.

Technique (Figs 25. 6A to D)

After obtaining the contrast fistulogram study, the fistulous tract is catheterized either with angiographic catheter (4F) or using venflon (18-20G). The catheter should be advanced close the inner opening of fistula. After flushing the catheter with 50% dextrose solution, the diluted glue preparation (1:1 or 1:2) is injected, starting from inside and gradually withdrawing the catheter outside, while continuously injecting the glue.

After the procedure, recatheterization of the tract is not done, otherwise the glue may get dislodged. If the fistula has not closed, another session of glue injection is tried. Sometime we may need 3-4 session to close the tract depending upon the length, diameter and degree of epithelialization of the tract.

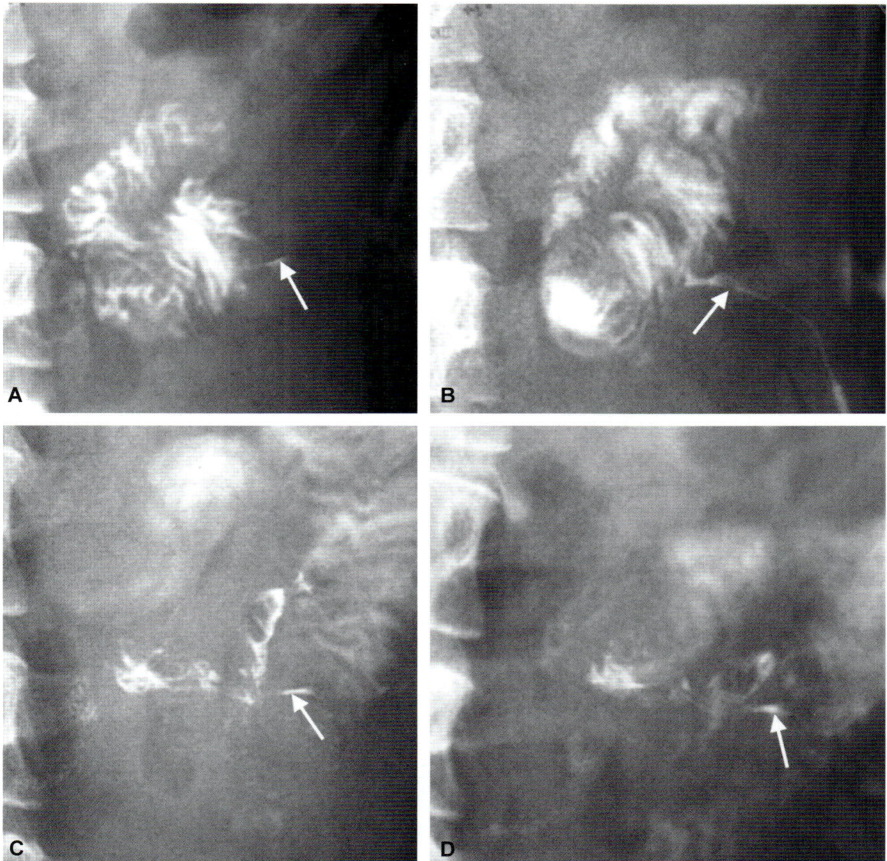

Figs 25.6A to D: Technique of enterocutaneous fistula closure with glue: Contrast study to show outline and length of the fistulous tract (arrow) (A, B). Following Glue injection, the cast of glue outlining the fistulous tract is seen (arrow) (C, D). The tract was completely obliterated on follow up

REFERENCES

1. Yang ZQ, Shin JH, Song HY, Kwon JH, Kim JW, Kim KR, Kim JH. Fluoroscopically guided percutaneous jejunostomy: outcomes in 25 consecutive patients. Clin Radiol. 2007 Nov;62(11):1061-5; discussion 1066-8. Epub 2007 Sep 4.
2. van Overhagen H, Ludviksson MA, Laméris JS, Zwamborn AW, Tilanus HW, Dees J, Hansen BE. US and fluoroscopic-guided percutaneous jejunostomy: experience in 49 patients. J Vasc Interv Radiol 2000 Jan;11(1):101-6.
3. Cope C, Davis AG, Baum RA, Haskal ZJ, Soulen MC, Shlansky-Goldberg RD. Direct percutaneous jejunostomy: techniques and applications—ten years experience. Radiology 1998 Dec;209(3):747-54.
4. Miller KS, Tomlinson JR. Sahn SA. Pleuropulmonary complications of enteral tube feedings, two case reports: review of the literature and recommendations. Chest 1985;88:230-33.
5. Wasiljew BK, Ujiki GT, Beal JM. Feeding gastrostomy: complications and mortality. Am J Surg 1982;143:194-95.
6. Shellito PC, Malt RA. Tube gastrostomy: technique and complications. Ann Surg 1985;201:180-95.
7. Gauderer WL, Ponsky JL, Izant AJ. Gastrostomy without laparotomy: percutaneous endoscopic technique. J Pediatr Surg 1980;15:872-75.
8. Ho CS. Percutaneous gastrostomy for jejunal feeding. Radiology 1983;149:595-96.
9. Tao HH, Gillies AR. Percutaneous feeding gastrostomy. AJR 1983;141:793-94.
10. Wills JS, Oglesby JT. Percutaneous gastrostomy. Radiology 1983;149:449-53.
11. Brown AS, Mueller PA, Ferrucci JT. Controlled percutaneous gastrostomy: nylon T-fastener for fixation of the anterior gastric wall. Radiology 1986;158:543-45.
12. Cope C. Suture anchor for visceral drainage. AiR 1980;135:402-03.
13. Celestin LR. Permanent intubation in inoperative cancer of the esophagus and cardia. Ann R Coll Surg Eng 1959;25:165-70.
14. Atkinson M, Ferguson R. Fibre-optic endoscopic palliative intubation of inoperable oesophogastric neoplasms. BMJ 1997;1:266-7.
15. Gray RR, Ho CS, Yee A, et al. Direct percutaneous jejunostomy. AJR Am J Roentgenol 1987;149:931-32.
16. Coleman CC, Coons HG, Cope C, et al. Percutaneous enterostomy with the Cope suture anchor. Radiology 1990;174: 889-91.
17. Frimberger E. Expanding spiral—a new type of prosthesis for the palliative treatment of malignant oesophageal stenosis. Endoscopy 1983;15:213-14.
18. Lee SH. The role of oesophageal stenting in the non-surgical management of oesophageal strictures. Br J Radiol. 2001 Oct;74(886):891-900. Review.
19. Neyaz Z, Srivastava DN, Thulkar S, Bandhu S, Gamanagatti S, Julka PK, Chattopadhyaya TK. Radiological evaluation of covered self-expandable metallic stents used for palliation in patients with malignant esophageal strictures. Acta Radiol 2007 Mar;48(2):156-64.
20. Patton JT, Carter R. Endoscopic stenting for recurrent malignant gastric outlet obstruction. Br J Surg 1997; 84:865-66.
21. Klose KJ. Nitinol prostheses for the treatment of inoperable malignant esophageal obstruction. J Vasc Intervent Radiol 1994; 5:899-904.
22. Spinelli P, Cerrai FG, Dal Fante M. Endoscopic treatment of upper gastrointestinal tract malignancies. Endoscopy 1993; 25:675-78.
23. de Baere T, Harry G, Ducreaux M, et al. Self-expanding metallic stents as palliative treatment of malignant gastroduodenal stenosis. AJR Am J Roentgenol 1997; 169:1079-83.
24. Pinto IT. Malignant gastric and duodenal stenosis: palliation by peroral implantation of a self-expanding metallic stent. Cardiovasc Intervent Radiol 1997; 20: 431-34.
25. Lopera JE, Brazzini A, Gonzales A, Castaneda-Zuniga WR. Gastroduodenal stent placement: current status. Radiographics. 2004 Nov-Dec;24(6):1561-73. Review.
26. Mauro MA, Koehler RE, Baron TH. Advances in gastrointestinal interventions: the treatment of gastroduodenal and colorectal obstructions with metallic stent. Radiology 2000; 215:659-69.
27. Kaw M, Singh S, Gagneja H, Azad P. Role of self-expandable metal stents in the palliation of malignant duodenal obstruction. Surg Endosc 2003; 17:646-50.
28. Rey JF, Romanczyk T, Greff M. Metal stents for palliation of rectal carcinoma: a preliminary report of 12 patients. Endoscopy 1995; 27:501-04.
29. Spinelli P, Dal Fante M, Mancini A. Rectal metal stents for palliation of colorectal malignant stenosis. Bildgebung 1993; 60(suppl 1):48-50.
30. Mainar A, Tejero E, Maynar M, et al. Colorectal obstruction: treatment with metallic stents. Radiology 1996;198:761-64.
31. Saida Y, Sumiyama Y, Nagao J, et al. Stent endoprosthesis for obstructing colorectal cancers. Dis Colon Rectum 1996;39:552-55.
32. Edmunds LH Jr. Williams GM, Welch CE. External fistulas arising from the gastro-intestinal tract. Ann Surg 1960; 152:445-71.
33. Fischer JE. The management of high out-put intestinal fistulas. Adv Surg 1975;9:139-76.
34. Reber HA, Roberts C, Way LW, Dunphy JE. Management of external gastrointestinal fistulas. Ann Surg 1978;188: 460-67.

35. Blackett RL, Hill GL. Postoperative external small bowel fistulas: a study of a consecutive series of patients treated with intravenous hyperalimentation. Br J Surg 1978;65: 775-78.
36. Soeter PB, Ebeid AM, Fischer JE. Review of 404 patients with gastrointestinal fistulas. Ann Surg 1979;190:189-202.
37. Miller WT, Sullivan MA. Roentgenologic demonstration of sinus tracts and fistulae. AJR 1969;107:812-17.
38. Lee YC, Na HG, Suh JH, et al. Three cases of fistulae arising from gastrointestinal tract treated with endoscopic injection of histoacryl. Endoscopy 2001;33:184-86.
39. Seewald S, Brand B, Omar S, et al. Endoscopic sealing of pancreatic fistula by using N-butyl-2-cyanoacrylate. Gastrointest Endosc 2004; 59:463-70.
40. Suga T, Akamatsu T, Kawamura Y, et al. Actual behaviour of N-butyl- 2-cyanoacrylate (histoacryl) in a blood vessel: a model of the varix. Endoscopy 2002;34:73-77.

Chapter Twenty-six

Interventional Radiology in Portal Hypertension

Naveen Kalra, Niranjan Khandelwal

There has been a significant change in the role of the radiologist in the management of portal hypertension in the last few decades. In the 1970s, the role of the radiologist was limited to determining the presence and cause of portal hypertension using angiographic techniques like splenoportography, arterioportography and transhepatic portography. Subsequently with the development of effective cross-sectional imaging tools like computed tomography (CT) and magnetic resonance imaging (MRI), the invasive imaging for portal hypertension diminished and progressively the focus changed from diagnostic to percutaneous therapeutic procedures. The primary goal in treating portal hypertension is reducing the portal venous pressure and thus helping treat its complications like variceal bleeding, refractory ascites or hydrothorax, hypersplenism, etc. When it is not possible to achieve the primary goal, palliative procedures can be offered to control the symptoms related to portal hypertension, which may be life threatening in certain cases.

The various portal interventions can be broadly classified as:

1. Interventions that reduce portal pressure:
   a. Transjugular intrahepatic portosystemic shunts (TIPS)
   b. Revision of occluded surgical and radiological portosystemic shunts
   c. Embolization of arterioportal fistulas
   d. Recanalization of occluded portal vein
   e. Partial splenic embolization
   f. Recanalization of hepatic venous outflow.
2. Interventions to palliate symptoms related to portal hypertension:
   a. Percutaneous transhepatic variceal embolization
   b. Balloon-occluded retrograde transvenous obliteration of gastric varices (BRTO).

TRANSJUGULAR INTRAHEPATIC PORTOSYSTEMIC SHUNT

TIPS refers to the creation of a portosystemic shunt by the transjugular insertion of an expandable metal stent between the hepatic and portal veins under image guidance. It was first performed by Colapinto and coworkers in 1982 in six patients and has been in use for the last two decades to treat the complications of portal hypertension, to control refractory ascites and treat Budd-Chiari syndrome.[1] The purpose of TIPS is to decompress the portal venous system and prevent its complications, including rebleeding from the varices. Pre-TIPS evaluation includes routine tests of liver and kidney function, as well as Doppler ultrasound, contrast enhanced CT or MRI of the liver. The procedure may be performed under conscious sedation and in case the procedure is going to be prolonged or the patient is hemodynamically unstable, then general anesthesia is preferred.

INDICATIONS OF TIPS[2]

- Acute variceal bleeding unresponsive to medical therapy (including sclerotherapy/banding)
- Secondary prevention of variceal bleeding
- Refractory ascites
- Portal hypertensive gastropathy
- Refractory hepatic hydrothorax
- Budd-Chiari syndrome
- Veno-occlusive disease

As TIPS, like a surgical shunt, has a risk of hepatic encephalopathy, liver failure and procedural complications, it is not used as a primary therapy for variceal bleeding, for which medical and endoscopic therapy is preferred. In refractory cases of esophageal as well as gastric and ectopic varices, TIPS has been effective in controlling rebleeding and is preferred to surgery especially in patients with poor liver function, though frequent re-interventions to maintain shunt patency is a disadvantage as compared to surgical shunts. The rebleeding rate after TIPS has been reported to be 19% (10-32 months follow-up), while that of surgical shunts has been reported to be ranging between 3 and 45%.[3] TIPS, unlike surgery, does not need general anesthesia, postinterventional intensive care, parenteral nutrition and immobilization. Recent developments like use of covered stents and simultaneous embolization of varices may improve efficacy and cost effectiveness of TIPS to such a degree that it may become comparable or even superior to surgery. TIPS is more effective than sclerotherapy in obliterating varices and reducing rebleeding events with various studies reporting an 7-23% incidence of rebleeding with TIPS as compared to a 45-66% rebleeding rate with sclerotherapy.[4] However the increase in survival is not significant.

Refractory ascites implies that sodium restriction and maximum diuretic therapy are unsuccessful in controlling ascites. In refractory ascites, TIPS has been found to be more effective as compared to peritoneo-venous shunts and may be used in patients who are intolerant of repeated large volume paracentesis. Various studies have reported a survival benefit in patients of refractory ascites treated with TIPS as compared to those treated with large volume paracentesis, with a 1- year survival of 77% as compared to 52% in the paracentesis group and is probably related to a general reduction of portal hypertension related risks.[5] Hepatic hydrothorax is also a complication of cirrhosis and due to the limited therapeutic options to treat this condition, TIPS is an important tool for its management.

Patients of Budd-Chiari syndrome with moderate severity of disease may be candidates for TIPS as patients with mild severity are better managed medically and severe disease is best managed by liver transplantation. Though porto-caval surgical shunts may also be effective in these patients, operations within the portal space are to be avoided as many of these patients may be eventual transplant patients.

CONTRAINDICATIONS OF TIPS[2]

Absolute

- Primary prevention of variceal bleeding
- Congestive heart failure (right atrial pressure > 20 mmHg)
- Multiple hepatic cysts
- Uncontrolled systemic infection or sepsis
- Unrelieved biliary obstruction
- Severe pulmonary hypertension (45 mmHg).

Relative

- Hepatoma, especially with central obstruction of all hepatic veins
- Portal vein thrombosis
- Severe coagulopathy (INR > 5)
- Thrombocytopenia of less than 20,000/cm^3
- Moderate pulmonary hypertension.

The steps of the procedure are explained in Figure 26.1. The first step of the procedure involves cannulation of the hepatic vein through transjugular approach. TIPS is usually performed via the right transjugular route as it provides the straight path to the hepatic vein openings. It is important to establish which hepatic vein is being used so that the intrahepatic puncture towards the portal vein is made in the appropriate direction. This can be done by using ultrasound or lateral fluoroscopy as the right hepatic vein is directed posteriorly while the middle hepatic vein is directed anteriorly on lateral view. About 3% of the population has a dominant inferior right hepatic vein. The right hepatic vein is dorsal and cephalad to the anterior superior branch of right portal vein, and is usually chosen for the shunt. After cannulation of the hepatic vein, hepatic venography is performed to ensure that the vein is large enough to provide an outflow tract of sufficient diameter (8-10 mm). The second step is the passage of a long needle from the hepatic vein, through the liver parenchyma into the

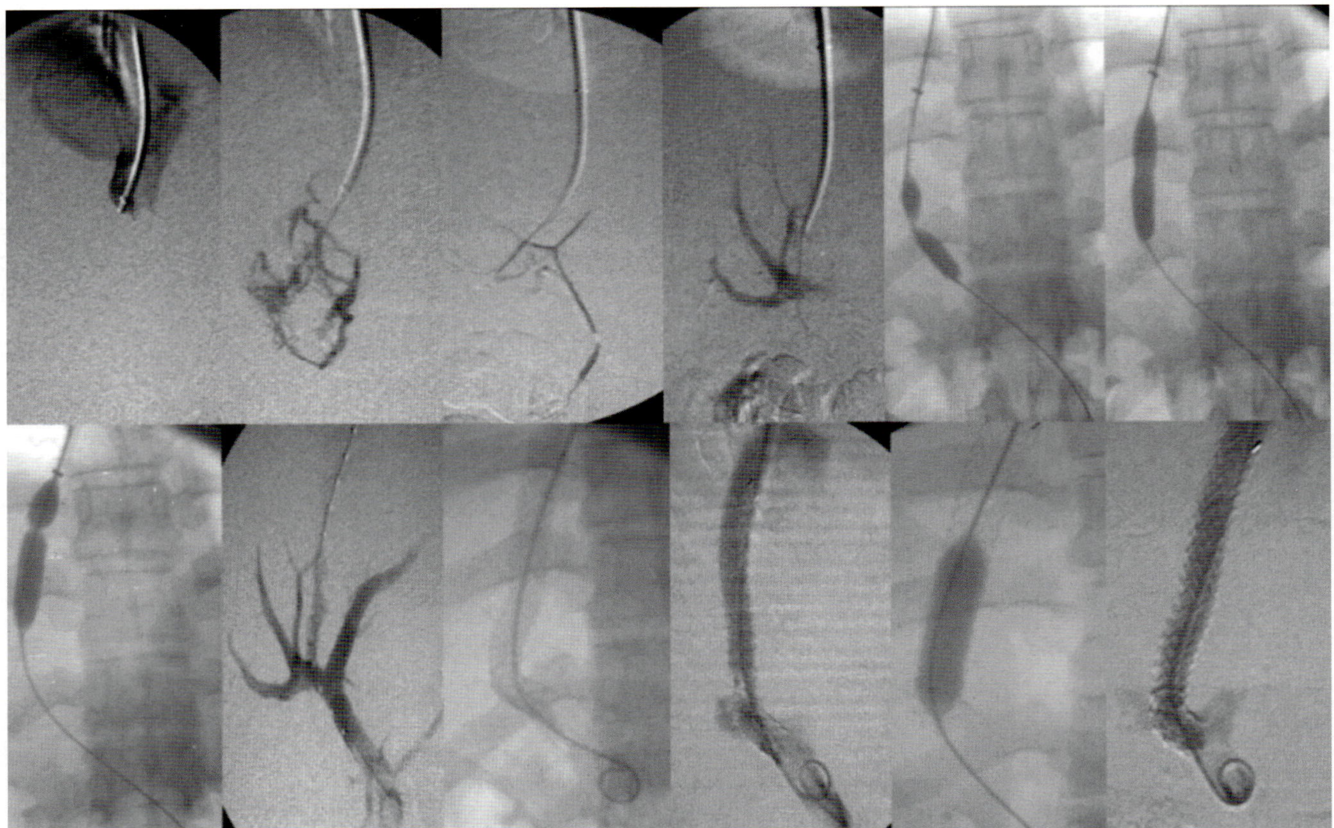

Fig. 26.1: TIPS technique. A needle sheath combination is placed across the hepatic parenchyma into the right portal vein from the hepatic venous side via the transjugular route. After doing a venogram via the hepatic venous side, the needle is advanced into the portal venous system. The needle is removed and the guidewire is passed into the portal venous system. A balloon catheter is passed over the wire and the balloon is placed across the hepatic tract and inflated to dilate the tract. A PTFE covered stent is placed across the hepatic parenchymal tract and dilated with the balloon to the optimum size. (*Courtesy: Dr SS Baijal, Department of Radiodiagnosis, Sanjay Gandhi PGIMER, Lucknow*)

portal vein. This is the riskiest step of the procedure. Different methods are used to select the site of puncture from the hepatic vein towards the portal vein. CO_2 injection and bony landmarks may be used to determine the level of portal vein. The right PV branch typically runs at the level of the 11th rib about 0.5-1.5 vertebral widths from the lateral border of the spine. Ultrasound may also be used to minimize the number of needle passes required to enter the portal vein. The site of portal venous access is critical as the portal vein bifurcation is extrahepatic in about one half of the patients and entry must be peripheral to this point to avoid the possibility of exsanguinating hemorrhage. When the right hepatic vein is used the needle is turned anteromedially for the right portal vein and when the middle hepatic vein is used the needle is directed posteriorly for the right portal vein or anteriorly for the left portal vein. Subsequently the portal vein pressure is measured and the baseline pressure gradients between the portal and hepatic veins are measured. A marking pigtail catheter is advanced into the main portal vein for venography for determining the suitability of the portal vein puncture. The third step involves balloon angioplasty, with dilatation of the parenchymal tract created by the needle. The last step is stent deployment to ensure patency of the tract. The ends of the stent should project for a short distance into the hepatic and portal vein to prevent displacement. However, extension of the stent too far into the hepatic or portal vein may make subsequent liver transplant difficult. The Wallstent was initially preferred because of its flexibility, ability to maintain its lumen around tight curves and cost factor but subsequently lost favor because of its shortening with expansion and suboptimal radioopacity. Gianturco Z and Palmaz stent have also been used for TIPS. The rigidity of the Palmaz stent makes it difficult to negotiate the tortuous parenchymal tract.[6] Most interventional radiologists now use the Viatorr PTFE- covered stents. Stents of various diameters are available with chances of shunt stenosis decreasing and encephalopathy increasing with larger size of stent.

A technically successful outcome including both creation of a shunt and decrease in portosystemic gradient to <12 mmHg is usually achieved in 95% of patients, while clinical success including resolution of complications of portal hypertension is achieved in 90% of patients.[7] There is some evidence that relative reduction of gradient (by 50% of baseline) may be sufficient to prevent variceal rebleeding. A portal pressure gradient of < 8 mm Hg may be required for control of refractory ascites.[7]

At the end of the procedure a portal venogram is performed to document shunt patency and nonvisualization of gastroesophageal varices. If the portosystemic gradient remains elevated despite use of a 12 mm balloon or if the varices continue to fill, embolization of varices should be done.

The immediate mortality rate of the TIPS procedure is 0-2%.[8] This may be higher for less-experienced operators. Early procedure-related death is due to extracapsular perforation with intraperitoneal bleeding, hepatic artery thrombosis with fulminant hepatic failure or acute right heart failure. The 1-year survival rate for TIPS varies for the indication for which the procedure is performed and is 48-90% when placed for control of bleeding varices and 48-76% when the indication is ascites.[9] Both the Child-Pugh score and a model using a bilirubin level of > 3 mg/dl (1 point), alanine aminotransferase level > 100 IU/L (1 point), pre-TIPS encephalopathy (1 point), and urgency of TIPS (2 points) have been successfully used to predict the mortality rates for TIPS(Emory score).[9] Recently the MELD (Mayo Endstage Liver Disease) score has been adopted to determine prognosis in patients who are candidates for TIPS or liver transplantation. This score is based on the serum bilirubin, creatinine, international normalized ratio and recent need for dialysis. The calculations can be done on the website (http://www.mayoclinic.org/gi-rst/mayomodel6.html). Early mortality post-TIPS is high in patients with Child-Pugh score greater than 12 (class C), Emory score greater than 4-5 or a MELD score greater than 18-25.

TIPS should be performed after weighing the severity of the complication from which the patient is suffering with the risk of the procedure and the likelihood of the patient surviving long enough to receive a liver transplant. In certain cases of relative contraindication such as portal vein thrombosis, TIPS may be carried out after attempted recanalization of the portal vein, while patients with a significant coagulopathy may be able to undergo TIPS following use of clotting factors or platelets.

COMPLICATIONS OF TIPS[2]

Complications	*Frequency(%age)*
TIPS dysfunction	
Thrombosis	10-15
Occlusion/stenosis	18-78
Transcapsular puncture	33
Intraperitoneal bleed	1-2
Hepatic infarction	1
Fistulae	Rare
Hemobilia	< 5
Sepsis	2-10
Infection of TIPS	Rare
Hemolysis	10-15
Encephalopathy	
New/worse	10-44
Chronic	5-20
Stent migration or placement into the IVC or too far into portal vein	10-20

TIPS dysfunction can be due to thrombosis, which usually occurs early and the cause of which may be leakage of bile into the shunt, hypercoagulable syndromes, or inadequate coverage of the TIPS tract with sufficient stents. More commonly, TIPS dysfunction may be due to pseudointimal hyperplasia within the parenchymal tract or within the outflow hepatic vein, leading to stent occlusion. The primary patency rates at 1,2,3,4 and 5 years is 25-66%, 5-42%, 21%, 13% and 13%.[10] The criteria of shunt dysfunction on Doppler ultrasound are absent flow, significant rise or fall in shunt velocity (> 50 cm/sec) compared with the first post-TIPS study, low-peak shunt velocity (< 50-90 cm/sec), high-peak shunt velocity (>190cm/sec), low main PV velocity (< 30 cm/sec), return of antegrade flow in intrahepatic PVs and reversed flow in the peripheral segment of the hepatic vein draining the shunt. Doppler has a sensitivity and specificity of 86% and 48% respectively[11] which indicates that an abnormal Doppler ultrasound is predictive of occlusion or stenosis whereas a normal ultrasound does not exclude TIPS dysfunction. Due to the air trapped in the graft fabric, Viatorr stent visualization is possible only days to weeks after deployment. As Doppler lacks the sensitivity and specificity to identify a significant number of patients with shunt dysfunction, recurrence of symptoms should be managed by shunt venography and intervention. Recently it has been shown that the use of Polytetrafluoroethylene covered stents (e.g. Viatorr) reduces the incidence of TIPS dysfunction, with a large series reporting a shunt patency rate of 86% as compared to 47% for bare stents.[12] The PTFE film minimizes transmural permeation of bile and mucin and thus prevents hyperplastic tissue ingrowth. The other major complication of TIPS is hepatic encephalopathy. It happens because the nitrogen-containing compounds produced by bacterial action in the gut are not metabolized by the liver before entering the circulation. This complication is more likely when the residual portosystemic gradient is less than 10 mmHg. However most patients respond to conservative medical therapy, with only rarely TIPS occlusion needed to control the encephalopathy. Percutaneous endovascular attempts have been made to manage hepatic encephalopathy induced by both surgical shunts and TIPS. Constraining stents and constraining stent grafts have been used to reduce shunt diameter. These devices have the advantage of not completely occluding the shunt but only diminishing the flow within the shunt by reducing shunt diameter.[13] Reduction stent grafts are superior to bare reduction stents in achieving an immediate significant increase in portosystemic gradient by constraining the shunt diameter and effectively managing TIPS induced hepatic encephalopathy refractory to medical treatment. All patients with TIPS should be considered transplant candidates and care should be taken to not extend the stents beyond the minimum necessary portions of the portal and hepatic vein, inferior vena cava junction, so as not to complicate the portal to portal vein anastomosis performed during transplantation.

Revision of Occluded Surgical Shunt

Recurrent variceal bleeding and/or hepatic encephalopathy may occur in upto 10% of patients treated with surgical shunts, with shunt stenosis being the most common cause of recurrent bleeding.[14] Percutaneous transluminal angioplasty is an attractive alternative method of therapy for shunt stenosis in appropriate patients and has significantly less morbidity as compared to shunt correction surgery.[14] Proper size of balloon is essential and use of a high pressure balloon should be avoided to prevent shunt rupture.

Arterioportal Fistulas

Arterioportal fistulas (APF) between the portal vein and the systemic arteries occur intra-abdominally and unlike the peripheral arteriovenous fistulas are not readily accessible for surgical treatment. The patients, when symptomatic, usually present with features of portal hypertension, cardiac failure or intestinal ischemia. APF may be congenital or acquired. When congenital they may be multiple and are usually secondary to hereditary telangiectatic diseases, arteriovenous malformations and aneurysms.[15] The acquired arterioportal fistulas may be a sequalae of blunt or penetrating trauma, iatrogenic injury such as ligation of an artery, percutaneous biopsy, cholangiography and splenoportography, or may be seen in hepatocellular carcinoma, cirrhosis or cavernous hemangiomas. The hepatic artery is the most common artery involved and the intrahepatic fistulas are commonly secondary to iatrogenic procedures and congenital vascular disorders, while the extrahepatic ones are usually as a result of trauma or ruptured hepatic artery aneurysms.[16] The splenic artery is the second most common artery involved, with most cases occurring from rupture of splenic artery aneurysms.[17] Superior and inferior mesenteric arterioportal fistulas are often iatrogenic or traumatic. Arteriography confirms the diagnosis with definitive demonstration of the fistula feeding vessel, the location and size of the shunt, the portal vein flow and the collaterals. Radiological intervention is now the therapy of first choice in all cases of arterioportal fistulas due to its reduced morbidity as compared to surgery and the repeated access availability. Small fistulas with slow fistulas are easier to treat but larger fistulas with higher flow are also no contraindication to endovascular treatment.[15] Selective and superselective cathetrization is done and various embolizing materials like coils and wires, isobutyl-2-acrylate, gelfoam and balloons have been used to occlude the fistulas.[18] In the absence of arterial access or for fistulas persisting after arterial embolization direct percutaneous injection or percutaneous transhepatic embolization may be done.[15]

Recanalization of Occluded Portal Vein and its Tributaries

5-10% of all portal hypertension cases are due to extrahepatic obstruction and one fourth of these cases are due to neoplasms such as hepatocellular carcinoma, pancreatic cancer and bile duct cancer invading and blocking the portal vein.[19] Portal venous stents may be placed in all of these carcinomas to resolve blockage of portal vein and alleviate the related symptoms.[20] Through percutaneous approach and using a cholangiographic needle a sheath is placed into the portal vein and the catheter is advanced beyond the stenotic site which is subsequently dilated using a balloon. The stent of appropriate size is then placed across the stenotic segment. The results are encouraging when the portal venous flow was blocked at the main portal vein with intact splanchic veins, while with involved splanchic veins the stent patency and prognosis are not favorable.[20]

Partial Splenic Embolization

Hypersplenism is a common complication of portal hypertension and has been symptomatically treated with splenectomy, splenic artery ligation and splenic embolization. Splenectomy has a high morbidity and considerable mortality rate, may result in postsplenectomy sepsis and destroy the chance to perform a subsequent portosystemic shunt. Splenic artery ligation, due to the development of subsequent collaterals is also not an effective method to relieve hypersplenism. In partial splenic embolization the supply is occluded more peripherally in the splenic parenchyma.[21] The splenic artery is selectively cannulated through the transfemoral route using a 4F catheter. The catheter is move forward so that the tip lies distal to the last pancreatic artery. Particulate material such as gelfoam is then injected to induce splenic infarction and induce fibrosis in 40-75% of splenic parenchyma.[22] The embolising agent such as gelfoam or PVA particles are soaked in antibiotic solution containing 1,00,000 units of penicillin and 40 mg of gentamycin. This procedure not only treats the hypersplenism in a convenient and non-invasive way, but also reduces the portal flow resulting in decreased portal pressure. Partial splenic embolization preserves the normal direction of blood flow through the splenic circulation, unlike total splenic embolization in which it is reversed.[21] This helps avoid the contamination of the infarcted spleen with gut bacteria and development of splenic abscess. Various complications such as splenic abscess, rupture, septicemia and pneumonia have been described with this procedure. However, the performance of partial splenic embolization instead of complete infarction of splenic tissue, proper antibiotic prophylaxis and postembolization care may reduce these complications significantly.[21]

Percutaneous Transhepatic Variceal Embolization

Percutaneous venous embolization has also been used to control acute variceal bleeding especially after failure of sclerotherapy or in cases of recurrent bleeding after sclerotherapy and is effective in controlling bleeding in 70-90% of patients.[23] The rate of survival after this procedure appears to be higher than that reported after conservative treatment. However, recurrent bleeding has been reported to occur in 37-65% of patients within a few months after embolization.[23] Three major collateral pathways from the mesenteric circulation to the splenorenal shunts are responsible for postsurgical variceal bleeding. The transgastric collaterals and the transpancreatic collaterals can be embolized through the transhepatic approach, while the transcolic collaterals are usually embolized through the transfemoral trans-shunt approach. Portal vein should be patent for carrying out the procedure. Shunt stenosis should be excluded before percutaneous venous embolization is performed. Prophylactic variceal embolization may be considered in patients in whom large collaterals develop postoperatively. Portal vein thrombosis is the major complication of this procedure.[24] Transcatheter variceal embolization also has limited use as an adjunct to TIPS placement.

Angiographic Vasopressin Infusion

Intravenous systemic vasopressin has been used to control variceal bleeding and the vasopressin is infused through the superior mesenteric artery at the rate of 0.1 mg/minute for 24 hours.[25] This causes reduced mesenteric blood flow with drop in portal pressure resulting in decompression of varices and subsequent thrombosis of bleeding site. Somatostatin can also be used to control variceal hemorrhage and has fewer complications as compared to vasopressin.[25]

Balloon-occluded Retrograde Transvenous Obliteration of Gastric Varices

Bleeding of gastric varices is a severe complication in patients with cirrhosis and though has a bleeding frequency lower than that of esophageal varices, the outcome is worse than in esophageal varices. Shunt surgery is usually contraindicated in these patients as they have poor liver function. Endoscopic sclerotherapy is also less effective in gastric varices as compared to esophageal varices with high early rebleeding rates. TIPS also has decreased success rate for gastric varices, with hepatic encephalopathy and shunt obstruction being other problems. Balloon-occluded retrograde transvenous obliteration of gastric varices has recently been reported as an effective new method for control of gastric varices with gastrorenal shunt and has a recurrence rate as low as 0-10%.[26,27] Worsening of esophageal varices due to obstruction of a large gastrorenal shunt is a problem with BRTO. The outflow vein for the varices is typically the left inferior phrenic/ adrenal to left renal vein for gastric varices and right gonadal vein for duodenal varices.These veins are selectively engaged with a diagnostic catheter. A 6-French balloon occlusion catheter is inserted into the gastrorenal shunt via the right femoral vein. Through the balloon catheter retrograde venography is performed with the balloon inflated to classify the varices and the collaterals. When the gastric varices are identified, a sclerosing agent (10 ml of 5% ethanolamine oleate and 10 ml of iopamidol) is slowly injected from the balloon catheter until the feeding veins from the portal or splenic vein are visualized.[26,28] After infusion of sclerosing agent, the balloon is kept inflated overnight and the catheter is removed next morning. Complex types of variceal communications require use of a microcatheter or initial partial splenic embolization to reduce flow through the shunts. The risks of using ethanolamine oleate include renal failure, pulmonary edema, and anaphylaxis. Intravenous haptoglobin may be given to prevent hemolysis-induced renal damage as it binds free hemoglobin.

Budd-Chiari Syndrome

In the past decade, percutaneous radiological management is becoming the procedure of choice for management of BCS. BCS can be acute, subacute or chronic. The acute form is uncommon and is usually due to extensive thrombosis. Thrombolysis is the first line of therapy and locoregional thrombolysis by selective catheterization as well as mechanical and hydrodynamic techniques has been used for removal of obstructing thrombus. If thrombolysis is unsuccessful portocaval shunt, either surgical or TIPS may be done. A series of seven cases treating acute BCS with TIPS reported a significantly less morbidity and mortality as compared to surgery.[29,30] The interventional treatment of Budd-Chiari has been dealt with in detail in the chapter on hepatic venous outflow tract obstruction.

Recent Advances

Recently Liu et al have used radiofrequency ablation (RFA) for treating patients with cirrhotic hypersplenism.[31] The mechanism of this procedure is similar to partial splenic embolization for hypersplenism. In a study of forty patients who were treated with splenic RFA and followed for 2 years, it was found that splenic and portal venous flow decreased and hepatic arterial flow increased significantly after the RFA procedure. This also increases liver regeneration in cirrhotics.

REFERENCES

1. Colapinto RF, Stronell RD, Birch SJ. Creation of an intrahepatic porto-systemic shunt with a Gruntzig balloon catheter. Can Med Assoc J 1982;126:267-71.
2. Boyer TD, Haskal ZJ. The role of transjugular intrahepatic portosystemic shunt in the management of portal hypertension. Hepatology 2005;41:386-99.
3. Luca A, DA'Amico G, La Galla R, et al. TIPS for prevention of recurrent bleeding in patients with cirrhosis: meta-analysis of randomized trials. Radiology 1999;30:612-22.
4. Cello JP, Ring EJ, Olcott EW, et al. Endoscopic sclerotherapy compared with percutaneous transjugular intrahepatic portosystemic shunt after initial sclerotherapy in patients with acute variceal hemorrhage. Ann Intern Med 1997;126:858-65
5. Sanyal A, Genning C, Reddy KR, et al. The North American study for the treatment of refractory ascites. Gastroenterology 2003;124:634-51.
6. Boyer TD. Transjugular intrahepatic portosystemic shunt: current status. Gastroenterology 2003;124:1700-10.
7. Haskal ZJ, Martin L, Cardella JF, et al. Quality improvement guidelines for transjugular intrahepatic portosystemic shunts. J Vasc Inter Radiol 2003;14:S265-70.
8. Karim V. Hepatic, splenic, and portal vascular systems. In Karim V (Ed): Vascular and Interventional Radiology. 2nd ed. Saunders, Elsevier, Philadelphia 2006;269-319.
9. Chalasani N, Clark WS, Martin LG, et al. Determinants of mortality in patients with advanced cirrhosis after transjugular intrahepatic portosystemic shunting. Gastroenterology 2000;118:138-44.

10. Sanyal AJ, Contos MJ, Yager D, et al. Development of psuedointima and stenosis after transjugular intrahepatic portosystemic shunts. Characterisation of cell phenotype and function. Hepatology 1998;28:22-32.
11. Owens CA, Bartolone C, Warner DL, et al. The inaccuracy of duplex sonography in predicting patency of transjugular intrahepatic portosystemic shunts. Gastroenterology 1998;114:975-80.
12. Bureau C, Garci-Pagan JC, Otal P, et al. Improved clinical outcome using polytetrafluoroethylene coated stents for TIPS: results of a randomized study. Gastroenterology 2004;126:469-75.
13. Maleux G, Verslype C, Heye S, et al. Endovascular shunt reduction in the management of transjugular portosystemic shunt induced hepatic encephalopathy: preliminary experience with reduction stents and stent grafts. AJR Am J Rontgenol 2007;188:659-64.
14. Ruff RJ, Chuang VP, Alspaugh JP, et al. Percutaneous vascular intervention after surgical shunting for portal hypertension. Radiology 1987;164:469-74.
15. Vauthey JN, Tomczak RJ, Helmberger T, et al. The arterioportal fistula syndrome: clinicopathologic features, diagnosis and therapy. Gastroenterology 1997;113:1390-401.
16. Vicq PH, Brissiaud JC, Manaa J, et al. Post-traumatic intraparenchymatous hepaticoportal fistula. Chirurgie 1986;112:578-83.
17. Watson WD, Bonta MJ, Bush CR. Splenic arteriovenous fistula causing massive ascites: a case report. Angiology 1986;37:36-40.
18. Bapuraj JR, Kalra N, Rao KLN, et al. Transcatheter coil embolization of a traumatic intrahepatic arterioportal fistula. Indian J Pediatr 2001;68:673-6.
19. Cohen J, Edelman RR, Chopra S. Portal vein thrombosis: a review. Am J Med 1992;92:173-82.
20. Yamakado K, Nakatsuka A, Fujii N, et al. Portal venous stent placement in patients with pancreatic and biliary neoplasms invading portal vein and causing portal hypertension: initial experience. Radiology 2001;220: 150-56.
21. Koconis KG, Singh H, Soares G. Partial splenic embolisation in the treatment of patients with portal hypertension: a review of the English language literature. J Vasc Interv Radiol 2007;18:463-81.
22. Spigos DG, Jonasson O, Mozes M, et al. Partial splenic embolization in the treatment of hypersplenism. AJR Am J Roentgenol 1979;132;777-82.
23. Lunderquist A, Simert G, Tylen U, et al. Follow-up of patients with portal hypertension and esophageal varices treated with percutaneous obliteration of gastric coronary vein. Radiology 1977;122:59-63.
24. L'Hermine C, Chastanet P, Delemazure O, et al. Percutaneous transhepatic embolization of gastroesophageal varices: results in 400 patients. AJR Am J Roentgenol 1989;152:755-60.
25. Gulati MS: Angiography and interventions in portal hypertension. In Berry M, Chowdhury V, Mukhopadhyay S, Suri S (Eds). Diagnostic Radiology: Gastrointestinal and hepatobiliary imaging, 2nd ed, Jaypee Brothers, New Delhi, 2004;402-23.
26. Punamiya SJ. Interventional radiology in management of portal hypertension. Ind J Radiol Imag 2008;18:249-55.
27. Ninoi T, Nishida N, Kaminou T, et al. Balloon occluded retrograde transvenous obliteration of gastric varices with gastrorenal shunt: long-term follow-up in 78 patients. AJR Am J Roentgenol 2005;184:1340-46.
28. Choi YH, Yoon CJ, Park JH, et al. Balloon occluded retrograde transvenous embolization for gastric variceal bleeding: its feasibility compared with transjugular intrahepatic portosystemic shunt. Korean J Radiol 2003;4:109-16.
29. Fisher NC, McCaVerty I, Dolapci M, et al. Managing Budd-Chiari syndrome: a retrospective review of percutaneous hepatic vein angioplasty and surgical shunting. Gut 1999;44:568-74.
30. Baijal SS, Roy S, Phadke RV, et al. Management of idiopathic Budd-Chiari syndrome with primary stent placement: early results. J Vasc Interv Radiol 1996;7: 545-53.
31. Liu Q, Kuansheng M, Song Y, et al. Two-year follow-up of splenic radiofrequency ablation in patients with cirrhotic hypersplenism: Does increased hepatic arterial flow induce liver regeneration? Surgery 2008;143: 509-18.

Index

A

B

C

D

E